Foundation Skills for Caring

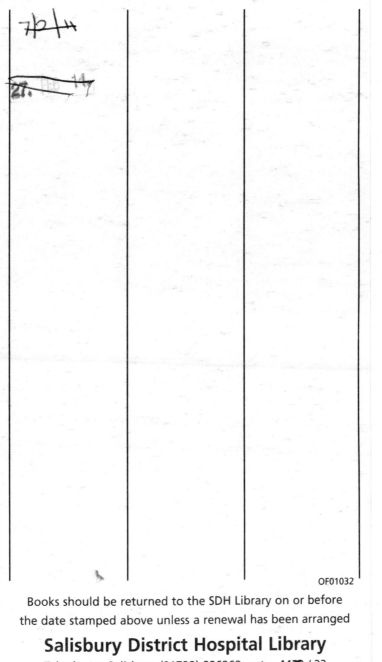

OF01032

How to use this book

Foundation Skills for Caring is a feature-rich textbook that has been developed with you, the student, in mind.

Each chapter begins with outcomes and concepts to help you plan your workload, and ends with a conclusion and reference section to support further learning. Throughout the rest of the book you'll find a wide range of innovative tools, all designed to help you become a capable and confident practitioner.

S **Scenarios**
Case studies which provide real-life situations for you to investigate

a **Learning activities**
Ideas to help you explore key issues, either individually or within your interprofessional learning group

e **Evidence-based practice boxes**
Examples of how best practice has been based on research

c **Professional conversations**
Practitioner perspectives to help you understand the roles of different professionals

t **Practice tips**
Advice to help you provide exceptional care

! **Professional alerts**
Warnings about potential pitfalls, to ensure you work safely and effectively

 Links to *Foundation Skills for Caring*
Cross-references to help you navigate between chapters in this book

Links to *Foundation Studies for Caring*
Cross-references to help you find relevant chapters in our sister theory volume

W **Web options**
Markers flagging up information that can be sourced online

W **On the websites**
Markers flagging up relevant material on our companion site

Foundation Skills for Caring

Using Student-Centred Learning

edited by Alan Glasper,

Gill McEwing and

Jim Richardson

palgrave

macmillan

First published 2009 by
PALGRAVE MACMILLAN

Palgrave Macmillan in the UK is an imprint of Macmillan Publishers Limited,
registered in England, company number 785998, of Houndmills, Basingstoke,
Hampshire RG21 6XS.

Palgrave Macmillan in the US is a division of St Martin's Press LLC,
175 Fifth Avenue, New York, NY 10010.

Palgrave Macmillan is the global academic imprint of the above companies
and has companies and representatives throughout the world.

Palgrave® and Macmillan® are registered trademarks in the United States,
the United Kingdom, Europe and other countries.

ISBN-13: 987-0-230-55269-2
ISBN-10: 0-230-55269-2

This book is printed on paper suitable for recycling and made from fully
managed and sustained forest sources. Logging, pulping and manufacturing
processes are expected to conform to the environmental regulations of the
country of origin.

A catalogue record for this book is available from the British Library.

10 9 8 7 6 5 4 3 2 1
18 17 16 15 14 13 12 11 10 09

Printed in the UK by
CPI William Clowes Beccles NR34 7TL

Contents

List of figures

List of tables

Acronyms and abbreviations

A&E	Accident and Emergency Department
ABPI	ankle brachial pressure index
ADSS	Association of Directors of Social Services
ANTT	aseptic non-touch technique
ASD	autistic spectrum disorder
AVPU	alert, responds to voice, pain or unresponsive
BDHF	British Dental Health Foundation
BMI	body mass index
BNF	British National Formulary
BP	blood pressure
bpm	beats per minute
BSI	bloodstream infection
BSL	British Sign Language
CAUTI	catheter-associated urinary tract infection
CGS	Glasgow coma scale
CHG	chlorhexidine gluconate
COPD	chronic obstructive pulmonary disease
CPAP	continuous positive airway pressure
CRBSI	catheter-related bloodstream infection
CVC	central venous catheter
CVP	central venous pressure
DH	Department of Health
EBL	enquiry based learning
ECF	extracellular fluid
EPUAP	European Pressure Ulcer Advisory Panel
EWMA	European Wound Management Association
GP	general practitioner
Hb	haemoglobin
HCP	healthcare practitioner
HDU	high-dependency unit
IBCT	incorrect blood component transfused
ICF	intracellular fluid
ICP	intracranial pressure
IP	implantable port
ISC	Intermittent self-catheterisation
IV	intravenous
LED	light-emitting diode
LTC	long-term condition
MHRA	Medicines and Healthcare Products Regulatory Agency
mm/Hg	millimetres of mercury
NHO	National Haemovigilance Office
NHS	National Health Service
NICE	National Institute for Clinical Excellence
NMC	Nursing and Midwifery Council
OAB	over-active bladder
PAT	pain assessment tool
PBL	problem-based learning
PCOT	point-of-care testing
PEA	pulseless electrical activity
PECS	Picture Exchange Communication System
PI	povodine iodine
PICC	peripherally inserted central catheter
PICU	paediatric intensive care unit
POAD	peripheral obstructive arterial disease
PPE	personal protective equipment
PVD	peripheral vascular disease
RCN	Royal College of Nursing
RCP	Royal College of Physicians
RN	registered nurse
ROSC	return of spontaneous circulation
SA	sinoatrial
SABRE	Serious Adverse Blood Reactions and Events reporting system
SCL	student-centred learning
SCRT	subcapilliary plexus refill time
SHOT	Serious Hazards of Transfusion reporting scheme
TPR	temperature, pulse and respirations
UTI	urinary tract infection
VAP	ventilator-assisted pneumonia
VF/VT	ventricular fibrillation/ventricular tachycardia
WHO	World Health Organisation

Notes on contributors

Joanna Assey, formerly Lecturer, School of Health Sciences, University of Southampton

Marion Aylott, Lecturer in Children's and Young People's Nursing, School of Health Sciences, University of Southampton

Carol Barron, Module Coordinator for Child Development, School of Nursing, Dublin City University

Neil Bloxham, Charge Nurse/Clinical Educator, Plymouth Hospitals NHS Trust

Mark Broom, Senior Lecturer, Faculty of Health, Sport & Science, University of Glamorgan

Pauline Cardwell, Practice Educator for Undergraduate Nursing Sciences, School of Nursing and Midwifery, Queen's University Belfast

Diane Carpenter, Lecturer, School of Health Sciences, University of Southampton

Margaret Chambers, Lecturer in Nursing (Subject Advisor Paediatrics), School of Nursing and Community Studies, University of Plymouth

Carol Chamley, Senior Lecturer Children's Nursing, School of Nursing, Midwifery and Healthcare, University of Coventry

Mary Clynes, Module Coordinator Children with Healthcare Needs and Professional/Contemporary Issues/Children, School of Nursing, Dublin City University

Matthew Cole, Chief Podiatrist, Plymouth Primary Care Teaching Trust, South and West Devon Health Community

Tim Coney, Lecturer, School of Health Sciences, University of Southampton

Yvonne Corcoran, Module Coordinator for Approaches in Nursing Practice, School of Nursing, Dublin City University

Doris Corkin, Teaching Fellow Undergraduate Nursing Sciences, School of Nursing and Midwifery, Queen's University Belfast

Alyson Davies, Team coordinator/Lecturer in Child Health, School of Health Science, University of Swansea

Pam Diggens, Lecturer School of Health Sciences, University of Southampton

Cheryl Dunford, Lecturer in Tissue Viability, School of Health Sciences, University of Southampton

Elaine Gibson, Medical Educational Specialist ConvaTec Limited, and Tissue Viability Nurse Specialist East Kent Hospitals University

Alan Glasper (ed), Professor of Nursing, School of Health Sciences, University of Southampton

Chris Hanks, Academic Lead in Health Studies - Care of Older People, School of Nursing and Community Studies, University of Plymouth

Tracey Harrington, Lecturer in Children's and General Nursing, School of Nursing, Dublin City University

Jan Heath, Skills for Practice Lead, Southampton University Hospitals NHS Trust

Deborah Heron, Lecturer in Nursing, School of Health Sciences, University of Southampton

Tim Jenkinson, Lecturer in Nursing (Adult), School of Nursing and Community Studies, University of Plymouth

Sharon Jones, Lecturer Adult Nursing, School of Nursing and Community Studies, University of Plymouth

Janet Kelsey, Senior Lecturer in Health Studies, Academic Lead for Child Health and Programme Lead for BSc Child Health Nursing, School of Nursing and Community Studies, University of Plymouth

Jessica Knight, Lecturer in Nursing, School of Health Sciences, University of Southampton

Veronica Lambert, Lecturer, School of Nursing, Dublin City University

Siobhan MacDermott, Module Coordinator for Nursing as a Research Based Profession, Practice Orientation Module and Children with Complex Healthcare Needs, School of Nursing, Dublin City University

Andrea McDougall, Paediatric Dietitian, Royal Belfast Hospital for Sick Children, Belfast Trust

Gill McEwing (ed) Senior Lecturer, Faculty of Health and Social Work, University of Plymouth

Patricia McGuinness, Staff Nurse, Children's Ward Daisy Hill Hospital Newry, Southern Health and Social Care Trust

Karen Merrick, Clinical Nurse Specialist, The Children's Hospital, Dublin

Steve Miles, Academic Practitioner, School of Health Sciences, University of Southampton

Diana Morris, Deputy Sister, Outpatients Department, St Michael's Hospital, The Royal Cornwall Hospitals Trust, Hayle

Philomena Morrow, Nurse Lecturer, School of Nursing and Midwifery, Queen's University Belfast

Colleen O'Neill, Module Coordinator Children with Neurological Disorders, School of Nursing, Dublin City University

Doris O'Toole, Clinical Placement Coordinator, Children's University Hospital, Dublin

Jan Orr, Clinical Skills Lecturer/Practitioner Faculty Health and Social Work, University of Plymouth

Rachel Palmer, Academic Practitioner, School of Health Sciences,, University of Southampton

Gareth Parsons, Senior Lecturer, Faculty of Health, Sport & Science, University of Glamorgan

Jennie Quiddington, Lecturer, School of Health Sciences,, University of Southampton

Sara Raftery, Module Coordinator Practice Care, School of Nursing, Dublin City University

Jim Richardson (ed), Head of Division, School of Health, Sport and Science, University of Glamorgan

Ross Sherrington, Academic Practitioner, School of Health Sciences, University of Southampton

Lucy Smith, Lecturer Practitioner, School of Health Sciences, University of Southampton

Anita Stuart, Senior Podiatrist, Seventrees Clinic, Plymouth

Emma Toms, Podiatry Service, Plymouth Primary Care Teaching Trust, South and West Devon Health Community

Lesley Wayne, Research Assistant, School of Nursing and Community Studies, University of Plymouth

Mike Weaver, Senior Learning Technologist, School of Health and Social Care, Bournemouth University

James Wilson, Lecturer, School of Health Sciences, University of Southampton

Michelle Wilson (Child Branch Student), School of Nursing, Midwifery and Healthcare University of Coventry

Acknowledgements

Every effort has been made to trace the copyright holders of third party material in this book. However, if any have been inadvertently overlooked, Palgrave Macmillan will be pleased to make the necessary arrangements at the first opportunity.

The publishers and authors wish to acknowledge the following for their kind permission to use copyright material:

Falmouth College of Art and Design, Royal Cornwall Hospital NHS Trust, for permission to reproduce Figure 3.5 Posters displayed in clinical areas to promote Improving Working Lives
Judy Waterlow for permission to reproduce Figure 10.2 Waterlow pressure ulcer prevention/treatment policy
Elaine Gibson, Tissue Viability Nurse Specialist, East Kent Hospitals NHS Trust, Education Specialist ConvaTec Ltd for permission to reproduce photographic images Chapter 10 Pressure Ulcer Care
Suzanne Cobb for permission to reproduce Figure 15.8 Brushing Teeth
Mosby publishers for permission to reproduce Figure 21.1 and Figure 22.2 Wong-Baker FACES Pain rating Scale
Jo Eland for permission to reproduce Figure 21.3 Eland Colour Scale
Kathy Mak for permission to reproduce Figure 25.9 Component parts of an intravenous set
BMJ Publishing Group for permission to reproduce Figure 30.1 Six step handwashing technique devised by Ayliffe et al (1978) ensuring that all parts of the hands are covered
Resuscitation Council (UK) for permission to reproduce Figure 36.1 Paediatric basic life support (for healthcare professionals with a duty to respond); Figure 37.1 Adult basic life support (for healthcare professionals with a duty to respond)
Mrs D Dooley and Staff Nurse P. McGuinness for permission to reproduce Figure 38.1 Framework for holding children still for clinical procedures

Photographs: Chapter 3 Communication Figures 3.2, 3.3, 3.4, 3.6, 3.7, 3.8, 3.9, 3.10, 3.12 © Gill McEwing, Figures 3.1, 3.11 © Jan Orr; Chapter 4 Communicating with Adolescents Figures 4.1, 4.3 © Gill McEwing, Figures 4.4, 4.5, 4.6 © Jan Orr; Chapter 10 Pressure Ulcer Care © Elaine Gibson; Chapter 11 Eye Care © Sara Raftery, Colleen O'Neill & Mary Clynes; Chapter 12 Mouth Care Figures 12.2, 12.4 © Gill McEwing, Figures 12.1, 12.3 © Mary Clynes; Chapter 13 Catheterisation and Catheter Care © Steve Miles; Chapter 14 Basic Foot Care and Managing Common Nail Pathologies © Matthew Cole; Chapter 15 Care of the Infant Figures 15.1, 15.2 © Marion Aylott; Figures 15.3, 15.4, 15.5, 15.6, 15.7 © Gill McEwing; Chapter 16 Vital Signs Figures 16.1, 16.2, 16.3 © Pam Diggens, Figures 16.4, 16.5, 16.6 © Gill McEwing; Chapter 17 Blood Pressure © Sharon Jones; Chapter 18 Pulse Oximetry © Sharon Jones; Chapter 19 Blood Sugar Measurement © Mary Clynes, Colleen O'Neill & Sara Raftery; Chapter 20 Neurological Assessment © Jessica Knight & Rachel Palmer; Chapter 23 Diabetic Foot Assessment © Anita Stuart & Emma Toms; Chapter 24 Assessing and Managing Hydration © Children's University Hospital, Dublin; Chapter 26 Enteral Feeding © Gill McEwing; Chapter 27 Preparation of Infant Feeds © Doris Corkin; Chapter 28 Routes of Medication Administration © Carol Barron; Chapter 29 Patient Controlled Analgesia © Mark Broom & Gareth Parsons; Chapter 32 Aseptic Technique and Wound Management © Kevin Campbell, Technical Manager for Clinical Education Centre, MBC, Queens University Belfast; Chapter 33 Central Venous Catheters © Janet Kelsey; Chapter 34 Blood Transfusion © Karen Merrick; Chapter 35 Oxygen Therapy and Suction therapy © Gill McEwing; Chapter 36 Basic Life Support: Child © Gill McEwing; Chapter 37 Basic Life Support: Adult © Jan Heath; Chapter 38 Clinical Holding for Care, Treatment or Interventions © Philomena Morrow; Chapter 39 Orthopaedic Procedures © Ross Sherrington

Pauline Cardwell, author of Chapter 32 Aseptic Technique and Wound Management, wishes to acknowledge and thank Carol Warwick, Tissue Viability Nurse, Royal Victoria Hospital, Belfast for her help and advice.

Introduction

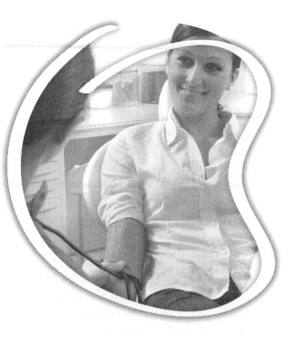

Alan Glasper, Gill McEwing
and Jim Richardson

Links to other chapters in *Foundation Skills for Caring*
  1 Fundamental concepts for skills
  3 Communication

Links to other chapters in *Foundation Studies for Caring*

Introduction
  1 Study skills
  2 Interprofessional learning
  5 Communication

Don't forget to visit www.palgrave.com/glasper for additional
online resources relating to this chapter.

This book addresses the skills and competences for practice that you will need in order to make the transition towards your chosen healthcare career. There is a companion volume to this book called *Foundation Studies for Caring* which covers the theoretical components of healthcare education, and the books share a companion website featuring many resources that will help you to acquire the knowledge and skills needed over the foundation component of your programme. At the heart of this *Skills* book is the quest to link theoretical knowledge to the real world of practice in which the patient or client holds primacy.

Foundation Skills for Caring is predicated on 'student-centred learning' (SCL) in which you, the reader, will take centre stage in the learning processes. If you are also working with the *Studies* book, you will be familiar with this approach and can move straight on to the next chapter. If you are new to SCL, read on to discover more about it, how it will help you learn and develop, and how you should use this book to your best advantage.

What is student-centred learning?

In this SCL-based book you will be asked to engage in scenarios and activities which encourage you to investigate, question and interact with new ideas and practices. Sometimes short case studies will be utilised to facilitate your learning. Often you will work and learn together with others on these activities in 'learning groups', some of which will be uniprofessional (such as mental health nursing) and some interprofessional, where you will learn with others such as physiotherapists or dieticians.

Exploring the patient's experiences to help you learn

Some of the healthcare skills detailed throughout this book use scenarios involving actual patient experiences; we call this a client-focused approach, and, in this book, it is done from an interprofessional perspective. This means that you can explore the scenarios (where used) and the clinical skills required by all healthcare professionals (such as hand hygiene) within the context of either nursing or other healthcare professions. Therefore, whichever healthcare path you choose to follow, these skills will have direct relevance for you and you will be able to apply them in your own practice setting.

Because this book takes a student-centred learning approach, it *involves* you in the learning process at every step, rather than simply listing facts. It is characterised by:

- Active learning: you will be invited to explore issues and gain further insights through local practice observations.
- Studying individually and in groups: debating issues with colleagues enriches and diversifies your understanding.
- Working through activities and seeking out and responding to questions and dilemmas, many of which you are encouraged to pose for yourself.

The aim of this and the companion book is to help you to embark on the road to becoming a professional nurse or other healthcare practitioner. For this reason the questions and activities that will guide your learning frequently place you in the role of, for example, the qualified nurse rather than of a student or care assistant.

This book and its sister volume will introduce you to a new and refreshing approach to learning about healthcare theory and practice. It is the ability of the healthcare professional to seek out answers and provide the best possible care that separates the registered practitioner from non-professional colleagues. Nurses and other health professionals need to be constantly aware of practice developments, often brought about by research findings, so their knowledge is ever-evolving. Developing the skills to access current information is key to professional practice, and it is these skills of enquiry that we hope to promote through the chapters in this book. They will help you understand and deliver evidence-based care to your clients.

The delivery of clinical skills in practice settings is underpinned by Florence Nightingale's constant rhetoric to her probationer nurses that they must 'first do the patient no harm'. 'Doing the patient no harm' reflects the mission of the national healthcare professional regulators (such as the Nursing and Midwifery Council) who are committed to public protection. The editors and authors of this book have endeavoured to ensure that regulatory educational skills requirements for healthcare students are fully embodied within its pages.

Learning through enquiry

In taking a client-focused approach we want you to be able to visualise the bigger picture – that is, the full healthcare environment – before being tempted to examine each piece of the jigsaw. This, we believe, is fundamental to appreciating the holistic and integrative nature of contemporary healthcare practice, which crosses professional boundaries in order to provide the best possible patient care. This places learning in context; it gives you the opportunity to experience the excitement and challenge of professional practice from a position of safety, whilst also acknowledging the frustrations that some days can bring. This reality, together with your own experiences drawn from practice, will enable you to seek out and understand the background and detail behind each application of a clinical skill event. Additionally we have prepared through the companion web pages other resources such as sequential photographs to allow you to see skills and their delivery within the context of healthcare practice. The process of investigation is often called being 'reflective', and this can be shown in a 'reflective cycle'. There are several examples of the reflective process, but the figure below shows an adaptation from Gibbs (1998).

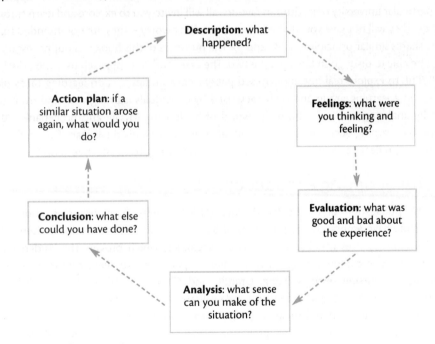

Figure I.1 The reflective cycle

It would be helpful to keep these reflective stages in your mind as you explore and make sense of the different scenarios, and the complex world of healthcare which unfold in the chapters of this book. Being reflective means getting in touch and keeping in touch with the way you and others practice.

Student-centred learning is an umbrella term which incorporates the following approaches:

- enquiry-based learning (EBL)
- problem-based learning (PBL)
- case studying
- action learning.

So what are these approaches to learning?

The modern history of the SCL movement began at the medical school at McMaster University in Hamilton, Canada. EBL/PBL found favour there as it was perceived by teachers to be an ideal medium for exploring the real world of patient care, where students could learn how to 'solve problems' and think critically. It is, however, important to understand that the term 'problem' encompasses 'enquiry', or the asking of questions about a particular subject. The enquiry may or may not be directly related to a patient problem as such (for example the specific illness or disease), but rather the learning issues to be explored.

This is particularly pertinent in higher education, where the emphasis has moved away from direct teaching to a more holistic use of the term 'learning'. Hence strategies to enhance learning opportunities, such as the use of EBL/PBL, have been adopted by many disciplines, including nursing and the other health professions. Additionally, many traditional boundaries between the healthcare professions are becoming increasingly blurred in response to changes in healthcare delivery (Humphris and Masterson, 2000) and students are expected to work flexibly across these interprofessional boundaries. This changing workplace environment now requires an innovative approach to healthcare education that facilitates greater understanding of the roles of different members of the interdisciplinary healthcare team. SCL is an innovative learning method which is suited to interprofessional healthcare education, as it challenges students to identify the ideas and skills they will need to tackle the complexities of healthcare delivery (Duch, Groch and Allen, 2001).

All of the learning approaches mentioned here are enquiry based. Whichever approach your particular university or institution favours, all will invite you to explore and learn through practice. They will not give you all the answers, but don't worry – they are not intended to.

EBL shares similar principles to PBL and for the purposes of this book it is not necessary for you to be able to distinguish between the two. The case-studying approach uses the principles of EBL/PBL to explore real but anonymised patient case studies. Action learning takes place similarly in a learning group and is characterised by individuals learning with and from each other by analysing real issues from the world of healthcare. McGill and Brockbank (2004) believe that learning occurs when an individual or groups of individuals learn from reflection and that this reflective learning in turn facilitates new learning from effective action.

Some reasons for adopting a model of SCL

Since the publication of *Fitness for Practice* (UKCC, 1999) many pre-registration nursing curricula have embraced the principles of SCL as a method of educating students. SCL based on enquiry uses genuine, real-life client scenarios, which provide the students with an opportunity to explore a range of issues directly pertaining to client care in a variety of contemporary nursing settings (Long, Grandis and Glasper, 1999). Exploration follows a systematic approach to enquiry, reflection and evaluation (Long and Grandis, 2000).

Learning is often undertaken as a group, with individual students taking on specific responsibilities for researching and gathering evidence to bring back to the team. This contributes to the group's overall collective understanding of the issue or problem being explored.

In a recent Canadian study of second year nursing students, Morales-Mann and Kaitell (2001) demonstrated that the factors which most influenced the levels of learning within the group were positive attitudes and group effort. Rhem (1998) believes that the reason why this method is prevailing within higher education institutions is that it orientates students towards strategies of 'meaning making' over simple fact collecting.

In this way the product of the group is greater than the sum of the parts, resulting in higher levels of attainment in which prior learning is valued and built upon. Additionally, this type of cooperative learning brings with it enhanced social skills (Connolly and Seneque, 1999) which are highly valued in the healthcare professions.

Perhaps more importantly, the linking of clinical skills (prized by practitioners) and theoretical knowledge (prized by academics) through the medium of SCL (O'Neil, Morris and Baxter, 2000) may bridge the theory–practice gap which has bedevilled the profession for so long. Morales-Mann and Kaitell (2001) have described this type of learning strategy as liberating the academic from the traditional roles associated with teaching. This is good news for you and your lecturers as you will both enjoy the process!

Acknowledging some challenges

Not all students find the approach easy; indeed some prefer a more structured didactic approach whilst others thrive on the freedom to explore, share and learn in a way that they feel reflects the way in which they will practise as professionals. A study by Glasper (2001) looked at a UK cohort of 15 children's nurses on completion of their three-year pre-registration programme. Using a nominal group technique, he identified five areas which students liked most about SCL and five that they liked least. Students valued the friendships and support generated by working as a group, and believed that SCL enabled them to share experiences, exchange views and gain confidence. They saw SCL as having made the group work 'exceptionally well'. Conversely, students also voiced their frustrations about a lack of structure, having to rely on others to pull their weight and then being provided with poor quality feedback by their peers from what they had researched.

Groups are usually led by tutors but can be led by students. Steele, Medder and Turner (2000), in a comparison of student-led versus tutor-led group work, identified a preference for student facilitators. In this study of second-year medical students, peer facilitators were given slightly higher ratings than academics, but it was noted by the investigators that peer-facilitated groups often took shortcuts in the SCL process.

You will need to use your skills in reflection to assess your own views of SCL, and take steps to address any problems.

Getting the most from this book

Because this is a different kind of textbook from many others, it is not encyclopaedic. We have selected certain clinical skills which we believe you are most likely to need to acquire during the foundation component of your healthcare programme and which will help you to address each of the Nursing and Midwifery Council (NMC) and other regulatory body outcomes (for entry to a particular field of practice programme). This book provides you with the opportunity to identify what you need to learn and to equip yourself with the necessary clinical skills foundations on which to build your own professional practice. It will help you explore and experience new ways of learning and to seek out pathways, whilst pointing you towards those resources which will help you to make sense of complex clinical issues. This is student-centred learning and we hope you enjoy the challenge. We think you will.

Getting started

In order to maximise and enjoy your learning and make the best use of your study time, read the next section carefully.

Each chapter in this skills book has expected learning outcomes; however, as an enquiring student, it is likely that you already have many questions about healthcare practice and how this relates to the practice of colleagues from other disciplines. When you start to read each chapter, you may identify with particular clinical or personal experiences which prompt you to question why you thought or reacted in a particular way, so make sure you note these. You may be exploring some topics for the first time with little or no previous experience, therefore not knowing what you do not know! For many students in healthcare this can initially raise some anxieties, but you are not alone! This is usual and part of the learning process.

There are prompts for learning in the form of questions and activities at regular points within each chapter. Some of these are best attempted before you read on as they will help you to identify how much you currently know, as well as the level and accuracy of existing knowledge. Sometimes, we do not appreciate what we have previously taken for granted until it is clearly brought to our attention – better in a book than in the clinical environment! The companion textbook to this volume, *Foundation Studies for Caring*, has been written to let you see the relationship between theory and practice, and by dipping into each you will begin to build up a picture of your world of healthcare. Additionally, the companion website allows you to further explore each chapter topic. The chapter writers have placed kite marked websites on each of the web-based presentations to allow you access to other types of learning material which you will find extremely helpful in your learning groups or action learning sets.

Your most important role as a healthcare student is to constantly question, to gain knowledge and to identify the evidence base that underpins accepted professional practice. Sometimes, you might discover that care might be based more on 'custom and practice' than evidence, and that there is a need to seek out the most informed sources rather than following tradition.

This book helps you to identify the areas of knowledge underpinning clinical skills that you may need to explore and the kinds of questions that you might choose to ask. Developing the confidence to ask questions is a very important part of being a healthcare professional who needs to be able to seek out information from patients and their relatives, often about sensitive or potentially embarrassing topics. All healthcare professionals need also to possess assertiveness and interpersonal skills so as to be able to appropriately question and sometimes challenge colleagues, whether they are from the same or other disciplines. Clearly, effective communication is immensely important both now as a student and in your future career.

Deciding what to focus on

It is also acknowledged that knowledge is constantly changing. This can be a troublesome idea when starting a new career with a vast amount to learn. However, once the overall picture is grasped and the foundations are laid, more complex issues can be tackled. This comes through reading and accessing other resources, and also from being an active observer and participant in clinical practice. Soon you will feel more comfortable in questioning accepted practice. As a student you are privileged to experience a wide range of practice environments and you will observe that care might differ between practitioners. Questioning the rationale for those differences, rather than accepting that this is 'just the way that it is done', will add to your repertoire of knowledge and skill. The manner in which questions are asked is likely to influence the response you receive!

Key points you may like to consider:

- Is this the appropriate time?
- Is this person likely to have the correct information or appropriate experience?
- Do I need permission to ask this person?
- How do I phrase the question; for example, to avoid offence or to ensure the question elicits a relevant answer?

Throughout the book you will be invited to seek the opinions of friends, relatives, patients and others, finding out their views related to different health issues. Getting into the habit of seeking others' opinions will help to develop the skills you will need throughout your professional career. Working in healthcare is a lifelong learning experience, which requires you to remain open to others' views and opinions.

Most textbooks are studied in isolation. However, it is well established that learning with others can contribute very positively to the learning experience, not only in being more interesting and satisfying, but also in extending ideas. Spending time thinking about practice is useful, but it is likely to be yet more productive if you can engage with others. They may identify aspects which you haven't thought about. Your views may be questioned and this may prompt you to think more laterally – to think the unthinkable!

As discussed, your university or college centre will normally provide you with opportunities for small-group learning in the form of a learning group or action-learning set and you may have additionally an interprofessional group in which you have membership. Perhaps you are also a member of an online learning group facilitated through one of the virtual learning platforms such as Blackboard or WebCT. You will certainly have access to email, and much of your collaborative leaning will be facilitated through this medium. Each chapter also presents a set of concepts. This list is not definitive. Again, as you approach the topic area in each chapter, you may have your own concepts to add to the list. When reviewing the concepts embodied within the chapters, view them as broadly as possible as this will enhance your understanding. For example, the concept of 'care' will be viewed differently depending on whether you are a patient, client, husband/wife, child, parent, friend, nurse, manager, doctor, physiotherapist, chaplain, undertaker or employer. Accessing the literature will also broaden and deepen your current understanding of each concept. Continually reflect on your personal experience, your current understanding and how new knowledge can change practice. It is through this process that improvements in practice are made.

Practising in a changing world of healthcare

The ways in which new healthcare practitioners are prepared for their unique role within health services has changed radically over the last few years. Different health professions now often learn together. There is now more flexible access as well as opportunities to 'step on' and 'step off' courses, as your individual learning needs dictate. This book hopes to introduce you to a way of learning that reflects and complements the diversity of this approach. Whether you embark on your studies in a college of further education or at university, we intend this book to act as an effective resource as you begin a career in healthcare.

Although the fundamental principles upon which healthcare is founded remain unaltered, the ways in which professionals practise, the roles they occupy with others and the public's expectation are constantly changing. In this century more than ever before, healthcare practitioners will have to adapt their practice to meet the needs of the increasing number of people who are living longer, well into old age. Nurses among others must find ways of providing the best care possible, yet be constrained by tighter costs and account for their every action.

Whilst research and new technologies will enable more and more dreams to be realised, lives to be saved and health to be optimised, some of the longer-established treatments will, as now, be found wanting. We have already entered the arena of the 'super bug'. There are new challenges; old diseases over which we previously had control are increasing again (for example tuberculosis), and the full impact on health from environmental change is yet to be realised. Smoking has increased dramatically amongst young women and we are yet to see the full impact of the rising tide of obesity in children and adults. The expectations and demands of modern living are leading to increased levels of stress, mental illness and suicide in all age groups. Conversely, many people who develop cancer are living much longer after treatment than they previously did and there is improved use of transplants and organ donation. No wonder public expectation constantly rises as the media proclaims that more and more is possible!

Aside from all this, new ways of caring for people within the community aim to more effectively support independence. This brings with it the challenge of taking acceptable risks when public protection must always be paramount. Healthcare professionals have to be able to make such difficult decisions daily. When things go wrong, more people then ever before will know their rights and will have the confidence to seek redress but, because the gap between wealth and poverty continues to widen, the professional's role in safeguarding the interests of the more vulnerable becomes ever more important.

As the boundaries of practice change, nurses and others will choose to extend their skills into new areas. Some will overlap with the skills of other professionals, and yet all will continue to use those skills which the public recognise and know as 'nursing', 'occupational therapy', 'physiotherapy' and so on. It is this mix of essential skills, knowledge and attitudes that is woven into the fabric of the healthcare professional and which is central to lifelong professional practice. It is these fundamental principles which will be introduced during the initial period of this book, and the way you understand them will influence the way you will practise in the future.

References

Connolly, C. and Seneque, M. (1999) 'Evaluating problem-based learning in a multilingual student population', *Medical Education* **33**(10), 738–44.

Duch, B. J., Groch, S. E. and Allen, D. E. (2001) *The Power of Problem Based Learning: A practical 'how-to' for teaching undergraduate courses in any discipline*, Stirling, VA, Stylus Publishing.

Gibbs, G. (1988) *Learning by Doing: A guide to teaching and learning methods*, Oxford, Further Education Unit, Oxford Polytechnic (New Oxford Brookes University).

Glasper, E. A. (2001) 'Child health nurses' perceptions of enquiry-based learning', *British Journal of Nursing* **10**(2), 1343–9.

Humphris, D. and Masterson, A. (eds) (2000) *Developing New Clinical Roles: A guide for health professionals*, Edinburgh, Churchill Livingstone.

Long, G., Grandis, S. and Glasper, E. A. (1999) 'Investing in practice: enquiry- and problem-based learning', *British Journal of Nursing* **8**(17), 1171–4.

Long, G. and Grandis, S. (2000) 'Introducing enquiry-based learning into pre-registration nursing programmes', in Glen, S. and Wilkie, K. (eds), *Problem-Based Learning In Nursing Programmes: A new model for a new context*, Macmillan (now Palgrave Macmillan), Basingstoke.

McGill, I. and Brockbank, A. (2004) *The Action Learning Handbook*, London, RoutledgeFalmer.

McMaster University (1996) *Tutor Handbook*, Hamilton, Ontario, McMaster University.

Morales-Mann, E. T. and Kaitell, C. A. (2001) 'Problem-based learning in a new Canadian curriculum', *Journal of Advanced Nursing* **33**(1), 13–19.

Newman, M. (2000) 'Project on the effectiveness of problem based learning (PEPBL)', PEBL [online] www.hebes.mdx.ac.uk/teaching/research/PEPBL/index.htm (accessed 2 January 2009).

Nursing and Midwifery Council (NMC) (2002) *Requirements for Pre-Registration Nursing Programmes. Section 3: Nursing competencies*, London, NMC, pp. 9–21.

O'Neil, P. A., Morris, J. and Baxter, C. M. (2000) 'Evaluation of an integrated curriculum using problem-based learning in a clinical environment: the Manchester experience', *Medical Education* **34**(3), 222–30.

Penfield virtual hospital (PVH) (2007) PVH [online] http://www.hud.ac.uk/hhs/departments/nursing/penfield_site/default.htm (accessed 2 January 2009).

Rhem, J. (1998) 'Problem-based learning: an introduction', *National Teaching & Learning Forum* **8**(1), December, NTFL [online] http://www.ntlf.com/html/pi/9812/pbl_1.htm (accessed 2 January 2009).

Schon, D. A. (1983) *The Reflective Practitioner: How professionals think in actions*, New York, Basic Books.

Steele, D. K., Medder, K. D. and Turner, P. (2000) 'A comparison of learning outcomes and attitudes in student versus faculty-led problem-based learning: an experimental study', *Medical Education* **34**(1), 23–9.

United Kingdom Central Council (UKCC) (1999) *Fitness for Practice*, London, UKCC.

Woods, D. R. (1994) *Problem-Based Learning: How to gain the most from PBL*, Hamilton, Ontario, McMaster University.

Chapter

1

Fundamental concepts for skills

Alan Glasper, Gill McEwing
and Jim Richardson

 Links to other chapters in *Foundation Skills for Caring*

 Links to other chapters in *Foundation Studies for Caring*

W Don't forget to visit www.palgrave.com/glasper for additional online resources relating to this chapter.

Introduction

This practical skills book and its companion website have been prepared to help you acquire some of the fundamental skills required for practice. Each skill will be presented with some essential theory and evidence base for the procedure. However, there are fundamental concepts that need to be taken into account when undertaking any procedure, and these will be discussed in this chapter.

Learning outcomes

This chapter will enable you to:

- understand consent for treatment and the capacity to consent
- discuss the need for privacy and dignity to be maintained during procedures
- the importance of risk assessment and patient safety
- explain the need for patient comfort
- be aware of the issues of safeguarding patients
- understand the role of documentation in healthcare procedures
- understand your own and other people's accountability in practice.

Concepts

- Safety
- Professionalism
- Caring
- Policies and procedures
- Legal aspects of healthcare.

Consent to treatment

The requirement for consent represents the legal and ethical expression of the human right to have one's autonomy and self-determination respected (McHale, Fox and Murphy, 1997). Its purpose is to protect and respect a patient's autonomy and to encourage meaningful decision making (DH, 2001e; NMC, 2002; Cable, Lumsdaine and Semple, 2003; Dimond, 2003).

A fundamental part of good practice is to obtain consent before providing care, and any healthcare professional who does not obtain valid consent may be liable to legal action by the patient and family, either in a civil or criminal offence of battery or in a claim for negligence (DH, 2001b).

Before any practical procedure is performed, the practitioner must ensure that a valid and meaningful consent is obtained before continuing with the procedure. This is required whenever a healthcare professional wishes to examine or treat any patient unless it is an emergency.

It must be remembered that consent needs to be given each time a procedure is performed and cannot be assumed to apply when a procedure for which consent has been given previously is repeated at a later time.

Valid consent

Consent is the patient's agreement for the healthcare professional to provide care (DH, 2001b). For consent to be valid the patient must have received sufficient information about the procedure, be competent to make the particular decision and not be under duress (Kennedy and Grubb, 2000; Aveyard, 2001; NMC, 2004; Montgomery, 2003).

All patients and clients have a right to receive information about their condition. You must be sensitive to their needs and respect the wishes of those who refuse or are unable to receive information about their condition. Information should be accurate, truthful and presented in such a way as to make it easily understood.

(NMC, 2002)

Consent can be given in a number of ways. The form of consent acceptable for a procedure will depend on the degree of risk involved, the treatment to be given and the clinical situation (Terry and Campbell, 2006).

Implied consent relates to behaviour of a patient, or in the case of a child the parent, that would indicate to the healthcare professional that he or she gives agreement for the procedure to be carried out. Implied consent usually applies for uncomplicated acts of care, such as assisting with personal hygiene. This may be given verbally but may also be non-verbal, such as the patient pulling up a sleeve to prepare for a blood pressure recording.

For healthcare procedures it may be difficult to distinguish between compliance and consent; therefore implied consent should not be relied upon and it is advisable to obtain express consent (Aveyard, 2002).

Express consent applies to both written and verbal consent which is required when a procure may involve an element of risk. The law does not specify when written consent is necessary (Kennedy and Grubb, 2000; Montgomery, 2003). When a procedure has more serious risks that may have major consequences, written consent is normally obtained. In these instances a consent form is used which states that the patient or parent is consenting to a clinical procedure that has associated risks. However written consent is only valid if all the elements above have been met (DH, 2001c). Although written consent provides evidence that the patient signed a form, the crucial factor is whether the consent was valid. There is no legal, ethical or professional distinction between the effectiveness of written, verbal and implied consent (Kennedy and Grubb, 2000; DH, 2001e; Dimond, 2003; Montgomery, 2003).

Express consent is achieved when all professionals involved in a procedure disclose adequate relevant information to enable the patient to make an informed decision. Tacit consent is when not all the relevant steps in the procedure are discussed and assumptions are made that, if patients agree to a particular procedure, they are therefore agreeing to the component parts without them being disclosed.

Information

An adult must be given adequate information about any treatment, disclosing its nature, purpose, associated risks and alternative treatments available. For children, the child and legal guardian need to understand the nature and purpose of the procedure (DH, 2001b) but this should be given in a way that meets the child's individual needs. The legal guardian should be provided with further information if required.

When performing nursing procedures, information should be provided describing the procedure, why it is necessary, the perceived benefits and risks, any available alternatives and the consequences of not performing the procedure.

Information may be given in a variety of ways, individualised to meet specific needs and circumstances, and is usually best given in steps and repeated at different stages to improve understanding (Kennedy, 2001). It should be honest and easily understood, and jargon should be avoided. The recipient should be given time to ask questions at any time before or during the procedure.

Voluntary

Consent must be voluntary, free from force, deceit, duress, overreaching or other ulterior forms of constraint (Terry and Campbell, 2006).

Capacity

Capacity is defined by the Mental Capacity Act (2005) as 'the everyday ability to make decisions or take actions that influence their life'. These decisions can be minor, everyday events or those that are less frequent and may have a major impact on the individual's life.

The Nursing and Midwifery Council (2002) states that you should presume that every patient and client is legally competent unless otherwise assessed by a suitably qualified practitioner. It is suggested that patients are legally competent if they have the capacity to understand and retain information about the procedure and can use this to make an informed choice. However those sectioned under the Mental Health Act (1983) may have their rights to consent restricted (www.departofhealth.gov.uk).

The Mental Capacity Act (2005) has been developed to support patient/clients/service users and also professional and lay users with issues related to consent, and to help clarify whether a person is capable of giving consent. It has five key principles:

- A presumption of capacity. Each person has the right to make his or her own decisions unless proven incapable.
- Individuals are supported to make their own decisions. People should be given practical help to make their own decisions.
- Unwise decisions do not mean that a person does not have the capacity to consent. Just because an individual makes unwise decisions – for example, dressing in an unusual way – this does not mean that person can be considered to lack capacity.
- Best interest. All actions (decisions) must be taken with the intention of the best interest for the individual at all times.
- Least restrictive option. Everything done for or on behalf of the person must follow the course that is least restrictive of his or her basic rights and freedoms.

The Mental Capacity Act (2005) also defines what is considered to be incapacity. People are deemed incapable when they are unable to make or communicate decisions because of an impairment or disturbance in the function of their mind or brain at the time a decision has to be made. An assessment that the impairment is sufficient can be made when they cannot demonstrate knowledge and understanding related to the issue or question they are being asked. An assessment process should be used and the Act gives some suggestions of criteria:

- failing to demonstrate relevant understanding of the information given to them when making a decision
- being unable to retain information relevant to the decision
- being unable to demonstrate that they can consider the pros and cons of information given to them
- being unable to communicate their decision by any means.

Following the assessment, if it is considered in the best interest of patients, a decision can be made for them and this will be considered a duty of care.

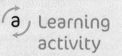

Learning activity

Look up Clause 5 of the Mental Capacity Act (2005) to understand how healthcare professionals are protected when making decisions in the best interest of the patient.

Consent when patients are less than 18 years old

A person under the age of 18 years is considered a minor and not an autonomous adult.

Consent by 16 and 17-year-olds is governed by the Family Law Reform Act (1969). They are presumed to have capacity to give consent to medical procedures unless the contrary is shown. In the United Kingdom except for Scotland, young people aged 16–18 can consent to treatment, but cannot necessarily refuse treatment intended to save their lives or prevent serious harm. If the patient refuses consent then those with parental responsibility, or a court, can give consent to treatment which is in the child's best interests. The British Medical Association (BMA) guidelines (2001) state that whilst young people's right to consent to treatment is now firmly established, their right to refuse it remains less certain. In Scotland if a child or young person is considered competent they may consent to treatment irrespective of age.

Children under 16 years old are presumed not to have capacity to consent unless they satisfy health professionals that they do have such capacity. However the common law case of Gillick (1985) established that a child less than 16 years old who does have capacity (is 'Gillick competent') can give consent for medical treatment. The Gillick case was about guidance on contraceptive advice and treatment to girls under the age of 16, but the case resulted in two outcomes. One was that it is lawful to provide contraceptive advice and treatment to girls under the age of 16 subject to certain guidelines (the Fraser guidelines). The other was that in certain circumstances children under the age of 16 can give consent in their own right (Gillick competence).

Larcher (2005) gives some guidelines to help in judging capacity. These include being able to:

- understand in simple terms the nature, purpose and necessity for the proposed treatment
- believe the information applies to them
- retain the information long enough to make a choice
- make a choice free from pressure.

Young people under 16 therefore may legally consent to treatment if they satisfy the criteria of competence and voluntariness. However competence is context related, and although the young person may have been able to give valid consent in one set of circumstances this does not necessarily apply in another situation. In law, it is the doctor's responsibility to assess competence, although other professionals with appropriate skills may be delegated to help (Larcher, 2005).

If a 'Gillick competent' child refuses a procedure, that does not mean that he/she lacks capacity. It may be due to anxiety, such as fear of the pain when having a dressing removed. In all cases effective preparation should be given, and where appropriate local anaesthetic, systemic analgesia or sedation can be offered.

When children are not 'Gillick competent' at least one person with parental responsibility should normally give consent. Those with parental responsibility are under a legal obligation to act in the child's best interests. If all those with parental responsibility refuse consent for a procedure that the doctors think is strongly in the child's best interests, then the doctors should involve the courts. In an emergency, if parental consent is not forthcoming and there is not time to involve the courts, act to save the child from death or serious harm.

For healthcare professionals it is important to be aware of who has parental responsibility. According to current law, a mother always has parental responsibility for her child. However fathers do not always have such responsibility. With more than one in three children now born outside marriage, some parents may be unclear about who has legal parental responsibility for their children (Directgov, 2008).

Living with the mother, even for a long time, does not give a father parental responsibility and if the parents are not married, parental responsibility does not always pass to the natural father if the mother dies.

- Those who have parental responsibility:
  - mothers and fathers married to mother
  - fathers not married to mother but who jointly register birth (after 1 December 2003)
  - adoptive parents
  - by a parental responsibility agreement with the mother
  - by a parental responsibility order, made by a court.
- Those who do not have parental responsibility:
  - fathers not married to the mother
  - step-parents.

Assent

Assent is an agreement given by a child who is not competent to give legally binding consent under current legislation. Assent should always be obtained from children by the healthcare professional to indicate that they are willing to participate, even when they are insufficiently mature to make a fully informed decision to consent (Callery, Neill and Feasey, 2006).

In an emergency

When treatment is necessary to preserve life or where the lack of capacity of the patient is permanent or likely to be long-standing, in the absence of a legal guardian it is lawful to carry out procedures that are in the best interest of the individual (DH, 2001e, 2002; NMC, 2004; Cable, Lumsdaine and Semple, 2003; Dimond, 2003; Montgomery, 2003). Best interests are not confined to medical best interests but include the patient's values and preferences when competent.

Responsibility for gaining consent

Consent is usually obtained by the individual performing the procedure. Oral consent is likely to be sought immediately before the procedure is carried out. In some circumstances it may not be possible for the professional carrying out the procedure to gain consent; in these circumstances another healthcare professional may be asked to do so on their behalf. The DH (2002) agrees that consent may be provided to another healthcare professional who has been specially trained for that area of practice.

Withdrawal of consent during a procedure

Consent can be withdrawn at any time during the procedure. If this should occur then it is best to stop the procedure and discover why the patient has withdrawn consent. The consequences of stopping should be explained to the patient. Allowing patients, whether adults or children, a feeling of control can help as sometimes the situation becomes overwhelming and they find it difficult to cope. Giving them a short break or a choice in how the procedure progresses may help them through the rest of it. If stopping the procedure is dangerous for the patient, this needs to be considered and clearly explained to the patient; if possible the procedure should be continued until the danger is over.

Risk assessment and patient safety

Adverse events occur in around 10 per cent of admissions to hospital or at a rate of an estimated 850,000 each year. They cost approximately £2 billion a year in additional hospital stays alone. Approximately 400 people die or are seriously injured in adverse events involving medical devices every year, and the NHS pays around £400 million in settlement of clinical negligence claims (DH, 2000). Adverse incidents occur when there is unexplained or unintended harm to the patient. A near miss is when an occurrence might have led to a patient being harmed but something prevented that from occurring and by chance alone no harm resulted.

Risk assessment is simply an examination of any procedure undertaken during your work that could harm yourself or others. It is an employer's duty under the Management of Health and Safety at Work Regulations (1999) to provide safety in the work place and to ensure that any risk is managed 'so far as is reasonably practicable'. Health professionals must cooperate with their employer in obeying health and safety regulations. Under the Nursing and Midwifery Council's Code of Conduct (2002: para 8) all registered practitioners must 'act to identify and minimise the risk to patients and clients' and 'work with other members of the team to promote healthcare environments that are conducive to safe, therapeutic and ethical practice'.

A risk assessment is a careful examination of the environment that could cause harm to people. Once a hazard has been identified, precautions need to be put in place to reduce the risk. It is a legal requirement to assess and minimise risk to anyone in a workplace (Hayes, 2007).

Within a hospital there is a health and safety department with a risk manager, and usually there are risk assessors on each care unit, but it is everyone's personal responsibility to raise awareness of potential hazards so they can be removed or the risk minimised.

The five steps to risk assessment

- Look for hazards.
- Decide who might be harmed and how.

- Evaluate the risks and decide if existing precautions are enough or if more should be done.
- Record your findings.
- Review and revise if necessary.

> **ⓐ Learning activity**
>
> Think of a situation you have been in and work through the five steps listed in the text to help you identify risk. Look up the following article, which will help you identify the questions you should be asking yourself about the situation: Dimond, B. (2002) 'Risk assessment and management to ensure health and safety at work', *British Journal of Nursing* **11**(21), 1372–4.

Common workplace injuries occur from manual handling, slips, trips and falls, and contact with harmful substances. For healthcare professionals the situation is constantly changing and risks should be evaluated when there are:

- new items of equipment
- new methods of working
- policy changes
- MHRA medical devices alerts
- challenging behaviour of patients or relatives.
- new chemicals in the workplace
- changes in the environment.

It must be recognised that there are increased risks when caring for pregnant mothers, children, the elderly and adolescents.

Most simple hazards can be identified and acted upon, and the risk resolved. Potentially serious hazards require formal recording on a risk assessment form – which should be available with instructions in your health and safety manual – and shown to your manager to action (Hayes, 2007).

A risk assessment should take place whenever you are carrying out a procedure, and guidelines should be followed at all times. Procedural guidelines should be updated frequently and must be evidence based. The professional performing the procedure should be trained and competent to do so.

> **ⓐ Learning activity**   W
>
> To find out more, visit the following websites: MHRA Medicines and Healthcare Products Regulations Authority: www.medical-devices.gov.uk; and NHS Plus Health at work: www.nhsplus.nhs.uk/law&you/employers_riskassessment.asp.

Dignity and privacy

The concept of the maintenance of dignity is central to good practice (Walsh and Kowanko, 2002). Whenever a procedure is planned and carried out in practice, the approach of the nurse is crucial to the patient and every effort should be made to ensure it is a positive and constructive experience. Nurses are advised through the Code of Professional Conduct (NMC, 2002) that they are 'personally accountable for ensuring that they promote and protect the interests and dignity of patients and clients, irrespective of gender age, race, ability, sexuality, economic status, lifestyle, cultural and religious or political belief'.

The concept of dignity is linked to Article 8 of the 1998 Human Rights Act, which emphasises that individual patients should be treated as persons, and that respecting their wishes and dignity is fundamental to quality care (Woogara, 2001). Dignity is defined as an individual's self-worth (Jacelon, 2003) and comprises individual and interpersonal attributes. It is partly imparted by others in the immediate environment but it also exists independently. There is increased difficulty when dealing with children as you must not only protect the dignity of the child in his/her present state but also consider the dignity needs of the individual that child may become (Reed et al, 2003).

The Essence of Care (DH, 2001a) identifies privacy and dignity as one of nine key areas of care. Privacy and dignity are also firmly embedded within the National Service Frameworks for adults and children.

(e) Evidence-based practice: perceptions of dignity

In a study by Walsh and Kowanko (2002) the perceptions of nurses and patients with regards to dignity were compared. The results for patients and health professionals had many similarities, including respect for privacy, not being exposed, not being rushed, having time to decide, being seen as a an individual and not an object, consideration for emotions and demonstrating respect.

(a) Learning activity

You have been asked to attend to the hygiene needs of an 80-year-old woman on a mixed gender ward who is not able to go to the bathroom. What would you do to ensure that the privacy and dignity of this lady is maintained?

The health professional should endeavour to maintain the patient's dignity throughout the procedure. Dignity needs to be considered throughout the three stages of the procedure: before, during and after completion.

Before the procedure healthcare professionals should introduce themselves, effectively communicate the elements of the procedure and offer any choices that may be available throughout its delivery, such as when and where it should be performed, and whether pain relief is required. This helps patients feel that their opinions are considered and that they have some control. The environment should be prepared, taking into account issues of safety and the age of the patient. Children should be told their parents can be present if they wish, and play and distraction equipment may need to be assembled.

Dignity is enhanced by ensuring that the patient (or child/family) is made aware that he/she is the most important person at that moment in time.

Throughout the procedure the patient should be made as comfortable as possible; effective communication should continue throughout, offering appropriate reassurance. Every effort should be made to ensure the body is not unnecessarily exposed or violated and the procedure is carried out in privacy.

After the procedure, communication with the patient continues to be of vital importance. Allow the patients to ask questions and express any concerns without feeling rushed. Make sure clothing is replaced appropriately and the patient is happy with his/her physical appearance before returning to the ward or having the curtains opened.

Privacy is the subject of one of the statements of the 1998 European Convention on Human Rights and violation of this by healthcare professionals must be avoided. Woogara (2001) highlights that respecting privacy is manifested in a multitude of ways, including the right to enjoy and control personal space and property, the right to confidentiality and the right to expect treatment with dignity.

Breaches of privacy can easily be avoided during nursing procedures by thorough preparation of the environment. Violation of privacy can occur when curtains are not shut properly or when people walk through curtains when procedures are taking place, thereby putting patients in a vulnerable state (Woogara, 2001). This can be prevented by clipping curtains together or by using a 'do not disturb' notice. The major area for concern within the realms of privacy is that of confidentiality. Whilst drawing curtains around a bed can successfully protect the patient's personal space, the curtains do not provide a barrier to sound, and confidential information can easily be overheard. The best environment to perform procedures is away from the ward area in a treatment room.

Comfort

The meaning of comfort is broad, complex and individualised (Tutton and Seers, 2003). Siefert (2002) defines comfort as 'a state and/or process that is individually defined, multidimensional and dynamic; it may be temporary or permanent and requires that one's needs be satisfied in the physical, psychological, social, spiritual and/or environmental domains within a specific context.'

It appears that comforted patients heal faster, cope better, require less analgesia, have shorter stays and are generally more satisfied with care (Walker, 2001; Kolcaba and Wilson, 2002). A patient will be comforted by meeting such needs as alleviation of pain or nausea. The health professional should try to enable patients to achieve a state of calm or contentment so they are able to manage pain or problems that cannot be removed. This is particularly relevant when a painful procedure is performed and discomfort cannot be avoided (Kolcaba and Wilson, 2002).

According to Robinson (2002), discomfort may have number of causes, including fatigue, loss of appetite, being too hot or too cold, pain, bowel distress, loss of bodily control, vulnerability, fear, embarrassment, stress or depression.

Comfort needs may be physical, psychospiritual, sociocultural or environmental. The specific needs within each of these dimensions vary according to the individual and the procedure to be performed. Concerns about physical comfort need pain control, which should be assessed and the management of it planned before the procedure commences. Psychospiritual comfort needs would be met through verbal or physical communication such as touch. Cultural sensitivity would be addressed to meet the sociocultural needs; this may also include the need for reassurance. Comfort needs may also include the appropriate management of odours and maintaining a safe environment.

Patients' comfort needs must be considered throughout all the stages of a procedure, taking account of their fears, their need for privacy, confidentiality and safety, and their physical state. The healthcare professional performing the procedure should help maintain the patients' comfort by showing that they are knowledgeable and competent in performing the procedure and that they have the necessary equipment and facilities available to provide high-quality care.

Safeguarding

It is essential that all healthcare professionals, whether they are caring for children or adults, are aware of the need to safeguard their patients/clients. Abuse can occur to individuals of any age: adults, children, and individuals with mental health problems or learning disabilities. The perpetrator may be the parent, the partner, the siblings or the individual's own children. A survey of 2111 people over 65 living in their own homes found that 2.6 per cent had experienced abuse or neglect during the previous year. Neglect by partners significantly increased over age 85, and O'Keeffe and colleagues (2007) suggest that this may be due to the increasing frailty of both partners, leading to an inability to continue to provide support for each other (ADSS, 2005).

The Department of Health (2000d: 8–9) defines a vulnerable adult as:

> a person who is or may be in need of community care by reason of mental or other disability, age or illness, and who is or may be unable to protect him or herself against significant harm or exploitation.

All children are considered to be vulnerable, and safeguarding children is the process of protecting them from abuse or neglect and preventing impairment of their health or development. Healthcare professionals have a duty to safeguard and promote the welfare of all children within their care (DH, 2003).

The healthcare professional must:

- be aware of risk factors and be able to recognise signs of abuse and neglect
- be familiar with the organisation's policies and procedures for safeguarding
- ensure the referral of concerns to social services or police (after discussion with a senior colleague)
- document concerns and any related issues
- not promise confidentiality.

When carrying out any procedure on an individual the following topics need to be considered:

- When dealing with a child, assess the parent's capacity to support and care for the child during the procedure.
- Implement an individual approach to ensure that the needs of the patient are respected and provided for. This would include topics discussed earlier in the chapter such as informed consent, dignity, privacy, comfort and safety.
- Reduce anxiety by effective communication and appropriate support.
- Ensure that the patient is not suffering abuse through the implementation of the procedure. Ensure that the procedure is necessary and that there is no alternative treatment.
- Ensure that procedures are carried out competently and efficiently in order to minimise pain and suffering.

During a procedure factors that might cause concern would include: the reported cause of injuries sustained not matching the injuries; a pattern of injuries of various ages; repeated visits to the emergency department or admissions to hospital; worrying behaviour demonstrated by the patient or the relatives.

It is important to share any concerns with other professionals and appropriate agencies. The safety of the patient is paramount and any concern should be acted upon swiftly.

Documentation

The importance of record keeping cannot be over emphasised, and for the provision of high-quality care accurate, complete and up-to-date records are vital (Moloney and Maggs, 1999). Good-quality record keeping provides satisfactory communication, allows for continuity of care and prevents omissions in care provision.

After the completion of all procedures, accurate documentation should be completed to demonstrate that the duty of care has been fulfilled.

There is no single model for record keeping. The best format is one produced to meet the needs of the environment and the patient through consultation with the users.

High-quality documentation helps protect the patient by:

- improving communication
- sharing information (in multidisciplinary teams)
- providing an accurate account of treatment/care
- helping detect problems/changes in condition
- promoting high standards of care
- promoting continuity of care.

(Guidelines for records and record keeping – NMC, 2002)

The content and style of healthcare records should be:

- factual, consistent, accurate
- written soon after the event
- providing current information on the care and condition of the patient
- up to date
- written clearly/permanently (and in a form that will be legible when photocopied)
- signed/timed/dated
- alterations – dated, timed, signed
- without the use of:
  - abbreviations
  - jargon
  - meaningless phrases
  - irrelevant speculation
  - offensive subjective statements
- consecutive – in the correct order and date

- with clear identification of problems and action taken
- with clear evidence of:
  - care planned
  - decisions made
  - care delivered
  - information shared
- written with involvement of the patient/carer
- understandable by the patient/carer.

(Guidelines for records and record keeping – NMC, 2002)

Accountability

Accountability is defined as the obligation to be answerable for your own judgements and actions (Martin, 2004). Qualified professionals are personally accountable for their actions and any omissions in their practice. They must also have the knowledge to be able to justify their decisions. As a student you should be practising under the supervision of a qualified practitioner who is professionally responsible for your actions or omissions. However you can still be called to account by the university or the law in response to your actions or omissions. You have the responsibility to make your patients aware you are a student, and patients have the right to refuse to allow you to participate in their care.

There will be times when you are not being directly supervised by a qualified professional. If an emergency situation occurs at this time you should not participate in any procedure for which you have not been adequately prepared.

Conclusion

Before commencing any procedure, you should consider the key concepts outlined in this chapter. The healthcare professional should act as the patient's advocate, safeguard vulnerable individuals, and ensure that consent is obtained and the patient's individual needs for comfort, privacy and protection of dignity are met whilst providing care. The professionals are accountable for their actions and should provide a safe environment, adhere to local and national policies and procedures, and ensure that accurate documentation is made to ensure continuity of care and patient safety and demonstrate that their duty of care has been fulfilled.

References

Association of Directors of Social Services (ADSS) (2005) *Safeguarding Adults: A national framework of standards for good practice and outcomes in adult protection work*, London, ADSS.

Aveyard, H. (2001) 'The requirements for informed consent prior to nursing care procedures', *Journal of Advanced Nursing* **37**(2), 243–9.

Aveyard, H. (2002) 'Implied consent prior to nursing care procedures', *Journal of Advanced Nursing* **39**(20), 1–7.

Beauchamp T. L. and Childress J. F. (2001) *Principles of Biomedical Ethics*, 5th edn, Oxford, Oxford University Press.

Beyea, S. (2005) 'Patient advocacy-nurses keeping patients safe', *Association of Perioperative Registered Nurses AORN Journal*, May, 1046–7.

British Medical Association (2001) *Consent, Rights and Choices in Healthcare for Children and Young People*, London, BMJ Books.

Cable, S., Lumsdaine, I. and Semple, M. (2003) 'Informed consent', *Nursing Standard* **18**(12), 47–53.

Callery, P., Neill, S. and Feasey, S. (2006) 'The evidence base for children's nursing practice', Chapter 14 in Glasper E. A. and Richardson, J. (eds), *A Textbook of Children's and Young Peoples*

Nursing, Edinburgh, Churchill Livingstone.

Department of Health (DH) (1983) *Mental Health Act*, London, DH.

DH (2000) *An Organisation with a Memory*, London, Stationery Office.

DH (2001a) *Essence of Care*, London, DH.

DH (2001b) *Good Practice in Consent Implementation Guide: Consent to examination or treatment*, London, DH.

DH (2001c) *Reference Guide to Informed Consent for Examination or Treatment*, London, DH.

DH (2001d) *The Report of the Public Inquiry into Children's Heart Surgery at the Bristol Royal Infirmary (1984–1995): Learning from Bristol*, London, DH.

DH (2001e) *The Royal Liverpool Children's Inquiry: Summary and recommendations*, London, Stationery Office.

DH (2002) *Model Policy for Consent to Examination or Treatment*, London, DH.

DH (2003) *Every Child Matters*, London, Stationery Office.

DH (2005) *Mental Capacity Act (2005)*, London, Department of Constitutional Affairs.

Dimond, B. (2003) *Legal Aspects of Consent*, Salisbury, Quay Books.

Dimond, B. (2005) *Legal Aspects of Nursing*, Harlow, Essex, Pearson Education.

Directgov (2008) http://www.direct.gov.uk/en/Parents/ParentsRights/DG_4002954 (accessed 26 December 2008).

Dyer, C. (1992) *Doctors, Patients and the Law*, London, Blackwell Science.

Family Law Reform Act (1969) S8 Age of Majority Act (NI), London, Stationery Office.

Gates, B. (1994) *Advocacy: A Nurses Guide*, London, Scutari Press.

Gillick v West Norfolk and Wisbech Area Health Authority [1985] 3 All ER 402 (HL).

Harrison, C., Kenny, N. P., Sidareous, M. and Rowell, M. (1997) 'Bioethics for clinicians 9: Involving children in medical decisions', *Canadian Medical Association Journal* **156**(6), 825–8.

Hayes (2007) 'Risk assessment', pp. 62–3 in Glasper, E., McEwing, G. and Richardson, J. (eds), *Oxford Handbook of Children's and Young People's Nursing*, Oxford, Oxford University Press.

Jacelon, C. S. (2003) 'The dignity of elders in an acute care hospital', *Qualitative Health Research* **13**(4), 543–56.

Kennedy, I. (2001) *Bristol Royal Infirmary Inquiry. Learning from Bristol: the Report of the Public Inquiry into Children's Heart Surgery at the Bristol Royal Infirmary 1984–1995*, London, Stationery Office.

Kennedy, I. and Grubb, A. (2000) *Medical Law*, 3rd edn, London, Butterworth's.

Kolcaba, K. (1992) 'Holistic comfort: Operationalizing the construct as a nurse-sensitive outcome', *Advances in Nursing Science* **15**(1), 1–10.

Larcher, V. (2005) 'Consent, competence and confidentiality', *British Medical Journal*, 330(12 February), 353–6.

Mains, E. D. (1994) 'Concept clarification in professional practice: dignity', *Journal of Advanced Nursing* 19, 947–53.

Malinowski, A. and Leeseberg Stamler, L. (2002) 'Comfort: exploration of the concept in nursing', *Journal of Advanced Nursing* 39, 599–609.

Martin, E. A. (2004) *Oxford Dictionary of Nursing*, Oxford, Oxford University Press.

Moloney, R. and Maggs, C. (1999) 'A systematic review of the relationships between written manual nursing care planning, record keeping and patient outcomes', *Journal of Advanced Nursing* **30**(1), 51–7.

McHale, I., Fox, M. and Murphy, J. (1997) *Healthcare Law Text and Materials*, London, Sweet and Maxwell.

Montgomery, J. (2003) *Healthcare Law*, 2nd edn, Oxford, Oxford University Press.

Nursing and Midwifery Council (NMC) (2002) *Code of Professional Conduct*, London, NMC.

NMC (2004) *The NMC Code of Conduct: Standards for conduct, performance and ethics*, London, NMC.

O'Keeffe, M., Hills, A., Doyle, M., McCreadie, C., Scholes, S., Constantine, R., Tinker, A., Manthorpe, J., Biggs, S. and Erens, B. (2007) *UK Study of Abuse and Neglect of Older People, Prevalence Survey Report*, London, National Centre for Social Research.

Reed, P., Smith, P., Fletcher, M. and Bradding, A. (2003) 'Promoting the dignity of the child in hospital', *Nursing ethics* **10**(1), 67–76.

Robinson, S. (2002) 'Warmed blankets: an intervention to promote comfort for elderly hospitalized patients', *Geriatric Nursing* **23**(32) 1–3.

Royal College of Nursing (2003) *Restraining, Holding Still and Containing Children and Young People: Guidance for Nursing Staff*, London, Royal College of Nursing.

Siefert, M. L. (2002) 'Concept analysis of comfort', *Nursing Forum* **37**(4), 16–23.

Terry, L. and Campbell, A. (2006) 'Legal aspects of child healthcare', pp. 317–29 in Glasper, A. and Richardson, J. A. *Textbook of Children's and Young People's Nursing*, Edinburgh, Elsevier.

Tutton, E. and Seers, K. (2003) 'An exploration of the concept of comfort', *Journal of Clinical Nursing* **12**(5), 689–96.

Walker, A. C. (2001) 'Safety and comfort work of nurses glimpsed through patient narratives', *International Journal of Nursing Practice* **8**(1), 42–8.

Walsh, K. and Kowanko, I. (2002) 'Nurses' and patients' perceptions of dignity', *International Journal of Nursing Practice* **8**(3), 143–5.

Woogara, I. (2001) 'Human rights and patients' privacy in UK hospitals', *Nursing Ethics* **8**(3), 234–46.

Chapter

2

IT skills

Mike Weaver

Visit www.palgrave.com/glasper to read our online IT Skills chapter. Packed with top tips and valuable advice on information management and Web 2.0 technologies, it will help prepare you for study in the digital age.

Part
I

Skills for communication

Chapters

Chapter

3

Communication

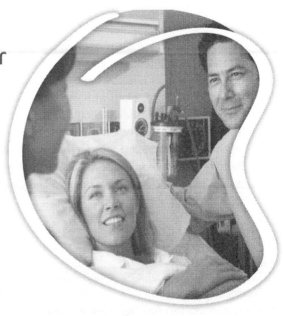

Jan Orr and Diana Morris

 Links to other chapters in *Foundation Skills for Caring*

4 Communicating with adolescents
5 Anxiety
6 Sign language
7 Breaking significant news
8 Breakaway skills
40 Last offices

 Links to other chapters in *Foundation Studies for Caring*

5 Communication
6 Culture
16 Safeguarding children
17 Safeguarding adults
28 Rehabilitation

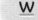 Don't forget to visit www.palgrave.com/glasper for additional online resources relating to this chapter.

Introduction

Effective communication is essential to healthcare delivery. Although we may think that communication should come naturally, it is not without challenge.

The provision of effective healthcare involves multiprofessional working. This can include many diverse teams, often with members from outside the traditional healthcare environments: for example, the voluntary sector, police and education. Multiprofessional working depends crucially upon good communication.

People are individual. Each of us has our own life experiences, pressures, morals and values. The diversity of people who access healthcare is vast. Barriers to communication can be endless. Effective communication in today's healthcare culture requires us to understand this and appreciate its importance.

Learning outcomes

This chapter will enable you to:

- explore effective communication
- understand the importance of multiprofessional team working
- identify different methods of communication

- recognise barriers to communication and explore client-centred methods of care delivery
- consider the nurse's professional responsibility.

Concepts

- Information giving
- Collaboration and partnership
- Social interaction
- Therapeutic relationships

- Safety
- Self-fulfilment
- Learning
- Value

- Respect
- Effects of poor communication.

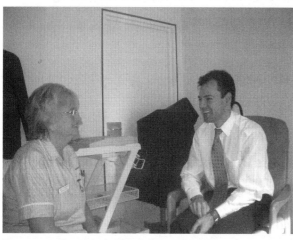

Figure 3.1 Communication is key to professional relationships

The chapter will also help you to develop key skills, including:
- professional responsibility
- care delivery
- interprofessional and interagency working
- barriers to communication
- methods of communication
- documentation.

(a) Learning activity

Before reading on consider why communication is important.

What is communication?

Communication is a daily process and often done without thinking. It appears easy when done well, but people often fail to communicate effectively. Communication takes time and requires engagement, empathy and the ability to listen and respond (Peate, 2006).

It can be defined as the way we transmit facts, feelings and meanings in order to fulfil goals. This process involves sending and receiving messages via symbols, words, signs, gestures, or other actions such as cues (Peate, 2006).

It involves a social interaction through messages by the transmission of information from one person to another. This can be verbal, non-verbal or both (Bailie, 2005).

Communication starts at birth when infants instinctively attempt to let adults know what they want and feel (Mathews, 2006).

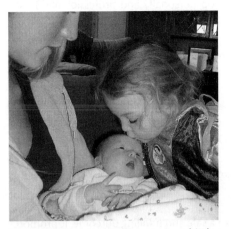

Figure 3.2 Communication starts at birth

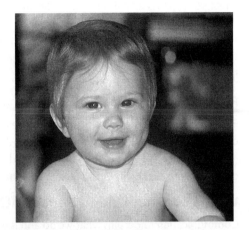

Figure 3.3 The social smile at six months

Communication in the healthcare setting

Howell (1982), cited in Sully and Dallas (2005), describes 'conscious and unconscious incompetence' as a communication model to demonstrate the acquisition of effective communication skills. It demonstrates that as we learn new skills, our ability to deal with situations changes. This model is particularly helpful in understanding how communication skills grow and improve with experience.

'Conscious and unconscious' communication model

Communication skills are transferable across different healthcare situations and circumstances. For example, a nurse working in intensive care does not need to be an expert to support a distressed relative.

However, the nurse may not realise how distressing the intensive care environment may be to the relative and, as a result, may not be able to offer appropriate sensitive support (*unconscious incompetence*).

The nurse could be aware that intensive care is distressing but does not know how to offer support (*conscious incompetence*).

Conversely, the nurse may be aware of the upsetting nature of the event and the feelings of the relative (*conscious competence*).

The nurse is then able to reflect on past experiences about the needs of the relative in this situation, and so can quickly decide what actions to take (*conscious competence*).

a) Learning activity

Imagine you have a clinical placement on a busy medical assessment unit. On your first day you are allocated your mentor Jed, a deputy ward manager with many years of experience working in medical assessment units. Under Jed's supervision you look after a 20-year-old female called Janet who has been admitted via her general practitioner with severe abdominal pain. Numerous investigative clinical tests have been carried out, and a diagnosis of leukaemia has been made. You are with Jed whilst Janet is told the news. Relating back to the 'conscious competence' model, how would you describe yourself in this situation? How do you think Jed would respond?

It is important to understand the theories and evidence base surrounding client/patient care. However, experiencing varying clinical situations gives the confidence and knowledge of how to deal with them effectively.

As a student and registered practitioner, you will find that reflection on practice is an effective way to learn about new skills and to develop personally and professionally. This is done by reviewing the situation or experience in order to describe, analyse and evaluate the experience: 'what went well, what could be better?' (Grandis et al, 2003). It is recommended that you undertake further reading about reflection (see for example Gibbs, 1998), discussed in the introduction.

Professional responsibility

The professional code of conduct for nurses is underpinned by the need for effective and collaborative communication at all times (NMC, 2008).

The *Essence of Care* (DH, 2001a) stated that all practicable steps must be taken to communicate effectively with patients and their carers.

Why is communication important?

Communication underpins what we do and is vital to a safe and fulfilling outcome. It promotes social interaction, and can make us feel wanted, special and important (Peate, 2008).

Effective communication is needed to promote a therapeutic relationship with the patient/client (Donnelly and Neville, 2008). Examples include:

- preparing an adult for a medical intervention
- listening to a worried patient
- discussing a discharge plan with an elderly patient
- planning client-centred actions to help a young person with mental health problems.

Communication is integral to safety. Consider, for example, an intensive care nurse coordinating a resuscitation team during a cardiac arrest. Each member of the team needs to know their role, otherwise life-saving intervention could be missed (Bailie, 2005).

Table 3.1 Effects of communication

Effects of good communication	Effects of poor communication
→ accurate identification of problems → patient/client satisfaction → patients/clients more likely to comply with their treatment and in their life style → quality care → job satisfaction → fewer clinical errors → fewer patient/client complaints	→ confusion → clinical incidents → poor staff morale → delayed patient/client discharge → complications such as infections, pressure ulcers → increased patient/client anxiety → complaints

[S] Scenario: a patient with senile dementia in A&E

Ann is 80 years old and has senile dementia. She lives at home alone with no living family. Her dementia has been becoming increasingly severe. Ann has been admitted to hospital with a fractured neck of femur as the result of a fall. In the Accident and Emergency Department, she is very distressed and continuously screaming. Ann has been given strong analgesia for pain and put into traction for comfort. Despite this she continues to scream. A registered nurse sits with her, holds her hand, explains to her what has happened and why she is in hospital, Ann becomes relaxed and talks to the nurse. The nurse is called away by the nurse in charge because the department is very busy. Ann becomes agitated again.

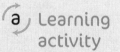

[a] Learning activity

Consider the communication needs in Ann's case. Do you feel that the nurses' actions were appropriate? Is there anything else you would have done?

⚠ Professional alert!

Working in the clinical setting can be stressful. The thought of endless clinical procedures that need to be done is daunting. When there is so much to do, the challenge of spending time sitting with patients can seem impossible, but taking the time to explain and reassure them is very important. This requires respect and trust from the practitioner, patient and the family/carers.

Did you consider Ann's privacy and dignity needs? Environmental factors can hinder communication and consequently the therapeutic relationship (Chinn and Meleis, 2005). Taking Ann to a more private and quieter area may help her to feel more relaxed.

Before undertaking any intervention it is important that informed consent is obtained from the patient. The patient needs to understand the nature and purpose of the procedure (Arnold and Underman-Boggs, 2007; DH, 2001b; Human Rights Act, 1998).

Barriers to communication

Communication is a complex process. Barriers can occur if the recipient has failed to understand the meaning or the importance of the message. The person transmitting the message may give too much or too little information. The use of jargon should be avoided as it can be very confusing (Peate, 2006).

Physical barriers to communication include:

- speech defects
- deafness
- poor vision
- developmental delay
- illness

- injury
- age
- dyslexia
- dyspraxia
- language difficulties

- tiredness
- poor diet
- dehydration

(Sully and Dallas, 2005).

⟳ a ⟳ Learning activity

Can you think of any other barriers to communication that you may come across in the healthcare setting?

Did you consider psychological and emotional reasons: for example bereavement, stress, anxiety, mental health problems

Other reasons could include:

- peer pressure
- time pressures
- lack of job satisfaction
- apathy
- distractions such as background noises.

To ensure that we fully meet the needs of the patient/client with barriers to communication, it is important to undertake a careful assessment. It can be helpful to involve the family, carers and close friends. However this must be with consent from the patient/client (Arnold and Underman-Boggs, 2007; NMC, 2008).

On the basis of the assessment, individualised actions can be planned in agreement with the patient/client. A range of communication methods may be required. For example, patients who do not speak English will need a translator, those with visual problems may need leaflets in Braille, and those with learning difficulties may need their carers to be present at all times.

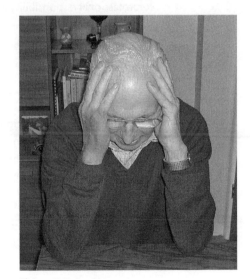

Figure 3.4 Anxiety

Clear, concise and factual documentation of the assessment and care plans are vital to ensure effective communication. This provides evidence that care has occurred and enables professional colleagues to continue individualised and evidence-based care. It is important that patients/clients have access to their nursing records. They should be involved in the documentation process, understand and be in agreement with it (Data Protection Act, 1998; NHS, 2006; NMC, 2004).

[S] Scenario: Why is John in a bad mood?

John is the carer of his elderly father, Paul, who was admitted to hospital because he is severely dehydrated. During the night Paul fell out of bed and sustained lacerations and bruises. John has been telephoned by the ward manager and the situation explained. John feels he has not been told the whole truth and not been given the opportunity to discuss the situation as the ward manager says she is too busy. John is furious that his father was not supervised and has threatened to take legal action.

---

[a] Learning activity

As a registered nurse what would you do in this situation?

In your answer consider ways in which communication occurs, including verbal and non-verbal communication. Did the ward manager fail to meet her professional responsibility and duty of care?

⚠ Professional alert!

Complaints often happen as a result of poor communication. Complainants are entitled to prompt, open, constructive, honest answers, and an apology where appropriate (DH, 2000; DH, 2004).

How to communicate effectively

The 'assertive communication' model described by Sully and Dallas (2005) looks at effective and ineffective ways to communicate with others.

Think about multiprofessional colleagues you have met in the clinical setting. Can you relate their behaviour to any of the examples of verbal responses outlined below?

'Assertive communication' model

A nurse named Chris is caring for a group of patients with orthopaedic problems. The physiotherapist, named Indigo, gives Chris a handover of her action plan. Indigo forgets to document this.

Passive behaviour: 'I'm not ok – you're ok'

When adopting passive behaviour, Chris speaks in a high-pitched, quiet voice with minimal eye contact. His sentences lack fluency, consistency and are hesitant. Chris may not say anything to Indigo but instead complain to his colleagues that she is incompetent.

Dialogue – 'Indigo, I'm sorry to bother you, I wasn't clear whether you wanted me to get the patient out of bed after lunch. I was wondering if you could document this, if that is OK.'

Manipulative behaviour: 'I'm ok, you're not ok, but I let you think you are'

Chris speaks softly, possibly seductively, or alternatively may speak louder than is appropriate. There is likely to be intermittent or continued eye contact, maybe reduced personal space (coming closer than is usual in such conversations). Once the task is finished the personal space is likely to be increased.

Dialogue – 'You're usually really good at getting difficult patients out of bed Indigo, would you like me to help you? I will then give you the relevant documents to complete.'

Aggressive behaviour: 'I'm ok, you're not ok'

Chris's body language may be rigid, over active, short and abrupt. Indigo is unlikely to expect him to communicate like this. There may be sarcasm and impatience in Chris's tone of voice. Eye contact is either a glare or avoidance, implying a disregard for Indigo. The communication comes as a demand rather than a request.

Dialogue – ' Indigo, you've forgotten to write in the patient's notes. You are always doing this. Can you do it now?'

Assertive behaviour: 'I'm ok, you're ok'

Chris makes eye contact with Indigo and gains her attention. Speech is clear, concise and non-accusatory. The tone of voice is moderate.

Dialogue – 'Indigo, I think you have forgotten to document your plan of care. Have you time to do it now?'

There are many models of communication, therefore further reading is recommended.

Improving Working Lives (DH, 2004) is a national standard introduced by the government. One of the aims was to raise awareness among employees in the National Health Service of the importance of working together. Posters have been produced and awareness sessions arranged locally to promote effective communication.

Part

I

(a) Learning activity

It is hoped that, for most of the time in your healthcare clinical work place, you will experience *assertive* behaviour. If this is not the case, think back to a situation where other behaviours were used, and reflect on why this happened.

⚠ Professional alert!

Working in the healthcare setting can at times be challenging and stressful. It is very important to treat patients, clients and colleagues with respect and dignity (Human Rights Act, 1998). We are all human beings, and under pressure we often say things in a way that we don't mean to. However to gain the trust and respect of our colleagues and patients/clients we need to think about how we communicate what we say, and about our non-verbal body language.

Figure 3.5 Posters displayed in clinical areas to promote *Improving Working Lives*

Reprinted with the permission of Falmouth College of Arts and Design, Royal Cornwall Hospital NHS Trust (2005).

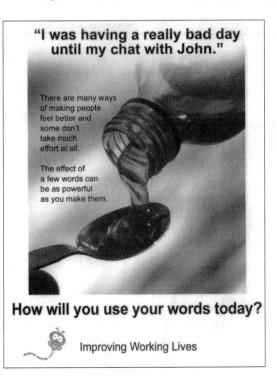

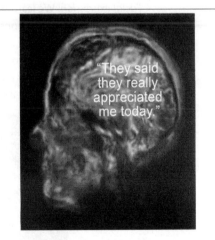

Peate (2006) describes nine types of non-verbal communication. They are:

- *Paralanguage*: the vocal cues that accompany language, the way we say words. This includes speech rate, intensity, pitch, modulation, articulation. The faster a person speaks, the more competent they may appear.
- *Kinesics*: communication through facial or body movements: for example, body gestures, nodding the head while listening, display of feelings such as frowning or raising eyebrows.
- *Occulesics*: associated with eye movements. Eye movements and gaze can be associated with culture.
- *Appearance*: can affect how a person is perceived. In *The Catherine Tate* show on the BBC, people with red hair are seen as antisocial. This of course is a fictional comedy show but does give an example of society's perceptions. www.bbc. co.uk/comedy/catherinetate.
- *Proxemics*: the distance people maintain while engaging with others. It can feel uncomfortable when someone stands too close or too far away.
- *Haptics*: involves touching. Touching occurs throughout the day, in hand shaking, hugging and kissing for example. Touch can convey many messages: positive feelings, reassurance, comfort. However cultural differences or personal feelings can make this a negative experience.
- *Olfactics*: the study of smell. Smell is a powerful memory aid. In addition, it can cause people to relate or disengage according to factors such as poor personal hygiene or a favoured perfume.
- *Chronoemics*: the way people react to time. Barriers to communication can occur because of time concerns. For example, if people need to pick their children up from school, this may make them seem agitated or anxious.
- *Facial expression*: We learn how to manage facial expression from childhood. Expressions may not always seem appropriate, for example if someone is yawning during a teaching session. This could be perceived as showing boredom, when in fact it may be difficult for students to concentrate because the room is too hot.

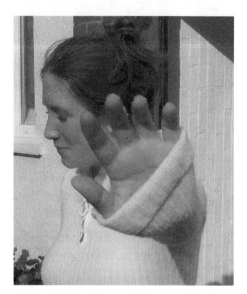

Figure 3.6   Kinesics

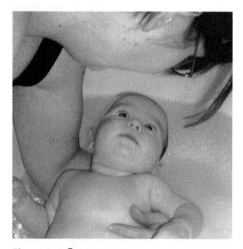

Figure 3.7   Eye contact

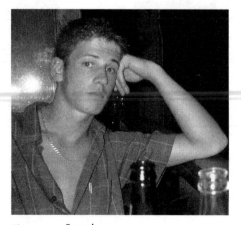

Figure 3.8   **Bored**

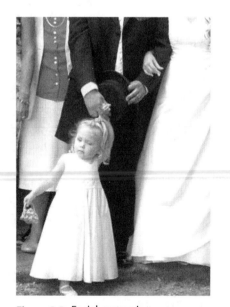

Figure 3.9   Facial expression

Part

> **a** Learning activity
>
> Think of the last time you had a conversation with a client. List any non-verbal communication strategies you used.
>
> Did your list include several of the factors mentioned above? Did you feel the communication between yourself and the client was positive? If it did not feel positive, was that because of any of those factors. In this case, how would you improve your use of non-verbal communication?

Multiprofessional team working

This forms a large and important part of work in the healthcare setting. Working in a collaborative partnership with the client/patient is integral to effective care delivery. To work effectively requires an understanding of each other's roles and responsibilities. When the team first meets, roles and responsibilities should be established to prevent confusion. An effective way to do this is by holding a meeting where action plans are documented. It is important to establish the routes and methods of communication within the team, as busy work schedules may make it difficult to get together for meetings (Arnold and Underman-Boggs, 2007; Darley and Edwards, 2002). Methods of doing this may include:

- telephone calls
- documenting in-patient and client records
- video conferencing
- meeting in different places in rotation, to balance out in a fair way the distances people have to travel.

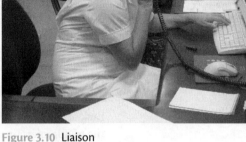

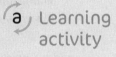
Figure 3.10 Liaison

> **a** Learning activity
>
> Can you think of any other methods of communication you have experienced in the clinical setting?

The multiprofessional team can be vast and diverse. For a registered practitioner, working as part of a team is an ongoing part of delivering patient/client care. The team often expands outside the clinical area (Arnold and Underman-Boggs, 2007). Take the case of Bronwyn, a student studying law at university who is being treated as an outpatient for breast cancer. The multiprofessional team involved in her care includes:

- breast-care consultant and other medical staff
- breast-care nurse specialist
- physiotherapist
- occupational therapist
- psychologist
- art therapist
- social worker
- voluntary self-help group
- general practitioner
- practice nurse
- phlebotomist
- pharmacist
- voluntary ladies' underwear fitter
- appliances officer
- Pilates teacher
- university occupational-health nurse advisor.

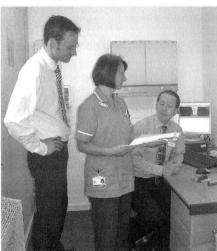
Figure 3.11 Multiprofessional working

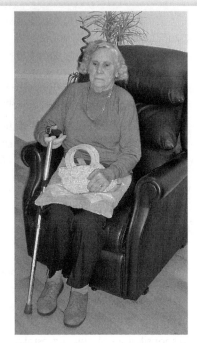

Figure 3.12 Jane

S Scenario: Jane is being discharged home.

Jane is aged 78 and has been in hospital for several weeks following cardiac surgery. She is delighted to be going home but her family are concerned that she lives alone and will not be able to cope. Social services have been involved but the family are unclear what the care package involves. The discharge date is imminent.

a Learning activity

As Jane's named nurse, what would you do in this situation? Think about the other professionals who may be involved.

⚠ Professional alert!

Lack of communication between the multiprofessional team can result in unsafe situations. Important information and actions could be missed or misinterpreted.

In this case Jane and her family need to be clear about the required after-care and medical follow-up. The nursing team caring for Jane should have gained an effective therapeutic relationship with her. Discharge planning should have started as soon as Jane was admitted so that Jane and her family fully understand the whole process of care and are prepared for her to go home. The care plan should be individual for Jane and she should be involved, along with her family if she wishes.

Conclusion

Communication is a vital ingredient in the delivery of client and patient-centred care. It is important to recognise barriers to communication and to realise that everyone communicates differently. Understanding the importance of this helps greatly in developing a rapport and a therapeutic relationship with the client/patient and their family/carers.

Involving patients/clients, and their families and carers (if appropriate), in decisions about their communication needs is very important for planning and delivering an individual care package.

Ensuring good communication within the multiprofessional team and involving all members throughout the patient/client's healthcare journey is also important. Think widely about who the team includes, as its members often come from outside the healthcare setting.

Documentation of your professional responsibility is vital so that communications can be properly shared with appropriate professional colleagues. This ensures that effective patient and client care is delivered.

Further reading

Bernard, M. (2000) *Promoting Health in Old Age*, Open University Press, Milton Keynes.

Department of Health (1999) *National Service Framework for Mental Health: Modern Standards and Models*, The Stationery Office, London.

Department of Health (2001) *Valuing People: A Strategy for People with Learning Disabilities*, The Stationery Office, London.

Glasper, E. A., McEwing, G. and Richardson, J. (2007) *Oxford Handbook of Children and Young People's Nursing*, Oxford University Press, Oxford.

Gibbs, G. (1998) *Learning by Doing: A Guide to Teaching and Learning Methods*, Oxford Further Education Unit, Oxford Polytechnic, Now Oxford Brookes University. (For information and advice on using reflection.)

References

Arnold, E. C. and Underman-Boggs, K. (2007) *Interpersonal Relationships: Professional Communication Skills for Nurses*, 5th edn, Saunders Elsevier, USA (see in particular pages 30–1).

Bailie, L. (2005) *Developing Practical Nursing Skills*, 2nd edn, Hodder Arnold, London (see in particular pages 42–59).

BBC (2007) *Catherine Tate Show*, www.bbc.co.uk/comedy/catherinetate.

Chinn, P. and Meleis, A.I. (2005) *The Essential Concepts of Nursing*, Churchill Livingstone, Edinburgh (see in particular pages 310–11).

Darley, M. and Edwards, C. (2002) *Managing Communication in Healthcare*, Balliere Tindall, Edinburgh (see in particular pages 93–5).

Data Protection Act (1998) www.information.commisioner.gov.uk.

Department of Health (2000) *The NHS National Plan: A Plan for Investment, A Plan for Reform*, The Stationery Office, London.

Department of Health (2001a) *Essence of Care: Patient Focused Benchmarking for Healthcare Practitioners*, The Stationery Office, London.

Department of Health (2001b) *Reference Guide to Consent for Examination or Treatment*, The Stationery Office, London.

Department of Health (2004) *Improving Working Lives: The NHS Plan. Putting People at the Heart of the Public*, The Stationery Office, London.

Donnelly, E. and Neville L. (2008) *Communication and Interpersonal Skills*, Reflect.Press.co.uk, Devon (see in particular pages 1–16).

Falmouth College of Art and Design and Royal Cornwall Hospital NHS Trust (2005) Posters to promote *Improving Working Lives*, Publications and Design Department, Royal Cornwall Hospital NHS Trust, Cornwall.

Grandis, S., Long, G., Glasper, A. and Jackson, P. (2003) *Foundation Studies for Nursing: Using Enquiry Based Learning*, Palgrave Macmillan, Basingstoke (see in particular pages 2–3).

Human Rights Act (1998) http://www.doh.gov.uk/humanrights/qa.htm.

Mathews, J. (2006) 'Communicating with children and their families', in A. Glasper and J. Richardson (eds), *A Textbook of Children's and Young People's Nursing*, 127–9, Churchill Livingstone, Edinburgh.

National Health Service (2006) *The Care Record Guarantee: Our Guarantee for NHS Care Records in England*, revised May 2006, www.connectingforhealth.nhs.ukcrdb.

Nursing and Midwifery Council (2004) *Guidelines for Records and Record Keeping*, NMC, London.

Nursing and Midwifery Council (2008) *The NMC Code Of Conduct: Standards for Conduct, Performance and Ethics*, NMC, London.

Peate, I. (2006) *Becoming a Nurse in the 21st Century*, John Wiley and Sons, Cornwall (see in particular pages 123–44).

Sully, P. and Dallas, J. (2005) *Essential Communication Skills for Nursing*, Elsevier Mosby, Edinburgh (see in particular pages 2, 94–102).

Chapter

4

Communicating with adolescents

Diana Morris and Jan Orr

Links to other chapters in *Foundation Skills for Caring*

3 Communication
5 Anxiety
6 Sign language
7 Breaking significant news
8 Breakaway skills

Links to other chapters in *Foundation Studies for Caring*

5 Communication
6 Culture
16 Safeguarding children
17 Safeguarding adults
22 Care of the adolescent
26 Mental health
27 Learning disability

Don't forget to visit www.palgrave.com/glasper for additional online resources relating to this chapter.

Part

I

Introduction

The aim of this chapter is to demonstrate the importance of communication with adolescents and how to achieve this effectively. Communication is a two-way process so how you listen is as important as the words used, the body language and manner of speaking. Good communication is central to working with adolescents, their families and carers (DES, 2005). This chapter will look at some barriers to effective communication with adolescents and some strategies that could be used to improve the clarity of communication between adolescents and healthcare professionals.

Learning outcomes

This chapter will enable you to:

- define adolescence
- outline the development of communication from childhood to adolescence
- discuss factors, in the context of healthcare, that have an impact on communication with adolescents and family
- focus an individualised communication strategy based upon family-centred needs

- use relevant literature and research to identify good practice
- be aware of adolescent life-limiting illness or disability and communication barriers
- be aware of current language trends.

Concepts

- Age range of adolescents
- Developmental age of adolescent
- Types of communication
- Types of communication behaviour
- Socioeconomic family dynamics
- Appropriate language, trends and body language

- Barriers to communication
- Peer pressure
- Speaking and listening
- Reading and writing
- Interpreting remarks
- Finding information and interpreting relevance

- Confidentiality
- Interaction
- Respect
- Breaking bad news
- Rapport

What is adolescence?

Adolescence can be defined as the process of growing from childhood to adulthood to establish one's identity. Differing definitions of the adolescent age range can be confusing. The World Health Organization (1995) definition states that the stage is commonly associated with physiological changes occurring with the progression from the appearance of secondary sexual characteristics (puberty) to sexual and reproductive maturity. The *National Service Framework for Children and Young People* states that adolescence is defined as ages 12–19 (DH, 2004). Within health and social care (to avoid confusion) the *National Service Framework* standard should be the model used.

Development

From the moment of birth a child instinctively attempts to communicate, focusing on its mother's face, crying for food or when uncomfortable. A baby continues to expand its methods of communication, and once at school a child's language development is increasingly influenced by the wider social, cultural experience and literacy (Glasper and Richardson, 2006).

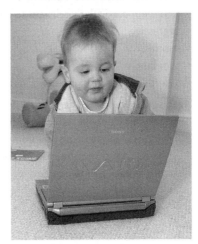

Figure 4.1
An instinct to communicate

a   Learning activity

Young children are given appropriate toys to encourage development and interaction. What is available in the hospital setting for the older child/adolescent?

Of the items you thought of, how many would aid communication?

Increasing diversity of experience influences social and moral development, characterised by a child's attitude and behaviour towards others (Glasper and Richardson, 2006). If language and literacy are not well established during earlier years, the ongoing development of good skills throughout adolescence could be problematic. The maturity of the adolescent is closely related to the levels of communication, and self-esteem problems may be related to school and family life. The onset of puberty can also impact on quality interaction with teenagers.

Remember, adolescent stress, either physical or emotional, can be exacerbated by traumatic experiences and can affect young people's maturity, beliefs, attitudes, health, behaviour and communication.

Types of communication

- *Verbal*: speech, tone.
- *Non-verbal*: a large percentage of feeling is communicated non-verbally via physical appearance, eye movements, utilisation of space, touch, facial expression and gestures.
- *Relational communication*: all behaviour has some message value and can be interpreted as caring or non-caring.
- *Digital communication*: using symbols (words are symbols).
- *Analogical communication*: involves representing something with a likeness and includes non-verbal communication.

Further examples of types of communication are found in the previous chapter.

a   Learning activity

Can you give examples of the different types of communication and where they might be used?

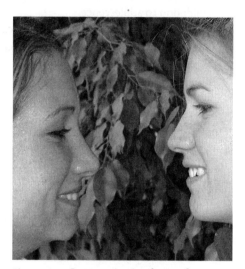

Figure 4.2 Communicating face to face

Types of communication behaviour

There are a variety of ways of behaving when we are communicating with others. The appropriate choice of behaviour is vitally important if we are to communicate effectively.

Behaviour is relevant to the communication needs of the adolescent, particularly as Carlowe (2007) reports, following a review by UNICEF, that adolescents in Britain are unhappy with life. Examples of this become evident in self-harming and eating disorders.

Consider these four different types of behaviour (as discussed in the previous chapter) which seem particularly relevant to adolescents (RSC, 2005):

- aggressive
- submissive
- avoidance
- assertive.

Aggressive behaviour offends or infringes someone else's rights. It is a display, perhaps both physically and verbally, of anger or dominance. It may be automatic or a one-off reaction to a particularly sensitive or threatening situation, or it might be triggered by 'the final straw'. Aggression can sometimes be an expression of fear, lack of self-esteem or the inability to control a situation in any other way.

Part

S Scenario: aggression in A&E

A 14-year-old boy attends the A&E Department with three friends. He has fallen and has possibly broken his arm. On arrival he is tearful, abusive and demanding immediate attention. His friends are equally noisy and encouraging his behaviour.

a Learning activity

Consider the reasons for his behaviour and how the situation could be handled sympathetically and effectively.

Submissive or accommodating behaviour allows the reduction of anxiety, guilt or fear by allowing views or thoughts to be misconstrued or ignored, or by being taken advantage of.

This type of behaviour is often instilled into children by parents, schools and hierarchical organisations. Traditional sayings such as 'don't rock the boat', 'let sleeping dogs lie', 'let it go over your head' have been commonly used. This is confusing to adolescents, showing no respect for their individuality. National standards in health and social care encourage user participation. The Royal College of Nursing Adolescent Forum is currently producing guidance for healthcare professionals working with teenagers, highlighting the importance of individual communication needs (Carlowe, 2007).

Avoidance behaviour is sometimes used to evade any confrontation.

Adolescents can be very adept at avoiding an uncomfortable situation, either through refusal to recognise a problem or by deliberately side-stepping confrontational situations. This is particularly evident in the adolescent in the healthcare setting; examples include taking drugs, substance misuse, unprotected sex, refusing to get a diagnostic test, not answering phone calls or avoiding socialising in certain places (RSC, 2005).

Assertive behaviour – What does the term 'assertive behaviour' mean to you? A method of getting what you want at the expense of others? Being in control and masterful? Being aggressive, domineering or bossy? Is it the mutual acceptance of other people's points of view or getting your own way?

Assertive behaviour means stating your own feelings whilst acknowledging the other person's point of view. It involves clear and steady communication, standing up for your rights and beliefs whilst looking for ways to resolve possible problems.

Many aspects of communication come down to not 'what' is said but 'how' it is said. Clear messages can be conveyed without saying a word but by using body language, and the meaning of a message can be altered by changing emphasis or tone of voice.

Adolescents may find this difficult. They may not immediately tell you how they feel, so getting to know the young person is integral to good communication. Consideration of body language and other non-verbal communication methods is also important.

⚠ Professional alert!

The nurse is the patient's advocate and should also consider professional responsibility (NMC, 2004).

a Learning activity

In your present clinical placement, can you think of any patients whom you could describe as being 'submissive' or showing 'avoidance behaviour'?

Did you feel the healthcare team communicated with these young people appropriately?

After reading and considering the types of behaviour, do you think you would communicate differently?

a Learning activity

Look at the photograph of a father and son (Figure 4.3) and consider their body language.

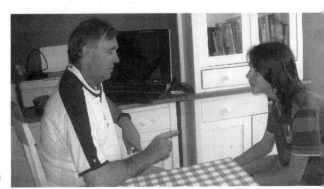

Figure 4.3
Father and son

Socioeconomic family dynamics

The early years of childhood greatly influence the attitudes of the adolescent. Social status can also be conveyed by language. In the United Kingdom the range of vocabulary can be indicative of the level of education attained. Dialect, accent, trendy words or specialist vocabulary in certain occupations and professions form almost a 'language culture'. In the medical profession it is important to use language and communication methods appropriate to the patient and carers (Montgomery and Hetherington, 2007).

Language trends

The 'in' words for adolescents change with time and vary regionally and nationally. This can be identified through television, radio, internet chatrooms and magazines.

Research at Lancaster University by Professor T. McEnry shows that 'yeah but, no but, yeah' is overused by adolescents today, and that a modern teenager has a knowledge of just 12,600 words compared with 25–34-year-olds who have command of approximately 21,400. The top 20 words used by adolescents (Care, 2007) are:

1	Me	8	Yeah	15	Of
2	I	9	That	16	It's
3	The	10	What	17	Oh
4	And	11	No	18	Is
5	It	12	In	19	Like
6	A	13	Know	20	On
7	To	14	He		

Learning activity

Make a list of the 'in' words or phrases that young people are currently using.

Have you found it easier or more difficult relating to young people who seem to have their own vocabulary?

Some adolescents are more comfortable when being nursed by younger practitioners because they are on the 'same wavelength', being nearer their own age. As a result they find it easier to relate and are more able to express themselves honestly (DIPEx, 2005). Do you agree with this statement?

Professional alert!

Consider the Professional Code of Conduct, confidentiality, ethical and legal issues. Effective communication should be individual to the adolescent, and consideration in relation to this is vital.

Barriers to communication

In an unfamiliar environment such as a clinic, hospital ward, accident and emergency unit or minor injuries unit to name a few, a usually articulate, confident young person may feel isolated and apprehensive, disorientated and confused. It should be remembered that an anxious person does not retain as much new information as normally. It is important for nurses to make time to talk with their patients. Student nurses are often encouraged to talk to those on the ward; this is a valuable time to build a rapport with your patient and find out if anything may be troubling him or her. This can be difficult if the patient does not wish to talk, but an act or word of kindness may be all that is needed to break down barriers (DH, 2004).

⚠ Professional alert!

Bearing in mind 'Gillick competence' (see Chapter 1), always consider the family needs of the adolescent and ask if the patient wants the family to be involved (DH, 2001).

⟳ Learning activity

Discuss with fellow students or other care professionals the barriers you may encounter when communicating with adolescents. Examples: the young person who won't talk; the adolescent who can't talk (maybe because of physical difficulty, language problems, cultural differences); fear; confidentiality issues causing conflict during an interview; distress as the adolescent may remind you of your own child or sibling; not knowing what to say.

Peer pressure

During adolescence it is very important to some to be part of the 'scene', to be liked and respected by a peer group. Examples could include being good at sport or watersports, the 'gothic culture', wearing the 'right' trainers and clothes, listening to particular music. In today's society the use of mobile phones, texting and emails is second nature and very important to many adolescents.

Key skills

To connect and communicate effectively with young patients the carer must listen carefully. Ask questions to verify the adolescent's story and listen for what is left unsaid by both parents and the adolescent. Pay attention also to the emotion behind the words. Use lots of eye contact and be ready to share information about yourself. Explain possible treatment options and ask about the

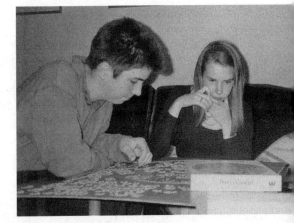

Figure 4.4 Puzzle

young person's preferences. You will need intuition and the ability to interact sensitively. Be confident in yourself when confronted with parents' distress. Whenever possible be empathetic (Healthcare Commission, 2007).

Parents of sick children of all ages can feel disorientated and confused and are often frightened by their lack of control in a clinical environment. Welcoming the adolescent patient and the family, discussing and explaining the action plan, with the immediate and long-term treatment and various options, are key parts of the care worker's job. Grandparents, siblings and other family members may also need support and information.

Guidelines for effective communication

- Use an appropriate manner.
- Convey warmth.
- Show respect.
- Convey understanding, interest, and empathy.
- Take time.
- Use open questions.

- Build on the other person's ideas.
- Make careful use of statements.
- Clarify and summarise.
- Maintain congruence between verbal and non-verbal communication.
- Use active listening.
- Practise ways to improve listening skills.

Pitfalls

- Do not appear bored/impatient/ threatening.
- Avoid being negative.
- Do not jump to conclusions.
- Do not pass judgement.
- Do not argue or disagree.

- Do not interrupt.
- Do not use multiple questions.
- Don't be distracting.
- Be aware of communication difficulties.
- Avoid lack of congruence between verbal and non-verbal communication.

⟳ Learning activity

In what ways would you adapt your communication where an adolescent:
- has a hearing impairment
- has visual impairment
- has a mental impairment
- is confused
- does not speak your language
- is aggressive
- is distressed?

S Scenario: admitting a 15-year-old accompanied by family members

A 15-year-old is admitted with symptoms of epilepsy. You have been asked to admit her. She has been accompanied by her mother, grandfather and younger sibling.

a Learning activity

With particular emphasis on communication skills, what do you need to consider during admission in this scenario? Consider: personal space, eye contact, trigger factors for seizures, her type of behaviour, any other problems, family dynamics, friends, anxiety, depression, bullying. Avoid being patronising.

S Scenario: patient does not wish parent to be present

An adolescent attends an outpatient clinic but does not wish the parent to be present during consultation.

a Learning activity

How would you deal with this situation?
    Consider: confidentiality, informed consent, NSF for children, the Human Rights Act, welfare of children in hospital, Fraser/Gillick guidelines (DH, 2001; NMC, 2004).

S Scenario: wound care

An adult, an adolescent and a young child need to have wounds cleaned and dressed.

a Learning activity

Considering all the issues previously discussed, what differences would there be in the way you tell a child, an adolescent and an adult about the procedure?
Do you find this activity easy?
    Do you use the same words for all the three age groups?

a Learning activity

Ask your colleagues to list things that would help get adolescents to 'open up'. Suggestions could include creating a family tree or drawing a circle of important people.

a Learning activity

Many wards do not allow mobile phones. Text messaging for adolescents is very important to keep in touch with their friends and family. How would you resolve this dilemma?
Do you allow adolescents to use their mobile? Consider:
- ward and hospital policy, health and safety, patients' rights, distress
- possible alternatives, such as a sitting room.

Many young people's wards are beginning to allow the use of mobile phones in certain areas since this is recognised as an important part of adolescents' communication needs.

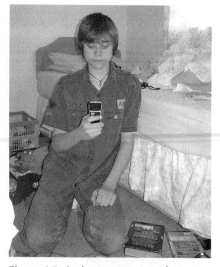

Figure 4.5 An important part of adolescents' communication needs

> ## [S] Scenario: communicating with whom?
>
> In a minor injuries unit the doctor is speaking to the parent and not to the young person. As the child/family advocate, consider an effective way to communicate with the young person.

Conclusion

During the writing of this chapter several young people were asked their views on communication.

They felt the most important aspects of communication were to be treated autonomously, to be listened to, to be respected and to be kept informed. They felt they knew their own rights and values, but disputed the claim about their limited command of just 12,600 words and that 'yeah but, no but' was among their commonest phrases.

In conclusion it would be wrong to typecast adolescents as a single stereotyped group. We need to consider each individual's level of development, socioeconomic family dynamics, barriers to communication, life-limiting illnesses or disabilities, and adjust communication accordingly. While there are specific issues to remember when dealing with adolescents, it is important to understand that every person is unique.

Further reading

International Transactional Analysis Association (ITAA) (n.d.) 'Transactional analysis', ITAA [online] http://www.tajnet.org/ta/index.htm (accessed 1 September 2007).

Johari Window (2006) 'Ingham and Luft's Johari Window model diagrams and examples', Businessballs.com [online] http://www. businessballs.com/johariwindowmodel.htm (accessed 1 September 2007).

UNICEF (2007) *Child Poverty in Perspective: an overview of child well-being in rich countries*, Innocenti Report Card 7, Florence, UNICEF Innocenti Reearch Centre.

References

Care, G. (2007) 'Yeah but no but . . .' *Vitality Matters*, August, 22–3.

Carlowe, J. (2007) Sex, drugs and rock'n'roll, *Nursing Standard*, May 9–15, 21–-3.

Department for Education and Skills (DES) (2005) *Every Child Matters: Common core of skills and knowledge for the children's workforce*, London, the Stationery Office.

Department of Health (DH) (2001) *Reference Guide to Consent to Examination or Treatment*, London, DH.

DH (2004) The National Service Framework for Children, Young People and Maternity Servicers, Standard 4, Growing up into adulthood, London, DH [online] wwww.dh.gov.uk (accessed 3 January 2009).

DIPEx (2005, October 17) 'The Spoon Room: Messages to future doctors', DH, Youth health talk teenage cancer [online] http://www. youthhealthtalk.org/EXEC (accessed 1 May 2007).

Glasper, A. and Richardson, J. (2006) *A Textbook of Children's and Young People's Nursing*, Edinburgh, Churchill Livingstone Elsevier.

Healthcare Commission. (2007) Improving Services for Children in Hospital, Healthcare Commission [online] http://www. healthcarecommission.org.uk/homepage.cfm (accessed 1 September 2007).

Montgomery, H., and Hetherington, J. (2007) 'Types of communication', pp. 984–5, in A. Glasper, A., McEwing, G. and Richardson, J. (eds), *Oxford Handbook of Children and Young People's Nursing*, Oxford, Oxford University Press.

Nursing and Midwifery Council (NMC) (2004) *Code of Conduct, Standards for Conduct, Performance and Ethics*, London, NMC.

Regional Support Centre, northeast, Scotland (RSC) (2005, April 21) 'Developing skills for personal effectiveness: communication skills', Joint Information Systems Committee [online] http://www.rsc-ne-scotland.ac.uk/ie (accessed 29 May 2007).

Rowe, J. (1999) 'Self-awareness: improving nurse–client interactions', *Nursing Standard*, November 10, 37–40.

World Health Organization (WHO) (1995) *Bridging the Gap*, Geneva, WHO.

Chapter

5

Anxiety

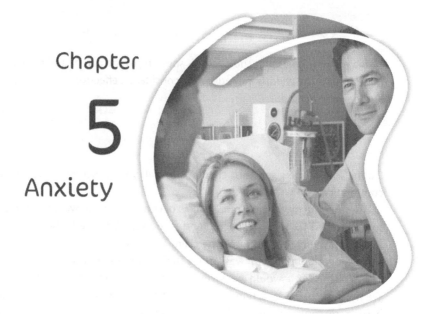

Margaret Chambers

 Links to other chapters in *Foundation Skills for Caring*

- 3 Communication
- 4 Communicating with adolescents
- 7 Breaking significant news
- 21 Pain assessment: child
- 22 Pain assessment: adult
- 40 Last offices

 Links to other chapters in *Foundation Studies for Caring*

- 5 Communication
- 15 Pain management
- 29 Loss, grief, bereavement and palliative care

W Don't forget to visit www.palgrave.com/glasper for additional online resources relating to this chapter.

Introduction

Anxiety – the subjective experience of persons undergoing a stressful encounter – is a common experience for most people during a healthcare episode, be that at the GP's surgery, in the community or in a hospital. Nurses are in the frontline of care giving and therefore must be able to recognise and manage anxiety. They require a repertoire of skills to support those who experience stress, at whatever level. The aim of this chapter is to highlight the importance of understanding anxiety and develop the skills required to manage the feelings of patients and clients in the healthcare setting

Learning outcomes

This chapter will enable you to:

- define the terms anxiety, stress and coping
- contextualise anxiety in the healthcare setting
- identify the causes of anxiety in patients and clients in healthcare settings
- determine methods of reducing anxiety in adults and children.

Concepts

- Anxiety
- Stress
- Coping
- Information
- Therapeutic relationships
- Communication
- Relaxation
- Stress immunisation
- Play

Stress

Stress has been defined as occurring where the demands of a situation outweigh the individual's ability to cope; it is both taxing and a potential danger to the well-being of the individual (Sorenson, 1994; Roberts, Towell and Golding, 2001). When an individual is confronted by stress, it causes a sense of anxiety. In addition stress has been linked to physical illnesses such as headaches, infections and asthma (Curtis, 2000) and to negative moods and depression (Brannon and Fiest, 1997). Stressors (threats) are those incidents affecting an individual that activate a stress response: that is, that are perceived as a threat by the individual.

There are a number of variables which affect the individual's response to stress. These include:

- the type of threat
- the length of time it lasts
- the intensity of the threat
- health status
- age, stage of developmental and cognitive maturity
- gender
- previous experience
- social support
- the individual's coping style
- available coping strategies.

Probably the best-known model of stress was developed in the 1980s (Lazarus and Folkman, 1984) and described the individual's response to stress.

> ### ⟳ⓐ Learning activity
>
> Consider the strengths and weaknesses of your understanding of the concept of anxiety. Identify opportunities and threats relating to your ability to recognise and manage anxiety in patients and clients in healthcare settings, across the age range.

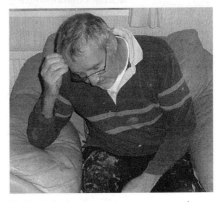

Figure 5.1 Anxiety, a common experience

a Learning activity

Consider a situation which caused you to feel threatened. What mental processes did you go through in order to appraise the level of the threat?

According to Lazarus and Folkman, when we are faced with threat we undertake two types of appraisal:

- *Primary appraisal*: how great is the threat we are facing?
- *Secondary appraisal*: how well can we cope with it?

If we consider a situation poses a threat that we cannot cope with effectively, then some level of stress will be experienced. Stress appraisals made in response to everyday events may differ from individual to individual (Lazarus, 1991). These differences relate to the perceived magnitude of the threat and the individual's perceived ability to cope with it, and to the personality traits of the individual (Forshaw, 2002).

Anxiety

Anxiety is the subjective experience of individuals undergoing stress, a specific and unpleasant experience in response to feelings of threat to the individual (Lau, 2002). Two forms of anxiety have been described (Curtis, 2000) that are important when considering the management of anxiety in the healthcare setting:

- *State anxiety* is defined as a feeling of alarm or dread that has arisen in a particular social situation.
- *Trait anxiety* is defined as a personality characteristic.

a Learning activity

Consider occasions you have experienced that have raised your levels of anxiety. How did you feel physically and emotionally on these occasions?

Consider people you know who demonstrate different levels of anxiety in the same situations. How would you describe their different personalities?

Many people experience feelings of anxiety in social situations that expose them to stress or feelings of threat. Some examples are:

- during visits to the doctor or the dentist, or when attending a hospital appointment
- when undertaking examinations or interviews
- when communicating with people who make them feel uncomfortable.

In these cases, and others like them, it is the situation they find themselves in that creates people's feelings of anxiety, which is a natural response to situational stress. Whilst all of us experience anxiety at times, there are some people who are natural worriers and this may have a significant impact on both their mental and physical health (Forshaw, 2002). Natural worriers demonstrate the personality trait of anxiety. In either case it may be argued that the level of anxiety experienced by an individual is directly related to that person's ability to cope with stress.

Coping

Coping with stress is defined as confronting and adapting to the threats with which individuals are faced (Keil, 2004). Lazarus and Folkman (1984) describe coping strategies as part of their model of stress. They suggest that individuals engage in a number of different strategies to reduce the anxiety which results from appraisals of threat. These strategies fall into two broad categories:

- *Problem-focused coping* relates to reducing the threat by changing the situation.
- *Emotion-focused coping* relates to dealing with the feelings of stress without changing the situation.

> **⟲ Learning activity**
>
> Return to the previous learning activity. Consider the problem-focused and/or emotion-focused strategies you used to manage the threat.

You may have described the feelings you experienced prior to taking your driving test. In this scenario the only problem-focused solution open to you might be to cancel the test! However there are a number of emotion-focused coping strategies that you could employ: for example you could use deep breathing or relaxation strategies to manage your feelings of anxiety and dread. You might use thought-stopping (see below), or desensitising techniques such as undertaking mock driving tests with your driving instructor.

Coping styles and coping strategies

Coping *styles* comprise both inborn and learned behaviours for coping through adaptation to the environment, and are relatively stable throughout life. They are typical ways of behaving that are related to personality or temperament. Coping *strategies*, which change with age and experience, are cognitive or behavioural methods employed to deal with stress (Ryan-Wenger, 1994). Coping strategies therefore are open to interventional changes, whilst coping styles, which are like personality traits, are not. Ryan-Wenger suggests that an individual's coping style may reduce the range of coping strategies employed by an individual when faced with threat.

A number of coping styles have been described. These include:

- *Avoidance versus vigilance*: avoidance is demonstrated by the individual's not wanting to know about the stressor and avoiding the feelings associated with it. Vigilance is demonstrated by a desire for knowledge about the stressor and a readiness to discuss it. Some individuals may demonstrate a combination of the two (Cohen and Lazarus, 1973).
- *Blunting versus monitoring*: blunters prefer unpredictability and utilise coping strategies that put psychological distance between them and the threat, whilst monitors favour predictability and use strategies for obtaining information (Miller, 1980).

Locus of control

Locus of control is a term used to describe an individual's perception of the cause of what happens to them. It was originally explained by Rotter (1966).

Rotter described two distinct types of people, those with an:

- *Internal locus of control*: people who feel in charge of their own lives.

> **⟲ Learning activity**
>
> Consider a number of people that you know. How do they explain the things that happen to them? For example, do friends who are fat blame themselves for eating too much of the wrong types of food or not doing enough exercise, or do they blame some other factor like their genes or their hormones?

- *External locus of control*: people who believe they are at the mercy or others or of chance (Forshaw, 2002).

A later development of the concept divides those with an external locus of control into two distinct groups: those who have an external locus directed at others (known as powerful others) and those who believe that whatever happens to them happens by chance.

The application of Rotter's theory to anxiety and stress management lies in the idea that having a 'fighting spirit' is negatively correlated with anxiety and depression, whilst fatalism, helplessness and anxious preoccupation are all related to lowered mood. Individuals who state that they can influence their own life events exhibit more successful coping strategies than those who do not (Curtis, 2000).

La Montagne (1984) studied the relationship between children's locus of control beliefs and coping skills following surgery. She showed that children with an internal locus of control tended to use more active coping behaviours such as information seeking, and further that children who were well informed demonstrated more active coping. Boyd and Joehnson (1981) also used Rotter's theory to inform their understanding of children's coping styles

Effects of stress and anxiety on the body

Selye (1956) described the physiological effects of stress upon the body, which he called the General Adaptation Model:

- *Stage of perceived stress*: the realisation that the individual is facing a threat.
- *Stage of alarm reaction*: noradrenaline and the stress hormone are released under the control of the sympathetic branch of the autonomic nervous system and affect the physiological status of the individual.
- *Stage of fight or flight*: the body is prepared to stay and face the stressor or to run away.
- *Stage of resistance*: the body adapts to the stressor. If the body has been unable to use the energy released to face the stressor or to run away, the body starts to recover. There is a reduction in activity in the autonomic nervous system but the adrenal cortex continues to release increased levels of corticosteroids since the threat remains.
- *Stage of exhaustion*: the resources of the body are reduced whilst the autonomic nervous system remains stimulated. This leads to poor functioning of the adrenal glands, leaving the body exposed to the development of physical manifestations of stress (Barker, 2007).

> **(a) Learning activity**
>
> Describe the immediate and long-term effects of increased autonomic nervous system activity upon the body.

The effects of anxiety and stress, initiated by the excitement of the autonomic nervous system and the release of noradrenaline and stress hormone are:

- In the short term:
  - tachycardia and palpitations
  - raised blood pressure
  - raised respiration rate
  - pupil dilation
  - constriction of blood vessels in skin
  - palmar sweating
  - tension in the muscles
  - decreased gastrointestinal activity
  - feelings of discomfort in the stomach ('butterflies').
- In the longer term:
  - headaches
  - hypertension
  - indigestion
  - anorexia
  - cardiovascular disorders
  - cancer
  - death (Curtis, 2000; Barker, 2007).

Managing anxiety in the healthcare setting

Anxiety has been identified as the subjective experience of individuals who are facing some sort of threat to their well-being. It is therefore to be expected that many experiences in healthcare settings will cause anxiety for most individuals. This may or may not be mitigated by the coping styles and/or strategies at their disposal. Since coping styles are innate or learned behaviours they are difficult to change. Nurses must therefore have a number of strategies available to help individuals to cope with stress in healthcare settings.

Returning to the work of Lazarus and Folkman (1984), there are two methods of adaptive coping: problem focused, which involves goal planning and action; and emotion focused, which involves managing the feelings of stress when there is no other way of finding a solution to the problem (Barker, 2007).

Problem-focused coping strategies

Problem-focused strategies involve breaking problems down into a number of smaller goals that can be managed more easily a step at a time. Once achieved, each step should be rewarded appropriately. Social support may be drawn upon in order to identify goals and sub-goals, and different perspectives on the problem (Barker, 2007) (see the scenario box right). Steps towards problem solving include:

1 Defining the stressor.
2 Setting realistic goals.
3 Examining alternatives.
4 Considering all other perspectives and motives.
5 Selecting an appropriate strategy.
6 Delineating necessary steps to reach goal.
7 Rewarding behaviour for having tried (Adams, 2004).

Part

> **S** Scenario: Problem-focused approach to fear of injection
>
> Joe is 7 years old and is visiting the outpatient department for a consultation following identification of hyperglycaemia and glucosuria. He has already experienced venepuncture at the GP's surgery and he is clearly very anxious about 'having a needle' again.
>
> How can you help Joe reduce his anxiety using a problem-focused approach?

Joe needs to develop coping skills to help him to manage his anxiety about venepuncture, other forms of blood-letting and injections, if his diagnosis is indeed diabetes mellitus. There are a number of problem-focused and emotion-focused coping strategies that can be mobilised to help him.

First you will need to take into account Joe's personal coping style, and discussion with him and his family will reveal whether he is avoidant or vigilant and whether he has an internal or external locus of control.

Using the model described by Adams (2004):

1 Define the stressor:

Help Joe to identify what it is about the venepuncture that he fears. Children of this age often have exaggerated fears about 'needles' (Carter, 1994) and misconceptions about the causes and treatment of disability and disease (Rushforth, 2006), which they may consider to be a well-deserved punishment for something they have done wrong. In addition they may have distorted understandings of medical equipment and internal body parts, including blood (Vessey, 1988; McEwing, 1996), and difficulties in the perception or expression of their pain experience (Twycross, 1998).

2 Set realistic goals:

The goal will be to have the procedure completed with a little distress as possible. Help Joe to understand that if he cooperates the procedure will be less stressful and will be over sooner, and suggest that he sits on his carer's lap during the procedure.

3 Examine alternatives:

Control or the lack if it is one of the stressors identified by patients in healthcare settings, and this is no less so for child patients and clients. Alternative goals for Joe could involve putting him back in control of the situation. This could mean allowing him to time the procedure, and giving him permission to watch (vigilant coping styles) or to be distracted (avoidant coping styles).

4 Consider all other perspectives and motives:

Consider the role of Joe's family and the play specialist in the management of the procedure.

5 Select an appropriate strategy:

- Help Joe to be in control of the situation by suggesting other coping strategies, including those mentioned in Step 3.
- Decide with Joe and his family how the procedure will be managed, how long it will take and what rewards Joe can expect for 'good' behaviour.

- Explain to Joe and his family how he can relax or be distracted during the procedure as appropriate.

6 Delineate necessary steps to reach goal:
- Explain the procedure to Joe and his family, using appropriate therapeutic play techniques.
- Manage Joe's pain experience by use of an appropriate analgesic cream or spray to the venepuncture site.
- Allow Joe to choose the timing of the procedure and go to the clinical area when he is ready.
- Allow Joe to sit on his carer's lap, using vigilance (inspection of the procedure) or avoidance (distraction from the procedure) as appropriate.
- Start and time the procedure according to Joe's needs.
- Offer a reward for Joe's having tried to cope with the procedure.
- Allow Joe the opportunity to re-live the experience through play activity.

7 Reward behaviour for having tried:
This should happen regardless of Joe's behaviour during the procedure and should reflect his trying rather than his success. It may take the form of putting Joe in control by allowing him to become the aggressor (by squirting water from a syringe at the offending healthcare professional!) or a simple poster for his bedroom wall. Whatever the reward, this should be decided in advance with Joe and his family.

Emotion-focused coping strategies

Emotion-focused coping strategies are about managing the feelings of anxiety provoked by stress (Barker, 2007). A number of these strategies are described in the literature.

Now try the learning activities related to the following two scenarios.

S Scenario: anxiety in preadmission

John is a middle-aged man who is to be admitted to hospital for a hernia operation. He comes to the preadmission clinic in a highly anxious state.

a Learning activity

Devise a programme of activities to help reduce his health-related anxieties using problem-focused coping strategies.

S Scenario: anxiety after diagnosis

Marie, aged 65, comes to the surgery in a highly agitated state. She has been diagnosed with breast cancer.

a Learning activity

How will you help Marie to manage her anxiety using problem-focused coping strategies?

Communication and information giving

A fuller explanation of communication and communication skills can be found in Chapters 3 and 4. However the value of these skills in reducing stress and anxiety requires further exploration. This is because information about healthcare procedures and treatments has been shown to enhance coping skills and reduce anxiety (Soares and Grossi, 2002; Field and

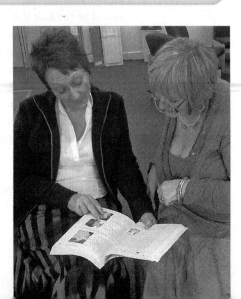

Figure 5.2 Information enhances coping skills

Adams, 2001; Richardson, Adams and Poole, 2006). For example, researchers have highlighted the importance of information giving and programmes of education for patients undergoing day surgery (Avis, 1994; Mitchell, 2000; Gilmartin, 2004) and elective surgery (Mitchell, 2003). In most studies it is patients and clients themselves who cite information as mitigating their stress, and written information to support verbal information is even more appreciated by them (Gilmartin, 2004).

There is some evidence that good information delivered at an appropriate developmental level is just as important for anxiety reduction in child patients (Glasper and Haggerty, 2006). This is evidenced by the success of therapeutic play techniques to explain, rehearse and re-live distressing medical experiences (Chambers, 2007) and of pre-admission preparation clinics, which are well established across hospitals in the United Kingdom.

It is important to remember the needs of those patients/clients who do not speak English as their first language, and you will also need to modify your approach in response to individual coping styles (Gilmartin, 2004).

a Learning activity

Consider the information needs of patients and clients in your clinical area. Devise a form of written information (fact sheet or information leaflet) to meet your patient/client's needs.

Stress immunisation techniques

Stress immunisation, sometimes referred to as stress inoculation or psychological immunisation, is a technique that can be used with both adults and children (Lau, 2002). Stress inoculation training (Meichenbaum and Cameron, 1983) is explored by Curtis (2000) and Forshaw (2002), who state that it takes the form of training through three stages:

- *Conceptualisation stage*: where individuals are educated about the body's response to stress and learn to analyse their own responses.
- *Skills acquisition and rehearsal stage*: individuals are taught to try out alternative responses, and to develop relaxation skills and other coping strategies.
- *Application stage*: individuals apply what they have learned to their behaviour and keep records of their responses.

Methods to desensitise children to prepare them for stressful healthcare encounters include therapeutic play techniques that introduce the child to stressful hospital equipment, materials and information, starting with the least alarming and moving to the most stressful. As children learn to handle and cope with the materials and equipment and become familiar with the environment, they grow in self-confidence and develop a sense of mastery (Glasper and Haggerty, 2006).

Physical activity

Exercise has been cited as a method of stress reduction which acts by reducing the levels of circulating adrenaline and allowing the individual to rest (Brannon and Feist, 2000). Curtis (2000) also claims that physical activity has psychological benefits, including the alleviation of stress and the reduction of anxiety. He argues that even a brisk walk can make an individual feel better and suggests that this may be due to the release of endorphins which produce a natural 'high' and act to elevate mood. Whilst exercise has been shown to reduce state anxiety, its effect upon trait anxiety is less clear (Curtis, 2000).

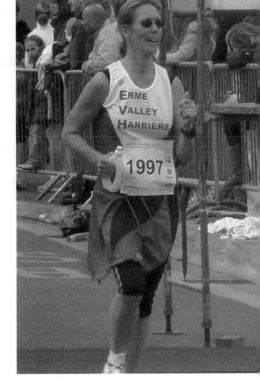

Figure 5.3 Exercise reduces stress

Relaxation

Relaxation techniques are used to reduce anxiety by rhythmically contracting and relaxing the body's muscle groups. Individuals learn to relax one muscle group at a time until the whole body is relaxed. This method of anxiety reduction is effective across all age groups and can be successfully taught to pre-school children (Poster, 1988). Relaxation lowers the level of circulating adrenaline, allowing rest and recovery by reducing the body's stress response (Brannon and Feist, 2000)

The first stage in the relaxation process is the preparation stage (Table 5.1).

Table 5.1 Relaxation techniques preparation phase

Action	Rationale
Prepare the environment by: → Choosing a non-stimulating, dimly lit and quiet place → Selecting a period when there will be no interruptions → Playing soothing background music as appropriate	To ensure an optimal environment for the relaxation process
Prepare the patient/client by: → Informing them of the purpose of the session → Informing them that they may stop the session at any time	Information reduces anxiety Respect for the patient/client's autonomy
Prepare self by: → Developing a calm and soothing voice → Speaking slowly → Being relaxed and comfortable	Optimise relaxation skills and techniques

Source: Poster (1988).

This is followed by teaching the technique to the patient/client and involves methods of relaxing the muscles and deep breathing techniques (Table 5.2).

Table 5.2 Relaxation technique

Action	Rationale
Ask the patient/client to lie back and get comfortable	Optimal state for relaxation to take place
Ask the patient/client to close their eyes and follow your instructions	Encourages the patient/client to focus on the relaxation process; avoids visual distraction
Ask the patient/client to take a deep breath, let it out slowly and then repeat	Allows oxygenation of the muscles; brings the focus to the breathing
Ask the patient/client to make a tightly clenched fist and then relax the muscles of the hand	Allows the patient/client to experience the feeling of relaxation in one muscle group
Repeat the muscle clenching and relaxing for all muscle groups rhythmically from the feet to the top of the head	Allows for gradual muscle relaxation of the whole body
Ask the patient client to empty their mind or think of some pleasant experience while they focus on the breathing and become calm	Allows the patient/client to focus on breathing and relaxed state

Source: adapted from Poster (1988).

Once individuals have mastered the technique in a safe environment, they can learn to relax under more stressful conditions when anxiety levels are high.

Although it has been stated that even preschool children can be taught how to relax their bodies, it is important to adapt the techniques to take account of their age and stage of cognitive development. For example, school-aged children may appreciate being coached to relax while using commercially produced taped sessions, and tape recordings of a mother's voice may have a soothing effect on toddlers and the very young.

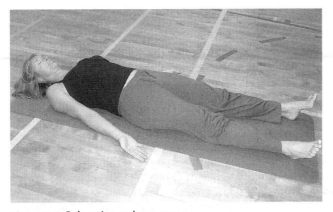

Figure 5.4 Relaxation reduces stress

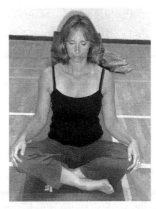

Figure 5.5 Meditation is an adaptation of the relaxation technique

An adaptation of the relaxation technique described by Curtis (2000) is known as mindfulness meditation. In this technique individuals are advised not to ignore unpleasant thoughts or feelings but rather to concentrate on them in a non-judgmental way. This promotes their ability to recognise the ways in which they see the world and produces relaxation through the discovery of the self (Curtis, 2000).

Other methods of emotion-focused coping

- Thought stopping:
  - This requires the individual to deliberately ignore or push away stressful thoughts. Postponing thought until after the event is a variation on the theme; for example, before a stressful healthcare encounter people might say to themselves 'by 12 o'clock tomorrow it will be over'.
- Positive self talk:
  - Individuals use positive messaging to themselves, such as 'I can do this' or 'I can cope with this situation'.
- Guided imagery:
  - Guided imagery is a technique that supports the use of the individual's imagination as a therapeutic tool. The individual is asked to focus on a pleasant experience and to concentrate on that image when faced with periods of stress or pain. Guided imagery can be successfully used with both adults and children (Burgess, 2001) and is often combined with relaxation for optimal effect.

Learning activity

Remember John from our earlier scenario? Devise a programme of activities to help reduce his health-related anxieties using emotion-focused coping strategies.

Learning activity

Consider Marie, our 65-year-old patient with breast cancer. How would you help her to manage her anxiety using emotion-focused coping strategies?

Conclusion

Anxiety is a common experience of individuals who are accessing healthcare provision and is the physical manifestation of the body's stress response. There are two types of anxiety: trait anxiety, which is a characteristic of the personality and therefore difficult to modify; and state anxiety, which is a response to situational stress and can be mitigated through interventions that develop skills for coping with stress.

The experience of anxiety differs from individual to individual according to personality traits, age and stage of development, and experience amongst other variables. Some stress may be good for individuals in that mastery of stressful experience promotes and enhances self-esteem and develops coping skills for the future. However, all healthcare professionals have a responsibility to support patients and clients who experience stress and anxiety which may have a negative effect on health and well-being.

References

Adams, N. (2004) 'Psychological interventions in chronic illness', in J. Sim and S. French (eds), *Physiotherapy: A psychological approach*, 3rd edn, 275–97, Butterworth Heinemann, Edinburgh.

Avis, M. (1994) 'Choice cuts: an exploratory study of patient's views about participation in decision making in a day surgery unit', *International Journal of Nursing Studies* 31, 289–98.

Barker, S. (2007) *Vital Notes for Nurses: Psychology*, Blackwell, Oxford.

Bennettt, P. (2000) *Introduction to Clinical Health Psychology*, Open University Press, Buckingham.

Boyd, H. F. and Joehnson, G. O. (1981) *Analysis of Coping Style: A cognitive-behavioural approach to behaviour management*, Merrill, Columbus, Ohio.

Brannon, L. and Fiest, J. (1997) *Health Psychology*, Brooks Cole, Pacific Grove, California.

Brannon, L. and Feist, J. (2000) *Health Psychology*, Wadsworth, Belmont, California.

Burgess, C. (2001) 'Complementary therapies: guided imagery and infant massage', *Paediatric Nursing* 13(6), 37–41.

Carter, B. (1994) *Child and Infant Pain: Principles of nursing care and management*, Chapman and Hall, London.

Chambers, M. A. (2007) 'The context of care in surgical nursing', in Chambers, M. A. and Joenes, S. (eds), *The Surgical Nursing of Children*, 1–13, Butterworth Heinemann Elsevier, Edinburgh.

Cohen, F. and Lazarus, R. S. (1973) 'Active coping processes, coping dispositions and recovery from surgery', *Psychosomatic Medicine* 35, 375–89.

Curtis, A. J. (2000) *Health Psychology*, Routledge, London.

Fields, L. and Adams, N. (2001) 'Pain management 2: the use of psychological approaches to pain', *British Journal of Nursing* 10, 971–4.

Forshaw, M. (2002) *Essential Health Psychology*, Arnold, London.

Gilmartin, J. (2004) 'Day surgery: patients' perceptions of a nurse led preadmission clinic', *Journal of Clinical Nursing* 13, 243–50.

Glasper, E.A. and Haggerty, E.A. (2006) 'The psychological preparation of children for hospitalisation', in Glasper E. A. and Richardson J. (eds), *A Textbook of Children's and Young People's Nursing*, 61–76, Churchill Livingstone Elsevier, Edinburgh.

Keil, R. M. K. (2004) 'Coping and stress: a conceptual analysis', *Journal of Advanced Nursing* 45(6), 659–65.

La Montagne, L. (1984) 'Children's locus of control beliefs as predictors of preoperative coping behaviours', *Nursing Research* 33, 76–85.

Lau, B. W. K. (2002) 'Stress in children: can children's nurses help?' *Pediatric Nursing* 28(1), 13–19.

Lazarus, R. S. (1991) *Emotion and Adaptation*, Oxford University Press, New York.

Lazarus, R. S. and Folkman, S. (1984) *Stress Appraisal and Coping*, Springer, New York.

McEwing, G. (1996) 'Children's understanding of their internal body parts', *British Journal of Nursing* 5(7), 423–9.

Meichenbaum, D. and Cameron, R. (1983) 'Stress inoculation training: toward a general paradigm for training coping skills', in Meichenbaum D. and Jaremko M. E. (eds), *Stress Reduction and Prevention*, 115–54, Plenum, New York.

Miller, S.M. (1980) 'When is a little information a dangerous thing? Coping with stressful events by monitoring versus blunting', in Levine S. and Ursin H. (eds), *Coping and Health*, 145–69, Plenum press, New York.

Mitchell, M. (2000) 'Psychological preparation for patients undergoing day surgery', *Ambulatory Surgery* 8, 19–29.

Mitchell, M. (2003) 'Patient anxiety and modern elective surgery: a literature review', *Journal of Clinical Nursing* 12, 806–15.

Poster, E. C. (1988) 'Stress immunisation: techniques to help children cope with hospitalisation', *Maternal-Child Nursing Journal* 12(2), 119–34.

Richardson, C., Adams, N. and Poole, H. (2006) 'Psychological approaches for the nursing management of chronic pain, Part 2', *Journal of Clinical Nursing* 15, 1196–1202.

Roberts, R., Towell, T. and Golding, J.F. (2001) *Foundations of Health Psychology*, Palgrave Macmillan, Basingstoke.

Rotter, J. B. (1966) 'Generalised expectations for internal versus external control of reinforcement', *Psychological Monographs* 80 (1, whole no. 609).

Ryan-Wenger, N. M. (1994) 'Coping behaviour in children: methods of measurement for research and practice', *Journal of Pediatric Nursing* 9(3), 183–96.

Rushforth, H. (2006) 'The dynamic child: children's psychological development and its application to the delivery of care', in Glasper A. and Richardson, J. (eds), *A Textbook of Children's and Young People's Nursing*, 146–63, Churchill Livingstone Elsevier, Edinburgh.

Selye, H. (1956) *The Stress of Life*, McGraw Hill, New York.

Soares, J. J. F. and Grossi, G. (2002) 'A randomised controlled comparison of and behavioural interventions for women with fibromyalgia', *Scandinavian Journal of Occupational Therapy* 9, 35–45.

Sorenson, E. S. (1994) 'Daily stressors and coping responses: a comparison of rural and suburban children', *Public Health Nursing* 11(1), 24–31.

Twycross, A. (1998) 'Children's cognitive level and their perception of pain', *Paediatric Nursing* 10(3), 24–7.

Vessey, J. (1988) 'Comparisons of two teaching methods on children's knowledge of their internal bodies', *Nursing Research* 37, 262–7.

Part

Chapter

6

Sign language

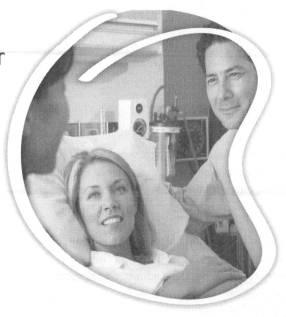

Joanna Assey

Links to other chapters in *Foundation Skills for Caring*

3 Communication
4 Communicating with adolescents
7 Breaking significant news

Links to other chapters in *Foundation Studies for Caring*

5 Communication
27 Learning disability

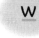

Don't forget to visit www.palgrave.com/glasper for additional online resources relating to this chapter.

Introduction

This chapter aims to give you knowledge and understanding of the skills required to support children's communication when they do not use words to communicate.

Learning outcomes

This chapter will enable you to:

- describe, with evidence-based reasons, the process for the use of the following as aids to communication:
  - some signing communication
  - symbols and pictures
  - objects
- understand and recognise signs, symbols, pictures and objects that may be useful when a child with communication difficulties is admitted to hospital.

- create a visual schedule to support the child with communication difficulties, especially in relation to those children who have autistic spectrum disorder (ASD).
- recognise areas on the ward where signs, symbols or pictures could be used to help children to find their way around the environment.

Concepts

- Children with communication difficulties
- Autism
- Signing
- Body language
- Visual schedules

Why do healthcare professionals need to be able to understand and communicate with children during their stay in hospital?

- to gain a more accurate understanding of the child's perspective
- because children are little experts in themselves and only they can offer certain information
- to assess any misunderstandings or gaps in knowledge
- to assess children's emotional attitude towards their condition
- to gain compliance with treatment
- to assess the child's own issues and problems with the condition and avoid assumptions about what psychosocial problems are present.

These skills may also help us understand more about treatment non-compliance and other issues. And finally, it is good practice. 'All Healthcare Professionals who work with children should have training in the necessary communication skills to enable them to work effectively' (DH, 2003b: 16).

Signing

Some children are unable to communicate verbally because of their developmental age, conditions such as autistic spectrum disorder (ASD) or learning disabilities, or because they have a hearing impairment. They require alternatives to verbal interaction to help them communicate their needs and to build relationships with others.

Communication forms the basis of our lives. It helps us understand and manage our world, build relationships and deal with problems. It generally involves speaking, using gestures and facial expression (and in many cases reading and writing). Any absence of these can result in confused or little communication taking place. To facilitate interaction with children who have communication difficulties, it is essential that other forms of communication are available.

t☆
Practice tip

- Remember to use body language, facial expression and voice tone to reinforce the message.
- Do not flood the child with language, signed or spoken.
- Give them time to process and time to respond.

When we are talking to children who have communication difficulties we should not speak in abstract terms but use very literal language. As we talk, our tone and body language are also important for understanding. Using gestures may help by giving visual cues about the meaning of the words. Gaining basic information about the communication needs of children, and producing a practical communication trail, can help children and healthcare professionals communicate with each other, especially about the care and treatment the children receive and you, as healthcare professionals, are giving.

'When I see it then I understand'

For children with communication difficulties, speech is no longer considered the ultimate means of interaction. Signing, symbols and other augmentative communication techniques are now viewed as acceptable alternatives.

Over the years many systems using signs, symbols and pictures as well as the spoken word have been developed, for example British Sign Language (BSL) Paget Gorman. The ones most commonly used for children with communication difficulties are Makaton, Signalong and Picture Exchange Communication System (PECS). Levett (1969) produced the first published example of visual communication to support spoken English. Makaton signing, developed from BSL, was first introduced in 1974. In 1976 some new words were introduced so that the system could be applied to children (Birkett, 1984).

> t☆
> ### Practice tip
>
> We as healthcare professionals often talk too fast when making requests or giving children information or instructions about their treatment. SLOW YOUR SPEECH DOWN.
>
> Some children may only pick up key words in a sentence. It is important to check that the child has understood the main idea of the message. USE KEY WORDS: use 'JOHN EAT' rather than, 'John come and sit down and eat your dinner'.

Total communication

Total communication is an approach that makes use of a number of modes of communication, including signed or auditory, written and other visual methods. What you use will depend on the needs and abilities of the child (Mayer and Lowenbraun, 1990). Total communication is about communicating in any way you can. It's not just about talking, it's about signing, pointing to pictures, symbols, photographs or objects. It's also about using gesture or body movement.

> Total communication is a communication philosophy – not a communication method and not at all a teaching method. ... Total communication is an approach to create a successful and equal communication between human beings with different language perception and/or production. ... To use total communication amounts to a willingness to use all available means in order to understand and be understood.
>
> (Hansen, 1980)

Introduction to some signing systems

It has long been recognised that children with communication difficulties can benefit from alternatives to spoken methods of communication such as PECS, unaided systems such as sign language, or signing systems such as Makaton (Walker, 1996) and eye pointing (Glennen and De Coste, 1997). Learning and using these systems will mean better communication between the child, parent and healthcare professional team, which will lead to better cooperation with treatment and help the healthcare professional to understand the child's condition and feelings about the treatment, and how the treatment is affecting the child, for example to determine whether the child is experiencing pain.

> t☆
> ### Practice tip
>
> It will be important if possible to obtain information about the child's communication style(s) prior to admission.
>
> This could be introduced in the information leaflet given before admission. This will provide all staff with the opportunity to familiarise themselves with the appropriate system.

What is signed language/communication?

Sign language is a combination of visual cues used to communicate, like hand positions, gestures and facial expressions, to send a message. The message is received visually and sometimes tactilely; signs may be enhanced by body language and facial expressions and other forms of communication. It was first developed as a means of communication for hearing-impaired individuals. Research suggests that using sign language along with speech is likely to accelerate a person's ability to speak (Kopchick, Rombach and Smilovitz, 1975; Miller and Miller, 1973).

There has been little research to establish which forms of signing are most effective, but systems can be supported by expert opinion or by asking the views of the children who use them.

t☆

Practice tips

Always check that children have understood what you have been saying. Get them to repeat or show you so that you can assess their understanding.

It is really important to work with parents or carers.

British sign language (BSL)

BSL is a visual-gestural language created and preferred by the British deaf community; it has its own vocabulary and grammatical structure. It is recorded as being used as early as the sixteenth century and is used in British schools for children who have hearing impairments (Magill and Hodgson, 2003). BSL was only recognised by the government in 2003 as the preferred language of people who are deaf. Most other signing systems have been adapted or developed from BSL. (See www.RNID.org.uk.)

W

Signalong

Signalong is a total communication system with over 12,000 signs where you use every clue to get your meaning across. It is a sign-supported system based on BSL and is designed to help children with communication difficulties particularly associated with learning disabilities. The signs are drawn and described by use of a consistent method that enables users to access vocabulary according to need. Developed by Kennard and Grove (1991) and first published in 1992, it offers a wide range and selection of signs to aid communication.

It is not necessary for every child to learn every signed word. Signs should be taught when the relevant meaning can be attached to them. Using Signalong's multi-pronged approach, most children of all abilities are able to sign before they are able to talk, provided signs are used consistently with speech. (www.signalong.org.uk.)

W

Makaton

Makaton, which has a vocabulary of 500–600 signs, suits children or adults with learning difficulties or brain damage. Its three creators were named *Margaret*, *Kathy* and *Tony*, hence Ma-Ka-Ton. This system is very different from BSL; it is not much more than a set of vocabulary items, whereas BSL is a full language with a complete grammar.

Those who have developed the Makaton vocabulary describe it as not just another signing system. As its name suggests, it is a vocabulary which has been specifically designed to provide a controlled method of teaching communication. It can be used for children (with or without learning disabilities) and other people with language difficulties in order to provide a basic means of communication. It is also used to encourage expressive speech wherever possible, and to develop an understanding of language through the visual medium of the signs and the logical structure of the sign language (Walker, 1996, 1978, 1973).

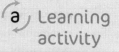 Learning activity

In your interprofessional learning group, try to role play a scenario in which a young client has a communication impairment that warrants the use of a signing system.

(e) Evidence-based practice

Powell (1999) undertook some research into the use of manual signs in the promotion of communication abilities in individuals with learning difficulties. He concluded that early communication skills are supported by the use of manual signs for those who are unable to express themselves verbally.

Crystal (1976) concluded that Makaton vocabulary contains all the essential features of a language. The use of Makaton vocabulary for teaching language to those who have a learning disability and other communication difficulties is therefore linguistically justified. It is clear that healthcare professionals exert an influence over the communication performance of their patients. It is also recognised that, as with spoken language, the receptive signed vocabulary is greater than the expressive (Walker et al, 1985; Birkett, 1984).

- Makaton is not a language but an aid to communication which aims to provide functional communication.
- It offers a multi-modal approach to communication with one mode facilitating another, providing a visual representation of language.
- Makaton is presented in two vocabularies: the Core Vocabulary and the Resource Vocabulary, and divided into nine stages (Makaton, 2005).
- Stage 1 is introduced to beginners. It provides basic concepts necessary for everyday living and is presented in stages of increasing complexity.
- Drawn signs will have the corresponding word(s) underneath, acting as an aid for the sign.
- It is important for words and signs to be used together and they need to clearly convey the meaning of the concept they represent.
- The Resource Vocabulary used in conjunction with the Core Vocabulary offers a wide topic-based resource covering life experiences. (www.makaton.org.uk.)

t☆ Practice tips

Healthcare professionals need to recognise that children's signs may not look like those in a textbook. Think how children sometimes mispronounce words.

Signs may also be modified due to physical problems.

It is really important to always speak when using symbols.

Symbols/Pictures

A symbol is a very simple line drawing that stands for one word or idea; for example, the symbol for a cup may not look like the one used at home but represents the idea of a cup. Because of their simplicity, symbols are easier to draw than most pictures. In many cases they stand for words whose meaning is easily understood (concrete concepts), and when you look at them you recognise them at once. Some people however will need to learn them by matching the symbol to the real thing or a photo. Other symbols, representing abstract concepts, are more difficult to learn. Using symbols can help people to understand the key words someone is saying or writing. It is important to avoid using sentences that need more than three symbols to show the main meaning as that can cause confusion.

There is a lot of software around that allows you to explore different uses of symbols. Examples include software by Picture Communication Symbols, by Mayer Johnson Incorporated, Widget, Makaton and PECS (www.pecs.org.uk) For more information about using other symbols go to www.easyinfo.org.uk.

t☆ Practice tip

Laminated signs/symbols/ pictures – for toilet, bath, shower and so on – around the ward will increase the feeling of safety and promote the child's independence in moving around.

Objects

Children with very limited understanding of language and/or with sensory problems may find words, symbols or pictures very difficult; sometimes using objects can help. Such an object can be anything from a favourite teddy bear or toy to a flannel or toothbrush that helps the child to understand what is happening around them, what it is that you want them to do next, where they may be going, who is going to be working with them and so on. Objects are chosen to be meaningful to the particular child. Usually they are items that the child comes into contact with in everyday life.

So why should we be using objects? Because they are easier to understand than words and pictures as they are part of real life. A spoken word is gone as soon as it has been said but people can hold an object for as long as they need to. This means they have more time to get the meaning from the object.

Objects can be used in many of the ways that speech, signing and photos can. When choosing objects you need to think carefully about:
- which object will represent what idea
- how big the object is
- whether it can be easily carried around
- where it will be
- how the child will access it.

The chosen objects can be used to help people understand and remember what is happening around them. They might find it helpful to hold, touch, smell or listen to objects. Objects can sometimes be used to communicate with other people, perhaps by choosing an object, by looking at it or picking it up, or perhaps by giving the object to someone else to show what the giver wants. More information about objects can be obtained from http://www.ace-centre.org. uk/html/resources/objectsref/resobja.html; http://callcentre.education.ed.act.uk.downloads/ quickguides/aac/objects.pdf; or http://www.sense.org.uk.deafblindness/communication/objref. htm.

Visual schedules

Hodgen (1995: 29) stated that 'A major function of communication is to give information' and a visual schedule may be helpful to ensure children have all the information they require about their day in hospital. 'Visual schedules help the child who has ASD and other special needs understand their world better' (Savner and Myles, 2000: 1). Many of us use calendars and planners to remind us of the things we have to do; individuals with ASD need visual schedules to better understand their day. Visual schedule systems provide easy and consistent cues about daily activities:
- They provide a structure that allows a child to anticipate what will happen next.
- By providing the child with a vision of his/her day, they reduce anxiety and promote calmness between transitions.
- They are especially important for children who have difficulties with communication.
- They are crucial in establishing an atmosphere of trust and security.
- Once established, they can also provide a structure for the child to begin to make some choice/decisions about care and treatment.

(C) Professional conversation

Mohammed, a foundation degree in health student, says, 'I was assigned to a learning disability special school for one of my first placements, and was not really looking forward to the placement. When I arrived I felt very inadequate as I was unable to communicate with the children I was working with. I took my mentor, who was an occupational therapist, to one side to let her know how I felt.

'She was really helpful and showed me an introduction to the picture exchange communication system (PECS).

'I was so delighted the next day when I used it for the first time with David, one of my allocated children. His smile let me know that he had understood me, and that was a real reminder to me that theory and practice should always be joined up!'

t☆ Practice tips

- Remember the child you are communicating with has difficulties.
- Don't flood the child with language, whether in speech, sign, symbol or picture.
- Give the child time to process the thought, and time to respond to you.

- Very few of us are signing experts.
- Try to produce signs as accurately as you can, but accept whatever efforts the child makes to communicate with you.
- Check with parents/carers about the child's style of signing and their own interpretations if they have them.

- It does not matter if the signs are not perfect, effective communication is what we want, especially when the child is in hospital.

a Learning activity

For one of your interprofessional learning group activities, debate the use of symbols and pictures as a method of communication with certain client groups.

Conclusion

Having worked through this chapter, you will have become aware of many of the challenges facing healthcare professionals when they are working with young people with communication difficulties. Central to the support available in such cases is the ability of the multidisciplinary team's members both to communicate with each other and to involve the child and family when delivering any intervention that requires a communication episode.

The healthcare professional has a duty to protect and safeguard the interests of young patients by giving them and their families the time and the information that they need in order to give assent and consent. Now reflect back on the outcomes which are set out at the beginning of this chapter, and consider how much you have learnt about using different communication strategies.

References

Birkett, E.M. (1984) *A Comparative Study of the Effects of the Makaton Vocabulary in the Language Stimulation Programme on the Communication Abilities of Mentally Handicapped Adults*, published thesis [online] www.makaton.org/research/birkett (accessed 7 July 2007).

Comforth, A., Johnson, K., Walker, M. (1974) *Makaton Vocabulary: Teaching sign language to the deaf and mentally handicapped*, Makaton [online] www.makaton.org (accessed 7 July 2007).

Crystal, D. (1976) *Child Language, Learning and Linguistics*, London, Edward Arnold.

Department for Education and Science (2004) *Every Child Matters: Change for children*, Nottingham, DFeS Publications.

Department of Health (DH) (2003a) *Every Child Matters*, London, DH [online] www.doh.gov.uk/nsf/children (accessed 7 July 2007).

DH (2003b) *Getting the Right Start: The National Service Framework for Children, Young People and Maternity Services, Part I: The*

NSF Emerging Findings consultation document [online] http://www.dh.gov.uk/en/Publicationsandstatistics/Publications/PublicationsPolicyandGuidance/DH_4006182 (accessed 26 February 2009).

Glennen, S. and De Coste, D. (1997) *Handbook of Augmentative and Alternative Communication*, San Diego, Singular Publications.

Hansen, B. (1980) *Aspects of Deafness and Total Communication in Denmark*, Copenhagen, The Center for Total Communication.

Hodgen, L.A. (1995) *Visual Strategies for Improving Communication, Volume 1*, Troy, Michigan, Quirk Roberts Publishing.

Kennard, G. and Grove, T. (1991) *Sign Along* [online] http://www.signalong.org.uk/wa/methodology/index.htm (accessed 27 July 2007).

Kopchick, G., Rombach, D. and Smilovitz, R. (1975) 'A total communication environment in an institution', *Mental Retardation*, 13, 22–3.

Levett, L.M. (1969) 'A method of communication for non-speaking severely subnormal children: trial results', *British Journal of Disorders of Communication*, 6, 125–8.

Magill R. and Hodgson A. (2003) *Start to Sign*, 3rd edn, London, RNID.

Makaton Development Vocabulary Project (MVDP) (2005) *An Introduction to Makaton*, Makaton [online] www.makaton.org/about/overview.htm (Accessed 20 July 2007).

Mayer, P. and Lowenbraun, S. (1990) 'Total communication use among elementary teachers of hearing-impaired children', *American Annals of the Deaf*, 135, 257–63.

Miller, L. and Miller, E. E. (1973) 'Cognitive-developmental training with elevated boards and sign language', *Journal of Autism Child Schizophrenia*, 3, 65–85.

Powell, G. (1999) 'Current research findings to support the use of signs with adults and children who have intellectual and communication difficulties', Makaton [online] http://www.makaton.org/research/powell99.htm (accessed 20 July 2007).

Savner, J. (1999) *Visual Supports in the Classroom*, video available from Autism Asperger Publishing, PO Box 27173, Shawnee Mission, Kansas 66283–0173.

Savner, J.L. and Myles, B.S. (2000) *Making Visual Supports Work in the Home and Community: Strategies for individuals with autism and Asperger syndrome*, Shawnee Mission, Kansas, Autism Asperger Publishing.

Sellars, G. (2006) 'Learning to communicate with children with learning disabilities', *Paediatric Nursing*, **18**(9), 26–8.

Walker, M. (1973) *An Experimental Evaluation of the Success of a System of Communication for the Deaf Mentally Handicapped*, London, University of London.

Walker, M. (1978) 'The Makaton vocabulary', in Tebbs, T. (ed.), *Ways and Means*, Basingstoke, Globe Education.

Walker, M. (1996) *The Makaton Core Vocabulary Revision, Symbols*, Camberley, Surrey, Makaton Vocabulary Development Project.

Walker, M., Parsons, F. S., Cousins, S., Henderson, R. and Carpenter, B. (1985) *Symbols for Makaton*, Camberley, Surrey, Makaton Vocabulary Development Project and EARO.

Chapter

7

Breaking
significant news

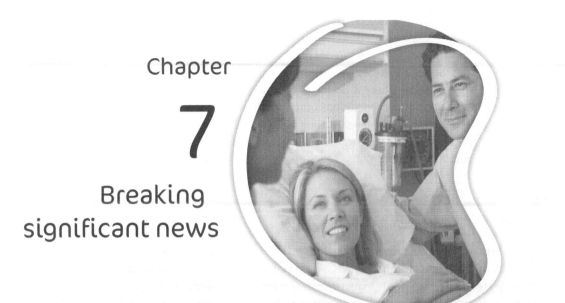

Jennie Quiddington

Links to other chapters in *Foundation Skills for Caring*

3 Communication
4 Communicating with adolescents
5 Anxiety
6 Sign language
40 Last offices

Links to other chapters in *Foundation Studies for Caring*

5 Communication
28 Rehabilitation
29 Loss, grief, bereavement and palliative care
31 Child emergency care and resuscitation
32 Adult emergency care and resuscitation

Don't forget to visit www.palgrave.com/glasper for additional
online resources relating to this chapter.

Introduction

Many healthcare professionals consider breaking significant news to be an aspect of care that belongs specifically to the medical profession. However there may be unexpected circumstances where a doctor is unavailable or the news pertains to other practitioners' expertise. On these occasions other healthcare professionals need to take the responsibility for delivering such news. Nursing staff may be asked to organise the meeting between the doctor and the recipients, so it is imperative that they know what is required to provide the best outcome.

Learning outcomes

This chapter will enable you to:

- define breaking significant news
- describe the conscious and unconscious factors that are activated, and recognise the manifestation of these factors in healthcare professionals and recipients when breaking significant news
- identify the principles of user-centred care in relation to breaking significant news to the recipients and their support network

- identify the relevant management activities when breaking significant news to a staff member and/or service user
- demonstrate the skills in breaking significant news to recipients and their support networks
- justify the skill of reflecting on the impact of your own attitudes and behaviour towards breaking significant news to the recipients and their support network.

Concepts

- Communication
- Emotion
- Anxiety
- Relationships
- Empathy and hope.

Some important definitions before we begin are:

- *Recipients*: the patients, their partners, relatives or patient-chosen supporters such as friends, work colleagues or healthcare professionals.
- *Location*: usually a room in the place of care. This could be in a hospital, doctors' surgery, private practice clinic or family home. However emergency care professionals may have to break significant news in less than optimum locations such as the roadside.

[S] Scenario: family background for role play learning activity

Filip Polinski is a 35-year-old psychology graduate and migrant worker from Poland. He has only been able to find employment in a local car-valeting firm since arriving in England. Due to low wages and high rents he has moved into the family home of his girlfriend Libby Pritchard, whom he has known for a year.

Libby shares the house with her parents Marcus and Elsa Pritchard, who are both 59 and met at primary school. They both trained as financial advisers, and got married 35 years ago shortly after qualifying. Marcus has worked in the same financial investment company all his adult life, and is planning to retire as he has found the latest management changes at work very difficult. Recently he has started to drink to excess, and to go out in the evenings alone. Elsa gave up work many years ago to look after their children,

Janet, 35, William, 29, and Libby, 25. She feels increasingly isolated since the family moved to a small rural village on the outskirts of the city where Filip and Marcus work. This isolation has been exacerbated by her recent diagnosis of coronary heart disease, which was completely unexpected despite years of unexplained physical symptoms.

Libby has an 8-year-old son called Jack from a previous relationship. He was born when she was still at school and Libby has required ongoing support from her parents for Jack's care. Jack's father has wanted no involvement with the child or Libby since he learned of the pregnancy. Jack started at a new school when the family moved home, and has found this difficult as the children in his class tease him over his obesity.

Libby and Filip share a love of art, and in fact met at the local art class. Libby recently graduated from the local university with a degree in commercial design, and was hoping to find her first full-time job. However she and Filip have just discovered that they are expecting their first child. The pregnancy was unplanned and the news has put their relationship under extra pressure. The family home is small, and with Filip's addition to the crowded household, things are becoming strained. There is also uncertainty as to whether Filip can remain in the country permanently.

Fortunately Filip, Libby, Jack, Marcus and Elsa get lots of support from William and Janet.

William works as a ranger in a conservation area and lives close by with his long-term partner, Andrew. Jack loves his uncles and enjoys accompanying William for walks through the conservation area.

Janet lives alone with her son Paul, who is 3 years old. He has very high support needs due to his learning disabilities. Since the death of her husband last year, Janet has been struggling financially and is faced with the prospect of having to sell her house.

'Bad news' is any information which is inauspicious and causes suffering or threat to an individual's view of his or her future. The problem confronting the healthcare professional is that it is often very difficult to anticipate how the news may be received by the recipients. To acknowledge this uncertainty the word 'significant' has been used, as this implies that the news may affect the recipients in ways than the news breaker may not initially consider. For example, following my delivery of a couple's eleventh child I relayed the news with delight and excitement that they had a beautiful baby girl. This was greeted with despair from the wife and rage from the husband, who immediately left the room. On exploring these responses with the tearful wife, I realised that a male was the only child that her husband would welcome and that until this son was produced she would have to continue having babies. Lacking knowledge of their history or hopes for a son, there was little chance that I could have anticipated their response.

A common approach to breaking significant news revolves around the following four statements:

- 'This is what we found ...'
- 'This is what happened ...'
- 'This is what is going to happen ...'
- 'This is what we're going to do ...'

This approach fails to consider the individuals' psychological and emotional responses to the news, or the need to empower the recipients to make their own decisions based on knowledge, personal experience and a constructive relationship with the healthcare professional. It takes considerable skill to break significant news in a manner that is recipient-centred, constructive and establishes a positive patient–carer relationship. Success in this activity will contribute to the recipient's ability to trust healthcare professionals in the future. Wondrak (1998) emphasises the importance of health workers being effective and confident in their daily communications with clients/patients in order to develop therapeutic relationships.

The conscious approach of the healthcare professional

The following are examples of the type of thoughts that may run through your mind as you approach the recipients, taking into consideration their circumstances, your personal beliefs and the environment. By reflecting on what belief lies behind each example, you can identify how it may affect your attitude or behaviour. This knowledge can help you deal with the situation more appropriately.

'I need to give information'

There is often a belief that this is a time purely for giving information, and that the more information we give, the less likely it is that there will be misunderstandings or that we will be accused of withholding information at some point in the future. This belief can lead to our overlooking the recipients' need for emotional support and opportunities to ask questions before the meeting ends.

'I think this must be great (or terrible) news'

It is easy to base our anticipation of the recipients' response to the news on our own hopes or fears, rather than waiting to observe and hear their personal response. As a result the manner of our delivery may be inappropriate for the recipient.

'I will withhold this information as you might not be able to take it and I fear making you upset'

Our expectation of the recipients' inability to cope with the news may be based on our own inability to cope with such news, and fear that if they cry we will also become tearful. To avoid this personal embarrassment, some healthcare professionals try to avoid breaking news that may elicit such a response. However recipients usually interpret the tears in our eyes as evidence that we are human and have compassion for their circumstances.

'I'm not the person to give this news, as I don't know enough about it'

This perception is often based on the unrealistic expectation that we must know the answers to all the questions that the recipients may ask on hearing the news, and fear that we will have to admit we do not know all the answers. If you have a good relationship with them you may be the best person to deliver such news, providing you have created an opportunity for access to those with more knowledge.

'I know more about this issue than the recipient'

As healthcare professionals we may assume that we have more knowledge about the patient's diagnosis and prognosis. However there are expert patients and their supporters who have lived with their condition for many years and may have accessed the most up-to-date research regarding the treatment and possible prognosis for their condition.

'I have only got five minutes to tell them and the corridor will have to do as the office is being used'

This is the response of the news breaker who has not planned the encounter and considered the effect of the news on the recipient, or is trying to fit the meeting in before attending to prescheduled tasks. The recipients are put at risk of public humiliation as they must respond to the news in a place frequented by other service users, their friends, relatives and healthcare staff. This lack of consideration will be experienced negatively by the recipients and may damage the relationship between them and healthcare professionals.

'I'm able to give hope when the situation is bleak'

Although this is a valuable attribute, it needs to be tempered with realism. We may attempt to be too upbeat because we fear the patient or their chosen supporters will not be able to deal with the reality of the prognosis. However, if our hopefulness is too extreme the recipients may experience betrayal when reality sets in.

Unconscious factors in healthcare staff and recipients

The following are examples of the hidden factors in the unconscious that may be activated as you approach the recipients. By examining what beliefs and experiences lie behind each example, you can consider how they are likely to affect attitudes and behaviour in both parties. Frequently these factors lead an individual to respond to the other parties as if they were the ones involved in their own past experience. This knowledge can help you be prepared for and manage unexpected responses in yourself and others.

Everyone has 'personal baggage' that affects the way they respond

Many healthcare professionals are drawn to this career as a result of encountering disability, long-term or fatal illnesses, and inappropriate relationships such as incest in their family or friends. If these experiences have been traumatic or unresolved through the mourning process, a person presenting with similar problems can trigger the past experience of the healthcare professional. The recipients, in turn, will bring their previous experiences of healthcare and others who have held power over them. Our professional status gives us great power and this may trigger behavioural and emotional responses that belong to the recipients' former experience.

Major barriers: social status, race, age, spiritual beliefs, gender and personal experience

These barriers may be linked to ignorance, prejudice and scapegoating. The underlying problem is usually linked to the person's lack of knowledge of (or negative personal experience at the hands of) a person or group who fits the same criteria as the person who is delivering or receiving news. It can be difficult to comprehend why a person makes particular decisions if we have not attained the same age and experience. But if we have suffered pain or neglect from a certain type of person or group, we may perceive that everyone with the same status, belief or gender will behave in the same way.

Subtle barriers: embarrassment, shame, fear, anxiety, amount of experience

Past negative experiences may make us want to avoid ever suffering the same feelings again. When an experience begins to trigger our unconscious memories we may do everything we can to move away from or block out the situation. This can result in not hearing what is said or in withholding information that may be pertinent to choosing care options. Bradshaw (2005) identifies 'toxic shame' as agony resulting in automatic defensiveness.

Inability to respond to the recipients' emotions or handle difficult family issues

Certain recipient emotions and experiences may trigger your past experiences and make an appropriate response more difficult. For example many people respond to aggression with fear and anger, but if you respond to a person's fear and tears with the same emotions it may be that a distressing past experience has been triggered in you. Inappropriate emotional responses can result from poorly managed relationships, particularly in childhood. Unresolved problems in family relationships may result in lack of experience when attempting to help others manage similar difficulties.

The news may affect our good relationship

The ability to form positive and constructive relationships with others is desirable. But if we avoid bringing reality into the relationship because we fear that will damage it, we will need to reflect upon our dependency on the relationship. As healthcare professionals we are employed to provide evidence-based care, not to seek friendship and support from our patients and their supporters.

Guilt: 'I encouraged them to think it would all be all right'

We may want to be seen as excellent healthcare professionals, but this unconscious need can lead us to give inappropriate advice or support. If treatment becomes ineffective we may be plagued with feelings of guilt, which can lead to inappropriate avoidance of the patient and his/her supporters. When giving reassurance, it is imperative that we never promise that 'it will be alright'; we can only provide realistic outcomes and possibilities.

> ### ⟲ⓐ⟳ Learning activity
>
> Read Sully and Dallas (2005) for more effects of unconscious processes in nurses and how they affect nurses' practice.

The optimum process of delivering significant news

Location

The optimum location is quiet, private and comfortable. You will need to manage the temperature to suit the recipients, and to check that the sun will not move into a position which causes irritation for anyone during the session. Optimum seating enables people to sit back and relax, but also to get out of the chair with minimal effort.

The location should allow you all to sit without barriers such as desks or tables, and offer personal space of approximately one metre around the body. The need for extra personal space usually increases with the level of distress, unless the individual desires closeness from a member of their support network.

You will need to anticipate how many people will be attending the delivery of news, as the location needs to be large enough to accommodate the patient's chosen support network. If the location cannot be changed it may be better to advise the recipients of this problem, so that they can choose who is to be present.

To enable an uninterrupted delivery of news and provide the recipients with time to respond to it, you will need to prevent intrusions. Turn off phones, put a 'Do not disturb' sign on the door and do not leave the recipients until the agreed time span has expired. Ask other staff members to take messages if anyone tries to contact you.

C Professional conversation

Saara, a first-year student nurse, says, 'I was working with my mentor during a shift and one of the patients called me over to his bed. He had been quite poorly and he was clearly concerned about his health. He asked me if he would be able to go home the next day, as had been originally planned when he was admitted for his minor procedure three days earlier. I knew from the morning report that he had developed a chest infection and could not possibly be discharged. I could not look him in the face and tell him, so I asked if he could wait a minute until my mentor – who was in another cubicle – returned. She told me I had done the right thing and she then took me with her to break the news of the delayed discharge to the patient. She was really good and very empathetic. The patient took the news very well and I realised that the way in which he had been told about the chest infection was an example of my mentor's skill in breaking significant news.'

Planning the session

Before you approach the patient or their support network, you need to plan how you are going the run the session and what information needs to be included. The setting of boundaries lets people know where they stand, and can contribute to a feeling of security if the boundaries are appropriate.

You need to schedule ample time for the delivery of news, questions that will come from the recipients, and your responses. It is best to set a time boundary for the session and to let them know the session is near completion at least five minutes before the end. This enables them to make the enquiries that they consider the most pertinent before you leave. Negotiate a time for breaking significant news that is suitable for the recipients, their support network and the healthcare professionals that may be involved in their care. If children are to receive news, their parents must be present at delivery.

Dias and colleagues (2003) observe that the effect of stress or surprise can make it difficult to remember information. Consider taping the session and giving the tape to the recipients before they leave, or give them written information which can be referred to later and can help to clarify complex matters. Consider ahead of time how the patient can receive future test results and what details you can provide about medical or surgical treatment, medication, in-patient and outpatient facilities, support networks and possible prognosis.

The presence of the chosen support network can be invaluable, but can inhibit the disclosure of issues which the recipient may only wish to discuss in private. You will need to consider whether their presence is appropriate at the time of delivery or whether you may need to allocate some time for the patient to talk with you alone. Sometimes partners or parents contribute to the problem, and where this is the case the recipient needs us to put down a boundary and prevent them attending the delivery of news.

Before the end of the session, establish the next appointment and the ground rules for how future discussions may proceed. Some recipients experience feelings of loss and abandonment when the healthcare professional leaves the location, so it is important to provide a contact telephone number to access support. Always inform other clinical staff that you are not available until the meeting is complete.

Skills for breaking significant news effectively

Set any time boundaries you have at the beginning of the conversation. For example: 'We have 30 minutes for this meeting. If you would like to meet again, we can book a time before we finish today.'

Prepare the patient to receive serious news by 'tolling the alarm bell'. For example: 'I am afraid I have some news that may be difficult to accept.' Always express compassion when delivering distressing information. This can be exhibited by using a gentle tone of voice, identifying that the recipient appears upset and expressing sadness that they have been affected this way.

Speak clearly to ensure they can hear as you deliver the news, avoiding complicated technical terms, jargon and abbreviations. It may be necessary to have an interpreter present if English is not the recipient's first language. As you deliver the news, assess the emotional responses as these will give you clues about the impact of your information. By giving information in small units you can assess whether the recipient is able to accept it or whether shock has made him/her start to withdraw from hearing more news.

Explore how the recipients feel about and understand your news. Identify where they have understood your information and gently educate where there are misconceptions. Exhibit sensitivity to the recipient's responses to the difficulties of the topic; avoid probing questions and give them sufficient time to consider and respond to the news. Respond appropriately to the recipients regardless of their emotional responses. If they express anger, avoid becoming defensive, and use empathy in an attempt to comprehend their emotional responses. If they feel we understand their distress our support will be more effective. Gavaghan and Carroll (2002) observe that recipients need to feel cared for by staff.

Session activities

During the session you may be confronted with a variety of responses to the news you are delivering. The following are areas you will need to consider and perhaps respond to in an attempt to deal with the issues.

You need to develop your own vocabulary so that the words you use feel comfortable for you, as well as being appropriate to the situation. Reflect on how you can ask questions without the patient feeling intimidated.

Establish how much the patient knows or wants to know at this time. This reveals the patient's assessment of the situation and enables you to identify misconceptions. The recipient may retain little of the news and may benefit from repetition with members of their support network present.

Try to create the opportunity to corroborate bad news rather than deliver it. If the recipient avoids acknowledging that there is a problem, this may indicate denial which needs addressing by the healthcare professional. The technique of delivering information in steps leading up to the bad news may result in the recipient being reluctant to ask questions, feeling unable to join in a discussion, or avoiding hearing important information. You may need to change your delivery technique to encourage participation from recipients. What they say or ask, and how they react to each piece of news, determines how much is said at any one time.

Be willing to discuss dying with recipients and their support networks as they may want information about physical or mental deterioration to be expected and what facilities are available when the patient approaches or reaches the time of death. Your clinical expertise makes you a valuable participant in any decisions they may want to make.

It is imperative that you offer options for treatment and care that the recipient and their support network can take with them after the meeting. This will enable them to maintain hope, give them information to consider once the shock of the news has subsided and allow them to make some decisions before you meet again.

Factors contributing to poor delivery of significant news

Healthcare professionals can be excessively blunt if the location or time available are not conducive to in-depth discussions. Failure to provide sensitivity, support, honesty and realism balanced with hope can lead to the recipient experiencing fear, anxiety and despair. Ptacek and Ellison (2000) discuss the healthcare professional's experience of breaking news.

Most patients want a diagnosis as well as a possible prognosis to enable them to start planning their lives with their support network. Concealing the incurable nature of their illness or treatment side-effects will prevent this necessary and healthy activity from taking place.

Failure to ask patients if they understand the information they are given can lead to them leaving the meeting having misunderstood or not heard the information. Family interference can take the form of a request that the patient not be told significant information or that the information is manipulated in some way. Both can harm the recipient–carer relationship and lead to a failure to utilise available treatment for the problem.

Reading Guggenbuhl-Craig (1999) will enhance your knowledge about the manifestations of power and control by healthcare professionals.

Words that hurt and words that heal

Identify words you can use to be able to convey the support and empathy all recipients require. Patients are not just looking for facts; they need believe that they have the ability to face the possible fight for life ahead of them, knowing you are working alongside them as they face their uncertain future. Patients and their support networks should never hear that 'there is nothing more to offer'. This ignores the importance of symptom management and creates a sense of abandonment by the healthcare profession.

The ability to maintain a consistent, relaxed, warm and open approach to whatever the recipient wishes to discuss is an essential skill for the healthcare professional.

Larson (2005) expects empathy to be expressed by all healthcare professionals. Empathy involves experiencing another's emotions as if they are an extension of yours. Empathetic responses let patients know you've understood how they feel. You need to communicate that you understand their position, hopes, ideals and feelings.

Positive responses to news

The way recipients receive the news may have implications for their future healthcare. Acceptance is often manifest as a desire to explore treatment options and become actively involved in the care programme. Decreased anxiety and uncertainty brings relief, and perception change manifests itself as hope that future results may be positive. There is realistic acceptance of the probable life span, yet a desire to live life at its optimum level. Accepting help to address emotional and spiritual issues and focusing on symptom management can lead to an enhanced patient–carer relationship.

Negative responses to news

You need to recognise and validate the patient's feelings as best you can, as shock, denial, sadness, frustration, fear, despair or anger can be manifest in rejection of our constructive information and/or members of their support network. Phrases such as 'there's no point' and 'I give up' demonstrate a recipient's negative approach to continuing care and may indicate the need for alternative treatment as well as other means of psychological support such as counselling. For example, depression could be treated with the help of medication, support groups or contact with people who have experienced the same problems and found their own methods for managing their lives constructively.

Age and level of depression may affect what the recipient wants to know. Elderly and child recipients often tend to want less information and have may little interest in decision making about their care or support. You may become aware that the recipient feels the information given is insufficient or confusing, yet fails to request more information or clarification. Recognition of negative reactions is a prompt that we need to inform other healthcare professionals about our concerns regarding the possible psychological responses or negative activities by the recipient.

Hope is a critical component of coping

Achieving realistic hopefulness is difficult even though we need to engender optimism regarding treatment. However we need a balance between hoping for the best and preparing for the worst. Emphasising hope can deny patients the opportunity to explore their wishes or fears, discuss dying, and consider how they want to continue their lives. By sharing hope, we align ourselves with the patient and provide much needed support. We don't need to share a patient's hopes or fears to respect, learn about and respond to them. Patients who feel that their life has real purpose and meaning are more able to cope with difficult news. Honesty, not false reassurance, is the best way to establish hope. For example we may be able to offer medication to offset pain or the effect of hallucinations when experiencing schizophrenia, even if we are unable to offer a cure for the underlying problem.

Some recipients find alternative therapies such as aromatherapy, reflexology, massage and psychotherapy give them a capacity for independent action away from mainstream healthcare. As healthcare professionals we need to ensure that the recipients are attending fully qualified practitioners of these alternative therapies who can act as other agents of therapeutic support.

Defining and exploring barriers

Once we have given the news, it may be important to explore what barriers patients have constructed that may inhibit their ability to make constructive use of our facilities and pharmacological, medical or surgical options. For example a lung cancer patient may feel guilty about smoking. We need to ask about this emotional burden, empathise with the patient's concerns and explore ways to alleviate the psychological pain.

Dias and colleagues (2003) note that relatives may request that certain information be withheld from the patient. We need to consider whether this request is in the patient's best interests by communicating with all members of the support network and the healthcare professionals involved.

'We want to protect the children so we won't tell them' is a common attitude from parents. However we need to support and enable the recipients to inform their family as this allows members to be prepared when physical or psychological changes occur in the patient. When information is provided to the relatives they may be empowered, have their misconceptions challenged or be able to embark on activities suited to a relative whose life expectancy has been shortened.

A fixed life expectancy can impair the remaining time for both the recipients and their support networks. It appears that uncertainty about when life ends may be a prerequisite for life to have meaning and value, as well as lowering stress and anxiety for all those involved in recipient care. We need to approach each case from an individual perspective as life expectancy can never be anticipated exactly.

Need to plan for future developments

We need to offer options, identifying what is possible and, once the plan is made, what activities it will entail. The choice must be made by the recipients, and regardless of how we feel about their decision we must be respectful of their wishes. Sometimes we may feel it is necessary to challenge their decisions, particularly if the barriers they erect prevent them from accessing treatment, but this needs a sensitive and empathetic approach.

Establish the next appointment and a format for how the discussions may proceed. Bad news may result in complex and seemingly insurmountable problems for the recipient and their support network. By encouraging people to prioritise problems you can ensure that they are dealt with in the most appropriate order. It may be more productive to tackle some problems during a later visit as this will give the recipient and their support network time to reflect on the news received and identify specific areas of concern. It will give the healthcare professional time to obtain more expert advice and the chance to include other members of the multidisciplinary team if they are required.

A reflection on the process of empathy

Reik (1937) proposes that we develop empathy as a capacity to share the experiences of others not just like our own but as our own.

Most people think of empathy as stepping into another person's shoes. The problem with that is you tend to go in as yourself, and as soon as you are there, start thinking about things that happened to you and how you felt when you experienced a similar situation to the recipient's. This mental response prevents you being open to what the recipient experiences.

Jung (1974) perceives empathy as the result of introjection of the object.

Introjection

This is a mental process that is an attempt to take into the psyche all forms of experience, such as art, travel, family relations, schooling, sport, partnerships, work, environment and ageing. The process of introjection may lie behind the ability to learn from experience.

Ability to empathise

We need experiences to be able to imagine what it is like to think or feel something. For example few of us will have experienced abdominal surgery, but most of us will have experienced some form of physical pain by the time we reach adulthood. We can use this knowledge of pain to start the process of empathy with a patient who is trying to cope with abdominal pain following surgery. Lack of experience due to age, lifestyle and beliefs may contribute to difficulty in empathising with others.

To avoid the error of thinking that the patient's pain is like my own, I make a conscious decision to envisage myself as sitting on my left-hand shoulder. From this place I can observe the patient's experiences with more detachment from my own experiences. I then try to draw into myself/introject the patient's experiences and see them solely from that person's perspective.

Another difficulty in empathising is that you need to have a fair degree of mental health, as drawing another person's experiences into yourself can be experienced as losing your own identity. This is why some patients with mental health problems and some with severe physical illness are unable to empathise with others.

Consequence of empathy

Money-Kyrle (1956) suggests that as patients speak we become identified with them by the process of introjecting them. Having understood them from the inside, we will re-project them and interpret what we have understood. This interpretation can enable us to understand why recipients feel and think as they do and help us offer suitable options for treatment or support.

Communication techniques

These techniques come from the counselling profession, and more skills can be gained from Chapters 3, 4 and 6 on communication. Practise these techniques with other healthcare professionals so that you all benefit from learning the skill:

- *Reflection*: repeat back key words that the person has said. This gives them the opportunity to say more, if they wish. It is important not to over use this technique as it can cause irritation.
- *Paraphrasing*: this is reformulating what the person has said and repeating it back to them. This may reveal hidden emotions that increase your understanding of the patient.
- *Clarification with the recipient*: checking that you understand correctly what the person said aids precision and avoids errors when responding to questions or documenting the meeting.
- *Summarising your news*: this improves understanding and may help if your news causes confusion. Repeating key points is often helpful and necessary.
- *Eye contact*: maintain regular eye contact, but again do not overdo this as it is very difficult to think clearly if you feel someone is staring at you. Position your chair so that you are not sitting directly opposite the recipient as this gives both of you the ability to look away from each other without having to obviously turn your bodies or heads.
- *Touching*: touching a person is a boundary issue, so do not assume that every individual finds being touched acceptable or desirable. Offer touch such as holding their hand, but develop ways of enquiring whether they will appreciate this gesture or find it an intrusion into their personal space. If they refuse your gesture, do not be tempted to touch them regardless of their emotional responses.

(a) Learning activity

This activity enables you to put into practice the theory gained through reading the chapter and references. In your interprofessional group you will role play a variety of family members in groups of three. Before you start, become familiar with the individual family member's history, needs and wants and then as a group select one of the mini-scenarios from the list below before you practise breaking the required news. These mini-scenarios, derived from the full family scenario given earlier, are to be used in your learning group for practising the skill of breaking significant news.

If you are delivering the news, you can make the choice as to whether you know the recipient's history or are unaware of it.

If you are the family member receiving the news, you must remember your family relationships and history leading up to the situation you are in.

The first student should play the role of the client and the second the healthcare practitioner breaking the news. The third acts as an observer and will complete the scoring grid detailed in Table 7.1, which helps them to assess whether their colleague has demonstrated the required skills when breaking news, and to offer feedback. Each student should practise playing each role (*as indicated in italics within each mini-scenario*).

- Janet has bought her son for assessment as she is finding him increasingly difficult to manage. You have been told that the assessment practitioner has unexpectedly gone off sick and will not be back for at least a month. *Convey this news to Janet.*
- Libby has come with her mother for her first antenatal scan. *You have been asked to inform her that there is evidence of a twin pregnancy.*
- William has come to pick up the results of his urine sample. *He needs to be informed that the results indicate evidence of a sexually transmitted infection.*

- *You need to start educating Jack and his family* that his diet needs to change to exclude excessive calories and that he needs to increase his daily exercise.
- Filip attended his GP's surgery complaining of feeling so depressed about his poor job opportunities and girlfriend's pregnancy that he feels like committing suicide. *You need to tell him that the GP has referred him for inpatient care at the local hospital.*
- Elsa has confided in you that she is worried that her husband is drinking too much and she is worried about his loss of interest in his work. You know that he has been diagnosed as having an alcohol dependency problem. *He has asked the staff to let his wife know as he can't face telling her on his own.*
- *You need to explain to Elsa* that she has to find ways of avoiding physical and emotional stress as this may exacerbate her heart problems.
- *You have been asked to inform Marcus* that his health check has revealed that he has high blood pressure, and that three work colleagues have complained that his breath frequently smells of alcohol and that he seems to have lost interest in his work. The doctor has diagnosed an alcohol dependency problem.
- You have found Jack crying in the waiting room and he has told you how he is teased at his new school by the other children and that his real Daddy doesn't want him. *You need to ensure that he feels better about himself before he leaves.*
- Libby has told you that she is afraid her new boyfriend will leave her if he knows about her twin pregnancy and she is thinking about having an abortion. *You need to enable her to feel more positive about her possible choices before she leaves the scanning department.*
- Janet admits she is terrified she is going to lose her home. She is in despair about how she is going to be able to find the money to support herself and her son. *You need to enable her to feel more positive about her possible choices before she leaves.*
- Andrew has confided in you that he made a stupid mistake by having sex with a total stranger two months ago. You are aware that William has been diagnosed with a sexually transmitted infection. *You need to enable Andrew to feel more positive about his possible choices before he leaves the department.*

Table 7.1 Student activity scoring grid

Criteria for breaking news	Achieved Yes/No	Feedback evidence
The location in which they are giving the news is identified and they position themselves appropriately to inform the patient		
They set a time boundary for the session		
Particular attention is paid to: gentleness of tone and sensitivity to patient's responses		
You see an attempt to empathise with the patient		
Delivery of news is at an appropriate speed and uses suitable words for the patient		
Patient's questions following delivery are managed constructively		
Able to give realistic hope during the session		
Able to formulate a plan with the patient for another meeting		
Enable the patient to feel ongoing support is available from staff		
Aid the patient to discuss and plan how they are going to inform their relatives		
Close the session in a positive and constructive manner		
Other good interventions observed		

References

Bradshaw, J. (2005) *Healing the Shame that Binds You*, Deerfield Beach, Florida, Health Communications.

Casement, P. (1995) *On Learning From the Patient*, London, Routledge.

Dias, L., Chabner, B. A., Lynch Jr, T. J. and Penson, R. T. (2003) 'Breaking bad news: a patient's perspective', *The Oncologist* **8**(6), 587–96 [online] http://www.breakingbadnews.co.uk/guidelines.asp (accessed 10 January 2008).

Gavaghan, S. and Carroll, D. (2002) 'Families of critically ill patients and the effect of nursing interventions', *Dimensions of Critical Care Nursing* **21**(2), 64–71.

Guggenbuhl-Craig, A. (1999) *Power in the Helping Professions* (Classics in Archetypal Psychology, 2), London, Continuum International Publishing Group.

Jung, C. G. (1974) *Psychological Types*, a revision by R.F.C. Hull of the translation by H. G. Baynes, Bollingen Series XX, Princeton, Princeton University Press.

Larson, E. B. (2005) 'Clinical empathy as emotional labour in the patient–physician relationship', *Journal of the American Medical Association* **293**(9), 1100–6.

Money-Kyrle, R. (1956) 'Normal counter-transference and some of its deviations', *International Journal of Psychoanalysis* 37, 360–6.

Ptacek, J. T. and Ellison, N. M. (2000) 'Healthcare providers' perspectives on breaking bad news to patients: assessment problems', *Critical Care Nursing Quarterly* **23**(2), 51–9.

Reik, T. (1937) *Surprise and the Psychoanalyst*, New York, E.P. Dutton and Co.

Sully P. and Dallas J. (2005). *Essential Communication Skills for Nursing*, Edinburgh, Mosby.

Wondrak, R. F. (1998) *Interpersonal Skills for Nurses and Healthcare Professionals*, London, Blackwell Science Ltd.

Part

Chapter

8

Breakaway skills

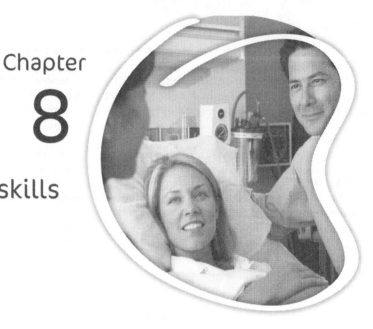

Diane Carpenter and
James Wilson

 Links to other chapters in *Foundation Skills for Caring*

3   Communication
4   Communicating with adolescents
5   Anxiety
6   Sign language

 Links to other chapters in *Foundation Studies for Caring*

4   Ethical, legal and professional issues
5   Communication
26   Mental health
27   Learning disability

W   Don't forget to visit www.palgrave.com/glasper for additional
online resources relating to this chapter.

Introduction

This chapter aims to give you the knowledge and understanding that underpin the skills of protecting yourself in an aversive or confrontational situation.

Learning outcomes

This chapter will enable you to:

- recognise signs of escalating aggression
- take appropriate action to maintain the safety of yourself and others by:
  - responding to early warning signs of aggressive behaviour by using verbal and non-verbal calming techniques
  - using non-aversive defensive interventions.

Concepts

- Aggression
- Mental health
- Communication
- Self-awareness

Welcome to the chapter on breakaway skills, which will introduce you to 'non-aversive defensive interventions'. Terminology changes frequently in health and social care provision and can be very confusing. There are other terms to describe the content of this chapter with which you may be more familiar, including:

- breakaways
- conflict management
- care and responsibility
- self-defence.

Basically they all mean the same thing, although 'care and responsibility' is a particular privately managed and regulated approach to the management of violence which is used in many prisons and NHS organisations, particularly within mental health settings. However, some healthcare practitioners, such as learning-disabilities nurses, reject this approach as not suitable for their client group. Student nurses are not required to become involved in restraint situations whilst in clinical practice, but they must attend an appropriate training course identified by their employer on completion of training. All such courses provide training in de-escalation techniques and the management of violence, as well as self-defence. In many clinical situations, however, healthcare students do need the knowledge and skills to help calm an escalating situation and to protect themselves from the threat of personal violence.

So why 'non-aversive defensive interventions'?

We prefer to use the term 'non-aversive' because the focus is on your personal protection in a clinical environment where you will be working with people with complex care needs. Although your primary aim is to protect yourself should you need to, it is likely that after an aggressive or violent event you will continue to care for the person involved, and will therefore need to maintain or resume a therapeutic relationship. It is possible to protect yourself skilfully in such a way that your responses are not perceived as aggressive (aversive).

Limitations of this chapter

W

As you read through this chapter and accompanying web material, you will be struck by how much of the guidance will appear to be common sense. The chapter includes a summary of commonly encountered errors made by health and social care staff. Taken in isolation the mistake may appear obvious and avoidable, but critical incident reviews have often highlighted a number of these occurring simultaneously as contributory or causative factors in an untoward event.

It should also be acknowledged that many errors occur as a result of an individual's stress response to an alarming situation. Self-awareness, reflective practice and focused training can help people to respond to such situations in a calm, skilful and controlled manner. This chapter should be seen as only one piece in the jigsaw and should be part of a wider package of training (Bowers et al, 2006; Hahn et al, 2006). Not all clinical areas provide specific training in non-aversive techniques, but where they do it is essential that you attend and complete these approved courses. Where such training is not provided, this chapter will contribute to a greater awareness of some of the basic principles which may aid you when confronted by an aversive situation.

Anger and aggression

It is important to differentiate between anger and aggression and to recognise that in some situations an angry response is perfectly justifiable; we have all experienced anger at some point in our lives.

> ⚠️ **Professional alert!**
>
> Aggression is NOT a justifiable expression of anger.

> **ⓐ Learning activity**
>
> Reflect upon:
> 1   a time when you have felt angry, and
> 2   a time when you have either witnessed or been the object of aggression.
> When you have done this, try to identify the differences between anger and aggression.

- *Anger* can be defined as a physiological and psychological response to a perceived threat (real or imagined). Other terms related to anger include fury, indignation and rage.
- *Aggression* can be defined as any offensive action, attack, or procedure which violates by force the rights of others.

Recognising escalating aggression

Sometimes the actual manifestation of an emotional response in one person may be misinterpreted by someone else. Fear and anger can appear very similar for example.

W

Aggression is expressed in different ways, most commonly identified by certain verbal and non-verbal behaviour. Have a look at the material on the companion website of one person engaging in verbal aggression and another using aggressive body language and behaviour.

> **ⓐ Learning activity**
>
> Recall a time when you or witnessed or were involved in a heated argument. Some of the signs you have already looked at will have been familiar to you, but how did you feel when the incident was happening?
> Write down your reflections.

You may have identified some of the more common physical feelings such as your heart rate increasing, your complexion changing and your mouth becoming dry. Your voice (or the voice of those you witnessed) may have been raised in volume and in pitch. These experiences are common to the fight, flight or freeze response.

As a person becomes increasingly aggressive, the situation can escalate until it reaches a point where you may perceive yourself to be in imminent danger. Hopefully, before this occurs, you will be able to employ some de-escalation techniques (see below) and calm the situation. An individual will rarely be calm one moment and violent the next. Along the journey to crisis there will usually be trigger factors which cause the person's behaviour to escalate towards violence. Knowing your patient, having a therapeutic relationship, and recognising the escalation signs can help you to prevent this from occurring. However, *sometimes a crisis cannot be avoided.*

- A *trigger* can be defined as something which starts a train of action.
- A *crisis* can be defined as a turning point, a decisive moment or an emergency.
- *Escalation* can be defined as a rapid increase in scale or intensity.

So far we have considered the signs of aggression in others and the feelings this engenders in us, but we also need to be aware of the environment in which we find ourselves. Environmental risk assessment is an essential and necessary skill, which we will return to later in the chapter.

Calming techniques

Being prepared for an aggressive outburst may prevent a crisis from occurring, not least because you are likely to feel more confident when there is less likelihood of your being taken by surprise. It is when patients are anxious or fearful that they are most likely to become aggressive. Having confident staff around them can provide sufficient reassurance to calm and de-escalate a situation. Physical interventions should only be used after calming techniques have been attempted and failed, and only by those fully trained to do so.

The law allows the principle of reasonable force to defend yourself. This is defined in terms of the minimum force necessary to remove yourself from imminent danger.

Examples of calming techniques

- Speaking with a calm voice at your usual speed or slower, and keeping the tone and pitch of your voice neutral (not raised or squeaky).
- Giving good eye contact but not staring. Fixing your gaze at a point in the middle of the person's brow may be helpful.
- Maintaining an open posture – not crossing your arms or hiding them behind your back, which may suggest to a patient that you are hiding a weapon or medication.
- Looking relaxed (even if you do not feel it). If you appear tense your aggressor may suspect you are about to attack.
- Listening. Try to understand what is happening, what the person is feeling. Don't be in a hurry to give advice. Initially focus on grasping a better understanding of the situation.
- Being sensitive to a person's self-esteem. Most people in emotional distress are feeling pretty helpless. A casual air or inappropriate humour could worsen the situation. Look for ways to restore the person's self-confidence.
- Identifying the person's feelings. Focus on what the person is feeling, and convey to them what you perceive that to be. This reflects an understanding and acceptance on your part of the nature of those emotions and beliefs. If you're unsure of what those feelings are, do not hesitate to acknowledge this fact. You may get some feedback that will clarify the issue.
- Avoiding a power struggle. This can only increase the anxiety level and cause further problems.
- Providing support. Most people in an emotional crisis are afraid of losing control. Offering support for the individual may help them deal with their problem without totally losing control.
- Not presenting consequences. In other words, do not threaten the person with what might happen if he or she hurts you.
- Personalising yourself. Let the aggressive individual know you are a person with a name. It is harder for someone to hurt you if they see you as a person and not an object, or for example as just 'a member of staff'.
- Dressing appropriately.

Some of these points will be discussed in more detail below.

One of the more difficult of the calming techniques to master is appearing calm even when you are not.

C Professional conversation

Rachel, a first-year nursing student, asked her mentor Geeta, 'I was on placement in an acute care setting when I witnessed one of the patients shouting in an aggressive manner at one of the healthcare support workers. He repeatedly asked the patient to "calm down", which didn't appear to help. What's the right thing to do in that kind of situation, Geeta?'

Geeta said, 'Nobody likes to hear people telling them to calm down, and it can inflame a situation. In situations like this it's important not to say "calm down" to someone in a state of high emotion, as this suggests that we don't take their situation seriously. Calmed down is the state where we want the patient to be; we need to use professional communication skills to facilitate this without being sucked into an argument.'

a Learning activity

Look in the mirror and practise a calm demeanour. Take a deep breath and relax your shoulders and then try again. We often hold our bodies in a tense posture without realising it.

Be prepared

In addition to the calming techniques considered above, there are several other important aspects to consider to help you be prepared should a crisis occur. One of these is to ensure you are wearing appropriate clothing.

Our choice of clothing sends signals about our attitudes, so careful thought has to be given to what we wear. We would recommend you consider the following points in a clinical environment where uniform is not worn:

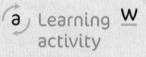

a Learning activity W

Visit the companion webpage for this chapter to investigate how clothing can be protective and/or provocative.

- Shoes should be flat soled and well fitting. Examples of poor footwear include flip-flops, stilettos and high boots:
  - Flip-flops make it difficult to run away from a dangerous situation.
  - Stilettos also hinder manoeuvrability and have the added problem that you are more likely to fall. Moreover, the heel could be used as a weapon.
  - High boots or those with steel toecaps can be associated with stereotypes of power and may be perceived as aggressive by the patient.
- Skirts and dresses come in a variety of forms from free flowing to very tight, and very long to very short. Some issues to consider are:
  - Free-flowing skirts can offer more material to be tugged at in a violent way. Elasticated waistbands can leave the wearer in an embarrassing state of half-dress if these are pulled.
  - Tight or short skirts (and low-cut tops) may be misperceived as inappropriately sexually provocative.
- Items of bric-a-brac such as necklaces, ties and body piercings could be ripped from your body during a crisis situation and either strangle you or cause additional painful complications.
- Long hair should be tied up or back so that it is not easy to grab hold of. Try to avoid pony tails.

Risk assessment

We have already discussed environmental risk assessment and you have identified potential hazards in a clinical environment. It is important that you continually assess the environmental risk and also the risk posed by individual patients. Constant assessment is particularly important for any patient in a mental health or learning disabilities service environment.

---

e Evidence-based practice box: risk indicators for violence

The Sainsbury Centre for Mental Health (Morgan, 2000) identifies the following as risk indictors for violence, although the list is not exclusive:

- previous incidents of violence
- previous use of weapons
- misuse of drugs and/or alcohol
- male gender, under 35 years of age
- known personal trigger factors
- expressing intent to harm others
- previous dangerous impulsive acts

- paranoid delusions about others
- violent command hallucinations
- signs of anger and frustration
- sexually inappropriate behaviour
- preoccupation with violent fantasy
- previous admissions to secure settings
- denial of previous dangerous acts.

If you identify a risk then be particularly vigilant in ensuring you keep yourself safe.

If you are visiting a patient in the community, follow the local policies and ensure that someone knows where you are at all times. It is unlikely as a student that you will be in the position of working alone, but should you find yourself in this situation – perhaps when you are near to qualification – then do not conduct an interview in the kitchen. There are too many potential hazards here such as knives or boiling water.

Be sensitive to the person's self-esteem. Most people who are losing or who have lost control feel pretty helpless underneath and use aggressive methods to attempt to regain this control. A casual tone or inappropriate humour could inflame the situation. Look for ways of restoring the person's self-esteem by maintaining a respectful manner towards them.

Do not create a power struggle. Try not to take an authoritarian stance – for example standing over a person with your arms folded or pointing your finger at them – as this is likely to increase their anxiety and create further problems. Remember that most people in an emotional situation are afraid of losing control and have a need for some kind of support and protection.

t
Practice tips

- Ensure that when you are in a room with another person who may become violent, you position yourself nearer the door.
- Where possible and appropriate, remove from the clinical environment any objects which may be used as weapons.

Elements for a violent incident

The following four elements are required for a violent incident to occur:

- a trigger
- a weapon
- a target
- high emotion.

---

a Learning activity

Give examples of what you would consider to comprise these four elements.

Stance

This is an extremely important aspect to behaving appropriately and keeping yourself safe in an untoward incident. When we think about the non-verbal messages that we transmit to others, one consideration is the way we stand. We refer to this as our stance.

Stance should include being mindful of the personal distance that you maintain between you and a potential assailant. You can't be hit if you are out of reach. The more distance between you and a potential assailant, the more reaction time you have and the better you can observe the person's body language.

A positive stance offers added protection; you are better balanced and you also appear confident. Aggressors are more likely to target someone who looks like a victim.

In a good stance the feet are approximately hip width apart with one foot in front of the other at a slight angle, with the foot bent slightly inwards. Practise this with a friend and give each other a *very gentle* push to ensure you have the position right and have a firm, stable stance. If you bend your knees slightly and turn slightly sideways you increase your resistance to being pushed over. Should you need to defend yourself from blows or kicks, you can put your arms up to act as a shield. Turning sideways also protects your vulnerable body parts from blows. Although receiving a thump to your bony bits is uncomfortable, it is preferable to being punched or kicked in the face, chest, stomach, loins or groin!

The legal position

This complex area could have a chapter dedicated to it on its own merit, but there are some guiding principles:

- Your personal safety is paramount. Always consider your surroundings and that your actions could have consequences for both yourself and the patient.
- There is no definition in law of what comprises reasonable force. This is judged by a court and depends on the situation as you perceived it to be and whether you used the minimum force you believed necessary to protect yourself and/or remove yourself from the situation.
- All verbal and physical aggression towards staff should be documented as required by your employer's health and safety policies and procedures.

Conclusion

This chapter has sought to distinguish between the normal emotional response of anger and the unacceptable aggressive response which may follow in some people. In most clinical areas there is a zero tolerance policy to aggressive behaviour, but clinical staff may on occasion have to cope with aggressive outbursts from patients, relatives or visitors. This chapter, therefore, has addressed the signs of escalating aggression and the environmental risk assessment necessary to minimise any harmful outcome. Calming techniques have been considered, including the need to increase one's self-awareness of aspects which may inadvertently inflame an aggressive outburst, such as provocative clothing and inappropriate footwear.

A suggestion has been made about an appropriate stance which will maximise your chances of protecting yourself in the event of an untoward aggressive episode occurring. The principle of reasonable force has also been considered. Above all, note that this chapter provides only a starting point in the management of aggression and cannot replace training in your own clinical environment.

Further reading

Carson, D. (1990) 'When taking risk is a management duty', *Health Service Journal* **100**(5221), 1464.

Carson, D. (1995) 'Calculated risk', *Community Care* 1092, 26–7

Irwin, A. (2006) 'The nurse's role in the management of aggression', *Journal of Psychiatric and Mental Health Nursing* 13, 309–18.

Rogers, P. and Vidgen, A. (2006) 'Working with people with severe mental illness who are angry', pp. 273–94 in Gamble, C. and Brennan, G. (eds), *Working with Serious Mental Illness: A manual for clinical practice*, 2nd edn, Edinburgh, Elsevier.

Ryan, T. (1999) *Managing Crisis and Risk in Mental Health Nursing*, Cheltenham, Stanley Thornes.

References

Bowers, L., Nijman, H., Allan, T., Simpson, A., Warren, J. and Turner, L. (2006) 'Prevention and management of aggression training and violent incidents on UK acute psychiatric wards', *Psychiatric Services* **57**(7), 1022–6.

Hahn, S., Needham, I., Abderhalden, C., Duxbury, J. and Halfens, R. (2006) 'The effect of a training course on mental health nurses' attitudes on the reasons of patient aggression and its management', *Journal of Psychiatric and Mental Health Nursing* 13, 197–204.

Morgan, S. (2000) *Clinical Risk Management: A clinical tool and practitioner manual*, London, The Sainsbury Centre for Mental Health.

Part

II

Skills for physical needs

Chapters

Chapter

9

Patient hygiene

Tim Coney

Links to other chapters in *Foundation Skills for Caring*

Links to other chapters in *Foundation Studies for Caring*

Don't forget to visit www.palgrave.com/glasper for additional online resources relating to this chapter.

Introduction

This chapter aims to highlight the principles of helping patients meet their personal hygiene needs. It covers many of the fundamental aspects of the professional's role in assessing these needs and where appropriate assisting patients as they maintain their personal hygiene. It provides a general overview of the nurse's role in this, and step-by-step procedures for bathing patients, providing nail, eye and hair care and for shaving male patients.

Learning outcomes

This chapter will enable you to:

- understand the practitioner's role in helping patients achieve their personal hygiene needs
- identify the indications for and describe the processes and procedures of:
  - giving a patient a bath
  - bed-bathing a patient
  - perineal care
  - nail care
  - eye care
  - care of the hair
  - shaving male patients.

Concepts

- Communication
- Infection control
- Universal precautions
- Assessment
- Evaluation
- Patient dignity and privacy
- Patient well-being
- Record-keeping

Helping patients meet their personal hygiene needs is one of the most fundamental aspects of care, and assisting patients in this way must follow an assessment and the development of an appropriate care plan (DH, 2003). Two aspects of hygiene which impact on the practitioner's role need to be considered. Firstly there are hygiene issues that relate to the individual who is delivering the care to the patient, which generally include the correct wearing of uniforms and any items of protective clothing such as disposable gloves and aprons when providing care to patients, and hand hygiene; these are covered in greater detail in Chapter 30 on 'Universal precautions'. Secondly there are the specific care interventions needed by patients who are unable to take care of their own personal hygiene needs. These interventions must be based on a nursing assessment of that patient.

Uniforms

Most National Health Service (NHS) trusts and other care organisations have a uniform policy or uniform guidelines which have to be adhered to. Uniforms and their associated policies are designed to offer protection as well as projecting a professional image that patients can recognise and easily relate to. The uniforms provided by organisations such as NHS trusts are not considered particularly glamorous by most staff, but they are designed to allow ease of movement and comfort rather than as fashion items. They should not be altered and care must be taken with additional items such as the wearing of badges and other symbols as these can pose risks of both personal injury and infection. Uniform policies also provide guidance on hair, particularly regarding its length and in which situations it should be completely covered, nails and nail polish, and the wearing of jewellery. These guidelines should always be adhered to in order to minimise the spread of infection and to protect the individual nurse and patient from injury. The wearing of single-use disposable aprons and gloves when assisting patients with their personal hygiene tasks is covered in Chapter 30 on 'Universal precautions'. The use of such items should be guided by any policies in force within the clinical area concerned, and by undertaking a personal risk assessment of the likelihood of contamination with bodily fluids.

Patient's personal hygiene

Helping patients meet their personal hygiene needs is a fundamental element of nursing care which is easily overlooked, or undertaken in a rushed manner. Assisting patients with their personal hygiene or providing patients with their daily hygiene routines is an important aspect of the nurse's role which is frequently delegated to unqualified healthcare assistants. In many cases this is acceptable and the various procedures will be performed adequately, but it is important to remember it is the nurse's responsibility to ensure these activities are properly supervised. Accountability for these nursing interventions remains with the registered practitioner (NMC, 2006), even though they may be undertaken by unqualified staff.

Many patients need help with their daily personal hygiene routines; this may be on a temporary basis or be a more permanent part of their care. Patients who have suddenly become ill or have suffered a minor injury which has incapacitated them temporarily may need some assistance with completing the most basic elements of personal hygiene such as washing and cleaning their teeth. Patients who have more permanent physical or mental disabilities, or have chronic and progressive conditions that lead eventually to physical disability, may in time become completely dependent on their carers for all aspects of personal hygiene. Nursing care should be based on an individual nursing assessment and be designed to help patients with their hygiene needs. Nursing interventions that help patients meet these needs should be sensitive to the impact this care may have on the patient's dignity, and privacy must be provided. Awareness of the embarrassment patients often experience when needing help with completing some of the basic aspects of their lives is an important aspect of these nursing interventions. You can read more about this in Chapter 3.

There are some common elements that need to be addressed when assisting patients to fulfil their basic hygiene needs:

- Find out what patients can do for themselves and agree any nursing intervention with them in order to encourage and assist them in completing these tasks; for example they may be able to wash their hands and face after using a commode or before eating, if a nurse provides the equipment and holds a bowl of water for them to use.

- Always gain informed consent before proceeding with any nursing intervention; take care to consider how this is obtained. 'Would you like me to help you with having a wash now?' may be a more appropriate way of communicating with a patient than 'I'm going to give you your bed bath now', which may leave the patient very little choice but to accept.

- Be aware of the loss of dignity and possible embarrassment patients may be feeling in having such basic tasks performed for them – often by someone much younger than themselves. This is particularly so for elderly patients who have been independent in respect of their own hygiene requirements before becoming ill.

- Involve the patient as much as you can; two nurses performing a bed bath on a patient should not be in conversation with each other and ignoring the patient. These techniques are highly personal and often embarrassing for patients. They are fundamental nursing care responsibilities and as such should not be delegated solely to unqualified, unsupervised healthcare workers.

- Undertake a risk assessment and make an informed decision about wearing a single-use disposable apron and gloves; hand washing needs to be considered and the disposal of any waste products – always adhere to the various policies regarding these issues. See Chapter 30 on 'Universal precautions' and organisational policies for guidelines.

- Show respect for the patient by addressing them by the name they prefer – informality may cause offence and if a patient wishes to be addressed formally this should be respected at all times.

Specific activities

Giving a bath

Many patients need help with bathing, and if they are physically unable to manoeuvre into and out of a traditional bath, specialist bathing equipment such as a side-entry bath will be needed.

⚠ Professional alert!

Patients from different cultural or religious backgrounds may have different values and requirements for their basic hygiene needs. Always check with the individual patients to prevent problems.

ⓐ Learning activity

Explain to a friend or colleague how you prepare to have a bath at home, and what aspects are important to you that make it a pleasurable event.

Now think of what you would ask a patient prior to preparing to bath them to ensure their comfort and safety.

Things to remember when bathing a patient.

- Newly arrived patients may not have had a bath for some time because of their physical immobility and the arrangements they have in their own homes. (Most domestic bathrooms are relatively small and do not have space to readily accommodate a mechanical hoist which may be needed to lower a patient who is immobile into a bath.) Daily bathing or showering may be part of the essential daily routine for the patient being cared for, and as such contribute to the individual's health and well-being. Inability to bath or shower regularly as a result of illness or injury may cause excessive body odour and reduce the skin's natural ability to provide one of the body's main defences against infection and disease. In addition bodily cleanliness improves self-esteem and is considered a basic human right (Young, 1991), which may have been compromised by the patient's inability to perform these tasks due to illness. However be aware of individual differences and preferences.
- The equipment needed may include the patient's own toiletries such as soap, towels and face cloths (which may be disposable wipes if preferred). Patients may request additional items they wish to be added to the bath water – but remember that many proprietary bath-water additions are oil based and may cause problems by making surfaces more slippery so that it is difficult to get the patient in and out of the bath; the use of such additions may create a dangerous situation. A risk assessment must be carried out before adding anything to the bath water.
- Consent will be required as with any other procedure.
- The temperature of the room and the bath water both need to be monitored.
- This is a highly personal and private activity during which the patient will be undressed. The door should be closed and all equipment should be gathered before starting, to avoid unnecessary disturbances.
- The patient should never be left alone.
- Encourage patients to do as much for themselves as possible.

ⓐ Learning activity

In certain circumstances in is necessary to attend to hygiene needs whilst the patient is in bed. Imagine you have been injured and require a bed bath; think of the aspects of the experience that would give you the most concern.

Bed-bathing patients

Two nurses should ideally be involved in bed-bathing patients so that the procedure can be completed quickly – thus avoiding the patient being exposed for a long period of time. One nurse should wash and the other dry to avoid leaving the patient wet for prolonged periods, which may cause excessive chilling (Pegram, Bloomfield and Jones, 2007).

Bathing and bed-bathing patients, in addition to making them feel more comfortable, also provides an opportunity to observe their general condition, such as skin reddening over pressure points, rashes and other abnormalities (Alexander, Fawcett and Runciman, 2006). This may also be a good time to engage patients in conversation in which they may well reveal essential information not previously noted. Bed-bathing often has to be adapted to suit the individual needs of the patient, or if only one nurse is working alone. Common issues that need to be addressed in bed-bathing include the use of soap or other proprietary skin cleansers in case the patient has an allergy or expresses a personal preference, the temperature of the water, and being aware of when in the procedure the water should be changed (Dougherty and Lister, 2004). Any policies on the wearing of appropriate protective clothing such as aprons and gloves provided by the organisation providing the care should be adhered to, as should the correct disposal of any waste and the laundering of soiled linen.

⚠ Professional alert!

Some NHS trusts have been heavily fined by their local authorities for sending clinical waste to landfill sites. Be aware of and adhere to the correct methods of waste disposal used by the organisation providing the care.

t ☆ Practice tip

Remember a bed bath is a potentially embarrassing procedure for the patient and the screens or curtains should be pulled around the bed area to ensure complete privacy. The procedure should not be interrupted. Remember that the curtains or screens around the bed area are not soundproofed and other patients may hear any conversations.

Part

II

Step-by-step procedure for bed-bathing patients

- Assess the needs of the patient.
- Plan the procedure with the patient and gain his or her consent.
- Offer a commode, bed pan or urinal before starting the bed bath.
- Collect the equipment needed:
  - two wash flannels (disposable wipes may be preferred)
  - two bath towels
  - soap or preferred skin cleanser
  - toiletry items (e.g. deodorant, hair brush, comb, razor, shaving foam)
  - bowl of warm water – check temperature
  - clean hospital gown, pyjamas/nightdress
  - clean bed linen
  - waste material receptacle
  - linen skip/laundry bag
  - disposable apron/gloves.
- Ensure privacy for the patient; make sure there are no drafts and that the bed is at the correct height, close doors and windows if necessary. Check the general environment around the bed for safety, moving obstacles such as chairs and lockers, and ensure the bed brakes are on.
- Wash hands and put on a disposable apron – paying heed to local policies (DH, 2006).
- Help the patient to remove clothes from the area being washed, ensuring the patient remains covered with a suitable sheet or blanket (Pegram et al, 2007).
- Position one of the towels across the chest to protect the area not being washed from splashes.
- Check if it is acceptable to use soap, especially on the face.
- Wash and rinse the top half of the body – commencing with the face and then the arms, hands and fingers, axillae and chest – with one nurse washing and rinsing and the other drying with the second towel, using a patting technique so as to avoid hard rubbing.
- Change the water, put on disposable gloves.

- Inform the patient you will be washing the genitalia and ask if they wish to do this for themselves with assistance if necessary (see the additional information on perineal care later in this section). Always use disposable wipes for this area (Potter and Perry, 2007).
- Change the water again and remove/change gloves if soiled.
- Wash, rinse and dry the legs and feet.
- Assist the patient to roll over and wash the back and then the bottom, using a disposable wash cloth or wipe – take care of any catheters or wound drains that may be present.
- Help the patient to dress in clean gown/nightdress or pyjamas.
- Change the bed linen and correctly dispose of the soiled linen removed from the patients bed.
- Help with teeth cleaning and mouth care (see Chapter 12).
- Offer to help shave male patients (see below).
- Clear away any remaining waste materials (see alert above); decontaminate and store the bowl according to local infection control policies (Marieb, 2004).
- Wash hands (DH, 2006).
- Document the procedure and care given (NMC, 2005).

Perineal care

Perineal care is normally undertaken as part of the routine bed-bathing procedure (Potter and Perry, 2007). Where incontinence is a problem, the patient has an indwelling catheter, has had genital surgery or has undergone childbirth, the perineum may become inflamed and sore (Potter and Perry, 2007). In such situations regular care is an important part of the patient's personal hygiene routine. As with other procedures patients may wish to perform this task themselves to reduce their embarrassment; in such cases the nurse's role will be to assist. In patients unable to manage this for themselves, the nurse will have to undertake this procedure for them. This will be a highly personal procedure which will include inspection and reporting any red areas or soreness, washing and drying the area if intact, using plain water to avoid excessive drying as a result of using soap (Dougherty and Lister, 2004). After washing and drying, the procedure may involve the application of any prescribed creams or ointments. If the patient has an indwelling catheter, this routine should include catheter care and toilet according to local procedures and policies (see Chapter 13).

Step-by-step procedure

Ensure patients have complete privacy and obtain their consent. Ascertain how much they can manage for themselves, and encourage them to do this with assistance. If patients are unconscious or have severely limited movements, the nurse will have to perform these tasks for them.

- The patient should be assisted into a supine (lying on the back, face or front upward) position to make this procedure easier to manage.
- Keep the patient draped with a towel on the lower abdomen and another under and over the upper thighs to avoid excessive wetting of the bed linen. Expose only the area being washed.
- It is important to remember that this can be an extremely embarrassing procedure, and preserving the dignity of the patient should be paramount.
- In most cases the use of soap is not recommended; the use of plain warm water should be sufficient to cleanse this area for most patients (Potter and Perry, 2007).
- A disposable apron and gloves should be worn for this procedure.
- In male patients gentle washing of the penis and scrotum will be necessary, holding the penis with a disposable wipe and encouraging the patient to undertake this for himself if possible.
- The procedure itself is carried out in a similar way to bed-bathing: by washing with a disposable wipe and then carefully drying the area, using a patting action rather than by

rubbing. Care must be taken to avoid contamination of the female genitalia with faeces if present, by washing and drying in a downward direction. In catheterised patients, catheter inspection and routine care as necessary are included as part of this procedure.

Nail care

Patients may ask for their toenails to be trimmed as part of their routine hygiene care. This is an issue for many elderly patients who may have been able neither to attend to their own foot and nail care for some time, nor to visit a chiropodist because of their physical limitations or immobility. Because of the potential risk of serious injury, especially where there are related peripheral circulatory problems, as in diabetic patients, care of the toenails should be undertaken by a podiatrist.

The policy of the organisation providing the care must be followed to protect the patients against injury resulting from inappropriate nail care (see Chapter 14 on Basic Foot Care and Managing Common Nail Pathologies).

Eye care

Eye care is described in detail in Chapter 11. Generally the eyes are kept moist and infection free by the production of tears (Booker and Nicol, 2003), and this may be absent or deficient in some patients. Performing eye care as part of the patients personal hygiene routine is restricted to cleaning the area around the eye with a swab moistened with normal saline (Bunker-Rosdahl and Kowalski, 2007). Great care must be exercised when performing this technique and the nurse must be sensitive to the patient who may be worried about sustaining an eye injury. Generally if performing this technique the eye is gently swabbed from the inner (nasal) aspect towards the outer aspect, using a single swab, which is then discarded. It is important that the equipment is then changed so that the second eye is not contaminated by swabs or fluid used on the first eye.

Care of the hair

Normal hair brushing or combing is something most patients are able to attend to for themselves; however hair should be brushed or combed for unconscious patients, and relatives often regard this as indicative of the quality of care being provided for their loved ones. Tidy clean hair is an outward sign that the patient has received appropriate nursing care for their personal hygiene needs. Hair washing may be needed for a number of reasons, as a part of the patient's normal hygiene routine or, for example to remove encrusted blood following a head injury. Hair washing is best performed by two nurses, and if possible should be undertaken in a bathroom area if the patient can be transferred to a suitable facility. In some cases it is acceptable to undertake this procedure using a bowl of water, shampoo and towels, with the patient's head extended over the end of the bed after removing the bed head. Generally hospital barbers have disappeared from NHS trusts; if there is one, arrangements can be made for hair cutting and styling as appropriate to the patient's wishes.

> **a) Learning activity**
>
> Let a colleague brush/comb your hair and then evaluate the experience.

Shaving male patients

Like hair care, face shaving is a very personal activity, and male patients often feel they have only completed their personal hygiene routines fully when their hair is tidy and they have been shaved. Successful face shaving is dependent on the contours of the face and the direction in which facial hair (stubble) grows. Men who shave have usually adopted a highly individual routine for completing the task and will have a preference for the type of shaving equipment they use, for example a wet shave or using an electric shaver. Helping a patient with shaving should consist of asking about what is needed and the shaving techniques favoured, and then helping the patient to undertake this for himself wherever possible. This may mean setting up the patient's own mains electric or battery-operated shaver (ensuring that it has been checked for safety according to local health and safety policies), or providing water and shaving cream/foam if a wet shave is required. If patients are unable to perform this procedure, a relative could be asked to help, or the nurse caring for the patient will have to undertake this procedure carefully and slowly in order to avoid cutting the patients face.

Conclusion

Helping patients meet their personal hygiene needs is one of the most fundamental aspects of nursing care, and assisting patients with their personal hygiene is an essential element of good nursing which should be developed in the early stages of training. These activities should not be regarded as non-nursing tasks, as planning, delivering and evaluating effective interventions for patients who find it difficult to maintain their personal hygiene involves a range of important nursing skills. Patients who have lost the ability to undertake some or all of the basic elements of maintaining their personal hygiene, either temporarily or permanently as a result of disease or injury, regard these nursing interventions as extremely important in helping them meet their day-to-day care needs.

References

Alexander, M. F., Fawcett, J. N. and Runciman, P. J. (2006) *Nursing Practice Hospital and Home: The adult*, 3rd edn, Edinburgh, London, New York, Oxford, Churchill Livingstone.

Booker, C. and Nicol, M. (2003) *Nursing Adults: The practice of caring*, Edinburgh, London, New York, Oxford, Mosby.

Bunker-Rosdahl, C. and Kowalski, M. T. (2007) *Textbook of Basic Nursing*, 8th edn, Philadelphia, Baltimore, New York, London, Buenos Aires, Hong Kong, Sydney, Toronto, Lippincott, Williams and Wilkins.

Department of Health (DH) (2003) *Essence of Care: Patient-focused benchmarks for clinical governance*, London, DH.

DH (2006) *The Health Act 2006, Code of Practice for the Prevention and Control of Healthcare Associated Infections*, London, DH.

Dougherty, L. and Lister, S. (2004) *The Royal Marsden Hospital Manual of Clinical Nursing Procedures*, 6th edn, Oxford, Royal Marsden Hospital/Blackwell.

Marieb, E. N. (2004) *Human Anatomy and Physiology*, 5th edn, Illinois, New York, Pearson Education, Scott Foreman Addison Wesley.

Nursing and Midwifery Council (NMC) (2005) *Records and Record Keeping*, London, NMC.

NMC (2006) *Code of Professional Conduct, Standards for Conduct, Performance and Ethics*, London, NMC.

Pegram, A., Bloomfield, J. and Jones, A. (2007) 'Clinical skills: bed bathing and personal hygiene needs of patients', *British Journal of Nursing* **16**(6), 356–8.

Potter, P. A. and Perry, A. G. (2007) *Basic Nursing Essentials for Practice*, 5th edn, St Louis, Missouri, Mosby.

Young, L. (1991) 'The clean fight', *Nursing Standard* **5**(35), 54–5.

Chapter

10

Pressure area care

Elaine Gibson and
Cheryl Dunford

Links to other chapters in *Foundation Skills for Caring*

9   Patient hygiene
30 Universal precautions
31 Wound assessment
32 Aseptic technique and wound management

Links to other chapters in *Foundation Studies for Caring*

3   Evidence-based practice and research
8   Healthcare governance
9   Moving and handling
10 Nutritional assessment and needs
12 Fluid balance in adults
13 Infection prevention and control
25 Care of the older adult – community
28 Rehabilitation
29 Loss, grief, bereavement and palliative care
00 Care of the adult – surgical

W   Don't forget to visit www.palgrave.com/glasper for additional
online resources relating to this chapter.

Introduction

This chapter aims to give you the knowledge and understanding of why pressure ulcers occur and how we can help prevent them. Assessment and treatment options for established pressure ulcers will also be included. The skills required to assess skin for damage and to grade skin damage will be described.

Learning outcomes

This chapter will enable you to:

- describe what pressure ulcers are and why they occur
- identify factors that place people at risk of developing them
- describe how to undertake the following with evidence-based reasons:
  - risk assessment
  - skin inspection
  - classification of skin damage (using the European Pressure Ulcer Advisory Panel grading scale).
- discuss measures required to prevent skin damage in terms of skin hygiene, use of pressure-relieving equipment, nutrition and wound management.

Concepts

- Communication
- Privacy and dignity
- Observation skills
- Safety
- Policy/guidelines
- Risk assessment
- Assessment tools
- Universal precautions
- Nutrition
- Mobility
- Pain management

What are pressure ulcers?

Pressure ulcers are areas of localised damage to skin and underlying tissue. They are the result of forces such as friction, shear and pressure being applied to the skin for periods of time. They usually occur over bony prominences such as heels, sacrum, hips and elbows where the soft tissue is compressed between the support surface and the bone; they can however, occur in other parts of the body where these forces are present. Pressure ulcers can develop as a result of lying or sitting on surfaces such as theatre tables and trolleys, wheelchairs, standard chairs and mattresses for long periods. This type of damage can also result from lying on catheter or drainage tubes or rolled up anti-emboli stockings.

Pressure ulcers can range from superficial damage involving little more than skin discolouration to deep ulcers which can extend down to tendon, muscle or bone.

What causes the skin to break down?

Skin is designed to withstand high pressures for short periods of time. However, tissue will start to break down when exposed to high levels or prolonged periods of pressure, combined with other forces such as friction and shear. Moisture will also hasten this breakdown. It is often the combination of these forces which causes the tissue to become distorted and leads to destruction.

It is important to recognise where these forces occur when nursing patients. Table 10.1 illustrates each force in turn.

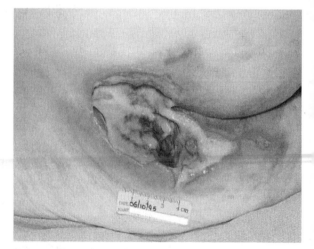

Figure 10.1 Pressure ulcer

Source: with kind permission of Elaine Gibson, Tissue Viability Nurse Specialist, East Kent Hospitals NHS Trust. Educational Specialist ConvaTec Ltd.

Table 10.1 Forces and their effects on skin

Force	Description	Example
Pressure	Downward force (patient's bodyweight) exerted onto a unit of area (e.g. buttocks). This is considered the major cause of pressure ulcers due to the occlusion of capillaries and other tissue structures that it causes. This will eventually result in tissue death (necrosis).	Lying on A&E trolley. Sitting in ward chair without adequate cushioning.
Shear	Shearing causes the different layers of tissue to move in opposing directions leading to disruption and separation of subcutaneous layers. Shear will intensify the effects of pressure. The elderly are more susceptible to the effects of shear as the amount of elastin in the skin (which gives skin its stretch) reduces with age. Shearing forces can cause small blood vessels to be kinked, stretched or torn, disrupting the blood supply.	Moving and handling of patients. Sliding down the bed or chair. Transferring from bed to chair where dragging occurs.
Friction	This force occurs when two surfaces are rubbed together, resulting in skin surface separation and loss. This damage is enhanced when moisture is present as this weakens skin. Friction usually presents as blistering.	Rubbing of straps or clothing on skin, armrests on elbows.

Part

II

Although we understand the mechanics of skin breakdown, there is still a lack of understanding of pressure ulcer development at the cellular, biochemical and genetic level (Clark, 2007). For this reason, it is vital to view each patient as an individual and to be vigilant when examining skin for damage.

> **ⓐ Learning activity**
>
> Think back to a patient you have known who needed help with mobility. How and when could the forces shown in Table 10.1 have been introduced?

How big is the problem of pressure ulcers?

Pressure ulcers are a significant problem in healthcare settings. Although they are more prevalent in elderly and immobile patients, they can occur in all settings including maternity, paediatrics and neonatal units.

A large European survey undertaken in 2003, which included the UK (Clark, Bours and Defloor, 2004), found that 18 per cent of hospital patients had some degree of pressure damage. Many patients with pressure ulcers are cared for in their own homes or in residential and nursing homes, and it is not known how large this number is. Various studies have identified that most pressure damage in hospital patients starts in the first few days following admission for an acute illness or enforced mobility (Versluysen, 1985; Torrance and Maylor, 1999).

Another estimate suggests that 400,000 people develop a new pressure ulcer each year in the UK (Posnett and Franks, 2007).

Pressure ulcers are very costly, both in terms of the pain and disruption to life that they cause and financially. A recent estimate of the cost has been given at £1.4–£2.1 billion annually (4 per cent of the total NHS spend), most of the cost being the additional nursing time that is required (Bennet, Dealey and Posnett, 2004). It must also be remembered that severe pressure damage can lead to the death of the patient.

Policies and guidelines

There are national and international guidelines on both the prevention and treatment of pressure ulcers. These are available electronically on the following sites:

- *The Management of Pressure Ulcers in Primary and Secondary Care: a clinical practice guideline*, 2005, Royal College of Nursing (RCN): www.rcn.org.uk/publications/pdf/ guidelines/rcn_guidelines.pdf.

W

- A quick reference guide is available from the RCN at: www.rcn.org.uk.
- *NICE Inherited Clinical Guidelines*, 2003 (with summary sheet and patient information leaflets), National Institute for Clinical Excellence (NICE): http://www.nice.org.uk.
- European Pressure Ulcer Advisory Panel (EPUAP), *Guidelines on Prevention and Treatment of Pressure Ulcers*, 1998 (currently under review): www.epuap.org.
- *The Essence of Care: clinical practice benchmarking programme* (DH, 2003, 2005) has also included pressure ulcer prevention as one of its benchmarks: http://www.doh.gov.uk/.

These will give you further information and advice on this subject.

> **a   Learning activity**
>
> Think back to any placements that you have had so far. Were you made aware of any policies and guidelines on pressure ulcers?

Preventing pressure ulcers

The most important aspect of preventing pressure ulcers is identifying those people at risk of developing them and then instigating preventative measures. Assessment is a key skill.

> **S   Scenario: an elderly patient with many mobility problems**
>
> Mrs Smith is 84 years old and lives on her own following the death of her husband four years ago. She has been admitted to hospital for treatment of an acute and severe chest infection. She has had rheumatoid arthritis for over 40 years and has hand and other small joint deformities as a consequence. She had a hip replacement eight years ago following a fall, but has become increasingly lame over the last five years and is now only able to walk short distances with the aid of a walking stick. While in hospital she has only been able to spend short periods of time sitting out, and her walking is now limited due to breathlessness and exhaustion.

Assessing risk

Determining whether a patient is at risk of developing pressure ulcers will require a number of skills such as:

- gathering information by talking to the patient, family and carers
- careful history taking
- observation of their skin
- observation of mobility
- information gathering relating to nutrition
- gaining insight into their understanding of pressure ulcers.

Before you begin your risk assessment, some underpinning knowledge about pressure ulcers is vital. There are a number of known intrinsic risk factors that will increase the risk of skin breakdown that you should be aware of. These include the following (NICE, 2003; RCN, 2005):

- reduced mobility/activity
- sensory impairment
- acute illness
- altered level of consciousness
- extremes of age
- vascular disease
- severe chronic or terminal illness
- previous history of pressure damage
- malnutrition or dehydration.

> **a   Learning activity**
>
> How many of these intrinsic factors do you think relate to Mrs Smith?

There are some specific groups of people who are more at risk than others. These include patients who are:

- elderly
- frail/terminally ill
- malnourished
- immobile
- sedated/anaesthetised
- presenting with spinal cord injuries
- presenting with neurological disorders
- presenting with fractured neck of femur.

Gathering information

It is important that you gather this information in a systematic way. There are a number of assessment tools available that have been developed over the years to assist with this process. The most commonly used within the UK are Waterlow (1988), Norton (Norton, McLaren and Exton-Smith, 1962) and Braden (Bergstrom et al, 1987). The Waterlow score is displayed below.

These tools work by providing the assessor with systematic list of known risk factors which are all allocated a score. When added together, these will provide a predictive numerical score.

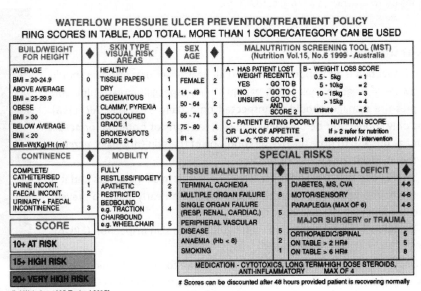

Figure 10.2
Waterlow pressure ulcer prevention/treatment policy

Reprinted with the permission of Judy Waterlow: www. judy-waterlow.co.uk

W

Please visit our companion website for up-to-date information about the Waterlow Pressure Ulcer Prevention/ Treatment Policy.

Although they are useful as part of the assessment process, there are many limitations with all scores currently available and it is therefore important to use them in combination with clinical judgement (RCN, 2005). Simply using a scale without knowledge and clinical skills (and the time and equipment to prevent pressure ulcers) will not have the desired effect (Halfens, 2000), as there is little evidence that using a risk tool or scale is better than clinical judgement (RCN, 2005).

Learning activity

If you are unfamiliar with the Waterlow score, try to allocate a level of risk for Mrs Smith with the information provided. If there are terms that you are unsure of, please visit the Waterlow website on www.judy-waterlow.co.uk in order to clarify these. This site will enable you to download a score card.

⚠ Professional alert!

When undertaking pressure ulcer risk assessments, always ensure that you explain to the patients what their risk is and what they can do to prevent skin damage.

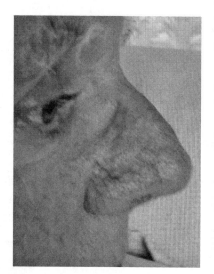

Figure 10.3 Reactive hyperaemia as a result of wearing glasses

Source: with kind permission of Elaine Gibson, Tissue Viability Nurse Specialist, East Kent Hospitals NHS Trust. Educational Specialist ConvaTec Ltd.

Skin inspection

Skin inspection is an important skill and all healthcare practitioners should be aware of what to look for. A patient's skin, especially areas vulnerable to pressure damage, should be inspected on a daily basis (EPUAP, 1998). Not only should you be observing the skin for signs of potential or actual damage but also to note the overall condition of the skin (dry, flaky, eczema, erythema and so on).

Exposure to pressure and other forces will result in skin changes and it is therefore important to be able to detect these at an early stage to prevent further damage and breakdown.

The following definitions are a useful guide to aid skin inspection (EPUAP, 1998):

- *Reactive hyperaemia*: this is the normal response to pressure which we all experience. It can be seen as a bright flush (erythema) of the skin associated with the release of an obstruction to the circulation and resultant increase in blood flow. In highly pigmented skin, this may appear as purplish/blue discolouration.
- *Blanching hyperaemia*: this again is a normal response and indicates that the circulation is intact. It can be seen as a reddened area that temporarily turns white or pale when pressure is applied with a fingertip. Blanching erythema over a pressure site is usually due to a normal reactive hyperaemic response.
- *Non-blanching hyperaemia*: this is indicative of damage to the microcirculation and is classed as Grade 1 pressure damage. There is an observable alteration to intact skin when compared with adjacent or opposite areas of the body. The ulcer appears as a defined area of persistent redness in lightly pigmented skin, whereas in darker skin tones it may appear with persistent red, blue or purple hues.

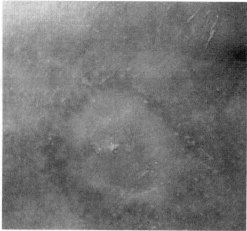

Figure 10.4 Blanching hyperaemia on a sacrum of a patient: simply by moving the patient and relieving the pressure the skin will recover. Early detection is the key to good management

Source: with kind permission of Elaine Gibson, Tissue Viability Nurse Specialist, East Kent Hospitals NHS Trust. Educational Specialist ConvaTec Ltd.

There may also be one or more of the following:

- change in skin temperature (warmth or coolness
- tissue consistency (firm or boggy feeling)
- sensation (pain, itching).

No colour change occurs to the hyperaemia when light finger pressure is applied. This indicates a degree of microcirculation damage. Blistering or swelling of the skin may also be present and the patient may complain of pain.

Incontinence lesions are often mistaken for pressure damage. They are associated with incontinence or diarrhoea and can lead to skin discolouration. The main differences are that they are not necessary on bony prominences and may be more purple in colour. The skin may be wet and/or oedematous (McDonagh, 2008).

- *Moisture*: Kelly (1994) suggests that even slight amounts of moisture can increase the risk of developing pressure damage by macerating the skin and decreasing its tensile strength, although he does not substantiate this statement with supportive research. The recent NICE guidelines (2003) also mention moisture as an exacerbating factor and highlight the need for this to be part of risk assessment. The EPUAP have in fact identified this within the Pressure Ulcer Prevention Guidelines (1998) in terms of maintaining and improving tissue tolerance. Bryant (2000) suggests that moisture may alter the resiliency of the epidermis to external forces as it may increase the risk of shear and friction forces. The existing body of knowledge remains inconclusive but what is clear is the importance of maintaining skin integrity.

The existence of a Grade 1 pressure ulcer or a moisture lesion is a significant factor in the development of a more severe ulcer (RCN, 2005; NICE, 2003; EPUAP, 1998). It is therefore important to correctly identify, report and record all Grade 1 pressure ulcers as rapid deterioration can occur (Donnelly, 2005).

Pressure ulcer risk assessment procedure

You will need:

- ward/practice pressure ulcer risk assessment documentation
- risk assessment tool (if used) e.g. Waterlow, Braden
- apron and gloves.

1. Observe previous documentation of risk and any documentation relating to status and change in medical condition.
2. Wash hands and put on apron (gloves may be required when inspecting skin if soiling is present or if required as part of infection control measures).
3. Introduce yourself to the patient, explain the rationale for assessment and what it will entail, and gain verbal consent before proceeding.
4. If the patient is able to communicate with you, begin assessment by gaining information on the patient's current health status. This includes how patients are feeling, ability to walk (activity) and to move by themselves (mobility), whether they have a temperature, are in pain, continence issues, and what their appetite is like. Information concerning the history of the current illness together with any longer-term conditions is of importance. In relation to nutrition, a history of recent weight loss may indicate some degree of malnutrition. If patients are unable to communicate, this information may be gained

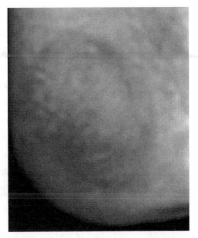

Figure 10.5 The skin remains red when touched. This is documented as a Grade 1 pressure ulcer

Source: with kind permission of Elaine Gibson, Tissue Viability Nurse Specialist, East Kent Hospitals NHS Trust. Educational Specialist ConvaTec Ltd.

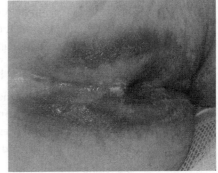

Figure 10.6 Moisture lesions will often present as a 'kissing' lesion (a mirror image). The wound margins are diffused and superficial, with red/pink/white patches associated with maceration (EPUAP 2005)

Source: with kind permission of Elaine Gibson, Tissue Viability Nurse Specialist, East Kent Hospitals NHS Trust. Educational Specialist ConvaTec Ltd.

Part

II

from relatives, carers or from medical/nursing notes. Always ask patients what they know about pressure ulcers.

5   Ensuring privacy by checking curtains and doors are closed and so on. Inspect the patient's skin all over, paying particular attention to areas prone to damage (spine, elbows, buttocks, hips, heels). To ensure dignity, this can be achieved by loosening or removing one item of clothing at a time (e.g. pyjama top then bottom). Any reddened areas will require further inspection (see Skin assessing section below). Your inspection may also require the use of touch to determine whether the area is painful, oedematous or warm to touch – this is particularly relevant if your patient has darkly pigmented skin. Always gain permission prior to this.

6   Remove apron/gloves and wash hands.

7   Document, date and sign findings in the appropriate place, together with dates for review.

8   If using a risk assessment tool, use findings to calculate score and level of risk. If not using a tool, assimilate findings to determine level of risk. Always discuss your findings with your mentor or the nurse in charge.

9   If the patient is found to be at any degree of risk or has evidence of pressure damage, then appropriate care plans and additional assessments/programmes (e.g. mobility, nutrition, pressure ulcer assessment) may need to be generated and implemented.

10   Pressure-relieving equipment may also be required. This information must also be documented and made known to additional members of the healthcare team.

11   Discuss your findings with the patients and their families/carers if appropriate. Information on what they can do to help protect their skin should also be provided; this may include written information (see practice tips below).

Assessing skin for hyperaemic response

Any reddened areas will need to be assessed for a hyperaemic response in the following way:

1   Ask the patient for permission to touch his/her skin.

2   Apply gentle finger pressure to the area for a few seconds.

3   Release your finger and observe colour change over the following few seconds.

Blanching (turning white or pale) indicates a normal circulation. If the skin does not change colour, this may well be indicative of skin damage.

The EPAUP suggest using small transparent pressure disks when assessing skin. These make it easier to observe if the red area blanches or not when pressure is applied.

Whenever skin inspection reveals any potential or actual skin damage, the first course of action is to reposition the patient off the area immediately (Gunnewicht and Dunford, 2004).

t☆
Practice tips

- Opportunities for undertaking skin inspection include when washing, moving or toileting patients (Gunnewicht and Dunford, 2004).
- Anti-emboli stockings must also be removed on a daily basis in order to inspect feet and heels.
- Wheelchair users may use a mirror to assist in skin inspection (NICE, 2003).
- Patient information leaflets are available from RCN and NICE websites or from phone lines.

⚠ Professional alert!

It is vital to update any assessment on a regular basis or when there is any change in the patient's condition. Most assessments are completed within the first few hours of admission, when available information may be limited. Your knowledge of particular patients will increase with time spent with them, so remember to update your assessment using this additional information.

The role of nutrition

Although poor nutrition may not be a direct cause of pressure ulceration, it is possible that impaired nutrition may increase tissue vulnerability to pressure (Mathus-Vliegen, 2001). It is a factor that can be readily influenced and will affect the body's ability to heal established pressure ulcers. Studies have shown that the nutritional status of both hospital and community-based patients is often poor (Strauss and Margolis, 1996).

Patients will require a nutritional assessment including measurement of weight, body mass index (BMI) and nutritional intake. A risk assessment tool such as MUST may be used. If malnutrition is indicated, nutritional intervention will be required. This should be achieved through enhanced normal feeding or if this is not possible by protein/energy-rich oral supplementation: in general, 30–35 kcal per kg body weight per day, with 1–1.5 g/kg/day protein and 1 ml per kcal per day fluid intake (EPUAP, 2003). A similar strategy is required for those patients with established ulcers. However, wounds which have a high exudates level may also have a high protein loss which will require replacing. Protein and calorie supplementation, along with the use of arginine, vitamins and trace elements with anti-oxidants effects appear to have a positive effect on healing (EPUAP, 2003).

Patients will require regular reassessment and adjustments made to the diet accordingly.

> ## Learning activity
>
> What sort of questions would you ask Mrs Smith about her diet to determine whether this could be increasing her susceptibility to pressure ulcers?

Part

II

Mobility and positioning

Immobility is a key factor in determining whether a patient will or will not develop pressure ulcers, so maintaining mobility is of great importance. Patients should be made aware of the importance of keeping mobile and active, and also of the need to avoid introducing shear and friction forces while doing this (e.g. not dragging heels up the bed). For those who are unable to maintain optimal mobility, regular and strict repositioning and a mobility programme will be required. This will need to take place on a regular basis, timed according to the individual patients' skin tolerance. The only reliable method of checking whether the repositioning programme is effective is to inspect the skin for signs of reactive and nonreactive hyperaemia.

> ## ⚠ Professional alert!
>
> Patients are a greater risk of developing pressure ulcers when sitting in chairs, as up to 70 per cent of their body weight is transferred through a relatively small surface area (the buttocks). They also tend to slip forward onto the sacrum. Patients also tend to sit out for long periods of time. In one study, the control group who had their sitting times restricted to less than two hours demonstrated a reduction in pressure ulcers, as well as a reduction in constipation, immobility and chest and urinary tract infections (Gerbhardt and Bliss, 1994).

Using pressure-relieving equipment

The function of pressure-relieving equipment is to increase the time a person is able to sit or lie down without causing tissue damage. There are currently over 8400 different types of pressure-relieving equipment available from 204 different suppliers! (DH, 2005). Some examples in common use are listed below.

Examples of pressure-relieving equipment

- replacement foam mattress
- alternating-pressure overlay system
- alternating-pressure mattress system
- electric-profiling bedframe
- foam cushions
- gel cushions.

Unfortunately, there is currently no conclusive research evidence to indicate which pressure reducing support surfaces are most effective (RCN, 2005). Selection must be made according to individual need and local availability. The RCN guidelines (2005) include a general consensus view that is shown in Table 10.2.

Table 10.2 Pressure-reducing equipment selection criteria

Pressure-reducing equipment selection criteria general consensus view (RCN, 2005) (based on EPUAP Grading classification)	
Grade 1 or 2 pressure ulcers	**Grade 3 or 4 pressure ulcers**
High-specification foam mattress and/ or cushion. *Plus* close observation of skin and repositioning regime.	Alternating-pressure mattress (overlay or mattress replacement) or sophisticated continuous low pressure system (low air loss, air fluidised). First choice should be an AP overlay.

Other factors may also need to be taken into consideration, including patient comfort, weight of the patient (all equipment will have an upper weight limit) and infection control considerations. All staff have a professional duty to understand how equipment works, and therefore instructions should be available and used at all times. Equipment should also be in good working order and not present an infection control risk. If patients require a particular type of equipment while in hospital, then this should also be available for their continued use in the community. It this is not the case, then a suitable substitute may be required. Bariatric equipment for use with patients who exceed normal working weight limits is also available from a number of companies.

Use of pressure-relieving equipment is an active intervention and therefore must be recorded in the patients' notes. Always explain to patients why they require equipment and how the equipment works.

It must be remembered that pressure-relieving equipment is not a substitute for good manual handling and skin care. Over reliance on equipment can prove detrimental (Maylor, 2004).

Skin care

The skin of the very old, very young or ill patients can be highly vulnerable, especially where moisture levels are increased (e.g. incontinence, perspiration, humidity or wound drainage). Incontinence is a major factor in the development of pressure ulcers. Good skin care is of vital importance to maintain skin integrity. Skin should be washed and dried carefully using mild products. Emollients and barrier creams may also be required. Thorough washing should always take place after all episodes of incontinence. The importance of skin care should be fully explained to patients who are able to care for themselves.

(a) Learning activity

What type of equipment would be suitable for Mrs Smith while in hospital? What factors would you take into consideration when deciding on equipment?

⚠ Professional alert!

Persistent moisture can cause erythema, maceration, incontinence, dermatitis and excoriation, which can be mistaken for pressure damage. Tape damage caused by repeated removal of adhesive tape can also be mistaken for pressure ulceration (Evans and Stephen-Haynes, 2007).

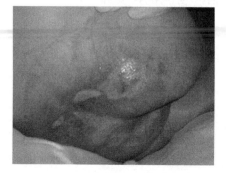

Figure 10.7 A moisture lesion combined with pressure damage

Source: with kind permission of Elaine Gibson, Tissue Viability Nurse Specialist, East Kent Hospitals NHS Trust. Educational Specialist ConvaTec Ltd.

Pressure ulcer grading

All too often, pressure ulcers do occur. It is important to recognise them at the earliest opportunity and to instigate a management plan. Hopefully this will also prevent further ulcers from developing. A number of pressure ulcer grading tools are available to help identify the extent of damage. The four-stage classification system developed by the European Pressure Ulcer Advisory Panel (EPUAP, 1998) is currently recommended by NICE (2005). This grading system is illustrated in Table 10.3.

Table 10.3 EPUAP pressure ulcer grading system

Grade 1	Non-blanchable erythema of intact skin. Discolouration of the skin, warmth, oedema, induration or hardness may also be used as indicators, particularly on individuals with darker skin.
Grade 2	Partial-thickness skin loss involving epidermis, dermis, or both. The ulcer is superficial and presents clinically as an abrasion or blister.
Grade 3	Full-thickness skin loss involving damage to or necrosis of subcutaneous tissue that may extend down to, but not through underlying fascia.
Grade 4	Extensive destruction, tissue necrosis, or damage to muscle, bone, or supporting structures with or without full thickness skin loss.

Part II

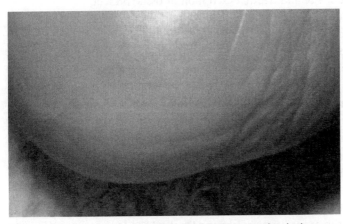

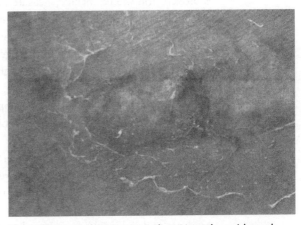

Figure 10.8 Grade 1 pressure ulcer: the heel remained red when touched lightly with a finger; more importantly the patient was complaining that his heel was sore

Source: with kind permission of Elaine Gibson, Tissue Viability Nurse Specialist, East Kent Hospitals NHS Trust. Educational Specialist ConvaTec Ltd.

Figure 10.9 Grade 2 pressure ulcer. Note the epidermal skin loss

Source: with kind permission of Elaine Gibson, Tissue Viability Nurse Specialist, East Kent Hospitals NHS Trust. Educational Specialist ConvaTec Ltd.

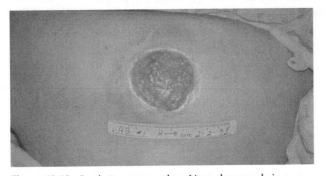

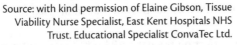

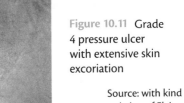

Figure 10.10 Grade 3 pressure ulcer. Note the muscle is exposed. Protecting the wound from trauma and infection by covering with an appropriate dressing is important.

Source: with kind permission of Elaine Gibson, Tissue Viability Nurse Specialist, East Kent Hospitals NHS Trust. Educational Specialist ConvaTec Ltd.

Figure 10.11 Grade 4 pressure ulcer with extensive skin excoriation

Source: with kind permission of Elaine Gibson, Tissue Viability Nurse Specialist, East Kent Hospitals NHS Trust. Educational Specialist ConvaTec Ltd.

Pressure ulcer grading is only appropriate for defining the maximum depth of tissue involved. It cannot be used in reverse order to describe wound healing (Defloor et al, 2006); for instance, a Grade 4 pressure ulcer cannot be termed a Grade 3 or 2 pressure ulcer as it heals. It should be referred to a Grade 4 pressure ulcer which is healing.

Full-thickness pressure ulcers (Grade 4) heal by replacing the same structural layers of body tissue they have lost with scar tissue. They tend to heal like a purse string, in that they heal from the wound margins and from the bottom up. They do not replace all the lost muscle, subcutaneous fat and dermis before they re-epithelialise (Leaper and Gottrup, 1998). This also means that the replacement tissue will always be vulnerable to breakdown in the future. Unfortunately deep tissue damage can sometimes occur beneath intact skin, which can be difficult to diagnose (Donnelly, 2005).

Learning activity

If you wish to develop your pressure ulcer grading skills, the EPUAP has an online quiz to help you. This can be accessed on www.epuap.org/puclas/index.html. You will be asked to look at a number of pressure ulcers and grade them according to their depth. This is a very worthwhile activity.

Wound management

A thorough wound assessment will need to be undertaken for any pressure ulcers where skin is broken. This should include measurement of size and depth, description of tissue present (e.g. slough, necrosis), odour and amount of exudate. The use of photography or wound tracings is recommended in order to measure size and evidence of healing.

The basic principles of wound management will need to be applied to the pressure ulcer. This will include appropriate and thorough wound cleansing and application of an appropriate dressing.

The optimum wound-healing environment should be created by using modern dressings such as hydrocolloids, hydrogels, hydrofibres, foams, films, alginates or soft silicones (RCN, 2005).

Dressings will be required for both protection, debridement of slough or necrotic tissue, and for exudate and odour control (Wickes, 2007)

Pressure ulcers commonly occur over the sacrum and heels which, due to the proximity to the anus and narrowness of the heel, makes them difficult areas to dress. The use of adhesive products or dressings cut to shape will make this easier (Gunnewicht and Dunford, 2004).

Pressure ulcers can also cause significant pain, which is often overlooked; this can result in increased anxiety and disturbed sleep. Pain should always be appropriately assessed and managed. Wound dressing change has been identified as the time of maximum pain (EWMA, 2005).

Having a pressure ulcer can have a negative effect on the patient's body image, and people with pressure ulcers can feel that they are losing their independence and dignity (Langemo et al, 2000). This needs to be acknowledged and the patient listened to and involved in as much as the care routine as is possible. Careful dressing selection can assist in eradicating leakage and odour.

Conclusion

There are few areas of healthcare where patients will not be at risk of pressure ulcers, and with increasing life expectancy the rate of occurrence is likely to rise. It must be remembered, however, that pressure ulcers are not bound to happen, even if the patient is assessed as being at high risk. As healthcare professionals, it is essential that we learn and take great care in our assessment and management skills. Learning the art of skin inspection and good skin care is important and worthy of your time. With so many international, national and local guidelines available, we all need be responsible in ensuring that both knowledge and practice is competent and up to date.

References

Bennett, G., Dealey, C. and Posnett, J. (2004) 'The cost of pressure ulcers in the UK', *Age Ageing* 33, 230–5.

Bergstrom, N., Braden, B., Laguzza, A. and Holman, V. (1987) 'The Braden scale for predicting pressure sores', *Journal of American Geriatrics Society* **38**(7), 748–52.

Bryant, R. A. (2000) 'Appendix B, Risk assessment scales', pp. 516–19 in Bryant, R. and Nix, D. (eds), *Acute And Chronic Wounds*, St Louis, Mosby.

Clark, M. (2007) 'Pressure ulcers', pp. 8–22 in *Skin Breakdown: The silent epidemic*, Hull, Smith & Nephew Foundation Publication.

Clark, M., Bours, G. and Defloor, T. (2004) 'A pilot study of the prevalence of pressure ulcers in European hospitals', in Clark, M. (ed.), *Pressure Ulcers: Recent advances in tissue viability*, Salisbury, Quay Books.

Defloor, T., Schoonhoven, L., Katrien, V. ,Westrate, J. and Myny, D. (2006) 'Reliability of the European Pressure Ulcer Advisory Panel Classification System', *Journal of Advanced Nursing* **54**(2), 189–98.

Department of Health (DH) (2005) *Arrangements for the Provision of Dressings, Incontinence Appliances, Stoma Appliances, Chemical Reagents and Other Appliances to Primary and Secondary Care*, London, DH.

Donnelly, J. (2005) 'Should we include deep tissue injury in pressure ulcer staging systems? The NPUAP debate', *Journal of Tissue Viability* 14, 5.

EPUAP (2009) *Pressure Ulcer Grading E-Learning and Self-Test* [online] www.puclas.urgent.be (accessed 9 February 2009).

Evans, J. and Stephen-Haynes, J. (2007) 'Identification of superficial pressure ulcers', *Journal of Wound Care* **16**(2), 54–6.

European Wound Management Association (EWMA) (2005) *Pain at Wound Dressing Changes: Position statement*, London, Medical Education Partnership Ltd (available from their website at www. Ewma.org).

European Pressure Ulcer Advisory Panel (EPUAP) (1998) *Pressure Ulcer Prevention and Treatment Guidelines*, Oxford, EPUAP.

EPUAP (2003) *Nutritional Guidelines for Pressure Ulcer Prevention and Treatment*, Oxford, EPUAP.

Gerbhardt, K. and Bliss, M. (1994) 'Prevention of pressure sores in orthopaedic patients: is prolonged chair sitting detrimental?' *Journal of Tissue Viability* **4**(2), 51–4.

Gunnewicht, B. and Dunford, C. (2004) *Fundamental Aspects of Tissue Viability*, Salisbury, Quay Books.

Halfens, R. (2000) 'Risk assessment scales for pressure ulcers: a theoretical, methodological and clinical perspective', *Ostomy Wound Management* **46**(8), 36–44.

Kelly, J. (1994) 'The aetiology of pressure sores', *Journal of Tissue Viability* **4**(3), 77–8.

Langemo, D.K., Melland H., Hanson, D., Olsen B. and Hunter S. (2000) 'The lived experience of having a pressure ulcer: a qualitative analysis', *Advances in Skin and Wound Care* 13, 225–35.

Leaper, D. J. and Gottrup, F. (1998) 'Surgical wounds', pp. 23–39 in Leaper, D. J. and Harding, K. G. (eds), *Wound Biology and Management*, Oxford, Oxford University Press.

Mathus-Vliegen, E. (2001) 'Nutritional status, nutrition and pressure ulcers', *Nutrition in Clinical Practice* 16, 286–91.

Maylor, M. (2004) 'Debating the relative unimportance of pressure-reducing equipment', pp. 59–64 in Clark, M. (ed.), *Pressure Ulcers: Recent advances in tissue viability*, Salisbury, Quay Books.

McDonaugh, S. M. (2008) 'Moisture lesion or pressure ulcer? A review of the literature', *Journal of Wound Care* 17(11), 4614, 466.

National Institute for Clinical Excellence (NICE) (2003) *Pressure Ulcer Risk Assessment and Prevention*, Clinical Guideline 7, London, NICE.

NICE (2005) *How to Put NICE Guidelines into Practice: A guide to implementation for organisations*, London, NICE.

Norton, D., McLaren, R. and Exton-Smith, A. N. (1962) *An Investigation of Geriatric Nursing Problems in Hospital*, Edinburgh, Churchill Livingston.

Posnett, J. and Franks, P.J. (2007) 'The cost of skin breakdown and ulceration in the UK', pp. 6–12 in *Skin Breakdown: The silent epidemic*, Hull, Smith & Nephew Foundation Publication.

Royal College of Nursing (RCN) (2005) *The Management of Pressure Ulcers in Primary and Secondary Care: A clinical practice guideline*, London, RCN.

Strauss, E. and Margolis, D. (1996) 'Malnutrition in patients with pressure ulcers: morbidity, mortality and clinically practical assessments', *Advances in Wound Care* **9**(5), 37–40.

Torrance, C. and Maylor, M. (1999) 'Pressure ulcer survey: part one', *Journal of Wound Care* **8**(1), 27–30.

Versluysen, M. (1985) 'Pressure ulcers in elderly patients: the epidemiology related to hip operations', *Journal of Bone and Joint Surgery* 67B, 10–13.

Waterlow, J. (1988) 'The Waterlow score for the prevention and management of pressure sores: towards a pocket policy', *Care Science and Practice* **6**(1), 8–12.

Wickes, G. (2007) 'A guide to the treatment of pressure ulcers from Grade 1–Grade 4', *Wound Essentials* 2, 106–13.

Chapter

11

Eye care

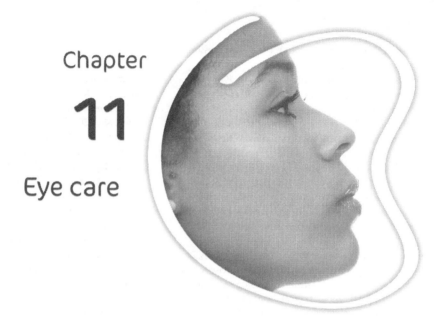

Sara Raftery, Colleen O' Neill
and Mary Clynes

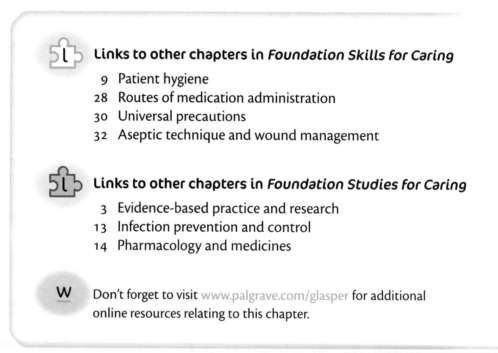

Links to other chapters in *Foundation Skills for Caring*

9 Patient hygiene
28 Routes of medication administration
30 Universal precautions
32 Aseptic technique and wound management

Links to other chapters in *Foundation Studies for Caring*

3 Evidence-based practice and research
13 Infection prevention and control
14 Pharmacology and medicines

W Don't forget to visit www.palgrave.com/glasper for additional
online resources relating to this chapter.

Introduction

This chapter aims to give you knowledge and understanding of the skills required to provide safe and effective eye care. Eye care involves a number of skills, including eye cleansing, eye irrigation, and the installation of eye drops and ointments. Under normal circumstances individuals can attend to their own eye care needs, but in certain situations assistance will be required. Assistance is needed in patients who are very ill or unconscious, postoperative patients, and patients who are unable to attend to their own needs due to a physical weakness or disability. Eye care is a fundamental aspect of care as lack of attention to the eye, or poor eye care, can lead to cross-infection and may damage the eye, sometimes irreversibly.

Learning outcomes

This chapter will enable you to:

- discuss the aims of providing eye care to a patient
- discuss the rationale for providing eye care to a patient
- describe the equipment required to carry out eye care
- prepare the patient for eye care

- describe how to carry out the following procedures:
  - eye cleansing
  - eye irrigation
  - installation of eye drops
  - installation of eye ointment.

Part

II

Core concepts

- Communication
- Infection control
- Universal precautions
- Record keeping
- Medication management
- Patient dignity
- Privacy

a Learning activity

Use the library and the internet to find a diagram of the eye. Identify the key structures relevant to the skills discussed in this chapter, eye irrigation and the installation of eye drops.

Looking in a mirror, identify these structures on your own eye.

Purpose of eye care

The aim of eye care is to:

- detect quickly any irritation, damage or disease of the eye and surrounding area
- prevent injury to the eye and surrounding area
- prevent eye infections
- treat eye infections
- prevent corneal damage in the unconscious patient
- relieve discomfort
- irrigate the eye to remove caustic substances from it.

a Learning activity

In order to understand fully the skills discussed in this chapter, research the following: the conjunctiva and the cornea.

Patients who may require eye care are:

- patients who are unable to attend to eye care themselves, e.g.:
  - those with physical inability or weakness
  - severely ill patients
  - postoperative patients
  - unconscious patients (Joyce and Evans, 2006)
- patients with eye infections or eye diseases who require the instillation of eye drops or eye ointments
- patients who have spillage of caustic substances into the eye (e.g. domestic cleaning agents) and require eye irrigation.

⚠ Professional alert!

For general eye care, a clean technique can be used. However, following eye surgery and in cases where there is damage to the eye, it is necessary to use aseptic technique when carrying out eye care (Dougherty and Lister, 2004).

S Scenario: emergency admission

James, a 37-year-old man, has splashed some cleaning fluid in his eye. He presents to the emergency department with pain and redness of the eye. He is quite anxious due to the discomfort and fear that his sight will be affected.

a Learning activities

- Reflect on the scenario above and imagine how James must be feeling.
- Think about what procedure will be required to remove any cleaning fluid remaining in his eye.
- Identify the equipment you will need for this procedure.
- How could you use your communication skills to reduce James's anxiety and reassure him?

General equipment required for eye care

You will need to collect the following:

- trolley or tray with:
  - sterile eye dressing pack
  - gallipot
  - non-shedding gauze swabs
- disposable waterproof towel
- cleansing solution
- 0.9 per cent sodium chloride (or other as advised)
- receiver for soiled gauze swabs.

t☆ Practice tip

Always ensure that there is a good source of light available when carrying out eye care. This will ensure that a thorough examination of the eye and surrounding structures can take place during the procedure. All findings should be clearly documented in the nursing notes.

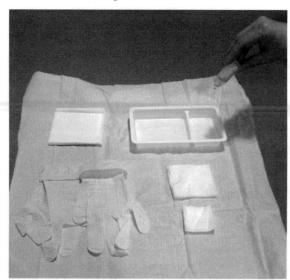

Figure 11.1 Equipment for eye care

Eye cleansing

Procedure for eye cleansing

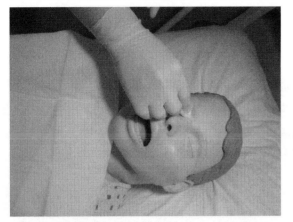

Figure 11.2 Swabbing the eye lid

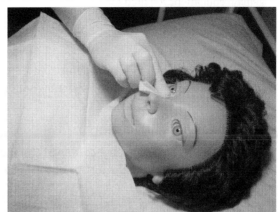

Figure 11.3 Swabbing the eye

1 Collect and prepare the necessary equipment so that you can carry out the procedure without unnecessary stoppages.

2 Ensure the patient's privacy to promote dignity.

3 Explain the procedure carefully to the patient to gain consent and cooperation and minimise anxiety.

4 Position the patient in a reclined position, ideally lying in bed with the head resting on pillows to maintain comfort and to ensure ease of access to the eyes.

5 Wash hands thoroughly using bactericidal handwash, and dry them to reduce the risk of cross-infection.

6 Open and prepare the required equipment.

7 Place disposable towel under the patient's head and around the neck in case of spillages.

8 Ask the patient to keep the eyes closed while the eyelids are cleansed to reduce any risk of corneal abrasion.

9 Moisten a non-shedding gauze swab with cleansing solution and clean the eyelid from the inner aspect to the outer aspect. Use each swab only once to reduce the risk of cross-infection. Repeat the procedure until all discharge has been eliminated.

10 Next, ask the patient to look up and swab the lower eyelid from inner aspect to outer aspect, using each swab once to reduce the risk of cross-infection. Repeat the procedure until all discharge has been eliminated.

11 Take care that the swab does not touch the cornea of the eye as this can cause damage.

12 Dry the eyelid carefully to remove moisture.

13 Ensure the patient is repositioned in the desired manner on completion of the procedure to promote comfort.

14 Remove and dispose of equipment to ensure safety.

15 Wash hands to reduce the risk of cross-infection.

16 Document the procedure in the nursing notes and report any findings to ensure a written record of nursing practice is maintained.

⚠ Professional alert!

- Eye care is only required when necessary (e.g. when there is discharge present) (Stollery, Shaw and Lee, 2005).
- When carrying out eye care, always treat the less affected eye first to minimise the risk of cross-infection.

t☆ Practice tips

- When cleansing the eye, always swab from the inner aspect (nasal corner) to the outer aspect of the eye. This ensures that discharge is swabbed away from the lacrimal apparatus and from the other eye, thus reducing the risk of cross-infection.
- If there is discharge which is difficult to cleanse, it may be useful to lay a wet swab over the eye for a short period to soften it (Stollery et al, 2005).

Eye irrigation

Equipment required for eye irrigation:

- general equipment required for eye care
- sterile 0.9 per cent sodium chloride or sterile water
- towel
- sterile receiver for irrigating fluid
- warm water (in a bowl) to heat irrigating fluid
- irrigating apparatus (irrigating flask or intravenous giving set).

Rationale for eye irrigation

Eye irrigation is required to remove corrosive substances that have spilled into the eye. It involves irrigating the surface of the eye with copious fluid to aid removal of the substance from the eye.

Procedure for eye irrigation

1 Collect and prepare the necessary equipment so that you can carry out the procedure without unnecessary stoppages.

2 Ensure the patient's privacy to promote dignity.

3 Explain the procedure carefully to the patient to gain consent and cooperation and minimise anxiety.

4 Warm the irrigation fluid to body temperature to ensure the fluid is comfortable for the patient when poured over the eye.

5 Position the patient in a well-reclined position, ideally lying in bed with the head resting on pillows to maintain comfort and to ensure ease of access to the eyes.

6 Incline the head to the side which requires eye irrigation, to avoid the irrigation solution or corrosive substance running down the face or into the other eye.

7 Wash hands thoroughly using bactericidal handwash, and dry hands to reduce the risk of cross-infection.

8 Open and prepare the required equipment.

9 Place disposable waterproof towel under the patient's head and around the neck in case of spillages.

10 If there is any discharge from the eye, clean the area using the procedure for eye cleansing.

11 Position the receiver below the affected eye and against the patient's cheek to collect the irrigation fluid as it drains.

12 Inform the patient that the eye will be gently held open as they will be unable to keep it open when the fluid is poured in.

13 Prepare the patient for the procedure by telling them when the irrigation fluid is about to be poured into the eye.

14 Pour a little irrigation fluid onto the patient's cheek initially so that they are familiar with the temperature and are comfortable with it.

15 Hold the irrigation apparatus above the eye, making sure it does not touch the eye, and direct the irrigation flow from the inner to the outer aspect of the eye to wash the corrosive substance away from the lacrimal apparatus and the other eye.

16 While maintaining a constant flow of irrigation fluid, ask the patient to look upwards, downwards, right and left to ensure the entire eye surface is irrigated.

17 Upon completion remove the receiver and dry the eyelids using dry, sterile, non-shedding gauze. Dry the patient's cheek and face using the towel to ensure patient comfort.

18 Reposition the patient in the chosen position of comfort.

19 Remove and dispose of equipment to ensure safety.

20 Wash hands to reduce the risk of cross-infection.

21 Document the procedure in the nursing notes and report any findings to ensure a written record of nursing practice is maintained.

⚠ Professional alert!

In some cases the patient will be prescribed anaesthetic eye drops prior to eye irrigation to minimise discomfort. If anaesthetic drops are required, instil these using the procedure for the instillation of eye drops (see below) and monitor their effectiveness prior to commencing the irrigation procedure.

a Learning activity

What is the function of the following structures surrounding the eye?
- eyelid
- eyebrow
- eyelashes.

Eye drops

Eye drops must be sterile. They are available in single-use applicators and multiple-application containers. When used in the home, multiple-application containers should be discarded after four weeks even if still partly full. When they are used in hospital wards, it is best practice to discard the bottle after one week (BNF, 2006). Each patient should have their own separate bottle which is labelled with the patient's name. If there are particular concerns regarding contamination, individual bottles should be used for each eye. When a patient has eye surgery, new bottles should be commenced postoperatively.

Eye drops frequently contain preservatives. There is an increased risk of contamination of eye drops in preservative-free solutions and when the eye is accidentally touched by the applicator during the installation of eye drops (Rahman, Tejwani and Wilson, 2006).

Eye drops must be stored according to manufacturer's instructions. Many products require refrigeration.

Equipment required for the installation of eye drops
- general equipment required for eye care
- prescribed eye drops.

> ### Practice tip
> If long-term eye medication is prescribed, it is important to promote independence by teaching the patient or carer to administer the prescribed drug (Holman, Roberts and Nicol, 2005).

Rationale for the installation of eye drops

Eye drops are liquid drug preparations which are introduced to the eye. They may be prescribed for a variety of reasons:
- Local anaesthetic eye drops can be used to alleviate discomfort following an eye injury or may be administered prior to procedures such as:
  - eye irrigation
  - removal of a foreign body from the eye
  - minor eye surgery
  - tonometry (measuring the pressure within the eye).
- Antibiotic eye drops may be prescribed to treat eye infections.
- Anti-inflammatory eye drops may be prescribed to treat inflammatory conditions of the eye.
- Eye muscle constrictors or dilators may be prescribed.
- Artificial tears may be prescribed to lubricate the eye when a patient has dry eyes.

Procedure for the installation of eye drops

1 Collect and prepare the necessary equipment so that you can complete the procedure without unnecessary stoppages.
2 Explain the procedure carefully to the patient to gain consent and cooperation and minimise anxiety.
3 Check the eye drops against the prescription to ensure:
   - The prescription is for the correct patient.
   - The prescription is fully completed and signed by a doctor.
   - The drug is correct.
   - The dose is correct.
   - The time the drug is to be administered is correct.
   - The drug has not expired.
   - The route for the drug administration is correct.
   - The eye to which the drug is to be instilled is correct.
   - The patient is not allergic to the drug.

   This will ensure that the medication is administered safely and accurately.

Part

II

4   Position the patient with the head tipped back and supported to maintain comfort and to ensure ease of access to the eyes.

5   Wash hands thoroughly using bactericidal handwash, and dry hands to reduce the risk of cross-infection.

6   If there is any exudate in the eye, cleanse the eye using the procedure for eye cleansing.

7   Gently shake the eye drop container to ensure even distribution of the drug (Stollery et al, 2005).

8   Taking care not to touch the cornea, use a non-shedding gauze swab to gently pull the lower eyelid downwards. The swab will absorb excess eye drops.

9   Ask the patient to look up and evert the lower eyelid to ensure correct placement of the eye drops on the conjunctiva and not on the cornea, which would cause the patient to blink.

10 Taking care not to touch the eye, hold the dropper just above the eye and place one drop into the lower conjunctiva.

11 Ask the patient to close the eye gently for approximately one minute to ensure the drug is absorbed (Stollery et al, 2005).

12 Wipe away any excess solution with the gauze to prevent discomfort and potential eye irritation.

13 Reposition the patient in the chosen position of comfort.

14 Remove and dispose of equipment to ensure safety.

15 Wash hands to reduce the risk of cross-infection.

16 Complete the drug prescription document to ensure accurate records of drug administration are maintained.

17 Continue to monitor the patient for effects and side effects of the prescribed drug.

> ### t ☆
> ### Practice tips
>
> If the patient is prescribed more than one eye drop preparation, leave approximately five minutes between each drug. This will prevent dilution and overflow which can occur if one drug immediately follows the other (BNF, 2006).
>
> Where an eye drop and eye ointment are both to be instilled, the eye drop should be administered first, as ointments are greasy and inhibit the absorption of the eye drop (Jamieson, McCall and Whyte, 2002).

Eye ointment

Equipment required for the installation of eye ointment:
* general equipment required for eye care
* prescribed eye ointment.

Rationale for the installation of eye ointment

Eye ointments are drug preparations which are introduced to the eye. They may be prescribed for a variety of reasons:
* Where a prolonged drug action is desired, eye ointments can be preferable to eye drops.
* Antibiotic eye ointments may be prescribed to treat eye infections.
* Eye ointments can provide a protective layer for the cornea.
* Eye ointments can offer relief if the eye or eyelid is inflamed.

Procedure for the installation of eye ointments

1   Collect and prepare the necessary equipment so that you can complete the procedure without unnecessary stoppages.

2   Explain the procedure carefully to the patient to gain consent and cooperation and minimise anxiety.

3   Check the eye ointment against the prescription to ensure:
   * The prescription is for the correct patient.
   * The prescription is fully completed and signed by a doctor.
   * The drug is correct.
   * The dose is correct.

- The time the drug is to be administered is correct.
- The drug has not expired.
- The route for the drug administration is correct.
- The eye to which the drug is to be instilled is correct.
- The patient is not allergic to the drug.

This will ensure that the medication is administered safely and accurately.

4   Position the patient with the head tipped back and supported to maintain comfort and to ensure ease of access to the eyes.

5   Wash hands thoroughly using bactericidal handwash, and dry hands to reduce the risk of cross-infection.

6   If there is any residual ointment or exudate in the eye, cleanse the eye using the procedure for eye cleansing.

7   Taking care not to touch the cornea, use a non-shedding gauze swab to gently pull the lower eyelid downwards.

8   Ask the patient to look up and evert the lower eyelid to ensure correct placement of the eye ointment.

9   Taking care not to touch the eye, hold the applicator just above the eye and deliver a line of ointment along the lower conjunctiva from the nasal corner in an outward direction.

10   Ask the patient to gently close the eye to distribute the ointment across the eye.

11   Wipe away any excess ointment with the gauze to avoid irritation to the peri-orbital skin.

12   To minimise any anxiety, inform the patient that there may be slight blurring of vision for a short period.

13   Reposition the patient in the chosen position of comfort.

14   Remove and dispose of equipment to ensure safety.

15   Wash hands to reduce the risk of cross-infection.

16   Complete the drug prescription document to ensure accurate records of drug administration are maintained.

17   Continue to monitor the patient for effects and side effects of the prescribed drug.

Conclusion

Eye care is an essential part of general care to ensure the patient's comfort. In certain circumstances eye care and treatments to the eye are performed when there is damage or infection in the eye. It is important that the healthcare professional has the skill to perform these competently and confidently to meet the patient's needs and to avoid further damage or discomfort.

References

British National Formulary (BNF) (2006) *BNF 52*, London, BMJ Publishing.

Dougherty, L. and Lister, S. (2004) *The Royal Marsden Hospital Manual of Clinical Nursing Procedures*, 6th edn, Oxford, Blackwell.

Holman, C., Roberts, S. and Nicol, M. (2005) 'Promoting healthy sight and eye care', *Nursing Older People* 17(1), 37–8.

Jamieson, E. M., McCall, J. M. and Whyte, L. A. (2002) *Clinical Nursing Practices*, 4th edn, Edinburgh, Churchill Livingstone.

Joyce, N. and Evans, D. (2006) 'Best practice: eye care for patients in the ICU', *American Journal of Nursing* 106(1), 72AA-72DD.

Stollery, R., Shaw, M. and Lee, A. (2005) *Opthalmic Nursing*, 3rd edn, Oxford, Blackwell.

Rahman, M. Q., Tejwani, D. and Wilson, J. A. (2006) 'Microbial contamination of preservative free eye drops in multiple application containers', *British Journal of Ophthalmology* 90(2), 139–41.

Part

II

Chapter

12

Mouth care

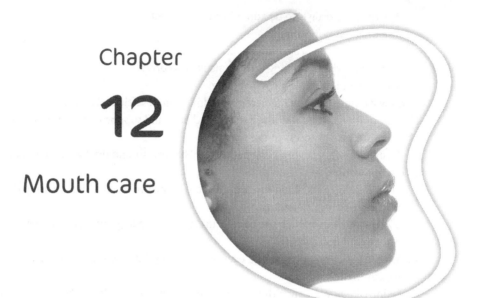

Mary Clynes

 Links to other chapters in *Foundation Skills for Caring*

 Links to other chapters in *Foundation Studies for Caring*

W Don't forget to visit www.palgrave.com/glasper for additional online resources relating to this chapter.

Introduction

Mouth care or oral hygiene is the provision of appropriate care to ensure that the tissues and structure of the mouth are in a healthy state. The condition of the mouth is not only an indicator of oral health but also of general health, and is a quality-of-life indicator (World Health Organisation, 2006). It can affect the patient's quality of life by interfering with eating and drinking and ability to talk with ease (Holman, Roberts and Nicol, 2005). A fundamental aspect of nursing is mouth care. A clean, fresh mouth promotes patient well-being and comfort. Mouth care involves oral assessment, appropriate mouth care, and evaluation and documentation of care. Oral assessment is necessary to ensure appropriate care implementation (Gilliam and Gilliam, 2006). Effective mouth care prevents potential infection, both oral and systematic, distress and discomfort to the patient (Xavier, 2000).

Learning outcomes

This chapter will enable you to:

- discuss the aims of mouth care
- discuss the rationale for providing mouth care
- describe the equipment required for mouth care
- describe how to carry out mouth care, with evidence-based reasons
- discuss the different type of cleaning aids and solutions used to provide mouth care.

Concepts

- Communication
- Infection control
- Universal precautions
- Assessment
- Evaluation
- Patient dignity and privacy
- Patient well-being
- Record keeping

Purpose of mouth care

The aim of mouth care is to:
- Prevent the build up of food and plaque on teeth and gums, thus preventing dental caries. Dental plaque is the accumulation of food particles, mucous and bacteria on teeth (Berry and Davidson, 2006).
- Prevent infection due to the build of bacteria in dental plaque. Aspiration of bacteria colonised from the oropharyngeal cavity can lead to the development of ventilator-assisted pneumonia (VAP), so mouth care is important is reducing the risk of VAP (Powers, 2006).
- Keep the mucosa clean, moist and intact.
- Keep the lips moist, smooth and pink, thereby preventing chapping of lips.
- Alleviate discomfort and promote well-being by refreshing the mouth.
- Prevent halitosis (bad breath).
- Maintain oral function.

S   Scenario: mouth care in a stroke victim

The following scenario introduces you to Anne, a 65-year-old lady who recently had a stroke. She has limited movement on the right side of her body. This is particularly distressing for her as she is right handed and she cannot do things for herself, including her own mouth care. She wears upper dentures and feels very self-conscious when these are removed. In addition to depending on healthcare professionals to look after her mouth care, Anne also finds since her stroke that some food particles remain in her mouth after eating and she is afraid she will develop halitosis.

Patients who may require mouth care

- patients who are taking reduced intake of fluids and nutrients, or who have not eaten or drunk for a period of time
- ventilated or sedated patients in intensive care units
- patients undergoing chemotherapy
- patients undergoing radiotherapy to the head or neck region
- patients on oxygen therapy
- elderly patients
- patients who are taking immunosuppressive medications.

⚠ Professional alert!

Before major surgery or any procedure with a risk of oral infection, an oral assessment should be carried out and infected gums or teeth treated (Greenstein, 2004).

Equipment

- clean tray
- plastic beaker
- bowl/receiver/kidney dish
- small-headed soft toothbrush
- toothpaste
- spatula
- pencil torch
- tissues
- denture cleaner
- piece of gauze to remove dentures
- container for dentures, with label
- clinical waste bag
- disposable gloves (non-sterile)
- apron
- lubricant for lips
- protective sheet or towel
- mouthwash if appropriate
- foam swabs if appropriate
- suction device if appropriate
- medication if prescribed, e.g. an antifungal agent if the patient has oral thrush (candida albicans).

A sterile mouth care pack may be used when intensive mouth care is needed for patients for whom tooth-brushing and mouthwashes are inappropriate (Jamieson, McCall and White, 2002).

⚠ Professional alert!

Toothpaste reduces the bacterial contamination of toothbrushes (Efstratiou et al, 2007).

Toothbrushes should be changed at least every three months or when there are signs of wearing of the bristles (Holman, Roberts and Nicol, 2005).

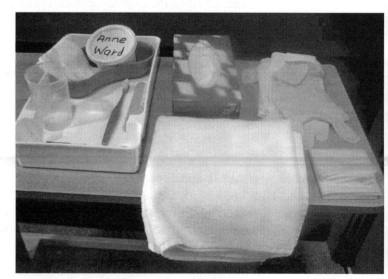

Figure 12.1 Equipment for mouth care

Procedure

1 Collect and prepare the equipment so that you can carry out the procedure smoothly and without unnecessary stoppages.

2 Wash hands and put on gloves and apron to prevent contamination with body fluids (saliva) and reduce the risk of cross-infection.

3 Explain the procedure to the patient in order to gain consent and cooperation.

4 Pull curtains around bed to ensure privacy. Mouth care is an invasive procedure and a potentially embarrassing interaction.

5 Ensure the patient is in a comfortable position, either in bed or sitting on a chair with a bowl in front of him/her.

6 If patient is unconscious, position on his or her side. Remove pillow and lower head of bed if possible, and support head. This ensures that secretions or mouthwash are drained out of the mouth by gravity and not aspirated into lungs. If it is not possible to lower the patient's head, keeping it to one side will allow fluid to flow out or pool in the side of the mouth where it can be suctioned away (Kozier et al, 2004). It is therefore necessary to have an oral suction device at hand to remove excess fluids that may pool in the side of the mouth.

7 Place towel or protective cover over patient's chest to protect clothes.

8 If the patient is unconscious, cover the bed with a waterproof cover and towel. Dentures of unconscious patients should be removed as they cause airway obstructions (Nicol et al, 2000).

9 If necessary ask or assist the patient to remove dentures so as to gain access to the oral cavity and view the area. It is important to involve the patient as much as possible in care in order to promote individualised care and independence. If the patient cannot remove the dentures, grasp the upper plate of the denture using a tissue or gauze piece at the front teeth with thumb and finger and move it up and down slightly to break the suction that holds the plate on the roof of the mouth. The lower plate can be removed by turning it so that one side is slightly lower than the other, thus ensuring that the lips are not stretched (Kozier et al, 2004).

10 The condition of the dentures should be observed, noting any stained, cracked or warped areas. Remember that the patient may be self-conscious when dentures are removed, so ensure privacy and be sensitive to the patient's needs.

11 Carry out an assessment of the patient's mouth and tongue, using a spatula and torch. The spatula helps to reveal areas hidden by the tongue. An assessment of the

mouth provides baseline data, monitors the effectiveness of treatment and identifies problems as they arise so that early intervention can occur. The use of an oral assessment tool is recommended to provide an accurate and comprehensive assessment of the condition of the oral cavity.

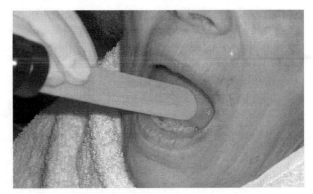

Figure 12.2 Mouth assessment

12 The assessment should involve checking the mouth for:
   • Inflammation and bleeding of the gums (gingivitis).
   • Ulcers and any white or yellow areas of the mouth and tongue indicating oral thrush (candida albicans). Antibiotics may affect the normal fora in the mouth, allowing the growth of harmful microbes such as candida (Adams, 1996).
   • Dental decay.
   • A white coating on the anterior tongue (furred tongue) and dry mucous membranes which indicate dehydration (Holman et al, 2005). The mucous membranes of the mouth should be pink and moist.
   • Quantity and consistency of saliva. The production of saliva can be reduced for a number of reasons. Many drugs (e.g. morphine, antidepressants, diuretics) can cause reduced saliva production (xerostomia), as can radiotherapy of head and neck which can damage the salivary glands. Anxiety and mouth breathing can also cause a dry mouth.
   • Halitosis.
   • Cracked, dry, ulcerated or bleeding lips.
   You also need to establish whether the patient has difficulty with chewing, swallowing or speaking.

13 Give the toothbrush to the patient or brush the patient's teeth using a small soft toothbrush and toothpaste. This removes adherent particles from teeth, tongue and gums. Moisten the toothbrush before applying a small amount of paste. Tilt the head of the brush against the teeth at a 45° angle so that the bristle tips are against the gumline and penetrate the gingival sulcus. Then move the brush back and forward using a vibrating motion from the

sulcus to the crowns. Repeat until the outer and inner surfaces of the teeth and sulci of the gums are cleaned. The biting surfaces are cleaned by moving the brush back and forth over them using short strokes (Kozier et al, 2004). Brush teeth carefully to avoid injury to gums and oral mucosa. Brushing should last three to four minutes (Garcia, 2004). The patient's own toothpaste and toothbrush may be used if available. The toothbrush is regarded as the best tool to remove dental plaque. Foam sticks are considered ineffective at removing debris and plaque from teeth and gums (Pearson and Hutton, 2002). They can be used to rinse or refresh the mouth and thus provide comfort.

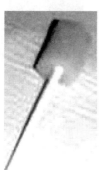

Figure 12.3 Example of a foam stick which can be used to rinse or refresh the mouth

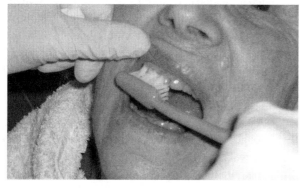

Figure 12.4 Tooth cleaning

14 Furring of the tongue can be removed by brushing the tongue with a soft toothbrush and toothpaste (Nazarko, 2006). This should be done gently to preventing gagging and subsequent vomiting.

15 Offer the patient a beaker of water and encourage vigorous rinsing of the mouth to remove debris and toothpaste from the mouth. Toothpaste remaining in mouth can have a drying effect on the mucosa (Beck, 2004). Explain to the patient that mouthwash should not be swallowed. If the patient is unconscious, place a curved dish such as a kidney dish against chin and lower cheek so that fluid can easily flow into it (Kozier et al 2004).

16 Floss teeth once a day to remove plaque and food particles from between teeth and under gumline (Clay, 2000).

17 Clean the dentures on all surfaces with a toothbrush and denture cleaning agent to remove food particles and plaque. Rinse well to remove traces of cleaning agent. Return them to the patient or place them in a container of water to ensure that they do not lose their shape by drying out. Ensure that the container is labelled with the patient's name and hospital identification number to prevent mix-ups.

18 Apply petroleum jelly to dried, cracked or ulcerated lips. This acts as an occlusive barrier which retains moisture (Gibson and Stone, 2004). Do not use petroleum jelly if the patient is receiving oxygen therapy because it may cause burns to the skin and mouth (Kozier et al, 2004).

19 Ensure the area around the patient's mouth is clean and dry, as fluoride residue may irritate the skin (Hampton and Collins, 2003).

20 Rinse the toothbrush and store dry at room temperature (Efstratiou et al, 2007).

21 Dispose of any waste material to maintain safety and prevent the spread of infection.

22 Document care provided and report any changes in condition to the medical team. The frequency of oral care is determined by oral assessment (Kinley and Brennan, 2004). However, Garcia (2004) recommends that oral care should be provided every two hours for intensive care patients, and every four hours or at least after each meal in other areas.

Mouthwashes

Chlorohexidine 0.1–0.2 per cent is an antibacterial mouthwash which inhibits the formation of plaque on the teeth (British National Formulary, 2005). It has an inhibitory action against gram-negative and gram-positive organisms and is effective for up to 12 hours (Berry and Davidson, 2006). However, its effectiveness in the prevention of chemotherapy-induced oral mucositis is questioned (Poting et al, 2006).

Chlorohexidine can be used two to three times per day and should be retained in the mouth for one minute before discarding (Greenstein, 2004). It may cause reversible brown staining of teeth and tongue. Chlorohexidine may be incompatible with some ingredients in

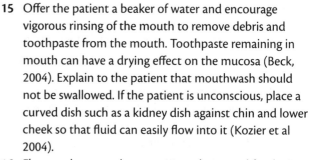

⚠ Professional alert!

There are many commercial mouthwashes available; however, their benefits are unclear.

toothpaste and so can cause an unpleasant taste in the mouth; it is therefore recommended that at least 30 minutes should be left between using the mouthwash and toothpaste (British National Formulary, 2005).

Water can be used as to moisten the mouth and to remove food particles and debris from the oral cavity. The use of small bottles of sterile water is recommended as hospital tap water may be a source of nosocomical infections (Anaissie, Prenzak and Dignani, 2002)

Sodium chloride can promote the healing of oral mucosal lesions; however, its tendency to cause dryness of the mouth limits its use (Berry and Davidson, 2006).

Providone-iodine may be used to treat oral mucosal infections but it does not inhibit plaque formation. It should not be used for longer than 14 days because of iodine absorption (British National Formulary, 2005).

Hydrogen peroxide may be used in the treatment of mouth ulcers, but it must be diluted to appropriate strength to prevent mucosal irritation (British National Formulary, 2005).

> ## Learning activity
>
> Use an internet search engine to find pictures of dental plaque.
>
> Find out if your workplace uses an oral assessment tool. Use an internet search engine to source an oral assessment tool and compare it with your workplace tool.

Conclusion

Most adults and children are able to perform their own mouth care, but some are unable to do so because of physical or cognitive disability or illness. It is an important part of daily hygiene, and in order to prevent infection and maintain the patient's comfort it is essential that the nurse is able to perform this fundamental skill competently.

References

Anaissie, E., Prenzak, S.R. and Dignani, M. (2002). 'The hospital water supply as a source of nosocomial infections: a plea for action', *Archives of Internal Medicine* **162**(13), 1483–92.

Adams, R. (1996) 'Qualified nurses lack of adequate knowledge related to oral health, resulting in inadequate oral care of patients on medical wards', *Journal of Advanced Nursing* 24, 552-560.

Beck, S. L. (2004) 'Mucositis', pp. 276–92 in Henke-Yarhoo, C., Hansen-Frogge, M. and Goodman, M. (eds), *Cancer Symptom Management*, 3rd edn, Sudbury, MA, Jones and Bartlett.

Berry, A. M. and Davidson, P. M. (2006) 'Beyond comfort: oral hygiene as a critical nursing activity in the intensive care unit', *Intensive and Critical Care Nursing* 22, 318–28.

British National Formulary (2005) *British National Formulary for Children*, London, BMJ Publishing UK.

Clay, M. (2000) 'Oral health in older people', *Nursing Older People* **12**(7), 21–6.

Efstratiou, M., Papaioannou, W., Nakou, E., Ktenas, L. A. and Panis, V. (2007) 'Contamination of a toothbrush with antibacterial properties by oral microorganisms', *Journal of Dentistry* 35(4), 331–7.

Garcia, M. (2004) *Oral Care of the Hospitalised Patient: Evidence-based care sheet*, Glendale, IL, Cinahl Information Sheets.

Gibson, F. and Stone, J. (2004) *Mouth Care Clinical Procedure Guideline*, London, Great Ormond Street Hospital for Children NHS Trust.

Gilliam, J. L. and Gilliam, D. G. (2006) 'The assessment and implementation of mouth care in palliative care: a review', *Journal of the Royal Society for the Promotion of Health* **126**(1), 33–7.

Greenstein, B. (2004) *Trounce's Clinical Pharmacology for Nurses*, London, Churchill Livingston.

Hampton, S., Collins, F. (2003) *Tissue Viability: A comprehensive guide*, London, Whurr Publishing.

Holman, C., Roberts, S. and Nicol, M. (2005) 'Promoting oral health', *Nursing Older People* **16**(10), 37–8.

Jamieson, E. M., McCall, J. M. and White, L. A. (2002) *Clinical Nursing Practices*, 4th edn, London, Churchill Livingston.

Kinley, J. and Brennan, S. (2004) 'Changing practice: the use of audit to change oral care practice', *International Journal of Palliative Nursing* **10**(12), 580–7.

Kozier, B., Erb, G., Berman, A. and Snyder, S. (2004) *Fundamentals of Nursing: Concepts, processes and practice*, 7th edn, Upper Saddle River, New Jersey, Pearson Prentice Hill.

Nazarko, L. (2006) 'Helping older people to maintain good oral hygiene', *Nursing and Residential Care* **8**(2), 57–60.

Nicol, M., Bavin, C., Bedford-Turner, S., Cronin, P., Rawlings-Anderson, K. (2000) *Essential Nursing Skills*, London, Mosby.

Pearson, L. S. and Hutton, J. L. (2002) 'A controlled trial to compare the ability of foam swabs and toothbrushes to remove dental plaque', *Journal of Advanced Nursing* **39**(5), 480–9.

Poting, C. M. J., Uitterhoweve, R., Scholte Op Reimer, W. and Van Achterberg, T. (2006) 'The effectiveness of commonly used mouthwashes for the prevention of chemotherapy-induced oral mucositis: a systematic review', *European Journal of Cancer Care* 15, 431–9.

Powers, J. (2006) 'Managing VAP effectively to optimise outcomes and costs', *Nursing Management* 37, 48B–48F (Supplement).

World Health Organisation (2006) *Oral Health in Aging Societies: Integration of oral health and general health*, Geneva, World Health Organisation.

Xavier, G. (2000) 'The importance of mouth care in preventing infection', *Nursing Standard* **19**(14), 47–51.

Chapter

13

Catheterisation and catheter care

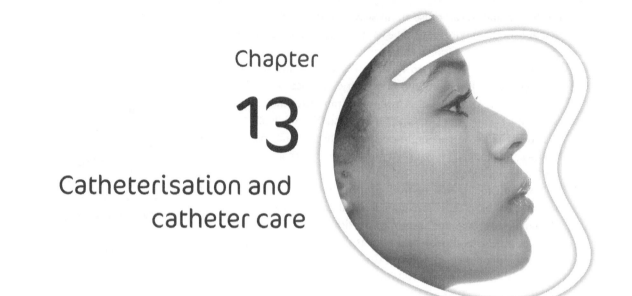

Steve Miles

Links to other chapters in *Foundation Skills for Caring*

Links to other chapters in *Foundation Studies for Caring*

W Don't forget to visit www.palgrave.com/glasper for additional online resources relating to this chapter.

Introduction

At any one time, 15–25 per cent of hospitalised patients in the UK will have an indwelling urethral catheter (Griffiths and Fernandez, 2005) and 80 per cent of all urinary tract infections are traced to indwelling catheters (DH, 2003). The risk of infection rises each day the catheter is in situ, and of those patients with a catheter 20–30 per cent will develop bacteriuria (bacteria in the urine); of those 2–6 per cent will show symptoms of a urinary tract infection. A small percentage, 1–4 per cent, will then go on to develop bacteraemia (bacteria in the bloodstream) and up to a third of these patients will die (Pratt et al, 2001). This demonstrates a direct causal link between catheterisation and mortality. It is for this reason that you must be aware of your role in preventing infections, and more importantly, ensuring catheters are only used for the correct reasons.

Catheter-associated urinary tract infections (CAUTIs) can easily be caused when a catheter is inserted with a faulty aseptic technique or when poor hygiene practice allows the migration of bacteria into the urethra and bladder, either on the outside surface of the catheter or via the drainage channel inside the catheter. This chapter will help you develop the skills to use catheters correctly.

Part

II

Learning outcomes

This chapter will enable you to:

- describe the reasons for insertion of an indwelling catheter or for a patient to pass an intermittent catheter
- understand the different needs of a patient with an indwelling urethral catheter and patients passing an intermittent catheter themselves
- advise on the most appropriate type of catheter for a patient with regard to choice of material and size
- advise on the most appropriate choice of drainage system for an indwelling catheter to suit a patient's needs
- recognise the problems that can occur with indwelling catheters

- advise patients and their carers on the day-to-day management of an indwelling catheter with particular regard to associated infection risks
- understand the need for accurate and comprehensive documentation relating to all aspects of the catheterisation
- describe the procedure for the following skills:
  - removal of an indwelling catheter
  - female catheterisation
  - taking a urine sample
  - emptying a urine drainage bag.

Concepts

- Catheters and when to use them
- Choosing the correct catheter and drainage system
- Catheter problems
- Patient education
- The importance of documentation
- Catheterisation skills

⚠ Professional alert!

Any urinary catheter held in place with a balloon, is known as a Foley catheter.

Catheters

A urinary catheter is a hollow tube which is inserted into the bladder in order to drain urine or instill fluids into the bladder. The urine drains via a number of openings ('eyes') at the tip of the catheter.

'Indwelling catheters' include an integral 'balloon' which, when inflated with sterile water, is retained in the bladder. There are two methods for inserting catheters:

- *Urethral*: the catheter is passed into the bladder via the urethra.
- *Suprapubic*: the catheter is passed into the bladder via an artificial opening on the abdomen which has been created for the purpose by a clinician. Ensure catheters used in this way are licensed appropriately (Medicines and Healthcare Products Regulatory Agency, 2001).

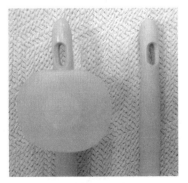

Figure 13.1 Urinary catheters

Intermittent self-catheterisation (ISC)

Intermittent catheters do not have an integral balloon and so cannot be retained in the bladder. They are inserted, usually by the patient, and removed once urine has drained.

This should be considered as first option if clinically appropriate and if the patient is able to manage the procedure (NICE, 2003). It can be used for drainage, where the patient may be completely dependent on this method to empty the bladder, for example patients with a spinal cord injury. It is also useful for those who may be able to pass some urine themselves, but may need to pass a catheter intermittently in order to completely drain the bladder, as in the case of intermittent urinary retention, multiple sclerosis or post surgery. ISC is also often used in the management of a 'stricture' of the urethra: a narrowing of the urethra, often due to injury, scar formation or a growth of abnormal tissue, (Blackwell, 1994) where a catheter may be passed once a week just to keep the urethra open.

There are a number of advantages for patients if this method can be adopted:

- fewer urinary tract infections
- less urethral trauma
- more positive body image
- ability to be sexually active
- improved quality of life
- increased independence.

In order for patients to catheterise successfully and safely, there must be a comprehensive assessment of their suitability and willingness to undertake this, as well as an education programme.

Reasons for catheterisation

Reasons will vary, depending on whether the catheterisation is to be short or long term (Table 13.1). In all cases it is reasonable to question whether the catheter is necessary and whether it is being used for the correct reasons. You should always estimate how long it will be necessary to use the catheter, and question whether intermittent catheterisation would be a viable alternative.

> **ⓐ Learning activity**
>
> Most manufacturers of intermittent catheters provide comprehensive information booklets for nurses and patients. Contact any of the following: Charter Healthcare, Rochester Medical, or Astra-Tech and ask for a booklet. Which do you think provides the information in the most clear, readable format?

> **⚠ Professional alert!**
>
> Intermittent *self*-catheterisation is a 'clean', not a sterile procedure, but patients must be taught that hygiene is paramount to avoid infections.

> **⚠ Professional alert!**
>
> The decision to catheterise should be a cautious one; only when clinical indications are met should a catheter be inserted.

Table 13.1   Short and long-term catheterisation

Short-term catheterisation	Long-term catheterisation
→ After surgery. → Accurate measurement of urine output in acute illness. → Urinary retention. → Determine residual urine (bladder ultrasound is the preferred method). → Allow irrigation of the bladder. → To bypass an obstruction. → To introduce medication directly into the bladder. → To carry out bladder function tests i.e. urodynamics.	→ Patients with neurological conditions i.e. spinal injuries, multiple sclerosis. → Bladder outlet obstruction if unfit for surgical repair. → Chronic urinary retention if ISC is not a suitable alternative. → Chronic incontinence, only if *all* other methods of management have been tried and proved unsuccessful. → If skin integrity is continually compromised and a catheter will alleviate this. → In some cases where it will improve a patient's quality of life, but only after discussion with the patient as to the risks involved, and in consultation with other healthcare professionals involved with the patient.

Sources: Getliffe (1996), Dougherty and Lister (2004).

Choice of catheter

The ideal catheter would have the following attributes:

- material as soft as possible for comfort but sufficiently firm for easy insertion
- largest size of internal drainage channel for the smallest possible external diameter.
- 'elastic recoil' so that, when the catheter is due to be removed, the balloon can be deflated to its original size, thus easing removal
- material which causes minimal tissue reaction
- inhibits, as far as possible, colonisation by bacteria
- resists encrustation by mineral deposits (covered later in the chapter).

A wide range of catheters is available and it is important that due consideration is given to the correct choice of product material, catheter size, length and balloon capacity, as well as patient comfort (Pratt et al, 2001).

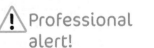

Learning activity

Many trusts, whether primary or secondary care, have a catheter policy. This gives guidance for all staff working in that trust on all aspects of catheterisation. Obtain a copy, and with colleagues compare the policies with those of other trusts.

Material

There are a variety of materials used for the manufacture of catheters. It is important to know which are for short-term use (seven days), medium-term use (28 days) and long-term use (12 weeks):

- PVC – quite rigid, mostly used for ISC catheters
- latex – often coated, e.g. teflon (medium term), hydrogel (long term), silicone, elastomer (long term)
- silicone – (long term).

Catheter size

The size of a catheter is represented by its 'Charriere' size (ch). Each unit is equal to 0.3 mm so, for example, size 12 ch = 4 mm external diameter. Internal diameters of the lumen (where urine drains) vary according to the manufacturing process.

Generally use size 12–14 ch for male and female urethral catheterisation. Any larger sizes via the urethra must only be used after obtainign further advice. Supra-public catheters are generally a larger size (16–18 ch).

Catheter length

- *Female*: 23–26 cm.
- *Standard*: 40–44 cm. This is used for men and also may be used for female wheelchair users, as this can reduce the risk of the catheter being pulled out when transferring from the wheelchair.
- *Paediatric*: 30 cm.

Balloon capacity

Always abide by manufacturers' recommendations, which are always printed on the packaging. Always inflate with sterile water.

Adult catheters: 10 ml.
Paediatric: 2–2.5 ml.
Only in certain specialised settings are larger capacity balloons used (Dougherty and Lister, 2004; Robinson, 2004).

⚠ Professional alert!

Always check that catheters are 'in date' and are stored according to manufacturers' recommendations, and test your patient for latex allergies,

⚠ Professional alert!

Wherever possible always use the smallest-size catheter.

Part

II

Choice of catheter support

Excessive movement of the catheter within the urethra can cause inflammation and trauma, predisposing the patient to infection, tissue necrosis, blockage of the urethral glands, bladder irritability and spasms (Hanchett, 2002).

Straps or adhesive attachments which are attached to the patient's thigh firmly secure the catheter and tubing (Figure 13.2). They act as a shock absorber, minimising the risk of trauma and should be used in all catheterised patients.

Choice of drainage system

When a drainage bag is attached to a catheter this makes a 'closed' drainage system. It is imperative that this closed system is maintained as much as possible. Disconnection should be kept to a minimum to prevent catheter-associated urinary infections (Pratt et al, 2001; NICE, 2003).

The reason for inserting the indwelling catheter has a direct influence on the choice of drainage system. For bed-bound patients, 2-litre 'night bags' directly attached to the catheter are the method of choice; these are either attached to the side of the bed or freestanding on purpose-made night-bag stands (Figures 13.3 and 13.4). The tap must not be allowed to come into contact with the floor due to the risk of infection. Follow manufacturers' recommendations regarding how often to change. This is usually every five to seven days.

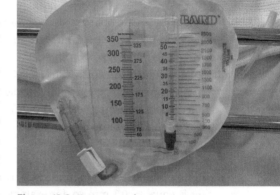

Figure 13.2 Catheter support

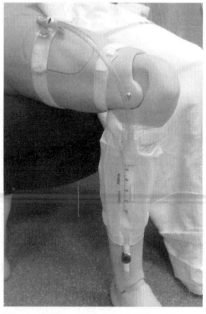

Figure 13.3 To accurately measure urine output: a urimeter enables urine volume to be recorded on an hourly basis

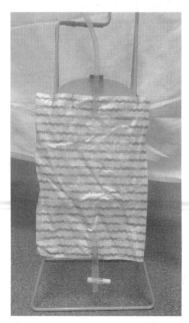

Figure 13.4 Re-usable 'night' bag

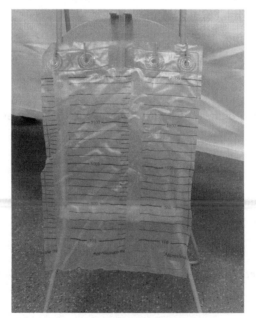

Figure 13.5 Single-use 'night' bag

Figure 13.6 Leg bag for mobile patient

For those patients who are more mobile and are using 'body-worn' bags (i.e. leg or thigh bags), single-use night bags are the product of choice. These are attached to the tap on the bottom of the body-worn bag, forming what is known as a 'link' system. The maintenance of a sterile, continuously closed urinary drainage system is central to the prevention of catheter-associated infection (NICE, 2003).

For those patients in hospital or a care home, or who have outside carers coming into the home after visiting other patients, this is the night bag of choice to reduce the risk of cross-infection (Pomfret, 2007).

Mobile patients

Leg bags of varying capacities, tube length and designs that can be worn on the calf, knee or thigh are available. There are also specialised products for wheelchair users and more active patients. Night bags are then attached to the outlet of the leg bag in order to drain urine overnight, without needing to break the closed drainage system.

Figure 13.6 shows the position of a leg bag with the top leg bag strap positioned above the knee.

Catheter valves

Historically, urine drainage bags have been fitted to the majority of patients, enabling the urine to drain continually into the bag. However, if the bladder is allowed to remain empty all of the time, the tone of the bladder muscle is compromised.

Catheter valves (Figure 13.7) are fitted to the end of the catheter itself, and when the valve is closed this allows the bladder to fill in the usual way. It is important that patients retain the sensation of 'fullness', the need to empty their bladders, so that they are aware of when to open the valve to drain the urine. It is also important that they have adequate bladder capacity, the cognitive awareness to comply with instructions and the dexterity to operate the valve.

It is vital to carry out an assessment on each patient to ensure he or she is able to manage this system. A urinary drainage bag can be fitted onto the end of the valve to allow drainage overnight.

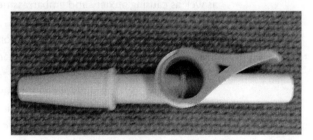

Figure 13.7 Catheter valve

Advantages

- Intermittent opening may help to retain bladder tone.
- It may play a part in flushing bacteria from the bladder (Addison and Rigby, 1998).
- There is some laboratory trial evidence that intermittent opening may increase the length of time before a catheter blocks with encrustation. (Sabbuba et al, 2005).

Contra-indications

- The patient is not properly sensitive to bladder fullness.
- Patient is unable to understand the principles and importance of regular opening.
- Patients have poor dexterity.
- Patients have been identified as at risk from 'ureteric reflux', where urine is able to travel back up the ureter from the bladder to the kidneys.
- There is renal impairment.
- There is uncontrolled 'detrusor (bladder) overactivity' where bladder spasms have not been controlled by any intervention. (Fader et al, 1997).

⚠ Professional alert!

Always seek a medical opinion to confirm a catheter valve is suitable for a patient.

Catheter problems

Infection

The presence of an indwelling catheter markedly increases the risk of a urinary tract infection. The longer the catheter stays in place, the greater the risk. It is estimated that the risk increases at the rate of 5 per cent each day the catheter is in situ (Pratt et al, 2001) and infection is inevitable for those with a long-term catheter (Getliffe, 1996). It is important to understand that this constitutes 'colonisation' by bacteria of the bladder and the urinary tract, and does not necessarily lead to a symptomatic urinary tract infection where antibiotic therapy would be required (Getliffe and Dolman, 2003).

Pain/discomfort

There are many reasons why patients may experience pain or discomfort. All should be investigated.

- Discomfort is often felt after insertion; this should reduce over 24 hours. The use of the anaesthetic gel on insertion helps to reduce this, and mild painkillers can be given.
- Ensure the smallest-size catheter has been used; larger catheters can block the para-urethral glands which usually lubricate the urethra.
- When free drainage is used, the bladder reduces to minimal size and the catheter tip and balloon can easily make contact and aggravate the bladder wall.
- Ensure drainage systems are well supported and do not cause tension.

Bypassing

Instead of the urine draining down the catheter lumen, urine can leak out around the outside of the catheter, resulting in wet clothes and wet bed as well as causing anxiety and embarrassment for the patient. There can a number of reasons for this occurring:

- *Twisted tubing*: this will prevent urine from draining into the catheter bag. Check tubing and re-align if necessary.
- *Constipation*: pressure exerted from the rectum can stop the catheter draining properly, causing it to bypass, so treat the constipation.
- *Debris*: this can physically block the drainage 'eyes' of the catheter (Rew, 2005). Normal shedding of cells from inside the bladder as well as mucus secretions need to be flushed out. Ensure adequate fluid intake, at least two litres a day.
- *Bladder spasm*: when the bladder muscle goes into spasm, the eyes at the catheter tip cannot deal with the resulting sudden increased demand to drain urine. Thus, this urine escapes between the outside surface of the catheter and the urethra, resulting in leakage. In some cases anticholinergic medication can be used to help relax the bladder.
- *Hydrostatic suction*: in some cases, if the catheter bag is positioned too low on the calf of the leg, a negative pressure at the catheter tip inside the bladder can draw bladder mucosa into the eyes of the catheter, thus blocking any flow of urine (Pomfret, 2000). Lift the catheter bag to see if drainage re-commences.
- *Encrustation*: approximately 50 per cent of long-term catheterised patients suffer with blockage of their catheters due to encrustation. Blockage occurs inside the drainage channel of the catheter and can be either partial or complete. The outer surface of the catheter can also be covered by mineral deposits known as struvite and calcium phosphates. These crystals form because the urine has become alkaline instead of acid as it usually is. This happens because commonly found bacteria

---

ⓐ Learning activity

Investigate what is meant by anticholinergic medication, used to treat over-active bladder (OAB). Name the most common ones used and compare their side-effects.

ⓐ Learning activity

For further discussion within your learning group, see Getliffe (1994) 'The characteristics and management of patients with recurrent blockage of long-term urinary catheters', *Journal of Advanced Nursing* 20, 140–9. Do you understand how encrustation forms?

such as *proteus mirablis* have colonised the catheter surface and multiplied. They produce an enzyme, urease, which plays a significant part in breaking down urinary urea, to release ammonia. It is this ammonia which turns the urine alkaline and so the crystals precipitate out and blockage can result (Getliffe and Dolman, 2003).

Patient education

Patients need the knowledge to look after their catheters and chosen drainage systems when they are at home.

- It is important that cleansing both of the meatus and of the catheter becomes part of their usual daily routine. This can be carried out with ordinary soap and water.
- Patients should ensure they wash their hands before and after emptying, or changing their bags or catheter valves.
- They should be taught how to position and secure the catheter and drainage bag appropriately.
- Leg bags should be emptied regularly, or whenever they are at most half full. An overfull leg bag will drag on the support mechanism and could exert undue pressure from the balloon on the base of the bladder.
- It is preferable to use single-use night bags which are discarded each morning. These reduce the risk of urinary infections. Drainable bed bags are often used for bed-bound patients and are an acceptable alternative as long as the link system is only broken between the catheter and the bag when the bag is changed.
- Patients need to know how to obtain further supplies and whom to call if problems occur.
- Those patients performing intermittent self-catheterisation have specific educational needs relating to technique, hygiene and advice on how many times a day to perform the procedure.
- The importance of adequate fluid intake should be stressed, not only to facilitate good drainage but also to reduce the risk of urinary infections.

Documentation

Not only do nurses have a duty to abide by record-keeping guidelines, but comprehensive, clearly written notes are an aid to communication and continuity of care between all health and allied professionals and also promote high standards of care (NMC, 2005).

Following catheterisation the nurse should include in the patient's notes:
- consent obtained
- reason for catheterisation
- date and time of catheterisation
- urethral or suprapubic catheterisation
- type of catheter, material, make, size, length, batch number and expiry date (this information is generally available as a sticker on the packaging which can be inserted into the notes)
- amount of sterile water inserted into balloon
- anaesthetic gel, amount used, make and batch number
- if any problems were experienced on insertion
- drainage system used
- amount of urine drained post catheterisation
- date of planned review, either for removal or change.

Clinical skills

These skills are reproduced here as a guide. At all times healthcare practitioners should ascertain whether there are local policies/protocols which must be adhered to in the area they are practising.

Part

II

a) Learning activity   <u>W</u>

'Skills for Health' is the Skills Council for the UK Health Sector. It has developed 'Competencies' to describe what individuals need to do, what they need to know and which skills they need in carrying out an activity. There are specific competencies related to the insertion and care of urinary catheters. Access the website at: http://www. skillsforhealth.org.uk/page.

Removal of catheter

In hospitals, catheters are often removed first thing in the morning so that if any problems occur with patients unable to pass urine, these can be dealt with during the daytime. Research has suggested that midnight removal may lead to a quicker return to normal continence and a reduced length of hospital stay (Griffiths and Fernandez, 2005). Patients may sleep better after the catheter is removed, less bothered by any resulting sensation within the urethra and less anxious about the expectation of nursing staff about passing urine.

The resources required will depend on whether the catheter is being removed permanently or being changed. If another catheter is to be inserted, check that those resources are also at hand. You will need:

- dressing pack containing sterile towel, galipot, foam swab or non-linting gauze, cleaning solution
- disposable apron and gloves
- syringe for deflating balloon
- syringe for urine specimen, and specimen container (if requested).

Procedure

1 Always check patient documentation first to ensure no problems were experienced when catheter was inserted as well as finding out how much water was inserted into the balloon at that time.

2 Explain the procedure to patients, and describe what symptoms they may experience once it is withdrawn, for example 'urgency and frequency' (regularly having to rush to the toilet to pass urine) and some discomfort. This is likely to resolve within 24 to 48 hours.

3 Hands must be washed and dried thoroughly, or cleaned with a suitable alcohol hand rub. Put on a clean disposable apron and gloves.

4 A catheter urine sample is not routinely required. If one is requested, see the section on 'Collection of a catheter specimen of urine', later in this chapter.

5 The meatus and the area of the catheter close to the meatal opening should be cleaned gently with saline, always swabbing away from the meatal opening.

6 Release any catheter support or catheter leg bag straps if attached to the patient's leg.

7 Insert an empty syringe into the catheter port and allow the water in the balloon to drain out. Any pulling on the syringe may collapse the inflation channel (Stewart, 2006) or may interfere with the balloon collapsing back to its former shape (Robinson, 2000; Daneshmand, Youssefzadeh and Skinner, 2002).

8 Once the water has drained from the balloon, inform the patient and gently and slowly pull the catheter out. Male patients may experience some discomfort as the deflated balloon passes through the prostate gland (Dougherty and Lister, 2004).

9 The meatus will once again need to be cleaned and everything then disposed of according to local trust policy.

10 Advise the patient of the need to maintain a good fluid intake, recording the amount of urine passed each time to ensure normal voiding.

11 Record in the patient's notes not only details of the procedure but also that urine has been passed since the removal of the catheter and the amount.

Female catheterization

You will need:

- sterile catheterisation pack containing gallipots, receiver, low-linting swabs, disposable towels
- disposable plastic apron
- disposable pad
- one pair non-sterile gloves
- one pair sterile gloves
- correct catheter and spare
- syringe with 10 ml sterile water unless catheter has pre-filled balloon
- 6 ml sterile anaesthetic gel
- syringe and universal specimen container and means of clamping tubing – if a urine specimen is required
- 0.9 per cent sodium chloride solution
- bactericidal alcohol hand rub
- catheter valve or drainage bag
- catheter support device.

Procedure

1 Explain the procedure to the patient and ensure that you have consent to continue, taking into consideration any language and specific communication needs (NMC, 2008).

2 Hands must be washed and dried thoroughly, or cleaned with a suitable alcohol hand rub. Put on disposable apron.

3 Place all the required equipment on the lower shelf of a dressing trolley and take it to the patient's bedside.

4 The patient will need to adopt the supine position with knees bent, hips flexed and feet resting about 60 cm apart. Ensure the patient's dignity by keeping the genital area covered until ready to commence the procedure.

5 Consideration must be given to any cultural sensitivities related to this intimate and invasive procedure. Ensure that a good light source is available.

6 Using an aseptic technique, open the catheterisation pack on the working area on top of the trolley. Once this is done, other, supplementary supplies can be opened and their contents placed within this sterile field.

7 Any cover that has been placed across the genital area can now be removed and a suitable disposable bed pad placed under the patients buttocks to provide protection to bedding.

8 Clean your hands once again using an alcohol rub, and put on non- sterile gloves.

9 Using the swabs from the catheterisation pack and 0.9 per cent sodium chloride, separate the labia minora so that the urethral meatus is seen and clean around the urethral orifice using single downward strokes. Once finished discard swabs and gloves appropriately and put on the sterile gloves.

10 An anaesthetic lubricating gel should be used, as evidence shows this not only reduces trauma to the urethra but the antiseptic properties can reduce the incidence of UTIs (urinary tract infections) (Kambal et al, 2004). Separate the labia minora and insert the nozzle into the opening of the urethra and squeeze the contents from the applicator. Abide by the manufacturers' recommendations as to length of time it should be left for it to be effective, usually three to five minutes.

11 Either place the disposable bowl from the catheterisation pack between the patient's legs to catch urine when it begins to drain, or attach the catheter to the urine drainage bag. These items are all within the sterile field but care should still be taken to ensure asepsis is maintained.

12 Keeping the labia parted with one hand introduce the tip of the catheter into the urethral orifice in an upward and backward direction. Advance the catheter 7–8 cm. Once urine begins to flow, either into the receiver or the urine drainage bag, inflate the balloon with the correct amount of sterile water, following the manufacturer's recommendations. Gently withdraw the catheter slightly, so it is felt to locate with the bladder neck sphincter.

Part

II

13 Connect to the chosen urine drainage bag and provide catheter support to ensure the catheter does not become taut when the patient is mobilising or when being moved in bed. In those patients who are suitable, a catheter valve may be fitted, ensuring that the bladder is drained before closure of the tap and giving detailed instructions on the management of the valve.

14 It is at this point a urine sample may be taken from the sampling port if that is indicated.

15 Ensure the patient is left comfortable, clean and dry, and measure what urine has drained into the bag for recording purposes.

16 Dispose of equipment according to trust policy.

17 Hands must be washed and dried thoroughly, or cleaned with a suitable alcohol hand rub. It is important to de-contaminate hands after removing gloves (NICE, 2003).

18 Details of the procedure and the outcome must be comprehensively recorded in the patient's notes.

Collection of a catheter specimen of urine

You will need:

- two swabs saturated with isopropyl alcohol 70 per cent
- device for clamping tubing
- sterile syringe
- universal specimen container
- disposable plastic apron
- one pair of sterile gloves.

Procedure

1 Explain the procedure to the patient and the reasons for taking the specimen, as well as gaining their consent.

2 Hands must be washed and dried thoroughly or else cleaned with a suitable alcohol hand rub. Put on a clean disposable apron and sterile gloves. NICE recommendations advise that where urine samples are obtained from a sampling port, an aseptic technique should be used (NICE, 2003).

3 Clamp the tubing below the access port until sufficient urine collects.

4 All drainage systems now have needle-free access ports which must be used (NICE, 2003).

5 Clean the access point with a swab saturated with 70 per cent isopropyl alcohol, and allow to dry.

6 Using the sterile syringe, aspirate the required amount of urine from the access port and place in an appropriate sterile container.

7 The needle-free access port should now be re-cleaned with a new swab saturated with 70 per cent isopropyl alcohol.

8 Unclamp the tubing and ensure the patient is comfortable.

9 Dispose of equipment; wash and dry hands thoroughly or use suitable alcohol hand rub.

10 Ensure container is labelled correctly and accompanied with the completed request form. It should be dispatched to the laboratory, as soon as possible after the sample is taken. Apply local guidelines regarding storage if it cannot be dispatched immediately.

11 Detail the procedure in the patient's notes.

Emptying a drainable urine collection bag

You will need:

- two swabs saturated with 70 per cent isopropyl alcohol
- clean/disposable jug
- non-sterile gloves
- disposable apron.

Procedure

1   Explain the procedure and gain the patient's consent.
2   Hands must be washed and dried thoroughly or else cleaned with a suitable alcohol hand rub. Put on a disposable apron and non-sterile gloves.
3   Clean the outlet valve with a swab saturated with 70 per cent isopropyl alcohol.
4   Open tap and allow urine to drain into the jug, ensuring it does not overfill and can be transferred to the appropriate place for disposal without risk of spillage.
5   Close the outlet valve and, using a new alcohol saturated swab, clean it once more.
6   Use a cover to transport the jug and dispose of the contents in accordance with local trust policy.
7   Dispose of equipment; wash and dry hands thoroughly or use suitable alcohol hand rub.
8   Note and document the amount drained if this is required for monitoring purposes, as well as any abnormalities.

[S] Scenario: deciding whether to catheterise

Mrs Joan Smith was admitted to her local district general hospital following a fall at home. Fortunately she did not suffer any trauma beyond bruises and abrasions. Having spent some time on the floor of her flat before she was found by a neighbour, she was suffering with hypothermia and tests revealed dehydration and an acute urinary tract infection. Rehydration therapy was commenced by intravenous fluids and antibiotics. Once her core temperature was within normal limits she was transferred onto Hardy Ward. Over the next two days she regained some of her strength and spirit but was troubled by urinary incontinence. This was mainly due to her having feelings of urgency but not being able to get to the toilet on time. The problem was worse at night and often resulted in a wet bed. This upset her greatly as she had never experienced incontinence before admission.

During report on her third day after a particularly upsetting night which resulted in her bed having to be changed three times, the night staff suggested that it might be better if she was catheterised: 'It would be easier for everyone all round.'

This notion was challenged by other staff who suggested a full continence assessment should be carried out. The assessment revealed that despite the initial intravenous fluids she received for 24 hours on admission, she had not been drinking very much and her fluid chart showed a negative balance over the last 24 hours. It was decided to keep a more comprehensive 'voiding diary' recording not only of all the fluids consumed but each individual void. This showed that she was voiding 12 times over a 24-hour period (normal 4–8) and only small amounts each time. Investigation also showed she had not had her bowels open for three days.

A care plan was completed to encourage adequate fluid intake commensurate with what was required for her weight of 10 stone (two litres) and a laxative to treat her constipation. Within two days she was feeling much better, voiding within normal limits and her constipation had been relieved.

This action by ward staff had averted the need for catheterisation which would have exacerbated Mrs Smith's problems and possibly delayed her discharge.

Within six days from admission she was discharged home and she promised that she would continue drinking two litres a day!

Conclusion

Catheterisation is often seen as a useful tool for the management of urinary incontinence. Where the necessity exists for the use of an indwelling catheter, this is because the benefits will outweigh the risks. For those where a catheter is an inappropriate choice, not only may it compromise the patient further, but it is often not without problems, and can have far-reaching, long-term, negative outcomes.

Further reading

Getliffe, K. and Newton, T. (2006) 'Catheter-associated urinary tract infection in primary and community health care', *Age and Aging* 35, 477–81.

Godfrey, H. and Evans, A. (2000) 'Catherisation and urinary tract infections: microbiology', *British Journal of Urology* 9(11), 682–90.

Parkin, J., Scanlon, N., Wooley, M., Grover, A., Evans, A. and Feneley, R. C. L. (2002) 'Urinary catheter "deflation cuff" formation: clinical audit and quantitative *in vitro* analysis', *BJU International* 90, 666–71.

Patel, M., Watts, W. and Grant, A. (2001) 'The optimal form of urinary drainage after acute retention of urine', *BJU International* 88, 26–9.

Pomfret, I. (1996) 'Catheters: design, selection and management', *British Journal of Nursing* 5(4), 245–51.

Pratt, R., Pellowe, C., Wilson, J., Loveday, H., Harper, P., Jones, S., McDougall, C. and Wilcox, M. (2007) 'Epic2: national evidence-based guidelines for preventing healthcare-associated infections in NHS hospitals in England', *Journal of Hospital Infection* 65 (February supplement), S28–S33.

Royal College of Physicians (RCP) (1995) *Report of a Working Party: Incontinence – causes, management and provision of service*, London, RCP.

Stickler, D., Jones, S., Adusei, G., Waters, M., Cloete, J., Mathur, S. and Fenely, R. C. L. (2006) 'A clinical assessment of the performances of a sensor to detect crystalline biofilm formation on indwelling bladder catheters', *BJU International* 98, 1244–9.

Woodward, S. and Rew, M. (2003) 'Patients' quality of life and clean intermittent self-catheterisation', *British Journal of Nursing* 12(18), 1066–74.

References

Addison, R. and Rigby, D. (1998) *A Guide for Patients: At home with your flip-flo catheter valve*, Bard – Patient Information Booklet.

Blackwell (1994) *Blackwell's Dictionary of Nursing*. Oxford, Blackwell Science.

Daneshmand, S., Youssefzadeh, D. and Skinner, E. (2002) 'Review of techniques to remove a Foley catheter when the balloon does not deflate', *Urology* 59 (1), 127–9.

DH (2003) *Winning Ways: Working together to reduce healthcare associated infection in England*, London, DH.

Dougherty, L. and Lister, S. (eds) (2004) *The Royal Marsden Hospital Manual of Clinical Nursing Procedures*, 6th edn, Oxford, Blackwell.

Fader, M., Pettersson, L., Brooks, R., Dean, G., Wells, M., Cottenden, A. and Malone Lee, J. (1997) 'A multicentre comparative evaluation of catheter valves', *British Journal of Nursing* 6(7), 359–67.

Getliffe, K. (1994) 'The characteristics and management of patients with recurrent blockage of long-term urinary catheters', *Journal of Advanced Nursing* 20, 140–9.

Getliffe, K. (1996) 'Care of urinary catheters', *Nursing Standard* 11(11), 47–54.

Getliffe, K. and Dolman, M. (eds) (2003) *Promoting Continence, A Clinical Research Resource*, 2nd edn, Edinburgh, Bailliere Tindall.

Griffiths, R. and Fernandez, R. (2005) 'Policies for the removal of short -term indwelling urethral catheters', *Cochrane Database of Systematic Reviews 2005*, 1. Art. No. CD004011. DOI: 10.1002/14651858.CD004011.pub2.

Hanchett, M. (2002) 'Techniques for stabilizing urinary catheters', *American Journal of Nursing* 102(3), 44–8.

Kambal, C., Chance, J., Cope, S. and Beck, J. (2004) 'Catheter-associated UTIs in patients after major gynaecological surgery', *Professional Nurse* 19(9), 515–18.

Medicines and Healthcare Products Regulatory Agency (MHRA) (2001) *Problems Removing Urinary Catheters*, London, MHRA.

NICE (2003) 'Prevention of healthcare-associated infections in primary and community care', NICE [online] http://www.nice.org.uk/nicemedia/pdf/Infection_control_fullguideline.pdf (accessed 15 October 2008).

Nursing and Midwifery Council (NMC) (2005) *Guidelines for Records and Record Keeping*, London, NMC.

NMC (2008) *The Code: Standards of conduct, performance and ethics for nurses and midwives*, London, NMC.

Pomfret, I. (2000) 'Catheter care in the community', *Nursing Standard* 14(27), 46–51.

Pomfret, I. (2007) 'Urinary catheterization: selection and clinical management', *British Journal of Community Nursing*, 12(8), 348–54.

Pratt, R., Pellowe, C., Loveday, H., Robinson, N. and Smith, G. (2001) 'The epic project: developing national evidence-based guidelines for preventing healthcare associated infections', *Journal of Hospital Infection* 47 (Supplement), S3–S4.

Rew, M. (2005) 'Caring for catheterised patients: urinary catheter maintenance', *British Journal of Nursing* 14(2), 87–92.

Robinson, J. (2000) 'Removing catheters', *Journal of Community Nursing* 14(12), 18.

Robinson, J. (2004) 'Fundamental principles of indwelling urinary catheter selection', *British Journal of Community Nursing* 9(7), 281–4.

Sabbuba, N. A., Stickler, D. J., Long, M. J., Dong, Z., Short, T. D. and Fenely, R. J. C. (2005) 'Does the valve regulated release of urine from the bladder decrease encrustation and blockage of indwelling catheters by crystalline Proteus Mirablis biofilms?' *Journal of Urology* 173(1), 262–6.

Stewart, E. (2006) 'Development of catheter care guidelines for Guy's and St Thomas's', *British Journal of Nursing* 15(8), 420–5.

Chapter

14

Basic foot care and managing common nail pathologies

Matthew Cole

Links to other chapters in *Foundation Skills for Caring*

9   Patient hygiene
23   Diabetic foot assessment

Links to other chapters in *Foundation Studies for Caring*

25   Care of the older adult – community
28   Rehabilitation
29   Loss, grief, bereavement and palliative care

Don't forget to visit www.palgrave.com/glasper for additional online resources relating to this chapter.

Introduction

With some knowledge and understanding, basic foot care can be easily undertaken. It is about providing the level of care otherwise capable individuals would undertake for themselves if they were able to.

It is often thought that for even the simplest of care tasks in the healthcare setting (cutting toenails and ensuring good hygiene), a specialist qualification is required but this is not the case. However, when nursing and caring for others, there is a need for a basic insight into a number of aspects of good clinical practice and skills.

This chapter aims to introduce you to the human foot: what is normal, what is abnormal and what may need specialist intervention, as well as how to undertake simple foot and toenail care. It does not cover everything but it will serve to ground you in some of the very basic foot health issues you will experience and see when caring for your patients.

Learning outcomes

This chapter will enable you to:

- recognise the appearance and key examination findings of a healthy foot compared with one affected by disease
- have a rudimentary understanding of the surface anatomy of the foot and the location of the pulses in the foot
- understand that systemic disease can manifest in the foot, leading to dysfunction and complications such as ulceration, and that these can have serious consequences for some patients
- recognise potential key symptoms and act appropriately to address common indicators of disease in the foot
- understand how key national guidance, local care pathways and arrangements can influence the management of some health conditions whose effects include those in the foot

- maintain a patient's basic foot hygiene and undertake safe, effective and appropriate nail care
- recognise the infection control issues in caring for a patient's feet and employ these in practice
- understand when not to cut a patient's nails but instead to undertake filing as an alternative or to take no action other than to refer on to an appropriate professional
- provide appropriate care for iatrogenic wounds, avoiding the potential to create dangerous tourniquet affects when toes are inappropriately dressed.

Concepts

- Adult and older person's foot health
- Holistic impact of poor foot health
- Chronic disease and aging in foot health
- Diabetes
- Anatomy
- Clinical risk assessment

- Personal care
- Patient-focused multidisciplinary working
- Infection control
- Ergonomics
- Dermatology
- Clinical emergency and urgent presentations

- National and local guidelines and procedures affecting clinical practice and decision making
- Self-directed learning
- Support learning from other chapters relating to the foot

The human foot

A healthy foot is warm to the touch (using the back of your hand), has skin that is intact and healthy looking, not dry or flaking (Springett and Merriman, 1995). The presence of hair on the feet (often on the toes, dorsum (top) of the foot and extending down from the leg) is a good indicator that the feet are in a healthy condition. There should be no swelling and the colour should not be red, blue/purple or very pale, although this is usually less evident in Negroid, Asian or Oriental skin (Springett and Merriman, 1995). Healthy toenails have a pinkish hue with a white free-edge – that being the part of the nail that gets cut.

Part

II

Many older people have common foot problems resulting from aging and the associated disease, deformity and disability caused by multiple long-term conditions affecting their general health (Helfand, 2004). Many will have deformity of the foot, which often presents as changes in the forefoot and toes.

Ill-fitting and inappropriate styles of footwear (including slippers) can cause an array of simple to limb-threatening foot health problems (Vernon et al, 2007). Such footwear is common in older people. Poor footwear is very definitely linked to pathological changes in the forefoot and to foot pain (Menz and Morris, 2005).

Arthritic conditions can deform the entire foot, also leading to difficulties with fitting footwear and with mobility, as can the effects of neurological dysfunction resulting from disease and injury.

Diabetes is commonly cited as causing significant complication in the foot and lower limb and can lead to ischaemic and neurological deficits in these regions. Many nurses therefore assume that they should not provide basic foot care for diabetic patients and must refer problems to a podiatrist, but this is not the case and they can provide simple care.

> ## a Learning activity
>
> Examine your own feet:
> - Try moving the joints in your foot and ankle through their range of motion.
> - Use a surface anatomy chart to identify sites on your foot and ankle.
> - Research the dorsalis pedis and posterior tibial pulses and find them on your foot – try finding them on other people's feet too.

> ## a Learning activity
>
> Use the library, internet and other sources to research the basic impact of diabetes on the foot and lower-limb:
> - What are the key effects?
> - What is the role of the podiatrist, nurse and doctor in the long-term management of patients with diabetes?
> - Research the disease processes and how they might present and impact on the foot health of patients who have diabetes.

Assessing the foot

Examine the feet and legs in plenty of light (preferably natural daylight) and have the feet in an easily accessible position. Having the people you are caring for on a bed or with their feet raised up on a reclining chair will allow you to access their feet with ease and prevent you having to bend excessively – remember to look after your back! Do not however, use a bed with a high footplate which would have to be leant over.

Start your check by looking at and feeling the feet from the lower end of the leg down across the ankle and around the heels. Remember to check the back of both heels. Then check the sole followed by the dorsum (top) of each foot, finally checking around and between each toe, making sure to check the 'webbing' – the area under the toes between the sole of the foot and the toes themselves.

> ## t Practice tip
>
> It is important to check the feet for obvious signs of injury and other common problems. Doing this regularly prevents simple problems becoming significant ones and should prevent some situations altogether – pressure ulcers on the heels of inpatients for example (Dougherty and Lister, 2004).

> ## t Practice tip
>
> It is good practice to check the feet daily day to identify any potential problems, especially for patients who are immobile, bed-bound or have neuropathy.

Check footwear for signs of damage and excessive wear. Remember to check inside the shoe for rough edges that may rub the foot or for pieces of debris and the like as the wearer may not be able to feel that anything is wrong. Footwear should be renewed regularly – although older people may be reluctant to do so, which can contribute to an increased risk of falls.

Indicators of clinical concern

Common problems are often very evident and the person you are caring for may well have noticed it or be complaining of pain, discomfort or other symptoms. Always ask people if they have had any problems since you last saw them, as they are often the ones best able to give you information about the condition of their feet but may be reluctant to trouble you, particularly in busy wards and care homes.

⚠ Professional alert!

Some people, particularly those with diabetes and neurological disorders, may have a sensory deficit in their feet and lower limbs, which means they may be unaware of changes and even of visually very obvious and significant problems such as ulcers – especially if they are on the soles of the feet where they may not be easily seen. Bear in mind that some conditions such as diabetes can also affect a person's eyesight.

Significant changes that can indicate a problem may be seen in Table 14.1.

Table 14.1   Changes in the foot which can indicate a clinical problem

Changes in temperature	➜ Inflammation with redness, heat and swelling combined with pain can indicate an injury or infection. Cellulitis is usually well demarcated (Parker, 2007). ➜ A sudden change to very cold, painful and pale-skinned leg with paralysis and paraesthesia can indicate a sudden ischaemic event requiring prompt medical intervention (Tidy, 2004).
Changes in colour	➜ A foot or leg which has suddenly become pale can indicate a significant circulation problem (see above). ➜ Redness can indicate inflammation – perhaps over an arthritic joint. Check that footwear is not rubbing to eliminate external causes which could lead to ulceration in 'at risk' feet. ➜ Dusky red-coloured subcutaneous streaks up the foot towards the leg in lines (lymphangitis) can indicate an infection that needs prompt attention (Centre for Cancer Education, 1997).
Changes in the skin	➜ Skin that has become thickened and hard (hyperkeratosis, callous) can indicate pressure points (Adams et al, 1989). ➜ Dry and cracked skin can indicate stress on the skin and a potential problem. ➜ Itching and scaling skin can indicate common problems such as Tinea Pedis – a fungal infection of the skin most commonly caused by dermatophytes (Hay, 1990).
Discharges	➜ Any exudate or bleeding etc, indicating a wound.

Indicators for prompt referral

Table 14.2, which is not an exhaustive list, outlines situations that would indicate the need for the patient to be promptly reviewed (this may depend on local arrangements and care pathways). Alternatively, consult a senior colleague in a care setting, or the patient's general practitioner in the community.

Table 14.2   Indicators for prompt referral

To a podiatrist	➜ Foot ulceration and other wounds.
	➜ Ingrowing toenails with a wound and hypergranulation tissue.
	➜ Cases of long-term neglect where foot problems are causing significant immobility, pain or ulceration or are hindering rehabilitation.
	➜ Amputees (partial or total foot and lower limb) for surviving limb interventions.
	➜ Patients referred to falls pathways for footwear and care advice and gait analysis etc.
To a podiatrist, vascular or other suitable MDT	➜ Sudden onset of discoloration, significant inflammation or swelling, numbness or pain of part or all of the foot/leg.

(c) Professional conversation

Deborah, a district nurse, says, 'My team were called in to see an older person who had not had any kind of healthcare input for years and hadn't seen a doctor for nearly 20 years. While she was generally quite well, she was self-neglected despite the best efforts of her two sons and had refused the help of social services.

'The patient was significantly overweight and her mobility was poor. She used the furniture to support herself while walking around the one room she lived in. For her, the biggest problem with moving around was the very real pain she was in because of the neglected state of her feet. She couldn't put on any shoes because of her very painful feet and overgrown toenails – they were literally inches long, and thick. Until we could do something to improve her feet we couldn't do much at all to get her mobile, help her look after herself better or reduce her risk of falls.

'She was very embarrassed and ashamed about the condition of her feet but after lots of persuasion she agreed to let a podiatrist visit her. The podiatrist gained the patient's confidence by talking to her for quite some time and was then able to provide her with the treatment she needed. The results were instant, and having put on a new pair of shoes the patient stood up and walked around with hardly any problems. She was so happy because for the first time in years she could stand up and move around without being in agony – in fact she was so happy she started to cry, which nearly set us all off.

' Inspired, I then went on the basic foot care course run by my trust and some weeks later tackled some similar toenails – although nowhere near as bad as this lady's – but it made a world of difference to the patient and I was really pleased with myself that I'd done it. For me it was about having the confidence, right tools and information to be able to do it, and the best thing is that patients can be treated quickly and easily by me, saving them time and discomfort. It also meant that I didn't have to spend time making referrals and phone calls, and I was saving the podiatrists the time they could be spending with someone who had a medical need for their skills.'

Part

II

t☆ Practice tip

Check local policy and care pathways as NHS Trusts usually have a process in place for appropriate referrals and multidisciplinary working, particularly around issues covered by National Service Frameworks and NICE guidelines.

Hygiene and washing feet

Good hygiene is paramount, so it is very important to keep feet clean. If patients are not being bathed or showered daily, it is important that the feet are washed every day:

1   Use tepid water and a mild soap, or if indicated other products suitable for sensitive skin or dermatological conditions.
2   Use a flannel or something soft to clean the feet, making sure to clean well between and under the toes, as this is a vulnerable area and often neglected. If the toes are deformed or difficult to separate, use a cotton bud to clean between them.
3   A soft nailbrush will remove any stubborn skin squames which have adhered to the skin, but be gentle and never use anything sharp to probe around and under the nails.
4   Feet should never be left soaking as this can draw out the natural skin oils, exacerbating problems with skin care and medical conditions.
5   Dry the feet thoroughly with a clean towel, paying careful attention to the areas between and under the toes. Rubbing the feet vigorously can damage fragile skin and could be painful for arthritic feet.

6   Having dried the feet thoroughly, apply any emollients or other such products as indicated in the care plan, making sure to avoid their use between the toes (unless using medicated products prescribed for such use). Always ensure the product is well applied and the skin is not left 'caked' in creams or other substances.

7   Always use clean hosiery made from natural materials such as cotton or wool which will allow the skin to 'breathe'.

8   Never use talc or other powders to aid drying as they can cause irritation to fragile skin and, once moist, form a paste which can soak against the skin, damaging it. This in turn can cause fungal and bacterial skin infections. Talc must not be used as an easy alternative to proper drying of the feet with a towel.

⚠ Professional alert!

Individuals who suffer from continence problems must have their feet cleaned and dried thoroughly when changing hosiery and footwear as a result of soiling from urine and faeces. It is not acceptable to apply hosiery to feet that have not been cleaned and dried properly in any circumstance, let alone when they are soiled in this way; it is considered to be neglect and must never be permitted.

Infection control: hands, feet and instruments

Whilst it is not necessary to wash people's feet prior to cutting their nails, it is advisable to remove any visible dirt with soap and water. However, if the feet are visibly unclean or soiled, then they should be washed and dried properly. A clean paper towel can be placed under the feet whilst cutting the nails, and the nail debris can be collected on this and disposed of in the clinical waste.

Hand hygiene is imperative and hands must be cleaned thoroughly, using an appropriate technique and following local procedures, both before and after any care is given. It is not always necessary to wear (non-sterile examination) gloves to cut and file toenails but you should follow local policy regarding their use and which type to use.

The basic instruments required are a pair of nail nippers and a foot dresser (a file). The nippers should be held as illustrated in Figures 14.2–14.5. Keep the wrist straight when using nippers and files to avoid potential strain (Health and Safety Laboratory, 2006).

Depending on the setting in which you are caring for your patient, and also on local policy, you may use either single-use disposable instruments or prepacked sterilised re-useable ones. After use, the single-use instruments must be disposed of in a sharps bin, whilst re-useable instruments must be decontaminated and re-sterilised either locally or centrally following the local procedures and policy (Department of Health, 2001a, 2001b).

© Professional conversation

Val, an infection control liaison practitioner, says, 'Single-use disposable instruments are just that – single-use. Single-use disposable nail cutters and files, like any other such instruments, should only be used on the one patient, the one time, and then disposed of. You can't keep them to be used again at a later date, even on the same patient – you never know who else might use them, and if the patients keep them they might lend them to someone else to use.

'The instruments can also act as a source of cross-infection and if left lying around could be contaminated with anything, including MRSA. Use them once and them put them straight in an appropriately sized sharps bin with a non-return lid or a trap in it to prevent them coming out or injuring someone.'

Some basic nail anatomy terms

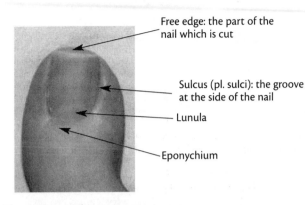

Free edge: the part of the nail which is cut

Sulcus (pl. sulci): the groove at the side of the nail

Lunula

Eponychium

Figure 14.1 Nail anatomy terms

Cutting and filing toenails

1 Make sure the feet are easily accessible – think of your back! Remember to have the person on a bed or at least with their feet elevated. Also make sure that there is plenty of light to work in.

2 Do not soak the feet prior to cutting the toenails. Rather than making things easier it will make the nails pliable and possibly uncomfortable to cut. It will also make them difficult to file properly.

3 Grip the nipper by the handles with the top arm against your fingers and the bottom arm in your palm (Figures 14.2 and 14.3).

4 The foot and toe can be held with the opposite hand (Figure 14.7).

5 Be careful not to twist or bend the nail, as this may be uncomfortable or cause pain.

6 Once the nipper has been placed correctly on the nail, cover the upper surface of the nippers with a finger from the opposite hand to prevent pieces of nail 'flying' out (Figure 14.8). There is a small risk of debris hitting the face or entering the eye so covering the nipper is important.

7 Do not cut the nails down into the sulci (the grooves at the sides of the nail), simply cut as straight across as possible following the shape of the end of the toe which will leave the nail with a marginal curve to it (Tollafield and Merriman, 1997). Likewise, do not put anything down the sides of a nail as this can damage it. There should be some free edge left after cutting so that the nail plate is clear of the ends of the sulci.

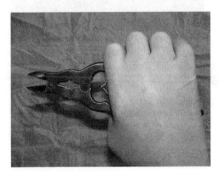

Figure 14.2 Gripping the nipper

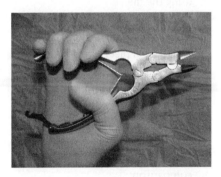

Figure 14.3 Gripping the nipper, fingers and palm

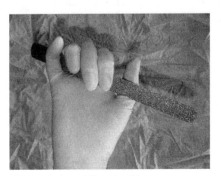

Figure 14.4 Holding the file

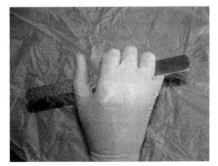

Figure 14.5 Holding the file, fingers and palm

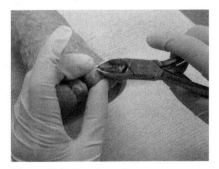

Figure 14.6 Cut the nail one part at a time

Part

II

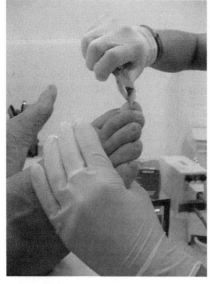

Figure 14.7 Grip the toes and foot with the opposite hand

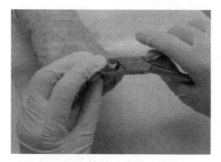

Figure 14.8 Cover the nippers when cutting but without touching the blades

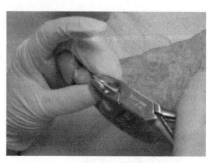

Figure 14.9 Gradually 'nip' along the nail, cutting off one piece at a time

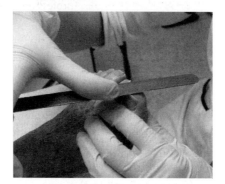

Figure 14.10 File the nails with pressure on the down stroke

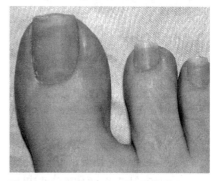

Figure 14.11 Example of nails before cutting

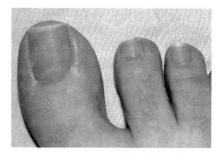

Figure 14.12 Same nails after cutting and filing

8   Be aware that nails are not always flat and occasionally skin tufts (angiokeratoma) may be present under the nail that should not be cut as they can bleed heavily (Tollafield and Merriman, 1997).

9   Hold the file between the little and fourth fingers and grip with the 2nd, 3rd and 4th fingers, using your thumb to put pressure against the nail (Figures 14.4 and 14.5).

10 File the free edge of the nail (Figure 14.10). When using the file, apply gentle pressure against the nail with your thumb on the file on the down stroke whilst moving the file back and forth from the top of the toe downwards so that the nail is filed in the one direction only. Do not file toenails from side to side as you would perhaps a fingernail. Sharp corners can be rounded off using the file.

11 To finish, check that there are no rough or jagged edges to the nails and that no pieces of cut nail have fallen into the spaces between the toes – which in some 'at risk' patients could cause trauma leading to a wound (Tollafield and Merriman, 1997). See Figures 14.11 and 14.12 for a before and after comparison.

Cutting thick nails

Use the nipper to take small pieces at a time, using the point of the nipper to 'break into' the nail. Cut using the flat side of the nipper to gradually 'reduce' the nail down. File the nail as above, but with thickened nails it is also possible to file them on the top to help smooth and further reduce the thickness. Do not however, over-file the top surface of a nail plate as this can cause it to become sore and you could even file through the nail exposing the nail bed beneath.

c Professional conversation

Kate, a specialist musculoskeletal podiatrist, says, 'I was on a ward one day assessing the surviving lower-limb of a patient who had just had the other leg amputated when I was approached by one of the nurses who wanted some help and advice. The nurse had recently been on a half-day basic foot care course organised by the podiatry service in my Trust and wanted some help with a patient she was caring for.

'The patient had some long, thick toenails and the nurse was anxious about cutting them but wanted to do it, having attended the course. We talked through how she was going to do this for her patient and whilst I observed she put her learning into practice.

'When she had finished caring for the patient, we talked about how she had found the experience; she was really happy and pleased with having done what she did. She found that by going through the process calmly and step by step, she had done what she thought she couldn't do and had a real sense of achievement. Once she had put her learning into practice, both she and the patient had something to smile about!'

Alternatives to cutting toenails

Some nails are too thick or difficult to cut. These can often be managed safely and effectively by filing, using a foot dresser or good quality emery board. This should be done whilst the nails are hard and dry, so do not soak them first. Using the same technique as described above, it is preferable to gently file the nails once per week.

Nails which should not be cut

In the following circumstances, professional intervention is initially required but after this such cases can be cared for using the techniques above:
- Onychogryphosis: thickened nails which are thick and deformed (Figure 14.13)
- Onychocryptosis: ingrowing toenails
- Onychomycosis: nails infected with fungi and yeast etc.
- dermatological conditions such as psoriasis when the nails have been affected
- nails which are bleeding, weeping or have an open wound.

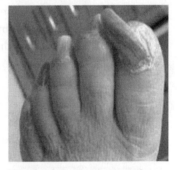

Figure 14.13 Gryphotic nails

a Learning activity

Use an internet search engine to find pictures of onychogryphosis, onychocryptosis and onychomycosis so you can recognise them.

Also find pictures of dermatological conditions that can affect toenails.

Nails which should not be cut but can be filed

The nails described below can be filed, which is best done when they are hard and dry and preferably on a weekly basis to keep them down, which is easier than trying to file through lots of nail:
- Diseased or deformed toenails of patients taking anticoagulants – although if the nails are not diseased or deformed, they can be cut and filed as for other patients.
- Involuted toenails (Figure 14.14) which curl around on themselves in the corners. Never cut these, but gently file ensuring the curled corners are never shorter than the sulci at the sides of the nail.

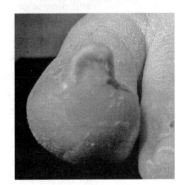

Figure 14.14 Involuted toenail

Patients with diabetes

There is no reason why patients with diabetes cannot have their toenails cut by someone other than a podiatrist – be that a carer, relative, nurse or doctor. It is an urban myth that nurses are not allowed to this. Provided you observe the advice and limitations given above, there is no reason for you not to cut the toenails of patients with diabetes (whilst taking extra care in those patients with identified risk factors such as ischaemia and neuropathy).

> ### (a) Learning activity
>
> Research the current National Institute for Health and Clinical Excellence (NICE) guidelines on foot care for patients with diabetes on their website: http://www.nice.org.uk.

Cuts created whilst cutting toenails

Cuts and abrasions created whilst cutting toenails seldom happen and are usually very slight. Where blood is present, normal infection control measures and personal protective equipment (PPE) should be used (Dougherty and Lister, 2004). Normally, suitable gloves and a plastic apron will suffice – but always follow local procedures. Simple 'nicks' can be dressed with a small plaster and this is normally entirely sufficient and can be left in place for 24 hours. Do not wrap any dressing completely around a toe as this can act as a tourniquet if the digit becomes swollen (Goslin, Tollafield and Rome, 1997).

If the cut is more significant gently cleanse the area and cover with a sterile non-adherent dressing and some dressing tape – remembering to apply the tape from the plantar surface to the dorsum of the toe only and not around it. Monitor as with all wound care.

Conclusion

Having studied the information and fully undertaken all of the learning activities in this chapter, you should have a basic grasp of the surface anatomy of the foot and the effects of some of the key disease processes which can put it at risk of clinical complications. You should now also be able to undertake a simple assessment of the foot and recognise when deformity and disease or other problems are affecting it – although you are not expected to diagnose and manage these manifestations.

However, the principle aim has been to enable you to provide a patient with appropriate basic foot hygiene and undertake basic nail care. In doing so you should now understand the importance of infection control, local and national guidance on a range of issues, when it is appropriate for you to undertake this care and when you should refer on or seek the input of senior colleagues.

In general, you will be able to undertake the physical care tasks detailed in this chapter for most of your patients, providing them with comfort and maintaining their personal care standards and dignity. The provision of any form of personal care is an essential part of caring for the patient, not just as another patient but as an individual and a person. It can promote a sense of health and comfort, which in turn can only help to promote the holistic well-being of the people you care for.

References

Adams, I., Whitting, M. F., Savin, J. A. and Branford, W. A. (1989) 'Skin and subcutaneous tissues', p. 92 in Neale, D. and Adams, I. (eds) *Common Foot Disorders: Diagnosis and management – a general clinical guide*, 3rd edn, Edinburgh, Churchill Livingstone.

Centre for Cancer Education, University of Newcastle Upon Tyne (1997) *Lymphangitis*, Centre for Cancer Education [Online] http://cancerweb.ncl.ac.uk/cgi-bin/omd?lymphangitishttp://cancerweb.ncl.ac.uk/cgi-bin/omd?lymphangitis (accessed 22 November 2007).

Department of Health (DH) (2001a) *Decontamination Programme: A protocol for the local decontamination of surgical instruments*, London, DH [Online] http://www.dh.gov.uk/en/Publicationsandstatistics/Lettersandcirculars/ Dearcolleagueletters/DH_4005492 (accessed 20 November 2007).

DH (2001b) *Single-Use Instruments For Tonsil and Adenoid Surgery*, London, DH [Online] http://www.dh.gov.uk/en/Publicationsandstatistics/Lettersandcirculars/ Dearcolleagueletters/DH_4009845 (accessed 20 November 2007).

Dougherty, L. and Lister, E. (eds) (2004) *The Royal Marsden Hospital Manual of Clinical Nursing Procedures*, 6th edn, Oxford, Blackwell.

Goslin, R., Tollafield, D. R. and Rome, K. (1997) 'Mechanical therapeutics in the clinic', p. 188–9 in Merriman, L. M. and Tollafield, D. R. (eds), *Clinical Skills in Treating the Foot*, Edinburgh, Churchill Livingstone.

Hay, R. J. (1990) *Fungi and Skin Disease*, London, Gower Medical Publishing.

Health and Safety Laboratory (2006) *Musculoskeletal Disorders in Podiatry and Chiropody Professionals*, HSL/2006/60, Health and Safety Executive.

Helfand, A. E. (2004) 'Foot problems in older patients: a focused podogeriatric assessment study in ambulatory care', *Journal of the American Podiatric Medical Association*, **94**(3), 293–304.

Menz, H. B. E. and Morris, M. E. (2005) 'Footwear characteristics and foot problems in older people', *Gerontology* **51**(5), 346–51.

Parker, S. (2007) *Cellulitis and Necrotising Fascitis*, Website of S. Parker, United Kingdom [Online] http://www.surgical-tutor.org.uk/default-home.htm?core/preop1/cellulitis.htm (accessed 22 November 2007).

Springett, K. and Merriman, L. (1995) 'Assessment of the skin and its appendages', p. 203 in Merriman, L. M. and Tollafield, D. R. (eds), *Assessment of the Lower Limb*, Edinburgh, Churchill Livingstone.

Tidy, C. (2004) *Limb Embolism and Ischaemia*, Egton Medical Information Systems Limited [Online] http://www.patient.co.uk/showdoc/40000242 (accessed 22 November 2007).

Tollafield, D. R. and Merriman, L. M. (1997) Operative techniques: appendages', p. 90–1 in Merriman, L. M. and Tollafield, D. R. (eds), *Clinical Skills in Treating the Foot*, Edinburgh, Churchill Livingstone.

Vernon, W., Borthwick, A., Walker, J., Hardy, B., Dunning, D., Denton, C., Drew. C. and Nunn, M. (2007) 'Expert group criteria for the recognition of healthy footwear', *British Journal of Podiatry* **10**(4), 127–33.

Part

II

Chapter

15

Care of the infant

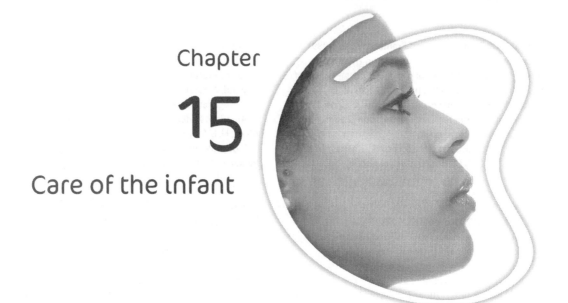

Marion Aylott

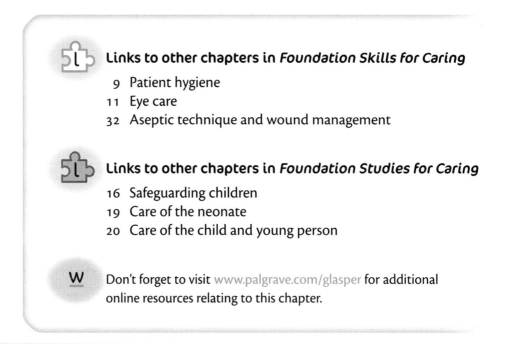

Links to other chapters in *Foundation Skills for Caring*

9   Patient hygiene
11 Eye care
32 Aseptic technique and wound management

Links to other chapters in *Foundation Studies for Caring*

16 Safeguarding children
19 Care of the neonate
20 Care of the child and young person

W   Don't forget to visit www.palgrave.com/glasper for additional online resources relating to this chapter.

Introduction

This chapter aims to give you knowledge and understanding of the skills required in providing safe and effective infant hygiene. Infancy is generally the period from birth until age 1 year. It is a time of enormous growth and change for children and families. Infants have health issues that are different from older children and adults, like nappy rash, cradle cap and a need for frequent feedings. The fundamental basis of much infant care, as we know it today, has evolved through many years of traditional and cultural customs. Respect for cultural beliefs and traditions is vital in gaining the confidence of mothers so that we can work together to bring about a standardised set of guidelines that will work in any situation worldwide. It is always difficult to introduce new guidelines, especially in an area where there does not seem to be an obvious problem with existing treatments. In some cases, cord care for example, there is overwhelming evidence to suggest that the increases in use of various baby products, alcohol wipes, dyes, creams and powders have only served to complicate matters.

This chapter on infant care concentrates on the importance of hygiene for staff and patients in reducing the risk of cross infection. With the introduction of modern matrons and directors of infection control, emphasis is focused on these practices in today's healthcare arena (Roberts, 2008). The chapter provides a practical risk control approach to the associated risks of basic nursing care and how these can be dealt with. One final note: the information and guidance contained within this chapter is provided with full-term infants specifically in mind. It is not meant to provide all the information you need to care for the infant.

Learning outcomes

This chapter will enable you to:

- describe with evidence-based reasons the procedure for the following infant hygiene skills:
  - hanging a nappy
  - swaddling
  - giving a sponge bath
  - umbilical cord care
  - bathing a baby
  - eye care
  - mouth care
- discuss possible hazards and problems associated with meeting infant hygiene needs, including standard precautions of infection control, safe moving and handling, and reference to their peculiar anatomy and physiology.

Concepts

- Infant
- Hygiene
- Infection control
- Safety
- Care
- Skin integrity

S   Scenario: an infant with omphalitis

You are caring for Tom who is a 4 kg term infant who has been admitted to your ward for IV antibiotics. He is febrile and has omphalitis (septic umbilical cord; see Figure 15.1). There is a pus-like discharge around the base of the cord, an offensive odour and some redness, warmth, swelling and tenderness around the cord. You reassure Hayley, Tom's mother, that even though his umbilical cord looks sore and painful, he isn't bothered by it and infection of the umbilical cord rarely becomes serious. But to manage the infection, she will need to keep the area clean and dry.

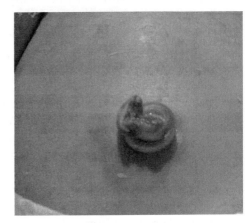

Figure 15.1 Omphalitis

W

a Learning activity

Current information and practice on umbilical cord care is at best confusing. An article by Trotter (2003) attempts to clarify the situation by explaining the physiology of cord separation and how different treatments affect this process, and reviewing the most up to date recommendations. Read this article online at www.sharontrotter.org.uk/rcm2003new.htm.

Changing a nappy

Until a child is toilet-trained, usually by 3 years of age, nappies are used to collect urine and bowel movements. An infant's soft and delicate skin needs special care. This is especially important as their bottoms are in frequent contact with moisture, bacteria and ammonia, and there is rubbing from the nappy (Darmstadt and Dinulos, 2000). Infants and toddlers are at risk of breached skin integrity as long as they are wearing nappies. Rashes and skin breakdown are much easier to prevent than to cure. Maintenance of skin integrity is achieved by:

- changing nappies frequently
- gentle cleaning
- patting skin dry
- if room temperature allows, laying the baby on a towel and leaving the nappy off for a while.

t ☆
Practice tip

Many infants need to be changed after feeding. Checking an infant's nappy as part of the feeding routine helps reduce the occurrence of nappy rash.

You will need:
- bowl
- changing mat
- non-sterile gloves
- apron
- appropriate size nappy
- during first 28 days:
  - cotton wool
  - warm water
- after 28 days:
  - cotton wool and warm water or
  - baby wipes
  - toy to keep the infant occupied
- nappy sack.

Procedure

1 Wash hands, put on gloves and apron (DH, 2003).
2 Use a changing table or changing mat placed on a surface at waist height. This prevents bending and back strain (Smith, 2005). Consider the infant's rolling ability when choosing a surface.
3 Have all equipment ready to hand; never leave an infant unattended, even for a brief moment.
4 Place the infant supine on the mat with the head turned to the right or left.
5 Open a clean nappy and set it aside in readiness.
6 Undo the tabs or pins of the dirty nappy. With disposable nappies, unfasten the tabs and fasten them back on themselves so they don't stick to the infant. Do not remove the dirty nappy yet – you still need it on so that you can finish the cleaning process. Cover a boy's penis with cotton wool or a wipe whilst cleansing to avoid getting splashed by unexpected urination.

7 Hold the infant's legs in one hand and pull the front of the nappy down with the other hand. If there is bowel movement in the nappy, use the front of the nappy to wipe most of the mess toward the back of the nappy. Folding under the dirty nappy and safe holding of the legs limit the spread of the excrement (Lijima and Ohzeki, 2006).
8 With the dirty nappy pressed flat under the baby, use cotton wool and warm water (for newborns) or wipes to gently cleanse the infant's nappy area.
9 Carefully and gently blot dry (DO NOT RUB) between skin folds and creases.
10 Lift the infant's legs and slide the dirty nappy out – set it away from the infant.
11 Place the clean nappy's top half under the infant's bottom and pull the other half up between the legs, which should be spread as widely as possible to ensure

comfort and avoid rashes (Kenner and Wright Lott, 2004). For boys, be sure to tuck the penis down so urine will flow down into the nappy instead of out of the top.

12 Secure the adhesive tabs or carefully pin the nappy corners snugly together. If using a cloth nappy, pin the nappy with your other hand between nappy and infant to avoid risk of a pinprick. Fasten the nappy snugly at both sides, but not so tightly that it pinches the infant's skin. You should be able to place at least two fingers between the nappy and the infant's abdomen.

13 Place the dirty nappy in the nappy sack and dispose of in a clinical waste bin (DH, 2003). Dispose of solid bowel movements in the sluice toilet before placing the diaper in the bin (DH, 2003). This helps decrease environmental odour.

14 Wash bowl with hot water and detergent, dry thoroughly with paper towels and store in a cool, dry area to prevent cross infection. Bacteria thrive in warm, moist and nutritious (dirty) environments (Campbell, 2006).

15 Remove gloves and apron and dispose of in clinical waste bin (DH, 2003).

16 Wash hands (DH, 2003).

17 Complete relevant documentation (NMC, 2008).

⚠ Professional alert!

A girl should be cleansed from front to back to avoid getting bacteria into the urethra (Chon, Frank and Shortliffe, 2001).

⟳ⓐ Learning activity   W

It is not unusual for infants to develop a thrush (candida infection) nappy rash after a course of antibiotics or an illness such as the common cold (see Figure 15.2). Go to the Department of Health website to research the advice they give: http://www.dh.gov.uk/en/Publicationsandstatistics/Publications/PublicationsPolicyAndGuidance/Browsable/DH_5289438.

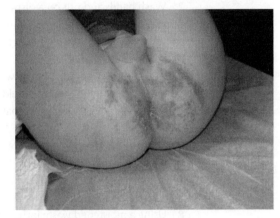

Figure 15.2 Nappy rash

Swaddling an infant

Swaddling infants, newborns in particular, gives them a sense of security, like the womb (Gavey, 2002). It often helps to comfort a distressed infant and can have a useful calming effect during procedures (Symington and Pinelli, 2003).

You will need a soft sheet or blanket.

Procedure

1 Wash your hands (DH, 2003).
2 Lay blanket or towel on a flat surface.
3 Fold one corner of blanket/towel down.
4 Lay the infant on the blanket with the head just above the fold. This keeps the face exposed.
5 Take right corner of blanket and gently wrap over infant's arm and tuck under opposite side.
6 Take bottom corner and fold upward over infant's feet and legs.
7 Take left corner of blanket and gently wrap over infant's arm and tuck around opposite side.

t★ Practice tip

Swaddling should be snug and secure, not loosely wrapped.

Giving a sponge bath

Sponge baths are required until the infant's umbilical cord falls off to prevent infection (DH, 2006). During any bathing an infant requires thermal protection since bathing can induce hypothermia through heat loss (Rudolf and Levene, 2006).

You will need:

- washcloth
- bowl with warm water (32–35 °C)
- soft hairbrush
- baby soap
- baby shampoo
- two towels
- plastic disposable apron
- non-sterile gloves
- nappy
- clothes.

Procedure

1 Ensure that the room is warm and that draughts are excluded by closing windows and doors for thermal protection before you begin.

2 Wash hands and put on a disposable apron (DH, 2003).

3 Have all of your supplies on hand so there is no temptation to leave the infant unattended at any time during the procedure (Lee and Thompson, 2007).

4 Check the temperature of the water in your bowl with the back of your hand or elbow. The water should feel neither hot nor cold (Young, 2004).

5 Lay the infant on a changing mat at a comfortable working height (hip height) (Smith, 2005).

6 Undress the infant and swaddle securely in a warm towel to prevent the infant from becoming cold (Lyon, 2004).

7 Use the dampened cloth with plain water only to wash the infant's face first (White and Denyer, 2006).

8 Using a moistened washcloth, begin to dampen the top of the infant's head. Place a tiny amount of baby shampoo on the washcloth and gently massage into the infant's hair. Rinse washcloth with clear warm water and wipe the soap from the infant's hair and head. Rinse and repeat to get all of the shampoo off the infant's scalp. Dry the infant's head with a towel.

9 Apply a small amount of a baby soap product to the washcloth and begin to gently work your way down the infant's body in sections. Pay special attention to creases under the arms, behind the ears, around the neck and, especially with a girl, in the genital area (White and Denyer, 2006). Rinse and dry as you go along to prevent the infant getting chilled.

10 Finally, put on gloves and cleanse the nappy area (DH, 2003).

11 Ensure that the infant is thoroughly dry. Lotions are not necessary. Furthermore, infant skin is extremely sensitive and the application of lotions may cause unnecessary discomfort due to skin reactions (Cowan and Frost, 2006).

12 Dispose of waste in a clinical waste bin (according to trust policy). Dispose of solid bowel movements in the sluice toilet before placing the diaper in the bin. This helps decrease environmental odour (Workman and Bennett, 2004).

13 Wash bowl with hot water and detergent, dry thoroughly with paper towels and store in a cool, dry area to prevent cross infection. Bacteria thrive in warm, moist and nutritious (dirty) environments (Marieb, 2004).

14 Remove gloves and apron and dispose of in a clinical waste bin (DH, 2003).

15 Wash hands (DH, 2003).

16 Complete relevant documentation (NMC, 2008).

t ☆
Practice tips

- Avoid sponge bathing immediately after a feed as there is a risk of inducing vomiting and discomfort (Lee and Thompson, 2007).
- Avoid eye area (see section on eye care below).
- Be sure to wash and dry thoroughly in all the infant's folds (neck, chin, behind ears) as these are areas where milk tends to collect.
- Avoid getting the umbilical cord wet (see separate section on cord care).

⚠ Professional alert!

Use this opportunity to assess not only the infant's skin condition but his/her overall behavioural response to care (DH, 2004).

Umbilical cord care

The umbilical stump represents a significant portal for infection (Furdon and Clark, 2002). Therefore, it is important to keep the stump clean so that it does not get infected (McConnell et al, 2004). The cord dries and falls off by a process known as dry gangrene usually by day 7 of life (see Figure 15.3).

You will need:

- non-sterile gloves
- disposable apron
- sterilised bowl
- cooled boiled water/ sterile water
- sterile gauze swabs
- waste bag
- changing mat.

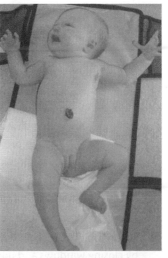

Practice tip

It is normal to see a few spots of blood or even a small discharge after the stump has fallen off. If however, the area around the belly button starts to look red and inflamed and the skin feels hot, then you should report these findings to a doctor (Anderson and Philips, 2004).

Procedure

1 Ensure that the room is warm and draught free so that the infant, particularly if newborn, does not get cold (Lyon, 2004).

2 Lie the infant supine on the changing mat and take off enough clothes to expose the cord stump but keep the infant warm (Chamley et al, 2006).

3 Dip gauze swab in sterile water/cooled boiled water and gently wipe around the stump (Zupan, Garner and Omari, 2004). Use a new piece of gauze or cotton bud each time to keep it as clean as possible (Breathnach, 2005) (see Figure 15.4). Do NOT rub or pull at the stump itself. Any of the black stump residue which remains should be left to fall off in time.

4 Once all the debris is cleaned away, use clean gauze to thoroughly dry the whole area (Worley, 2004).

5 Leave the stump exposed to the air as long as possible so that it can heal and fall off, a process known as dry gangrene (Zupan et al, 2004).

6 Report signs of inflammation (redness, oedema, tenderness, discharge) of the tissues surrounding the cord to a doctor immediately as these signs are indicative of omphalitis (WHO, 2008).

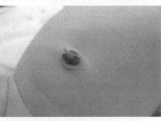

Figure 15.3 Healing the umbilical cord by the process known as dry gangrene

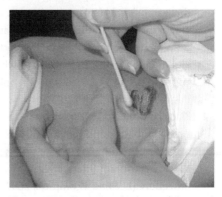

Figure 15.4 Cleansing the base of the cord

⚠ Professional alert!

Only cleanse the stump if clinically indicated by presence of debris (Zupan et al, 2004).

Giving a bath

Proper skin care and bathing helps maintain the health and texture of an infant's soft and delicate skin while providing a pleasant experience (Noonan, Quigley and Curley, 2006). Contrary to popular thought, most infants do not need a bath every single day. With all the nappy changes and wiping of mouth and nose after feedings, most infants only need to be bathed two or three times a week or every other day (DH, 2006). Bathing more frequently may lead to dry and irritated skin (Noonan et al, 2006). Current recommendations direct that infants, particularly in the neonatal period (first 28 days), should not be bathed routinely for thermal protection and not before the cord stump has fallen off (DH, 2006).

Part

II

You will need:

- washcloth
- infant soap product
- baby shampoo (tear-free formula)
- two towels
- bath with 5–8 cm deep warm water (32–35 °C)
- cotton balls
- clean nappy and clothing.

Procedure

1 Ensure that the room is warm and draughts are reduced by closing windows and doors; infants have a large surface area to body weight/volume ratio and therefore lose heat quickly (Chamley et al, 2005).

2 Wash hands and put on disposable apron (DH, 2003).

3 Fill the bath, paying attention to warmth, depth and moving, and handling. Fill the bath with the cold water turned on first (and off last) to avoid scalding yourself or the infant. The water should be comfortably warm, 32–35 °C, to prevent hypothermia or thermal injury (scalds) (Bull, 2007). It is recommended that the temperature of the water is tested by dipping your elbow in the water – the water should feel neither hot nor cold (Young, 2004). The bath depth should be approximately 5–8 cm to prevent accidental drowning (Lee and Thompson, 2007) and reduce the weight of the bath when carrying it to the appropriate surface. Ideally two people should undertake this manoeuvre (Smith, 2005).

4 Place bath on a stable surface at waist height, usually a table or bath stand (Smith, 2005). Ensure items to be used are near at hand so that there is no temptation to leave the infant unattended at any time during the procedure (Lee and Thompson, 2007).

5 Undress the infant and swaddle in a towel with only the face exposed. This helps to maintain the infant's body temperature and promotes comfort.

6 With the infant nursed on your lap, begin by cleansing the face, avoiding the eyes (eye care is undertaken separately and discussed later) with either a clean washcloth or cotton-wool balls and plain water from the bath. Soap is not recommended for use on infants' faces as their facial skin is particularly sensitive and prone to reaction (Cowan and Frost, 2006). Dry the face using a blotting as opposed to rubbing action (Suddaby, 2005).

7 If you wish to wash the infant's hair, expose the head only and hold the infant securely along your arm with the head supported in your hand. Gently dampen the infant's hair with water from the bath. Use your cupped free hand or a jug to help you do this. Avoid inadvertent splashing of the eyes.

8 Apply a small amount of baby shampoo, equivalent to no more than a 10-pence piece, to the infant's hair. Massage the scalp gently. Rinse the soap from the infant's hair and head. Rinse and repeat to get all of the shampoo off the scalp. Immediately, dry the infant's head with the towel as greatest heat loss is from the head, which represents one-third of the body surface area (Tortora, 2005).

9 Add baby bath if used as recommended by the manufacturer. Excess use causes the skin to dry out and may irritate the skin, causing or exacerbating eczema (Cowan and Frost, 2006).

10 Undress the infant from the towel, holding the infant securely with one arm under the shoulders and holding the far arm, with the other hand supporting the infant and holding the far thigh. Whilst speaking encouragingly, lower the infant gently into the water feet first and gently lower the rest of the body into the bath. Most of the body and face should be well above the water level for safety (Lee and Thompson, 2007) (see Figure 15.5). This manoeuvre reduces the risk of accidentally dropping or causing injury to the infant.

11 Cup water gently over the infant with your hand, doing so frequently to keep the infant warm. Wash the infant, paying special attention to creases under the arms, behind the ears, around the neck, and, especially with a girl, in the genital area (Samaniego, 2003). Have fun, but avoid splashing the floor as a wet floor poses a safety hazard (Hilton, 2004). Be mindful of the infant's body temperature and the time spent in the bath for thermal protection (DH, 2006).

12 An infant is very slippery when wet and mobile so, using the same procedure as above, gently lift the infant out of the bath and onto a towel in your lap (Lee and Thompson, 2007). See Figure 15.6.

13 Carefully dry the infant, paying particular attention to skin creases (back of neck, armpits, groins) to

prevent soreness (Samaniego, 2003). Dress the infant as appropriate and settle in a cot.

14 Ideally two people should carry the bath to a sink (Smith, 2005) and safely empty it of water.

15 Clean the bath with water and detergent, dry thoroughly with paper towels, and store in a cool, dry area to prevent cross infection. Bacteria thrive in warm, moist and nutritious (dirty) environments (Jamieson, McCall and Whyte, 2002).

16 Dispose of clinical waste and apron appropriately. Wash hands (DH, 2003).

17 Document procedure and any observations made, for example condition of infant's skin and reaction to the bathing experience (NMC 2008; DH, 2004).

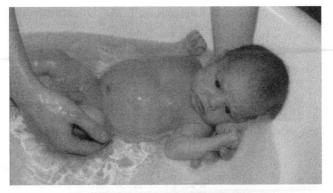

Figure 15.5 Holding the infant securely in a bath

(a) Learning activity   W

For simple video instruction on how to bathe and thoroughly dry an infant, and change a nappy, go to the following website http://uk.youtube.com/watch?v=8ayFXfY890E and http://uk.youtube.com/watch?v=I96Snk9jy_c&feature=related

⚠ Professional alert!

Talcum powders should be avoided as there is a potential risk of aspiration (DH, 2006). However, if a parent specifically requests it, apply it safely as follows: put the powder in your hand and then apply it to the infant's skin. Shaking powder into the air releases dust and talc which can make it hard for the infant to breathe.

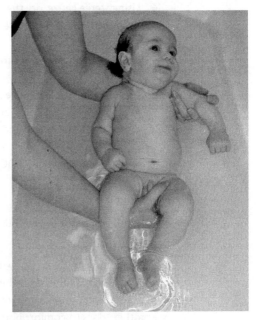

Figure 15.6 Safe handling of the infant in and out of a bath

Eye care

Mild ophthalmia, frequently referred to as 'sticky eye', is especially common in the early neonatal period. In the first few weeks of life an infant does not secrete tears, which are protective and usually prevent contamination of the eyes (Lissauer and Fanaroff, 2006). In this early period the infant is at risk of contamination of the eyes through dust and bacteria. Other predisposing factors include prematurity and/or illness, which lower an infant's resistance to infection (McGuire and Fowlie, 2005). The term 'ophthalmia neonatorum' is used to describe inflammation (redness and discharge) of the eyes of an infant within 28 days of birth. This is often due to chemical irritation caused by use of chemically irritant shampoos, wipes, lotions or soaps, and usually clears spontaneously (Johnson, Flood and Spinks, 2002).

t☆ Practice tip

Only perform eye care when clinically indicated: that is, when the eyes are 'sticky'. Eye care itself has the potential to introduce infection to the eyes (although the risk is small if eye care is carried out properly).

Part

II

You will need:

- non-sterile gloves
- apron
- cooled boiled/sterile water
- eye pack containing sterile galipot and sterile gauze (or equivalent)
- waste bag.

Procedure

1 Wash your hands and put on non-sterile gloves and apron (DH, 2003).
2 Swaddle the infant for security (Fern, Graves and L'Huiller, 2002).
3 Using cooled boiled or sterile water, moisten the sterile gauze and cleanse in a single sweep action, starting from the bridge of the nose and gently wiping outwards towards the ear (Mandell, Bennett and Dolin, 2004). Repeat this action with a fresh piece of gauze until the area around the eye is clean.
4 Using sterile gauze, dry the eye with the same action, using a single sweep action starting from the bridge of the nose and gently wiping outwards towards the ear (see learning activity below).
5 Repeat this process four times daily or until the eye improves.
6 Dispose of all clinical waste as appropriate (DH, 2003).
7 Remove gloves and apron and dispose of in a clinical waste receptacle. Wash your hands (DH, 2003).
8 Document the procedure, any observations made and the infant's response to it (NMC, 2008).

⚠ Professional alert!

If the 'sticky eye' does not improve or if redness is noted:

- Take a swab for microscopy culture and sensitivity.
- Inform the doctor.

⟳ⓐ Learning activity

Cleansing a sticky eye
Tom, pictured right is clearly distressed during this procedure, as evidenced by his facial expression, crying and leg extension. What might you recommend that Hayley, his mother, does to comfort him during this procedure?

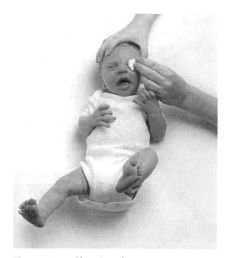

Figure 15.7 Cleaning the eye

Mouth care

Typically, we do not think of cavities or gum disease in connection with infants. But in fact, oral diseases begin very early, from the time bacteria begin to live in the oral cavity. As new teeth erupt and the diet of the infant becomes more sophisticated, bacteria continue to produce acids and toxins that are harmful to hard and soft tissues in the mouth. The nurse must endorse appropriate use of topical and systemic fluoride (BDHF, 2005) and provide and promote early vigilant preventive oral hygiene for the infant.

t☆ Practice tips

- You might find it useful to swaddle the infant to keep helpful little hands out of the way until you feel confident (Fern et al, 2002).
- Toothpaste use itself reduces the bacterial contamination of toothbrushes. But ensure toothbrushes are replaced every month to maintain the health of the bristle fibres (Efstratiou et al, 2007).
- Use this health promotion opportunity to educate parents and siblings about oral care (NMC, 2008).

You will need:
- non-sterile gloves
- apron
- small, soft toothbrush
- fluoride toothpaste
- cup with cooled boiled water/sterile water
- damp clean washcloth.

> ⚠ **Professional alert!**
>
> Even before an infant has teeth, after feeding wipe out baby's mouth with warm washcloth or gauze.

Procedure

1 Provide privacy.
2 Wash hands and put on gloves and apron before providing personal care. Use standard precautions (DH, 2003).
3 Sit with the infant on your lap, with their back against your front at a 45° angle, whist supporting the infant's head by cradling the chin in your hand to prevent choking, enabling you to reach their top and bottom teeth more easily (Selwitz, Ismail and Pitts, 2007).
4 Put a towel or a protective cover over the infant's clothing to ensure that it is kept clean and dry.
5 Wet the toothbrush with water and apply a dab of fluoride toothpaste about 0.5 cm long onto the centre of a small soft toothbrush (Douglass, Douglass and Silk, 2004). Talk encouragingly to the infant about what you are about to do. You may need to raise the top lip or lower lip with your fingers of your non-dominant hand to expose the teeth.
6 Whilst talking encouragingly to the infant about what you are doing, brush the teeth in small circular motions, a section at a time, focusing on the junction between the gingiva and the teeth. Gently brush all surfaces of the teeth, gums, tongue and cheeks (BDHF, 2005). Allow the infant to spit out excess toothpaste, or wipe it away with a clean washcloth. Rinsing is discouraged because

residual fluoride toothpaste on the teeth helps prevent caries (Selwitz et al, 2007).
7 Clean and dry the skin areas around the mouth as fluoride residue may irritate the skin (Hampton and Collins, 2003).
8 Rinse the toothbrush thoroughly under a running tap of potable (drinking) water and store in a dry environment at room temperature (Efstratiou et al, 2007). Clean or dispose of all other equipment as appropriate (DH, 2003).
9 Remove gloves and apron and dispose of in a clinical waste receptacle. Wash your hands (DH, 2003).
10 Document the procedure, any observations made and the infant's response to it (NMC, 2008).

> ⚠ **Professional alert!**
>
> The following observations must be reported (Selwitz et al, 2007):
> - sores, redness or bleeding of the mouth, on the gums, cheeks or lips
> - pain during mouth care
> - coating of the tongue or cheeks, for example thrush
> - loose or broken teeth
> - bad breath.

When brushing the sides of teeth, tilt the brush so that the bristles come in at an angle, pointed partially toward the gums (Figure 15.8). This will allow the bristles to clean the tooth all the way down to the gums. Use gentle pressure and a circular motion, since the area where the tooth meets the gum is rounded.

Once the back teeth start to come in, you may need to pull the lips and cheeks back to reach all of the areas of the teeth.

Be sure to clean the chewing surfaces of back teeth also. The fissures (grooves) on these surfaces are best cleaned with a scrubbing motion.

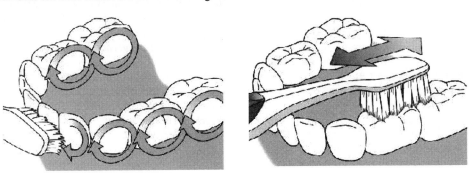

Figure 15.8
Brushing teeth

Reprinted with permission of Suzanne Cobb.

Part
II

C Professional conversation

Kate, Tom's community health nurse, says, 'I visited Tom and his mum, Hayley, at 8 months of age, soon after the eruption of his first tooth. Hayley asked me how she could best help his teething. I was able to give her some practical guidance relating to Tom's teething, and took this opportunity to discuss his dental health needs. In brief, I explained that tooth decay is the most common disease of childhood. It is five times as common as asthma and seven times as common as hay fever (BDHF, 2005).

- Oral flora colonise the mouth soon after birth.
- It is a myth that cariogenic bacteria colonise only after the tooth erupt.
- Tooth decay can begin as soon as the teeth erupt at 6–10 months of age.
- Tooth decay bacteria are transmitted from parents or other primary caregivers to the infant through fingers, shared eating utensils, cleaning a dummy with mother's saliva and so on.
- Tooth brushing should begin with the eruption of the first tooth.'

Conclusion

Infants who are clean and well cared for will benefit from a healthier beginning to life (Parker, 2004). Healthcare staff, particularly nurses, are often in a position to ensure these vital needs are met in a safe environment. A cookbook will not make you a great cook, and no book or chapter in a book will make you a great infant care nurse. But every cook starts out with a few basic recipes and techniques to which they add with further education, training and experience. This chapter has put forward guidance on just some of the clinically relevant skills that you are likely to use every day to ensure infant hygiene. Put simply, this chapter has sought to promote infant health through effective hygiene

References

Anderson, J. D. M. and Philips, A. G. S. (2004) 'Management of the umbilical cord: care regimes, colonisation, infection and separation', *Neonatal Reviews* 5(4), 155–9.

Breathnach, A. S. (2005) 'Nosocomial infections', *Medicine* 33(3), 22–26.

British Dental Health Foundation (BDHF) (2005) *Children's Teeth*, London, BDHF [online] http://www.dentalhealth.org.uk (accessed 9 February 2009).

Bull, L. (2007) 'A study of accident and emergency department attendances by infants under 1 in London: an epidemiology study', *Journal of Neonatal Nursing* 13(i), 19–23.

Campbell, J. (2006) *Campbell's Physiology Notes for Nurses*, London, Whurr Publishing.

Chamley, C. A., Carson, P., Randall, D. and Sandwell, M. (2005) *Developmental Anatomy and Physiology of Children: a practical approach*, Edinburgh, Elsevier and Churchill Livingstone.

Chon, D. H., Frank, C. L. and Shortliffe, L. M. (2001) 'Pediatric urinary tract infections', *Pediatric Clinics of North America* 48, 1441–59.

Cowan, M. E. and Frost, M. R. (2006) 'A comparison between a detergent baby bath additive and baby soap on the skin flora of neonates', *Journal of Hospital Infection* 7, 91–5.

Darmstadt, G. L. and Dinulos, J. G. (2000) 'Neonatal skin care', *Pediatric Clinics of North America* 47(4), 757–82.

Department of Health (DH) (2003) *Winning Ways: Working together to reduce healthcare associated infection in England*, London, DH.

DH (2004) *National Service Framework for Children, Young People and Maternity Services*, London, DH.

DH (2006) *Birth to Five*, London, DH.

Douglass, J. M., Douglass, A. B. and Silk, H. J. (2004) 'A practical guide to infant oral health', *American Family Physician* 70, 2113–22.

Efstratiou, M., Papaioannou, W., Nakou, M., Ktenas, E., Vrotsos, I. A. and Panis, V. (2007) 'Contamination of a toothbrush with antibacterial properties by oral micro-organisms', *Journal of Dentistry* 35(4), 331–7.

Fern, D., Graves, C. and L'Huiller, M. (2002) 'Swaddling the newborn', *Newborn and Infant Nursing Reviews* 2(1), 3–8.

Furdon, S. A. and Clark, D. A. (2002) 'Assessment of the umbilical cord outside the delivery room', *Advances in Neonatal Care* 2(4), 187–97.

Gavey, H. B. (2002) 'Responding to babies' needs through holistic care', *Nursing Standard* 16(21), 33–7.

Hampton, S. and Collins, F. (2003) *Tissue Viability: a comprehensive guide*, London, Whurr Publishing.

Harold, S. K., Tamura, T. and Colton, K. (2003) 'Reported level of supervision of young children while in the bathtub', *Ambulatory Pediatrics* 3(2), 106–8.

Hilton, P. (2004) *Fundamental Nursing Skills*, London, Whurr Publishing.

Jamieson, E. M., McCall, J. M. and Whyte, L. A. (2002) *Clinical Nursing Practice*, 4th edn, Edinburgh, Churchill Livingstone.

Johnson, P., Flood, K. and Spinks, K. (2002) *The Newborn Child*, 9th edn, London, Elsevier.

Kenner, C. and Wright Lott, J. (2004) *Neonatal Nursing Handbook*, St. Louis, Miss., Saunders.

Lee, L. K. and Thompson, K. M. (2007) 'Parental survey of beliefs and practices about bathing and water safety and their children: guidance for drowning prevention', *Accident Analysis and Prevention* 39, 58–62.

Lijima, S. and Ohzeki, T. (2006) 'Bacterial contamination on the hands of nursing staff in the most basic neonatal care', *Journal of Neonatal Nursing* 12, 53–8.

Lissauer, T. and Fanaroff, A. (2006) *Neonatology at a Glance*, Oxford, Blackwell.

Lyon, A. (2004) 'Applied physiology: temperature control in the newborn infant', *Current Paediatrics* 14, 137–44.

Mandell, G. I., Bennett, J. E. and Dolin, R. (2004) *Principles and Practice of Infectious Diseases*, 6th edn, London, Churchill Livingstone.

McGuire, W. and Fowlie, P. W. (2005) *ABC of Preterm Birth*, Oxford, BMJ Publishing.

Marieb, E. N. (2004) *Human Anatomy and Physiology*, 6th edn, San Francisco, Addison-Wesley.

McConnell, T. P., Lee, C.W., Couillard, M. and Sherrill, W.W. (2004) 'Trends in umbilical cord care: scientific evidence for practice', *Newborn and Infant Nursing Reviews* 4(4), 211–22.

McManus, J. (2001) 'Skin breakdown: risk factors, prevention and treatment', *Newborn and Infant Nursing Reviews* 1(1), 35–42.

Noonan, C., Quigley, S. and Curley, M. A. Q. (2006) 'Skin integrity in hospitalised infants and children: a prevalence survey', *Journal of Pediatric Nursing* 21(6), 445–53.

Nursing and Midwifery Council (NMC) (2008) *Code of Professional Conduct*, London, NMC.

Parker, L. (2004) 'Infection control: maintaining the personal hygiene of patients and staff', *British Journal of Nursing*, **13**(8), 474–8 [online] http://www.internurse.com/cgi-bin/go.pl/library/article.cgi?uid=127 86;article=BJN_13_8_474_478 (accessed 9 February 2009).

Roberts, S. (2008) 'Meeting the personal hygiene needs of the hospitalised child', *British Journal of Healthcare Assistants* 2(5), 214–16

Rudolf, M. and Levene, M. (2006) *Paediatrics and Child Health*, 2nd edn, Oxford, Blackwell.

Samaniego, I. A. (2003) 'A sore spot in pediatrics: risk factors for pressure ulcers', *Pediatric Nursing* 29(4), 278–82.

Selwitz, R. H., Ismail, A. I. and Pitts, N. B. (2007) 'Dental caries', *The Lancet* 369, 52–8.

Smith, J. (2005) *The Guide to the Manual Handling of People*, 5th edn, London, Backcare.

Suddaby, E. C. (2005) 'Skin breakdown in acute care pediatrics', *Pediatric Nursing* 31(2), 132–48.

Symington, A. and Pinelli, J. (2003) 'Developmental care for promoting development and preventing morbidity in preterm infants (Cochrane Review)', *Cochrane Database Systematic Review* 4, Article No. CD001814.

Tortora, G. J. (2005) *Principles of Human Anatomy*, 10th edn, Danvers, Wiley.

Trotter, S. (2003) 'Management of the umbilical cord: a guide to best care', *RCM Midwives Journal* 6(7), 308–11 [online] http://www. sharontrotter.org.uk/rcm2003new.htm (accessed 9 February 2009).

White, R. and Denyer, J. (2006) *Paediatric Skin and Wound Care*, Aberdeen, Wounds UK.

World Health Organisation (WHO) (2008) *Care of the umbilical cord: a review of the evidence*, Geneva, WHO [online] www.who.int/rht/ documents/MSM98-4/MSM-98-4.htm (accessed 9 February 2009).

Worley, C. (2004) 'Quality of life – part 1: Using the holistic caring praxis in skin and wound care', *Dermatology Nursing* 16(6), 527–8.

Workman, B. A. and Bennett, C. L. (2003) *Key Nursing Skills*, London, Whurr Publishers.

Young, A. E. (2004) 'The management of severe burns in children', *Current Paediatrics* 14, 202–7.

Zupan, J., Garner, P. and Omari, A. A. A. (2004) 'Topical umbilical cord care at birth', *Cochrane Database of Systematic Reviews* 3, Article No. CD001057. DOI: 10. 1002/14651858. CD001057.pub2.

Part

II

Skills for physiological assessment

Part III

Chapters

Chapter
16

Vital signs

Pam Diggens

 Links to other chapters in *Foundation Skills for Caring*

 Links to other chapters in *Foundation Studies for Caring*

 Don't forget to visit www.palgrave.com/glasper for additional online resources relating to this chapter.

Part
III

Introduction

The aim of this chapter is to enable you to develop knowledge and understanding of the techniques required in taking and recording a patient's temperature, pulse and respiration rate. Together with blood pressure these are considered the vital signs. The measurement of these vital functions provides important information regarding the health status of the patient and allows efficient monitoring of their condition. The use of appropriate sites, methods and equipment is important in order to gain accurate readings.

Learning outcomes

This chapter will enable you to:

- describe the procedure for assessing patients' vital signs, using evidence-based reasons
- discuss factors that can influence a person's temperature pulse and respirations, supporting this with relevant evidence

- identify and provide a rationale, using an evidence-based approach in your selection of equipment and sites to assess these vital signs
- identify reasons to undertake patient's temperature, pulse and respirations.

Concepts

- Equipment selection
- Body sites

- Normal values
- Factors that affect vital signs

- Regulation of vital signs

Temperature, pulse and respirations (TPR)

Measurements of a patient's temperature, pulse and respirations are techniques that you may find are collectively referred to as 'observations' or 'vital signs'. There is debate about using these terms interchangeably, since it is argued that taking patients' observations requires more than just performing one of the above techniques (Joanna Briggs Institute, 1999). The term vital signs traditionally refers to taking patients temperature, pulse, respirations and blood pressure (BP) (Castledine, 2006) and will be the focus of this chapter, as opposed to observations.

> Monitoring vital signs is often viewed as one of the more mundane aspects of nursing care, and is frequently devolved to healthcare assistants and nursing students. However, their immense value in patient care should not be overlooked.
>
> (Davidson and Barber, 2004: 42)

Consent

You need to ensure that you gain consent from patients prior to undertaking these techniques. This will require you to explain why you need to take their temperature, pulse and respirations and what is involved, so that patients have all the information necessary in order to give their consent (NMC, 2004). Read Chapter 1 for more information.

Temperature regulation

In normal health, irrespective of the body's external environment, the human body is able to constantly maintain its temperature between 35.8 °C and 38.2 °C, with an average temperature of 37 °C plus or minus 0.5 °C. This is achieved by the body's temperature control centre in the hypothalamus, which constantly maintains homeostasis by balancing the amount of heat lost with the amount of heat produced. There are several physiological mechanisms that aid heat production, including vasoconstriction, sympathetic nerve stimulation, skeletal muscle activity and the secretion of thyroid hormones. Heat loss also occurs in several ways:

conduction/convection, radiation and evaporation (Marini and Wheeler, 2006; Marieb and Hoehn, 2007).

The control centre is extremely sensitive to slight changes in temperature which are detected by receptors in the body. These receptors transmit impulses to the hypothalamus so that adjustments can be made to maintain homeostasis. Peripheral thermoreceptors are located in the skin and mucous membranes, whilst central thermoreceptors are located in blood vessels and internal structures. There are two centres, one for heat loss and the other for heat production. The hypothalamus acts as a sensor which activates either one of these centres in response to impulses from the thermoreceptors (Marieb and Hoehn, 2007; Marieb, 2004).

When thermoreceptors detect a rise in body temperature they send impulses to the hypothalamus, which activates the heat loss control centre. This centre then causes peripheral blood vessels to dilate, resulting in an increased volume of blood flowing through them. This enables more heat to be lost though the skin, a mechanism known as radiation. Additionally, sweat glands are activated to increase perspiration, also causing heat to be lost from the body. The overall effect is for the temperature to decrease.

Conversely, if body temperature is detected as being too low then thermoreceptors transmit this information to the hypothalamus. This time the hypothalamus activates the heat production control centre to conserve heat. This occurs by blood vessels constricting to reduce the amount of blood flowing through them, thus preventing further heat loss through the skin. Shivering also occurs as this increases skeletal muscle activity, which produces heat. This all contributes to increasing body temperature.

If the body's responses are insufficient to maintain homeostasis and energy reserves are utilised, the body can become exhausted and hypothermia may become life threatening. This can occur very rapidly.

Abnormal temperature

It is important to recognise any abnormal values in order to ensure they are reported to a qualified nurse. When a patient's temperature is lower than 35 °C the condition is termed hypothermia. This can be fatal if not treated, and younger children and elderly people may be more susceptible to this. There are three classifications of hypothermia, graded according to the patient's temperature, see Table 16.1 (Carlson, 2009). A lower temperature causes a slower metabolic rate and cellular activity. Patients with hypothermia may have decreased vital signs as their metabolic rate and cellular activity decrease (Marieb and Hoehn, 2007).

Table 16.1 Classification of hypothermia

Classification of hypothermia	Temperature range
Mild hypothermia	32 °C–35 °C
Moderate hypothermia	28 °C–32 °C
Severe hypothermia	25 °C–28 °C

Source: Carlson (2009).

The term hyperthermia refers to an elevated body temperature which is higher than the normal range. An increased temperature affects metabolism by increasing the body's metabolic rate. This in turn causes an increase in heat production. If untreated it can lead to heat stroke, which can be fatal, so it is vital that a higher than normal temperature is reported and action taken. It is important to understand that patients who have a fever will also have an elevated temperature, often as a result of infection, which is known as referred hyperthermia. This means that the body attempts to fight the infection by resetting the temperature sensor in the hypothalamus to a higher setting (Marieb and Hoehn, 2007). However, it must be remembered that there may be other causes for this.

a Learning activity

How might a patient look and feel who has a temperature higher than the normal range? Compare this with a patient who has a lower than normal temperature.

Factors that affect temperature

There are several factors that can affect daily fluctuations in body temperature. These are: the circadian rhythm, age, exercise, food/drink intake, hormones, drugs/medication, stress, ovulation and exposure to environmental extremes in temperature.

Generally, in health, a person's temperature fluctuates throughout the day; this is known as the circadian rhythm. A person's temperature often rises during the evening and is lower during the early hours of the morning (Marieb and Hoehn, 2007). As people age they become more sensitive to extremely hot or cold environments which can affect body temperature. Hormones can affect our body temperature; for example, women's temperatures can be raised during ovulation. During exercise, muscle activity and metabolic rate increase, causing the production of heat which will increase body temperature. Various medications can also affect temperature; for instance Paracetamol reduces temperature. Stress can have an impact on our nervous, immune and endocrine systems, and hence body temperature, due to increased action from the autonomic nervous system. Hot and cold food and drink may also affect our temperature, and it is important to allow sufficient time after meals and drinks before taking a patient's temperature. Environmental climates where individuals may be exposed to extreme temperature conditions may result in individuals developing heat stroke or hypothermia. Infants/children and elderly people may be more susceptible to climatic changes (Perry and Potter, 2002).

a Learning activity

Consider how the following two patients' temperature might be affected:
- an elderly patient who has been sitting near an open window on a cold winter's day
- a young adult patient admitted with a chest infection.

Recommended body sites for taking temperature

Despite debate concerning site used and variation in temperature at different sites (Woodrow, 2006a), the four main sites of the body where it is generally recommended to take a person's temperature are: oral, axilla, tympanic and rectum (Dobbins, Adams and Hewson, 2004). Ideally, to determine which site is most appropriate you should assess patients individually. However, depending upon the type of thermometers available in your clinical area you may have limited choice (NICE, 2007).

Types of thermometer

Although there are now numerous types of thermometer available (Woodrow et al, 2006), the ones most commonly used are digital, electronic and various chemical strips. The choice of the most appropriate thermometer will vary depending upon the patient's condition and what types of thermometers are available in your clinical area of practice. Evidence remains inconclusive regarding which type of thermometer to use (Woodrow et al, 2006).

There are a variety of temperature-sensitive, chemical liquid crystal strips which you place on the individual's forehead; however their accuracy and recording range is limited (Marini and Wheeler, 2006). This type of strip can be reused but may have a lower accuracy level. Additionally, some chemical strips can be placed orally or axillary and are intended for single use only (Crawford, Hicks and Thompson, 2006), minimising the risk of cross-infection. The Tempa-dot thermometer is an example of a chemical thermometer with a specific temperature range; therefore it may not detect temperatures outside this (Stanhope, 2006).

Tables 16.2 to 16.5 provide information to assist you in making an appropriate choice of site and thermometer. These are only guidelines and if you are in any doubt seek advice from your mentor or qualified nurse.

Table 16.2   **Taking temperature orally**

Not routinely recommended in children under 5 years (NICE, 2007).

Advantages	Disadvantages
Close to the receptors that quickly detect rapid changes in temperature (thermoreceptors), so changes are detected quicker here.	Affected by temperature of food or drink recently taken by patients.
Quick and easy site to take temperature from.	Has to be in correct position under the tongue to be accurate.
Records temperature quickly.	Not appropriate for patients having difficulties breathing or unprotected airways, or who cannot tolerate an oral thermometer.
	Not routinely recommended for infants.

Table 16.3   **Taking temperature rectally**

Not routinely recommended in children under 5 years (NICE, 2007).

Advantages	Disadvantages
Most accurate site (needs to be inserted at least 3.5 cm into rectum).	More uncomfortable, embarrassing and invasive for patients.
	More time-consuming.
	Faeces in rectum may produce false measurement.

Table 16.4   **Taking temperature axillary**

Advantages	Disadvantages
Suitable for patients who have difficulties breathing, unprotected airway or cannot tolerate an oral thermometer.	Not as close to major blood vessels, therefore a less accurate and reliable measurement.
	Skin surface temperature varies more with temperature changes of environment.
	Can be uncomfortable for patients with restricted mobility of arm/shoulder joints and therefore difficult to keep in place.

Table 16.5   **Taking temperature tympanically**

Advantages	Disadvantages
Less invasive	Technique can be difficult to master
Simple to use	Poor technique can produce inaccurate measurement
Comfortable for patient	
Records temperature quickly	

Taking a patient's temperature

Irrespective of thermometer type used, where possible and in accordance with the manufacturer's operator manuals, place a disposable cover on the thermometer's probe to minimise the risk of cross-infection. Cutter (1994) observes that inadequately cleansed thermometers are a risk and need to be cleaned, even when they have plastic sheaths. Once you have selected the appropriate site, ensure the thermometer stays inserted or in place for the specified duration according to the operator's manual to provide an accurate measurement. Dispose of the probe or plastic strip in the correct manner (NICE, 2003) in accordance with your clinical area's cross-infection and prevention, health and safety protocols. Ensure your patient is always left in a dignified and comfortable position. Correctly record the measurement on relevant charts or documentation (NMC, 2002) and if there are any abnormalities report them to a qualified member of staff.

Procedure for taking an oral temperature

Place the thermometer in the patient's mouth. Ensure it is in either the right or left posterior sublingunial pocket as this is more sensitive to changes and hence a more accurate site (Nicoll, 2002).

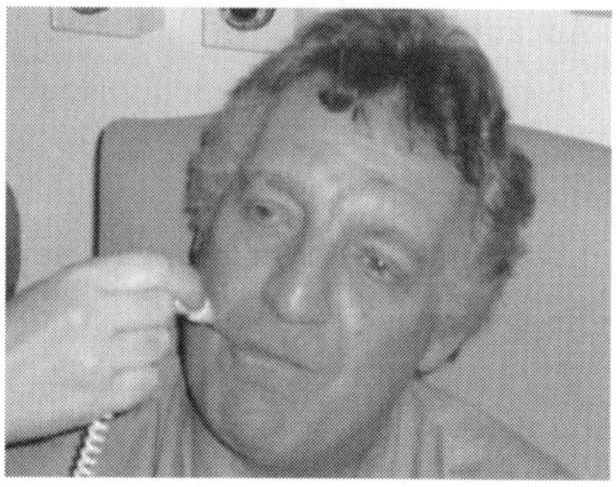

Procedure for taking a rectal temperature

To provide a more accurate measurement insert at least 3.5 cm of the thermometer into the rectum (Perry and Potter, 2002).

⚠ Professional alert!

The rectal method should not be routinely used in children under 5 years of age due to risk of trauma (NICE, 2007).

Procedure for taking an axilla temperature

Place the thermometer under the armpit in the centre. Get the patient to place their arm firmly against the thermometer to ensure it is central, and enable a more accurate measurement.

Consider if the patient is sweating: does this make a difference?

Procedure for taking a tympanic temperature

Ensure the patient's head is stabilised to prevent the probe being inserted too far, which can cause discomfort or trauma. Consider asking the patient to relax their head back onto a pillow if sitting in a chair. This helps stabilisation and can increase the patient's comfort.

For adults, place the tip of the probe into the auditory canal by firmly but gently pulling the ear (pinna) up and back (Figure 16.2). This straightens the canal so that the infrared sensor is lined up on the ear drum (Jarvis, 2004).

⚠ Professional alert!

The circadian rhythm will affect body temperature, which can be at its highest in the evening. You may need to take this into account when taking a patient's temperature (Carroll, 2000).

Figure 16.1 Taking an oral temperature

t☆ Practice tip

To provide consistency always try to obtain subsequent measurements from the same site and side (Holtzclaw, 1990).

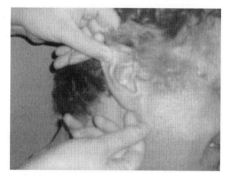

Figure 16.2 Pulling the ear (pinna) up and back

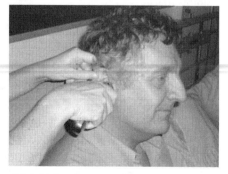

Figure 16.3 Insertion of tympanic thermometer

⟲a Learning activity

Consider what type of thermometer and site you would use to obtain a temperature measurement in each of these situations:
- an unconscious adult admitted with hypothermia
- a breathless patient with a respiratory problem
- a patient with an ear infection.

Regulation of heart rate

Although there are other factors that can influence heart rate, the body's main regulator is the autonomic nervous system. This is composed of two divisions; the sympathetic and parasympathetic nervous systems. Each system causes a different response on the rate of the heart by transmitting impulses to the sinoatrial (SA) node, a mass of minute cells located in the heart's right atrium. The SA node has the ability to generate impulses inherently, which is why it is often termed the heart's 'pacemaker'.

Impulses are transmitted continuously from both systems to the SA node. The parasympathetic system transmits impulses which have an inhibitory effect on heart rate, consequently slowing it down. Conversely, the sympathetic system has an excitory effect and therefore speeds the heart rate up. An average resting heart rate in a healthy adult is about 78 beats per minute (bpm), which is lower than the SA node's inherent ability to generate about 100 impulses per minute. This is attributed to the parasympathetic system having a greater influence on the heart rate than the sympathetic system. The parasympathetic system is therefore more dominant.

Factors that affect heart rate

There are various physical, neural and chemical factors that affect the heart rate and consequently the pulse rate (Marieb, 2004). Some of the physiological factors that can affect pulse rate include age, gender, exercise and temperature (Perry and Potter, 2002; Marieb, 2004)

As we get older our heart rate (and hence pulse) slows (Marieb, 2004) so it is important to recognise that the range for normal heart rate will depend upon the patient's age. Generally, males' pulse rates are lower than females' (Jarvis, 2004). Exercise also causes the sympathetic nervous system to increase the heart rate, which consequently increases the pulse rate. It is also useful to recognise that a patient's temperature can affect the pulse rate; in cold conditions heart and pulse rate are decreased (Marieb, 2004).

Pulse

As the heart beats, blood forced into the aorta causes arterial pressure to increase, resulting in expansion of arterial blood vessel walls. As arterial pressure falls, the arterial walls contract. This continual expansion and contraction can be palpated (felt) and is referred to as the pulse. In general, it is an accurate reflection of heart rate (Perry and Potter, 2002; Marieb and Hoehn, 2007; Jarvis, 2004). When we palpate a pulse, there are important features to determine when monitoring this vital sign; these are rate, rhythm and amplitude (Massey, 2006).

- *Rate*: refers to the number of beats palpated in one minute and reflects the rate (speed) at which the heart is beating. Normal rate is 60–100 bpm for an adult (Jarvis, 2004; Marieb and Hoehn, 2007). Tachycardia is a term used when the heart rate and hence pulse rate is greater than 100 bpm; conversely a rate slower than 60 bpm is referred to as bradycardia (Marieb, 2004).
- *Rhythm*: a regular (normal) pulse has an equal interval of time between each pulse. The rhythm may be regular or irregular. Irrespective of this, the pulse rate should always be palpated for one full minute (Castledine, 2006). Irregular beats when palpated will feel random rather than having equal time between them. In some patients, the pulse may be felt as having a pattern of irregular beats. This is then referred to as regularly irregular. This differs from irregular pulsations, although it is irregular. As well as informing a qualified nurse, if the pulse is irregular remember to write 'irregular' on the observation chart, and if necessary document the patient's notes. Further investigations, such as an electrocardiogram may be necessary to establish what type of heart rhythm it is.
- *Amplitude (strength)*: reflects the strength of beats. It is determined by palpating the pulse and noticing if it feels strong, weak or normal (Massey, 2006). When palpating a normal

Part

III

pulse, apply a moderate amount of pressure in order to feel it. However, be careful as too much pressure applied will obliterate the pulse so it will not be felt. A weak pulse will be more difficult to feel as it is easily obliterated when applying minimal to moderate pressure. In comparison, a bounding pulse is very forceful and is not easily obliterated when pressure is applied (Marieb and Hoehn, 2007)

It is important to recognise changes in amplitude, as this provides information about individuals' health. However, this is a difficult technique as some changes in amplitude are much harder to identify than others. Therefore it will take time and practice to gain the clinical experience required to identify differences in amplitude.

Body sites where arterial pulse can be palpated (felt)

There are various other sites where you can palpate an artery to obtain a pulse: apical, carotid, temporal, brachial, radial, femoral, popliteal, posterior tibial and dorsalis pedis (Perry and Potter, 2002). The most commonly used site for taking a patient's pulse is at the radial artery (Massey, 2006). In emergency situations the pulse may be more difficult to palpate at the radial site, and then the carotid or femoral are often used.

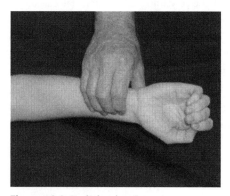

Figure 16.4 Radial pulse site

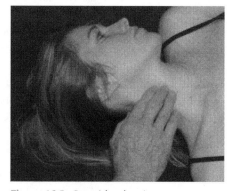

Figure 16.5 Carotid pulse site

Dorsalis pedis   Femoral   Posterior tibia

Popliteal   Temporal   Carotid

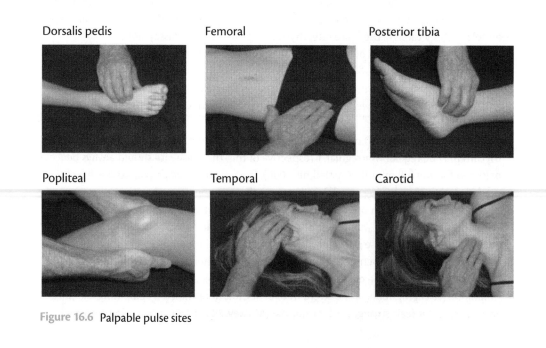

Figure 16.6 Palpable pulse sites

Taking a radial pulse

1   Use the fingertips (not pads) of your first two or three fingers as these are more sensitive (Massey, 2006).

2   Locate the radial bone, then move fingertips slightly down away from the bone. The radial artery is palpated more easily near the bone.

3   Press gently against the radial artery and palpate the radial pulse. Too much pressure can obliterate the pulse from being palpated (Perry and Potter, 2002).

4   Count the number of beats palpated for 60 seconds (Castledine, 2006) as this provides time to detect any abnormalities.

5   Record pulse measurement correctly on appropriate chart; remember to state on chart if pulse is irregular and which site was used. The chart enables a record to be made of measurements obtained, which will provide information to detect trends and gather information about any abnormalities.

⚠ **Professional alert!**

Do not use your thumb for a radial pulse as the pulse in your thumb may obliterate a radial pulse (Perry and Potter, 2002).

⚠ **Professional alert!**

The radial procedure is suitable for patients aged 2 years or more. For younger patients, you need to ask your mentor/trained staff to show you what to do.

t☆ **Practice tip**

If you are having trouble palpating the radial pulse, get the patient to bend the wrist slightly backwards. If you are in the correct position and are having difficulty palpating the pulse, you may have to apply more or less pressure with your fingertips. This may take a bit of time to practice – don't worry. If you are in the clinical area, ask your mentor/trained staff to help.

Respirations

Normal respirations should be quiet, audible sounds which are equal in depth and evenly paced (pattern), except in very young children who can have a rapid rate. Respiration occurs involuntarily, but we have voluntary control – hence the ability to hold our breath. It is for this reason that it is sometimes easier to take the pulse first and then change to counting respirations without making it obvious to the patient. When taking a patient's respirations it is important to determine the rate, rhythm and depth (Woodrow, 2006b).

The term eupnea refers to a normal respiratory rate (Jevon and Ewens, 2002) and in adults is between 10 and 18 breaths per minute (Woodrow, 2006b). A slower than normal rate is known as bradypnea whilst a rate greater than normal is called tachypnea.

Within the respiratory centre located in the medulla part of the brain there are nerve cells called neurones. Some of these are inspiratory neurones responsible for breathing in, and others are expiratory neurones that control expiration. Generally breathing out happens automatically and requires no effort and for this reason is known as a passive process. However, when one breathes out forcefully during expiration, this process becomes active as effort is required.

ⓐ **Learning activity**

If patients are having difficulty breathing how might they look? How would you recognise that breathing is difficult for them? Compare this with a patient breathing normally.

Factors that affect respiration

There are a variety of factors that can affect respirations. These include exercise, pain, smoking, certain medications and body position. During exercise there is an increased demand for oxygen, so the rate and depth of respirations increases. Pain can also alter the respiration rate and rhythm, as can injury, particularly if it is in the chest region. Changes in the pulmonary system of the lungs may occur due to smoking, causing respiratory rate to be increased. Certain medication, such as treatments used in general anaesthetics, may cause the respiratory rate and depth to be decreased. Consider patients who are slumped in their

Part
III

beds/chairs or lying flat; this may restrict how much their lungs can move and expand during inspiration and expiration (Perry and Potter, 2002).

⚠ Professional alert!

A change in respiration rate, in conjunction with changes in heart rate, can often be an early indicator that there is a deterioration in the patient's condition. Any abnormalities should be reported immediately as the patient may be at risk of deteriorating.

Taking respirations

1 Ask patients to bend their arm and place it across their chest, then place your fingers on the wrist as if you are taking their radial pulse. This enables you to feel their chests moving up and down as they are breathing in and out. With some patients, their chest movement is very clear to see. As you become more experienced you may be able to see the chest visibly rise and fall (Perry and Potter, 2002).

2 Count the rate (number) of respirations (one respiration is a breath in and out) for 60 seconds to provide enough time to detect any abnormalities.

3 Observe depth (volume) of respirations to detect any difficulties breathing, such as deep or shallow breathing.

4 Observe pattern of respirations to detect any breathing that is abnormal: that is, not relaxed or evenly paced (Woodrow, 2006b).

5 Record rate on chart; document any abnormalities for depth and pattern so that trends can be detected and information gathered about any abnormalities (NMC, 2002).

t☆
Practice tip

For infants/young children, count abdominal movements.

Conclusion

It is evident that monitoring vital signs is an important component of holistically assessing the patient. There are a variety of factors to consider prior to undertaking these procedures in order to ensure that the most appropriate equipment and sites are used for each individual. Take into consideration any factors that may affect patients' vital signs and note any abnormal values obtained. It is also important when undertaking these activities to recognise individual responsibility for reporting and if appropriate documenting all relevant information.

References

Carlson, K. K. (ed.) (2009) *AACN Advanced Critical Care Nursing*, Canada, American Association of Critical Care Nurses, Saunders, Elsevier.

Carroll, M. (2000) 'An evaluation of temperature measurement', *Nursing Standard* **14**(44), 39–43.

Castledine, G. (2006) 'The importance of measuring and recording vital signs correctly', *British Journal of Nursing* **15**(5), 285.

Crawford, D. C., Hicks, B. and Thompson, M. J. (2006) 'Which thermometer? Factors influencing best choice for intermittent clinical temperature assessment', *Journal of Medical Engineering and Technology* **30**(4), 199–211.

Cutter, J. (1994) 'Recording patient temperature: are we getting it right?' *Professional Nurse* **9**(9), 608–12.

Davidson, K. and Barber, V. (2004) 'Electronic monitoring of patients in general wards', *Nursing Standard* **18**(49), 42.

Dobbins, H., Adams, G. and Hewson, D. (2004) 'Homeostasis', pp. 127–51 in Mallik, M., Hall, C. and Howard, D. (eds), *Nursing and Knowledge and Practice: Foundations for decision making*, 2nd edn,

China, Baillere Tindall.

Dougherty L. and Lister S. (2004) *The Royal Marsden Hospital Manual of Clinical Nursing Porcedures*, 6th edn, Oxford, Blackwell.

Holtzclaw B. (1990) 'Temperature problems in the post-operative period', *Critical Care Nursing Clinics of North America* **2**(4), 589–97.

Jarvis, C. (2004) *Physical examination and Health Assessment*, 4th edn, Philadelphia, USA, Saunders.

Jevon, P. and Ewens, B. (2002) *Monitoring the Critically Ill Patient*, London, Blackwell Science.

Joanna Briggs Institute (1999) 'Best practice: evidence based practice information sheets for health professionals', *Vital signs* **3**(3), 1–6.

Marieb, E.N. (2004) *Human Anatomy and Physiology*, 6th edn, San Francisco, Benjamine Cummings Publishing.

Marieb, E. N. and Hoehn, K. (2007) *Human Anatomy and Physiology*, 7th edn, Pearson International Edition.

Marini, J. J. and Wheeler, A. P. (2006) *Critical Care Medicine: The essentials*, 3rd edn, Lippencott Williams and Wilkins.

Massey, D. (2006) 'Clinical assessment part 1: inspection, palpation and percussion', *British Journal of Cardiac Nursing* **1**(1), January, 7–11.

National Institute of Clinical Excellence (NICE) (2003) Home page [Online] http://www.nice.org.uk/nicemedia/pdf/Infection_control_fullguideline.pdf (accessed 9 February 2009).

NICE (2007) Home page [Online] http://www.nice.org.uk/nicemedia/pdf/CG50FullGuidance.pdf (9 February 2009).

Nicoll, L. H. (2002) 'Heat in motion: evaluating and managing temperature', *Nursing* **32**(5), s1–12.

Nursing and Midwifery Council (NMC) (2002) *Guidelines for Records and Record Keeping*, London, NMC.

NMC (2004) *The NMC Code of Professional Conduct: Standards for conduct, performance and ethics*, London, NMC.

Perry, A. G. and Potter, P. A. (2002) *Clinical Nursing Skills and Techniques*, 5th edn, USA, Mosby's.

Stanhope, N. (2006) 'Temperature measurement in the phase 1 PAC Journal of PeriAnesthesia Nursing* **21**(1), February, 27–36.

Woodrow, P. (2006a) 'Practice update: clinical skills with older people – taking tympanic temperature', *Nursing older People* **18**(1), February, 31–2.

Woodrow, P. (2006b) 'Practice update: clinical skills with older people – recognising acute deterioration', *Nursing Older People* **17**(5), July, 31–2.

Woodrow, P., May, V., Buras-Rees, S., Higgs, D., Hendrick, J., Lewis, T., Whitney, S., Cummings, C., Boorman, P., O'Donnell, A., Harris, P. and McHenry, M. (2006) 'Comparing no-touch and tympanic thermometer temperature recordings', *British Journal of Nursing* **15**(18), 1012–16.

Chapter

17

Blood pressure

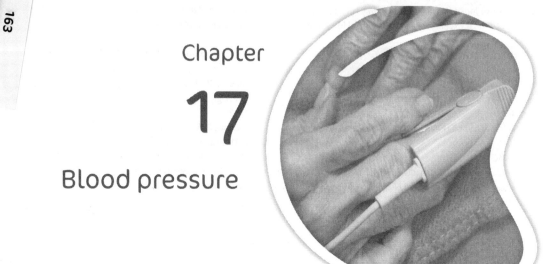

Sharon Jones

Links to other chapters in *Foundation Skills for Caring*

16 Vital signs
36 Basic life support: child
37 Basic life support: adult

Links to other chapters in *Foundation Studies for Caring*

14 Pharmacology and medicines
21 Care of the acutely ill child
23 Care of the adult – surgical
24 Care of the adult – medical
31 Child emergency care and resuscitation
32 Adult emergency care and resuscitation

W   Don't forget to visit www.palgrave.com/glasper for additional
online resources relating to this chapter.

Introduction

The aim of this chapter is to provide you with knowledge and understanding of the skill of blood pressure measurement in an adult environment. The recording of blood pressure (BP) is one of the main physiological measurements used to monitor and diagnose a patient's condition. Blood pressure is usually measured on admission to hospital, with subsequent monitoring to observe for changes. Additionally, patients may have their blood pressure recorded and monitored by their general practitioner or practice nurse, or may self-monitor at home. It is essential that measurements are accurate; error in measurement of BP has been well documented (Armstrong, 2001; Carney et al, 1999). Healthcare workers who are involved in measuring a patient's BP must be aware of the risks that inaccurate recordings may cause to the patient's future treatment and diagnosis.

Blood pressure measurement can be a key indicator of a person's health, although it should not be considered in isolation from other parameters of health. Consequently, a full assessment of a patient should be undertaken in the event of illness or traumatic injury. It is important that healthcare staff are aware of factors that can influence blood pressure readings, and take reasonable steps to limit these where possible.

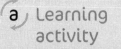

Learning activity

Before reading the chapter, jot down what you understand by the term 'blood pressure'.

Learning outcomes

This chapter will enable you to:

- describe how normal blood pressure is maintained
- recognise the differences between diastolic and systolic pressures
- briefly describe the factors that influence change in blood pressure
- describe the five auscultatory sounds that are identified when recording a blood pressure
- discuss the factors that influence blood pressure readings

- describe with evidence-based reasons the procedure for measuring an adult's blood pressure
- identify potential causes of error and discuss the importance of accuracy when performing this assessment
- define hypertension
- identify the role of the healthcare team in managing a patient with hypertension
- use relevant literature and research to underpin the clinical skill of blood pressure recording.

Part

III

Concepts

- Adult nursing – monitoring blood pressure
- Relevant anatomy and physiology
- Health and safety issues
- The evidence base underpinning clinical skill

- Auscultatory and oscillometric monitors
- Indicator of health
- Role of healthcare professionals

Anatomy and physiology

Blood pressure (BP) is the pressure exerted by the circulating blood against the walls of the blood vessels (Tortora and Derrickson, 2006). The term blood pressure usually refers to pressure within the arteries, the blood vessels that transport blood away from the heart. There are pressure gradient differences to the BP throughout the circulatory system, and this drives the blood through the body (Marieb and Hoehn, 2007). Blood pressure varies with the strength of the heartbeat, elasticity of the arterial walls, volume and viscosity of the blood, and a person's health, age and physical condition. The cardiac output and the peripheral vascular resistance influence the maintenance of normal BP (Tortora and Derrickson, 2006). Peripheral resistance is altered by the viscosity of the blood, vessel length and, more frequently, by blood vessel diameter. The major determinants of peripheral resistance are small-diameter vessels, known as arterioles. In response to neural and chemical controls, arterioles can dilate to decrease blood pressure or constrict to increase blood pressure (Tortora and Derrickson, 2006).

Learning activity

Review your understanding of the cardiac cycle. What does cardiac output refer to?

The terms systolic and diastolic pressure refer to the differences of the pressure of the blood. Systolic blood pressure is the peak pressure of the blood in the arteries caused by the ventricle contracting (systole). Diastolic pressure, which indicates the blood vessel resistance, is the minimum pressure of the blood against the wall of the vessel following closure of the aortic valve (Marieb and Hoehn, 2007).

The difference between the systolic and diastolic pressures is known as the 'pulse pressure', which is the throbbing pulsation felt in an artery during systole (Marieb and Hoehn, 2007). Another term you will meet is the 'mean arterial pressure'. This is the average pressure required to push blood through the circulatory system.

Cardiac output x total peripheral pressure = mean arterial pressure

Blood pressure is regulated by three mechanisms: the baroreceptor reflex, renin-angiotensin system and aldosterone release.

- *Baroreceptor reflex*: changes in arterial pressure are detected by baroreceptors, which send messages to the medulla of the brain stem. Through the action of the autonomic nervous system, the medulla adjusts the mean arterial pressure by altering the speed and force of the heart's contractions and the total peripheral resistance.
- *Reinin-angiotensin system*: the kidneys initiate this complex system. In response to a drop in blood volume or arterial pressure they release the enzyme renin; this forms angiotensin I, which is converted into angiotensin II. Angiotensin II is a powerful vasoconstrictor. This increases low arterial blood pressure by increasing peripheral vasoconstriction and stimulating aldosterone production.
- *Aldosterone release*: aldosterone stimulates sodium retention and potassium excretion by the kidneys. Sodium retention leads to an increase in the fluid volume, indirectly increasing arterial pressure.

Once the BP reaches a normal level the body stops producing renin, hence stopping the renin–angiotensin–aldosterone cycle.

Measuring an adult's blood pressure

There are two main methods of recording BP: direct and indirect. The most accurate method is direct, intra-arterial recording. However, this is an invasive technique that requires penetrating the skin and measuring inside the blood vessel. Invasive methods are usually performed in areas where patients require constant monitoring, such as high dependency units and theatres. The indirect method is more commonly used, measuring the BP in the brachial artery of the arm. There are various ways to indirectly measure BP:

- sphygmomanometer with stethoscope
- sphygmomanometer with Doppler
- sphygmomanometer with palpation
- automated monitors.

Learning activity

Identify the methods of recording blood pressure used in your practice area. What is the most common method, and why? Review the evidence underpinning this method.

Practice tip

When taking blood pressure, ensure patients are not sitting with their legs crossed – this gives a falsely high reading.

Monitors

There are two main types of BP monitors: auscultatory and oscillometric.

Mercury and aneroid devices are types of auscultatory monitors, using sound for measurement. Due to concerns regarding the safety of medical devices containing mercury (Commission of the European Communities, 2005) it is likely that these will be phased out (Medicine and Healthcare Products Regulatory Agency, 2006). Aneroid devices, whilst accurate, are susceptible to damage that is not necessarily apparent to the user (O'Brien et al, 2001). Therefore it is essential that they are regularly calibrated.

Oscillometric, or automated, devices rely on the variations of pressure in the cuff caused by the pulse of the artery. The height and frequency of changes determine the BP measurement. It is important that the cuff is placed directly over the artery to ensure an accurate reading. The manufacturer's instructions must be followed when using these devices, ensuring that they are calibrated and maintained regularly.

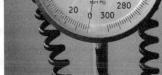

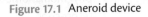

Figure 17.1 Aneroid device

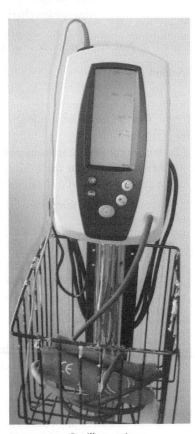

(a) Learning activity

Discuss the manufacturer's instructions that are supplied with the device with your mentor; find out who is responsible for calibrating and maintaining the devices, and how this is monitored in the practice area.

t☆ Practice tip

When using automated devices to record BP, always ensure you palpate the pulse to feel the strength and regularity. Any abnormalities should be recorded and reported to the registered nurse or appropriate health care professional.

Cuff size

The cuff is usually made of a durable material, and local policies relating to cleaning of the cuff between patient uses must be adhered to. Within the cloth sheath is an inflatable bladder; it is important that the bladder inside the cuff covers at least 80 per cent of the circumference of the upper arm.

Figure 17.2 Oscillometric or automated device

If the cuff size is too large or too small, the BP will be underestimated or overestimated respectively (O'Brien et al, 1997). The BHS Working Party (Williams et al, 2004) recommends that a cuff containing a bladder with the dimensions of 35 x 12 cm would be most suitable for the majority of adults and lessen the greater risk of overestimating the BP. However, it would be more appropriate to have different cuff sizes for patients with either larger or smaller arms (Table 17.1).

Figure 17.3 Position of bladder cuff

Part

III

Table 17.1 Cuff sizes by patient size

Cuff size	
12 x 26 cm	standard adult size
12 x 40 cm	obese adult size
10 x 18 cm	small adult size

Source: O'Brien et al (1997).

Procedure: manual blood pressure measurement

You will need:

- sphygmomanometer
- stethoscope
- observation chart.

t☆ Practice tip

Equipment checks:

- manometer – visibility of meniscus, calibration
- cuff – condition, length and width of inflatable bladder
- inflation/deflation device – any malfunctions, control valve
- stethoscope – condition and cleanliness.

Table 17.2 Action and rationale when taking a manual blood pressure measurement

Action	Rationale
1. Wash hands.	To reduce risk of cross-infection.
2. Explain procedure to the patient and assess level of understanding.	To gain informed consent and ensure patient understands the procedure.
3. Ensure the patient is positioned comfortably, and has been rested for approximately three minutes if supine or seated and one minute if standing.	To gain an accurate reading.
4. Remove tight clothing, support arm horizontally at heart level.	Overestimation of the systolic and diastolic pressures can occur if the arm is lower than mid-sternum. Underestimations can occur if the arm is raised above this level.
5. Avoid talking throughout the procedure.	To enable accurate recording of Korotkoff sounds.
6. Use a sphygmomanometer cuff of appropriate size, one that covers approximately 80 per cent of the circumference of the upper arm.	A too narrow or broad cuff could give an inaccurate reading.
7. Apply the cuff with the centre of the bladder positioned over the line of the brachial artery approximately 2 cm above the elbow.	To obtain an accurate reading.
8. Position the manometer at eye level, ensuring it can be easily observed by the practitioner.	To avoid risk of injury through straining or twisting the practitioner's back and allow accurate reading of manometer.
9. Locate the brachial pulse and inflate the cuff until the pulse cannot be felt. Wait for 15–30 seconds before continuing to measure the blood pressure.	This provides an estimation of the systolic pressure and avoids error in reading.
10. Inflate the cuff 30 mm Hg higher than the estimated systolic pressure.	The blood is prevented from flowing through the artery by the pressure exerted.
11. Position the stethoscope over the brachial artery; ensuring it does not come into contact with the tubing of the cuff (Figure 17.4).	Contact with the tubing may produce artefactual sounds.
12. Lower mercury column slowly (2 mm per second).	If you deflate the cuff too rapidly you may not hear the sounds accurately.
13. Observe the needle of the dial as it is lowered and listen for Korotkoff sounds.	The systolic pressure is the level when repetitive, clear tapping sounds first appear for at least two consecutive beats. The diastolic pressure is the level where the sounds disappear.
14. Read blood pressure to the nearest 2 mm Hg.	To avoid 'digit' bias (O'Brien et al, 1997).

Action	Rationale
15. Record the systolic and diastolic pressures, noting which arm was used, and compare with previous readings. Report irregularities to senior practitioner.	To maintain a record and allow changes in the patient's condition to be monitored.
16. Remove the cuff and ensure patient's comfort.	Continuity of care.
17. Clear away equipment and clean according to local policy.	To minimise the risk of cross-infection.

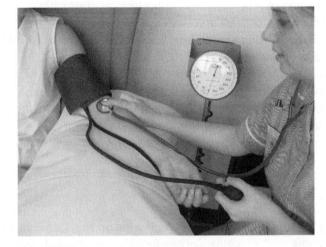

t☆
Practice tip

Always remember to document which arm was used for measurement as well as the time of day.

Figure 17.4 Stethoscope positioned over brachial artery

Korotkoff sounds

The five auscultatory, or Korotkoff, sounds that are identified when recording a BP are defined as follows:

- *Phase 1*: the first appearance of faint, repetitive, clear tapping sounds that gradually increase in intensity for at least two consecutive beats. This is the systolic BP.
- *Phase 2*: a brief period may follow during which the sounds soften and acquire a swishing quality. An auscultatory gap may occur here in some patients; this is where sounds may disappear altogether for a short time.
- *Phase 3*: the return of sharper sounds, which become crisper and regain, or even exceed, the intensity of Phase 1 sounds. The clinical significance, if any, of Phases 2 and 3 has not been established.
- *Phase 4*: the distinct, abrupt muffling sounds, which become soft and blowing in quality.
- *Phase 5*: the point at which all sounds finally disappear completely. This is the diastolic pressure, although this is under debate, and current recommendations suggest that both Phase 4 and Phase 5 should be recorded (Beevers, Lip and O'Brien, 2001).

a Learning activity

Practise listening for the Korotkoff sounds when carrying out blood pressure recordings; make a note of the measurements at which you hear the phases, and ask your mentor to help you to distinguish these on subsequent readings.

Hypertension and hypotension

Blood pressure is usually recorded in terms of millimetres of mercury (mm/Hg), which traditionally referred to the height of a column on the sphygmanometer. However, due to risks of toxicity associated with mercury use, the unit of measurement for blood pressure is currently under discussion by the British Hypertension Society Workforce, with suggestions for introducing the Système International (SI) unit, the kilopascal (Beevers et al, 2001).

Part
III

Hypotension in adults is generally defined as a systolic blood pressure of less than 100 mm/Hg (Marieb and Hoehn, 2007). This is often attributed to individual variances, but this should not lead the healthcare worker to dismiss such an observation, particularly where there is a risk the patient may be suffering from circulatory shock. Patients with malnutrition may have chronic hypotension due to anaemia and low levels of blood protein. Their BP is lower because of their lower blood viscosity (Marieb and Hoehn, 2007).

Orthostatic, or postural, hypotension also contributes to low blood pressure, and should be investigated further. Orthostatic hypotension is more common in the elderly, because of slower response to postural changes of the sympathetic nervous system (Marieb and Hoehn, 2007). This is usually characterised by a low systolic blood pressure on standing, and can be accompanied by feelings of dizziness.

Hypertension, or raised blood pressure, is considered a major risk factor for cardiovascular disease. It has been estimated that 20 per cent of the current population is either being investigated or receiving treatment for hypertension (Elliot, 2002). In line with recent European guidelines, the British Hypertension Society's classifications have changed (Williams et al, 2004), clearly outlining blood pressure levels for the diagnosis of hypertension.

> **(a) Learning activity**
>
> Consider the precautions that patients should be advised to take if they have orthostatic hypotension.

(e) Evidence-based practice: standard BP targets

Williams and colleagues (2004) note that there is limited evidence indicating optimal targets for blood pressure lowering, but acknowledge that the Hypertension Optimal Trial (HOT) provides the best evidence on optimal targets (Hansson et al, 1998). Consequently, the British Hypertension Society (Williams et al, 2004) continues to recommend an 'audit standard' blood pressure target of </−150/90 mm/Hg for patients undergoing treatment.

However, this audit standard target is the minimum standard of care for high-risk individuals, and a blood pressure target of </−140/98 mm/Hg is recommended for most patients. NICE guidance (2006) and the Joint British Societies (2005) refer to an optimal target of </−140/85 mm/Hg, with additional lower targets for higher-risk individuals, also indicated by the British Hypertension Society.

There are many factors that influence the BP of adults; these include age, anxiety, smoking, meals, time of day, temperature and sleep. It has been noted that some patients are affected by what is termed 'white-coat syndrome' (O'Brien et al, 2001). This refers to the elevation of a person's blood pressure on encountering a doctor – although this could also occur in the presence of a nurse – leading to suggestions that ambulatory blood pressure measurement may be more accurate (Owens, Atkins and O'Brien, 1999). To overcome this potential error it has therefore been suggested that ambulatory monitoring of BP may give a more accurate reading (Williams et al, 2004).

> **(a) Learning activity**
>
> Using a web-based search engine, enter the words 'causes of hypertension'. Consider your findings in relation to patients you may have cared for with known hypertension.

If an adult is suspected of having hypertension, a diagnosis should not be confirmed unless their systolic blood pressure is recorded at greater than 140 mm/Hg on at least three separate occasions over a two-month period (NICE, 2002; National Service Framework, 2000). It is also recommended that routine measurements of BP for all adults should be undertaken at least every five years until the age of 80 years. Adults who are considered at greater risk should be monitored annually (Williams et al, 2004)

Conclusion

Blood pressure is one of the main physiological measurements used to monitor and diagnose the patient's condition. Whilst it is generally accepted that there are 'normal' values for blood pressure measurements, it must be remembered that the value can vary from person to person, and even moment to moment. The circulatory system is complex, and it is noted that there are many physical and physiological factors that influence arterial pressure. Healthcare practitioners responsible for undertaking this recording must ensure that their practice is up-dated and their competence with this skill maintained to deliver safe, evidence-based care at all times.

References

Armstrong, R. S. (2001) 'Nurses' knowledge of error in blood pressure measurement technique', *International Journal of Nursing Practice* 8, 118–26.

Beevers, G., Lip, G. Y. H. and O'Brien, E. (2001) *ABC of Hypertension*, 4th edn, London , BMJ Books.

Carney, S. L., Gillies, A. H., Green, S. L., Paterson, O., Taylor, M. S. and Smith, A. J. (1999) 'Hospital blood pressure measurement: staff and device assessment', *Journal of Quality Clinical Practice* **19**(2), June, 95–8.

Commission of the European Communities (2005) *Communication from the Commission to the Council and the European Parliament: Community strategy concerning mercury* (COM/2005/20) [online] http://eur-lex.europa.eu/lexUriServ/site/en/com/2005/com2005_0020en01.pdf (accessed 10 July 2007).

Elliot, H. (2002) 'Epidemiology, aetiology and prognosis of hypertension', *Medicine Student Edition* **30**(7), 127– 30.

Hansson, L., Zanchetti, A., Carruthers, S. G., Dahlof, B., Elmfeldt, D. and Julias, S., for the HOT Study Group (1998) 'Effects of intensive blood pressure lowering and low-dose aspirin in patients with hypertension: principal results of the hypertension optimal treatment (HOT) randomised trial', *Lancet* 351: 1755–62.

Joint British Societies (2005) 'Joint British Societies' guidelines on prevention of cardiovascular disease in clinical practice', *Heart* 91, Supplement 5, v1–v52.

Marieb, E. N. and Hoehn, K. (2007) *Human Anatomy and Physiology*, San Francisco, Pearson Benjamin Cummings.

Medicine and Healthcare Products Regulatory Agency (2006) 'Blood Pressure Management Devices', DB20006 (03), MHRA [online] www.mhra.gov.uk (accessed 10 July 2007).

National Institute of Clinical Excellence (NICE) (2002) 'Management of type II diabetes: management of blood pressure and blood lipids, (Guideline H inherited)', NICE [online] www.nice.org.uk (accessed 5 July 2007).

NICE (2006) *Hypertension: Management of hypertension in adults in primary care*, Clinical Guideline No. 34, London, NICE.

National Service Framework (2000) *National Service Framework for Coronary Heart Disease*, London, Stationery Office.

O'Brien, E., Petrie, J. C., Littler, W. A., de Swiet, M., Padfield, P. D., Dillon, M. J., Coats, A. and Mee, F. (1997) *Blood Pressure Measurement: Recommendations of the British Hypertension Society*, 3rd edn, Plymouth, UK, BMJ Publishing Group.

O'Brien, E., Waeber, B., Parati, G., Staessen, J. and Myers, M. G. (2001) 'Blood pressure measuring devices: recommendations of the European Society of Hypertension', *British Medical Journal* **322**(7285), 531–6.

Owens, P., Atkins, N. and O'Brien, E. (1999) 'The diagnosis of white coat hypertension by ambulatory blood pressure monitoring', *Hypertension* **34**(2), 267–72.

Tortora, G. J. and Derrickson, B. (2006) *Principles of Anatomy and Physiology*, 11th edn, Hoboken, New Jersey, Wiley and Sons.

Williams, B., Poulter, N. R., Brown, M. J., Davis, M., McInnes, G. T., Potter, J. F., Sever, P. S. and Thom, S. (2004) *British Hypertension Society guidelines for hypertension management2004 (BHS-IV)328*, 634–40 www.bmj.com (accessed 3 October 2008).

Part

III

Chapter

18

Pulse oximetry

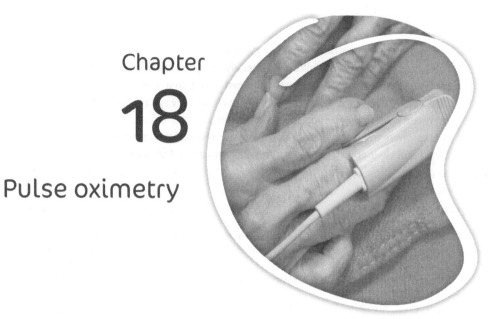

Sharon Jones

 Links to other chapters in *Foundation Skills for Caring*

16 Vital signs
17 Blood pressure
36 Basic life support: child
37 Basic life support: adult

 Links to other chapters in *Foundation Studies for Caring*

19 Care of the neonate
21 Care of the acutely ill child
23 Care of the adult – surgical
24 Care of the adult – medical
30 Emergency care and interventions
31 Child emergency care and resuscitation
32 Adult emergency care and resuscitation

W Don't forget to visit www.palgrave.com/glasper for additional
online resources relating to this chapter.

Introduction

The aim of this chapter is to provide you with an understanding of pulse oximetry and facilitate development of recording a patient's oxygen saturation level through this non-invasive technique.

Learning outcomes

This chapter will enable you to:

- demonstrate an understanding of how oxygen is carried by haemoglobin
- demonstrate an understanding of oxygen saturation
- identify the clinical signs of hypoxia
- describe the procedure for recording a patient's oxygen saturation level, with evidence-based reasons
- briefly describe the factors that influence oxygen saturation readings

- recognise the limitations of pulse oximetry
- identify potential causes of error and discuss the importance of accuracy when performing this skill
- use relevant literature and research to underpin the clinical skill of pulse oximetry.

Concepts

- Adult nursing: monitoring oxygen saturation
- Relevant anatomy and physiology
- Health and safety issues
- The evidence base underpinning clinical skill

- Oximetry monitors
- Indicator of health
- Role of healthcare professionals

The body requires a continual supply of oxygen and the elimination of carbon dioxide to sustain life; this essential exchange is a key function of the respiratory system, in conjunction with the circulatory system. Profound hypoxaemia (insufficient oxygen in the blood) can result in death in minutes (Hanning and Alexander-Williams, 1995), so it is essential that healthcare staff can recognise clinical symptoms and initiate appropriate treatment immediately.

The percentage of oxygen delivered in such circumstances may be dependent on the urgency of the patient's condition, or can be determined by undertaking arterial blood gas measurement (Pa O_2) or pulse oximetry to determine the percentage required. Pulse oximetry is a non-invasive method of monitoring patients, allowing for a range of different parameters to be assessed (Hill and Stoneman, 2000). Oxygen saturation is recorded by attaching a light-emitting probe to either a fingertip or earlobe, and measuring the changes in light absorption through a microprocessor. While it is not a new method of patient monitoring in intensive care and theatre settings, its use has become more common in general hospital and community environments (Capovilla, 2000), and is more frequently measured alongside traditional parameters of temperature, blood pressure, pulse and respiratory rate.

A pulse oximeter measures the oxygen saturation of haemoglobin in arterial blood; this is the amount of oxygen being carried in the haemoglobin, not the amount being delivered to the cells of the body (Woodrow, 2000). Oxygen saturation is symbolised as SpO_2. Additionally, the pulse oximeter can record the pulse rate and estimate the systolic blood pressure, although the latter is not so common.

> ### ⟲a Learning activity
>
> Review the observation charts of ten patients in the placement area; how many of them have had their oxygen saturation measurement recorded? Note variations in the measurements and consider reasons for these.

Part

III

Procedure for pulse oximetry

Equipment:
- oximeter
- sensor – finger/ear or forehead tape
- observation chart.

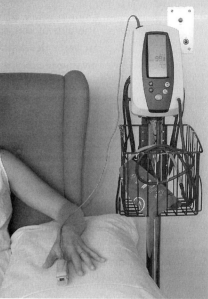

Figure 18.1 Finger probe in position

Table 18.1 Action and rationale for pulse oximetry

action	Rationale
Explain the purpose of the intervention to the patient and gain consent prior to procedure.	To ensure the patient understands the procedure and provides informed consent.
Position the patient comfortably, and ensure the area for the probe is clean.	To ensure accuracy of reading.
Wash your hands.	Apply universal precautions to all nursing interventions.
Select an appropriate site for the probe and attach correctly (see Figure 18.1).	Pulse oximetry relies on an adequate pulsating vascular bed.
Switch the pulse oximeter machine on.	To avoid error with reading.
Check the probe sensor detects the pulse and that it corresponds with the patient's pulse. The display panel will usually give a graphical indication of this, or a beep emitted in time with the pulse.	To ensure the pulse is detected for accuracy of monitoring.
Record the oxygenation saturation level and document in patient's notes.	To provide a written record of the patient's saturation level.
Report abnormal reading to a senior member of the healthcare team.	To maintain safety of patient.
Remove the probe sensor, clean area if adhesive used and check condition of the probe site.	Probes can cause discomfort due to pressure.
If continuous monitoring required, check the probe placement area and reposition at least two-hourly or as clinically indicated.	The heat source can cause burns if directly placed on skin rather than nail.
Re-position patient as required.	To maintain patient comfort.
Clean and store equipment according to local policy.	To prevent cross contamination and to maintain equipment and prevent accidental damage.

Oxygen saturation

The amount of oxygen that is delivered to the tissues is influenced by tissue perfusion, the amount of haemoglobin present in the blood and the saturation of haemoglobin by oxygen (Woodrow, 1999). However, pulse oximetry only measures oxygen saturation. Oxygen saturation is a measure of how much oxygen the blood is carrying, as a percentage of the maximum it could carry. Oxygen is carried in the blood in two ways:

- *Dissolved in plasma*: oxygen does not dissolve very easily in water, and therefore plasma carries only 3 per cent of all oxygen in the blood (Tortora and Derrickson, 2006). Measurement is from an arterial blood gas sample.

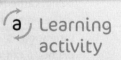

Learning activity

Review the factors that promote O_2 binding to and dissociation from haemoglobin.

- *Attached to haemoglobin*: haemoglobin is the primary carrier of oxygen in the arterial blood, transporting approximately 97 per cent from the lungs to the tissues (Marieb and Hoehn, 2007).

Thus oxygen in the blood stream is bound mainly to haemoglobin, and forms oxyhaemoglobin.

$$Hb \quad + \quad O_2 \xrightarrow[\text{Dissociation of } O_2]{\text{Binding of } O_2} Hb - O_2$$

| Reduced haemoglobin (deoxyhaemoglobin) | Oxygen | | Oxyhaemoglobin |

Figure 18.2 Formation of oxyhaemoglobin

Red blood cells contain haemoglobin (Hb). A haemoglobin molecule is made up of four protein chains, known as a globin. Within each globin is a molecule of haem, which is the iron-containing portion of Hb (Marieb and Hoehn, 2007). The Hb molecules contain four iron atoms, each capable of combining with an oxygen molecule. Within a single red blood cell there are over 600 million Hb molecules.

One haemoglobin molecule can carry a maximum of four molecules of oxygen, providing 100 per cent oxygen saturation (Marieb and Hoehn, 2007). However, full saturation (100 per cent) is not usually achieved when breathing air, so it is estimated that saturation levels in a healthy adult are approximately 97 per cent (Schutz, 2001).

One of the greatest advantages of pulse oximetry is that it allows for both intermittent and continuous assessment of oxygenation, without the need for invasive measurement through arterial puncture and arterial blood gas analysis (Hanning and Alexander-Williams, 1995). Cyanosis, a blue-purple colour visible in the skin, nail beds and mucosal membranes, is one of the indicators of severe hypoxia that occurs when the saturation of haemoglobin falls below 70 per cent (Woodrow, 1999). Patients at risk of hypoxia can be monitored quickly with pulse oximetry, giving an early indication of decreasing saturation levels, and hence allowing for prompt treatment.

> **(a) Learning activity**
>
> List the signs and causes of hypoxia. Can you identify patients who may be at risk of developing hypoxia?

Part III

(e) Evidence-based practice: monitoring and recognition of risk

Although pulse oximetry is not one of the traditional vital signs used for monitoring patients, it is now recommended that oxygen saturation is recorded with other physiological observations at the time of admission or initial assessment (NICE, 2007), and throughout the monitoring of an acutely ill or 'at risk' patient. Oxygen saturation measurement is considered as an important early predictor of deterioration and should be included as a core parameter (NICE, 2007). The National Confidential

Enquiry into Patient Outcome and Death (NCEPOD) (2005) attributed the mortality of acutely ill patients to delays in recognising that 'at risk' patients were becoming acutely unwell and the institution of appropriate therapy. Subsequently, NICE (2007) has stated that staff should be appropriately trained to undertake the relevant procedures and understand the clinical relevance of the readings.

Pulse oximetry: the mechanics

Two light-emitting diodes (LEDs) send red and infrared light through a pulsating arterial vascular bed; standard sites for this are the finger tips (Hanning and Alexander-Williams, 1995), although the ear lobes, bridge of nose or forehead may also be used if appropriate for the patient. A probe sensor is placed on the selected site and measures the transmitted light as it passes through the pulsating vascular bed to the photo detector on one side of the probe sensor. The infrared light is absorbed by the oxyhaemoglobin and the red light by reduced haemoglobin. The degree of light absorption is determined by the oxygen saturation of the blood. The measurement is then displayed on the oximeter screen.

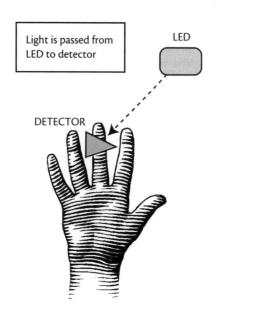

Light is passed from LED to detector

LED

DETECTOR

Figure 18.3 Pulse oximetry

> **⚠ Professional alert!**
>
> Remember to move the oximeter probe regularly – at least at 1–2-hourly intervals to avoid the potential risk of burns.

Pulse oximeter

The term 'pulse oximeter' is generally used to describe the whole unit, which consists of a microprocessor and a peripheral probe. There are a wide variety of microprocessor units, many displaying a visual digital waveform (plethsymograph) and an audible pulse (Hill and Stoneman, 2000). Thanks to technological advances the majority of units are reliable, with little interference due to either motion or electromagnetism on the pulse oximeter function (Hill and Stoneman, 2000). Pulse oximeters have an accuracy of approximately ± 2 per cent above an oxygen saturation of 70 per cent (Aitkenhead et al, 2007). Accuracy below this saturation level is not known due to ethical considerations regarding trials.

> **↻ⓐ Learning activity**
>
> Review your understanding of pulse oximetry; what does it NOT measure?

> **t☆ Practice tip**
>
> When the pulse oximeter is first applied there will be a short delay while the microprocessor 'averages' the saturation values and pulse rate.

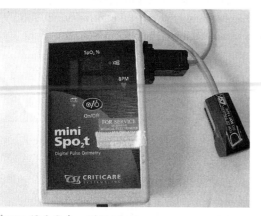

Figure 18.4 Pulse oximeter

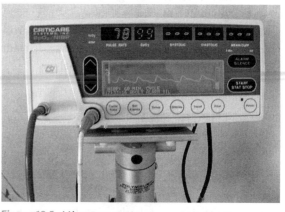

Figure 18.5 Microprocessor

Most oximeters have an audible alarm which alerts healthcare staff if the patient's saturation level falls below a certain level. The default settings on many oximeters are wide, and should be adjusted for individual patients. Alarms can provoke anxiety in the patient so lower alarm settings of 93–95 may be suitable for patients with saturation rates of above 95 per cent. Caution must be used when setting lower alarm limits to avoid unnecessary risk to the patient, (Woodrow, 1999).

As with all monitoring devices, it is essential that healthcare staff are aware of their responsibility regarding the use and maintenance of the equipment. Additionally, with oximetry, staff should have the understanding and ability to interpret waveforms, troubleshoot problems and correctly interpret the data (Capovilla, 2000).

Wave forms

Oximeters that display a visual digital waveform can enable perfusion to be determined. A normal waveform should be smooth and steady (Figure 18.7), and there should be correlation of the patient's pulse rate and heart rate (Capovilla, 2000). There is a risk that the actual heart rate may be underestimated in patients with irregular rhythms as measurement of the pulse is taken from the probe site (Woodrow, 1999); to avoid error the radial pulse, and where necessary the heart beat, should be measured independently.

Any abnormalities noted should alert the healthcare staff to question the accuracy of the displayed value and take appropriate action to maintain the safety of the patient.

> ### a Learning activity
>
> Review the different types of oximeters that are available in the practice setting. With your mentor, read the manufacturer's instructions regarding 'troubleshooting problems'.

> ### a Learning activity
>
> After gaining informed consent, record the heart rate of a patient who is being monitored with a pulse oximeter; does the heart rate correlate with the pulse rate?

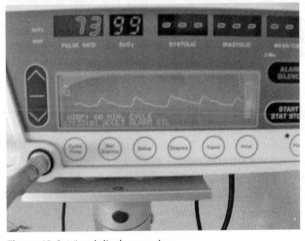

Figure 18.6 Visual display monitor

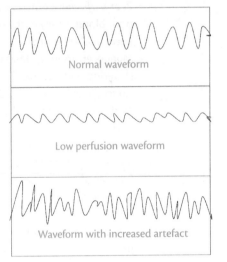

Normal waveform

Low perfusion waveform

Waveform with increased artefact

Figure 18.7 Simulations of pulse oximetry waveforms to illustrate normal and problematic patterns

Probe sensor

There is a range of probes available for use on various sites, although the finger probe is the most common. Whilst the microprocessor unit may be fairly robust, the probes can be easily damaged and care must be taken to protect them. Probes should be cleaned according to local policy; dirty sensors may alter the light absorption of the contact probes and affect the accuracy of the reading. Tape must not be used to hold probes in place, except on the manufacturer's instructions, to avoid the risk of pressure damage (Medicine and Health Product Regulatory Agency, 2001).

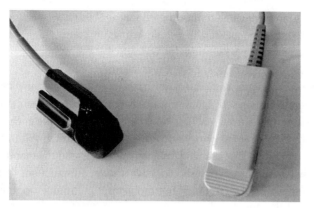

Figure 18.8 Finger probes

⚠ **Professional alert!**

The probe should not be placed on the same arm as a sphygmomanometer cuff as perfusion may be impaired (Hanning and Alexander-Williams, 1995)

As the pulse oximeter measures the amount of light transmitted through arterial blood, readings may be affected by anything that absorbs light (Aitkenhead et al, 2007), for example bilirubin, dark skin, dried blood and/or intravenous dyes. In these situations arterial blood gas analysis may be a more appropriate measurement that will minimise the risk of error due to an inaccurate reading. Whilst it is recommended that nail polish is removed, with the patient's consent, evidence suggests that this does not significantly affect readings (Rodden et al, 2007).

Limitations of oximetry

Although the advantages of pulse oximetry have contributed to the monitoring of critically ill patients, there are limitations to be noted:

- *Poor perfusion*: oximetry measures light absorption over a number of pulses. If there is a poor blood supply in the monitored area then the readings will not be reliable. Note: this is particularly relevant in the critically ill patient.
- *Motion*: errors in readings may be caused by excessive movement, including exercise, shivering, and tremors due to Parkinson disease or seizures.
- *Anaemia*: pulse oximetry does not measure haemoglobin levels; therefore anaemia will not be detected (Simon and Clark, 2003).
- *Carbon monoxide*: readings in the presence of carbon monoxide will be falsely high due to the inability of the pulse oximeter to differentiate it from carbon monoxide-saturated haemoglobin (Woodrow, 2000). Sources of carbon monoxide include cigarette smoke, car exhaust fumes and fires.
- *Venous pulsation*: if the probe is secured too tightly, or if a sphygmonometer cuff is applied to the same arm as the finger probe, there is a risk that venous pulsations may be created in the monitored area, leading to inaccurate readings. Right-sided heart failure also causes venous pulsations.
- *Hypercapnia*: carbon dioxide cannot be measured by pulse oximetry. Arterial blood gas analysis is used to measure carbon dioxide levels (Woodrow, 2000).

t☆
Practice tip

Oxygen saturations alone will not give a clear indication of the patient's condition – the measurement must be used in the context of the whole person.

Conclusion

In an age of rapidly advancing medical technology the pulse oximeter provides a rapid estimation of oxygen saturation and pulse rate through non-invasive means. It is important to remember that pulse oximeters do not provide assessment of haemoglobin concentration, cardiac output, oxygen consumption, sufficiency of oxygen or efficiency of oxygen delivery to the tissues. However, the use of pulse oximetry is becoming notably more common and can provide an early indication of hypoxia in a patient. In conjunction with other parameters such as blood pressure, pulse, respiratory rate and temperature, pulse oximetry can support the healthcare team in delivering timely and appropriate intervention for patients who are either acutely ill or at risk of deteriorating. As with all aspects of care delivery, it is essential that healthcare staff maintain their competence and proficiency to support the delivery of safe, effective, evidence-based practice.

References

Aitkenhead, A. R., Smith, G., Rowbotham, D. S. and Smith, A. (2007) *Textbook of Anaesthesia*, Edinburgh, Churchill Livingstone Elselvier.

Capovilla, J. (2000) 'Non-invasive blood gas monitoring', *Critical Care Nursing Quarterly* **23**(2), 79–86.

Hanning, C. D. and Alexander-Williams, J. M. (1995) 'Fortnightly review: pulse oximetry: a practical review', *British Medical Journal* 311, 367–70.

Hill, E. and Stoneman, M. D. (2000) 'Practical applications of pulse oximetry', *Update in Anaesthesia* **11**(4) [online] www.nda.ox.ac.uk/wfsa/html/u11/u1104_01.htm (accessed 6 July 2007).

Marieb, E. N. and Hoehn, K. (2007) *Human Anatomy and Physiology*, San Francisco, Pearson Benjamin Cummings.

Medicine and Health Product Regulatory Agency (2001) *Tissue Necrosis Caused by Pulse Oximeter Probes*, SN 2001 (08), MHRA [online] http:// www.mhra.gov.uk (accessed: 23 December 2008).

National Confidential Enquiry into Patient Outcome and Death (NCEPOD) (2005) *An acute problem? A report of the National Confidential Enquiry into Patient Outcome and Death (NCEPOD)*, London, NCEPOD.

National Institute of Clinical Excellence (NICE) (2007) *Clinical Guideline 50: Acutely ill patients in hospital*, London, NICE.

Rodden, A. M., Spicer, L., Diaz, V. A. and Styer, T. E. (2007) 'Does fingernail polish affect oximeter readings?' *Intensive and Critical Care Nursing* 23, 51–5.

Schutz, S. (2001) 'Oxygen saturation monitoring by pulse oximetry', pp. 77-82 in Lynn-McHale, D. J. and Carlson, K. K.(eds), *AACN Procedure Manual for Critical Care*, 4th edn, Philadelphia: W.B. Saunders.

Simon, S. B. and Clark, R. A. (2003) '(Mis)Using pulse oximetry: a review of pulse oximetry use in acute care medical wards', *Clinical Effectiveness in Nursing* 6, 106–10.

Tortora, G. J. and Derrickson, B. (2006) *Principles of Anatomy and Physiology*, 11th edn, New Jersey, Wiley and Sons.

Woodrow, P. (1999) 'Pulse oximetry', *Emergency Nurse* **7**(5), 34–9.

Woodrow, P. (2000) *Intensive Care Nursing*, 2nd edn, London, Routledge.

Chapter

19

Blood sugar measurement (using a glucometer)

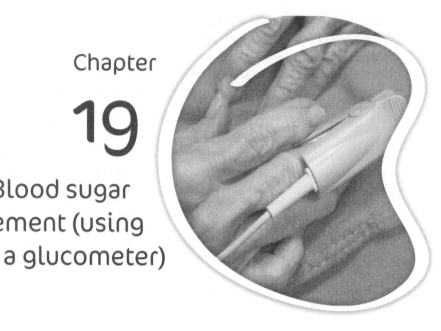

Mary Clynes, Colleen O'Neill and Sara Raftery

Links to other chapters in *Foundation Skills for Caring*

Links to other chapters in *Foundation Studies for Caring*

W Don't forget to visit www.palgrave.com/glasper for additional online resources relating to this chapter.

Introduction

In the human body the sugar concentration in the blood is controlled, with the normal limits being about 4–6 mM (mmol). Glucose levels are lowest in the morning and before the first meal of the day; they rise after a meal for a few hours and then return to normal limits. Failure to maintain blood glucose in the normal range leads to conditions of persistently high blood glucose known as hyperglycaemia, or, when the glucose is too low, hypoglycaemia.

Monitoring a patient's blood glucose can be a part of the care management required for any patient who may have difficulty maintaining blood glucose within normal limits. This chapter will identify the clients who may require this procedure and explain how to perform it efficiently and safely.

Learning outcomes

This chapter will enable you to:

- discuss the rationale for performing blood glucose measurement
- describe the equipment required to perform blood glucose measurement
- prepare the patient for the procedure
- describe care of the blood glucose monitor
- describe how to carry out blood glucose measurement.

Concepts

- Communication
- Infection control
- Universal precautions
- Patient education
- Patient dignity and privacy
- Report writing
- Quality assurance

Blood glucose measurement

Blood glucose measurement is a procedure to establish the level of glucose in the blood. It may be carried out under the following circumstances:

- In diabetic care to monitor blood glucose levels. The readings can enable the medical team to adjust insulin levels (Alexander, Fawcett and Runciman, 2006). It has the advantage of showing diabetic patients whether their blood glucose is high or low, unlike a urine test which only indicates high blood sugar (Burden, 2001).
- To detect hypoglycaemia (low blood sugar) or hyperglycaemia (high blood sugar).
- To monitor patients on parenteral nutrition to ensure that blood glucose levels are within acceptable limits. It is important to be aware that hyperlipidaemia (raised blood lipids) may alter blood glucose reading.
- To monitor patients who are taking hypogylcaemic medications.
- To eliminate diabetes mellitus as the cause in patients who present in an unconscious state (Skinner, 2005).

⚠ **Professional alert!**

Blood glucose levels are measured in mmol/l. The normal range for an adult is 4.5–5.6 mmol/l, for a child 3.4–5.6 mmol/l, and for a neonate 2.6–5.0 mmol/l (Skinner, 2005). The acceptable range, which may vary with individual patients, should be determined by a doctor and recorded in the patient's notes (Jamieson, McCall and White, 2002).

Part **III**

[S] **Scenario: fear of needles**

Sarah, a 15-year-old girl, has been recently diagnosed with diabetes. She does not like blood and needles. The importance of maintaining her blood sugars within a range has been explained to her. She is shocked to discover that she will have to check her blood sugar levels a few times a day and administer her own insulin injections.

Routine monitoring using a hand-held blood glucose monitor is a quick and convenient means of obtaining blood glucose values. It can be used by the nurse at the patient's bedside or the patient can be instructed in self-use. This is referred to as point-of-care testing (POCT). It facilitates holistic care and timely treatment (RCN, 2005). However, there is a significant risk that errors may occur when using POCT (Dougherty and Lister, 2008).

As mentioned earlier, there may be considerable variations in blood glucose levels depending on the time of day the sample is taken. They are lowest in the morning before breakfast (Blann, 2006), rise immediately after a meal and fall to fasting levels about two hours later (Skinner, 2005).

Capillary blood is used to measure glucose levels when using a blood glucose monitor, and gives a whole blood measurement of glucose. Laboratory-tested blood gives plasma glucose levels. Glucose is more concentrated in plasma, so plasma levels will be higher than whole blood capillary levels (Dungan et al, 2007). Some modern blood glucose monitors are capable of reporting either whole blood or plasma glucose levels (*Diabetes Forecast*, 2007). Therefore, it is important that the nurse records the correct reading.

Blood glucose monitors

Various kinds of blood glucose monitors are available. They vary in size, testing speed, amount of blood needed for the test, ability to store test results in memory, cost of meter and reagent/test strips. It is important to follow the manufacturers' instructions for storage and blood monitoring technique. Compatible test/reagent strips should be used. Monitors should be calibrated according to the manufacturers' guidelines to ensure an accurate result.

Contra-indications

Staff need to be aware that certain conditions may give false results, and in those instances a laboratory measurement using a venous blood sample is required.

Results may be affected by the following:
- dialysis treatment
- hyperlipidaemia
- severe dehydration
- high and low haematocrit values
- high bilirubin values
- peripheral circulatory failure
- intravenous infusions of ascorbic acid (Vitamin C)
- patients receiving intensive oxygen therapy (MHRA, 2005).

Equipment

- blood glucose meter
- test/reagent strips
- a spring-loaded finger pricking device and sterile lancets
- cotton wool balls
- non-sterile gloves and apron
- sharps bin
- record sheet
- receptacle for waste material.

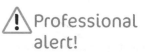

(a) Learning activity

Reflect on how it might feel to be diagnosed with a lifelong condition.

How can you use your communication skills to reassure Sarah about her fears of blood and needles?

Identify the equipment Sarah will need to monitor her blood sugar level.

⚠ Professional alert!

Proper quality assurance and training in the use of blood glucose meters are essential for patient safety (MHRA, 2005). The use of blood glucose meters by untrained staff or without the use of quality control procedures can lead to misleading results, adversely affecting the treatment of patients.

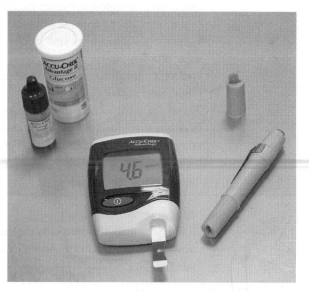

Figure 19.1 Meter and equipment

Procedure

1   Collect and prepare the equipment in order to carry out the procedure smoothly and without unnecessary stoppages.
2   Ensure that you are familiar with how the equipment works. Only practitioners who are specifically trained should use the monitor (MHRA, 2005).
3   Before carrying out the procedure, ensure that the blood glucose monitor is checked and is in working order to ensure accuracy of result. Check that that test/reagent strips have not expired and make sure they are suitable for use. When opening a new container record the date of opening, as strips may need to be used within a certain time once opened (Jamieson et al, 2002).
4   Wash hands and put on gloves and apron to prevent contamination with blood and reduce the risk of cross-infection.
5   Explain the procedure to the patient in order to gain consent and co-operation (NMC, 2008). Discuss any concerns or queries with the patient to minimise patient anxiety.
6   Ask patient to wash hands with soap and water prior to taking sample so as to reduce skin microbial load. Warm water dilates the capillaries and increases blood flow. Provide assistance as appropriate. Alcohol wipes should not be used to clean the puncture site as alcohol interferes with test/reagent strips and repeated use toughens skin (Smith, Durell and Martin, 2004).
7   Ask the patient to sit or lie down to ensure patient safety – some patients may feel faint when a blood sample is taken.
8   Select a suitable puncture site. The side of the finger or the side of the heel are potential sites. Avoid using the back of the heel and the fingertip to reduce pain and prevent damage to underlying nerves. Sites should be varied to reduce the risk of infection from recurrent punctures, to prevent the areas becoming hard and to reduce discomfort (Roche Diagnostics, 2004).

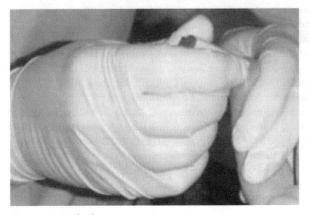

Figure 19.2 The lancet

⚠ Professional alert!

If a sample is taken from an alternative site such as the forearm, make sure that meter and reagent/test strips have been validated for this purpose, and be aware that results may differ from finger tip samples (MHRA, 2005). This is because blood glucose recordings in the finger tips show changes in glucose levels more quickly than other parts of the body (FDA, 2005).

9   Insert the lancet into the spring-loaded device.
10 Remove the protective cap.
11 Place the sterile lancet firmly against the selected area and press the release button to obtain a blood sample. The lancet will immediately puncture the skin.
12 Gently squeeze the finger or heel to produce a sufficient sample of blood to ensure accuracy of result. Avoid massaging blood from the puncture site as this may result in damage to the tissues and the subsequent seepage of tissue fluid will give a false result (Skinner, 2005).
13 If necessary position the finger in a downward position to aid the flow of blood.

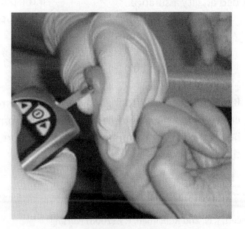

Figure 19.3
Taking a sample

14 Ensure that there is sufficient blood to cover the reagent/test strip. Do not smear or spread the blood on the strip.
15 Continue in accordance with the manufacturer's instructions as the procedure may vary depending on the type of monitor.
16 Read and record the result as soon as it is displayed on the monitor to ensure accuracy. The nurse must know the normal blood glucose range so that abnormalities can be recognised and treatment provided as appropriate.
17 Apply cotton wool to the puncture site and apply pressure to prevent further bleeding and to prevent haematoma formation.
18 Dispose of the lancet in the sharps bin to reduce the risk of injury.

19 Dispose of waste appropriately to prevent the spread of infection.

20 Ensure bleeding has stopped and the patient is comfortable.

21 Remove and dispose of gloves.

22 Wash hands or clean with bactericidal solution to prevent cross-infection.

23 Store the monitor and reagent/test strips according to the manufacturer's instructions.

24 The frequency of blood glucose monitoring will be dictated by the patient's medical condition.

25 Document the blood glucose level and report any abnormal findings to relevant personnel.

(a) Learning activity

Go to the Medicines and Healthcare Products Regulatory Agency website (www.mhra.gov.uk) and access their publication *Point of Care Testing Blood Glucose Meters: Advice for healthcare professionals*.

Find out what type of blood glucose monitor is used in your department and refer to the manufacturer's instructions for recommended quality assurance.

⚠ Professional alert!

If a significantly abnormal reading is obtained when performing blood glucose measurement and the patient is asymptomatic, check the following:

- Were the patient's hands washed prior to the test?
- Was the blood sample sufficient and correctly applied to the test strip?
- Are the reagent strips compatible with the blood glucose monitor?
- Have the reagent strips expired or are they damaged?
- Does the calibration code in the meter correspond with the reagent strips in use?

When all of the above have been checked and rectified, repeat the test. If the patient's blood glucose result is still abnormal, report the findings to medical staff immediately.

Conclusion

Blood glucose monitoring is an essential element in providing care for patients who have erratic blood glucose. It may need to be performed for a number of medical reasons either in hospital or in the community. Patient comfort and accuracy are fundamental to performing this task.

References

Alexander, M., Fawcett, J. N. and Runciman, P. J. (2006) *Nursing Practice Hospital and Home: The adult*, 3rd edn, London, Churchill Livingstone.

Blann, A. (2006) *Routine Blood Tests Explained: A guide for nurses and allied health professionals*, Keswick, M& K Update Ltd.

Burden, M. (2001) 'Diabetes blood glucose monitoring', *Nursing Times* **97**(8), 36–9.

Diabetes Forecast (2007) 'Blood glucose monitoring and data management systems', *Diabetes Forecast* **60**(1), supplement, RG36–51.

Dougherty, L. and Lister, S. (2008) *The Royal Marsden Hospital Manual of Clinical Nursing Procedures*, 7th edn, London, Blackwell Publishing.

Dungan, K., Chapman, J., Braithwaite, S. S. and Buse, J. (2007) 'Glucose measurement: confounding issues in setting target for inpatient management', *Diabetes Care* **30**(2), 403–9.

Jamieson E. M., McCall J. M. and White L. A. (2002) *Clinical Nursing Practices*, 4th edn, London, Churchill Livingston.

Medicines and Healthcare Products Regulatory Agency (MHRA) (2005) 'Point of care testing blood glucose meters: advice for healthcare professionals', MHRA [online] www.mhra.gov.uk/ publications (accessed 1 May 2007).

Nursing and Midwifery Council (NMC) (2008) *Advice: consent*, London, NMC [online] www.nmc.org (accessed 5 January 2009).

Roche Diagnostics (2004) 'Accu-Chem Safe T-Pro Plus: information leaflet', East Sussex, Roche.

Royal College of Nursing (RCN) (2005) *Competencies: An education and training competency framework for capillary blood sampling and venepuncture in children and young people*, London, RCN.

Skinner, S. (2005) *Understanding Clinical Investigations: A quick reference manual*, London, Balliere Tindall.

Smith, S. F., Durell, D. F. and Martin, B. C. (2004) *Clinical Nursing Skills: Basic to advanced skills*, 6th edn, New Jersey, Pearson Prentice Hall.

US Food and Drug Administration (FDA) (2005) *Diabetes Information Glucose Meters and Diabetes Management*, FDA [online] www.fda. gov/diabetes/glucose (accessed 1 May 2007).

Chapter

20

Neurological assessment

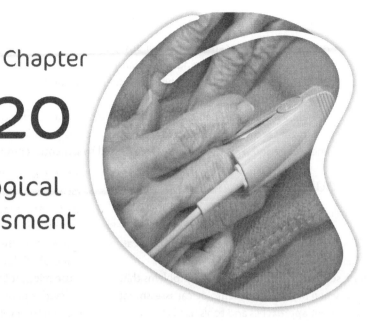

Jessica Knight and
Rachel Palmer

 Links to other chapters in *Foundation Skills for Caring*

16 Vital signs
36 Basic life support: child
37 Basic life support: adult

 Links to other chapters in *Foundation Studies for Caring*

14 Pharmacology and medicines
19 Care of the neonate
21 Care of the acutely ill child
23 Care of the adult – surgical
24 Care of the adult – medical
28 Rehabilitation
30 Emergency care and interventions
31 Child emergency care and resuscitation
32 Adult emergency care and resuscitation

 Don't forget to visit www.palgrave.com/glasper for additional online resources relating to this chapter.

Introduction

Assessment is an essential aspect of any patient's health journey, as it allows the healthcare practitioner to monitor trends and plan patient care. Neurological assessment requires the development of specialised techniques and understanding of the nervous system. The various stages or components of the neurological assessment have been segmented in this chapter to help you flow through the material and develop an understanding of the evidence base. It is highly recommended that direct supervision is provided for all practitioners until their knowledge and skills levels have been assessed by a mentor competent in this area.

Learning outcomes

This chapter will enable you to:

- describe the procedure for completing a neurological assessment
- recognise some possible difficulties and problems that can occur when performing a neurological assessment
- discuss different approaches and tools used in neurological assessment

- appreciate the importance of the underpinning anatomy and physiology of the nervous system
- use relevant literature and research to inform the practice of nursing
- begin to develop recognition of the deteriorating patient through the assessment process.

Concepts

- Assessment of conscious level
- Glasgow coma scale
- AVPU (alert, responds to voice, pain or unresponsive)

- Pupil assessment
- Vital signs
- Limb strength
- Sensation

- Painful stimuli
- Documentation
- Infection control, e.g. hand washing
- Consent

Performing a neurological assessment

Neurological assessments are performed for a number of reasons in clinical practice, such as following a head injury or a fall, when a patient is unresponsive, after anaesthesia or to obtain a base line with new admissions. Within the neurological assessment there are several components:

- level of consciousness
  - AVPU
  - Glasgow coma scale (GCS)
  - Pain/noxious stimuli
- vital signs
- pupil assessment: size and reaction to light
- limb strength (power)/movements
- sensation.

Equipment that you will need to perform a neurological assessment

- neurological assessment charts, e.g.
  - AVPU
  - GCS
  - vital signs chart
  - limb strength and sensation charts
- pen torch
- equipment for vital signs.

> **a** **Learning activity**
>
> Using a web search engine such as Google/Google Academic, put in the search words 'unconsciousness' and 'altered level of consciousness' to see what information might be available on this subject. Consider how you are going to filter and manage the volume of material that you could read.

Neurological assessment chart

The results of assessment of the central and peripheral nervous system are often documented on a single chart. It shows trends visually and provides concise information about the patient's neurological condition, encompassing level of consciousness, vital signs, pupil response, limb strength and sensation.

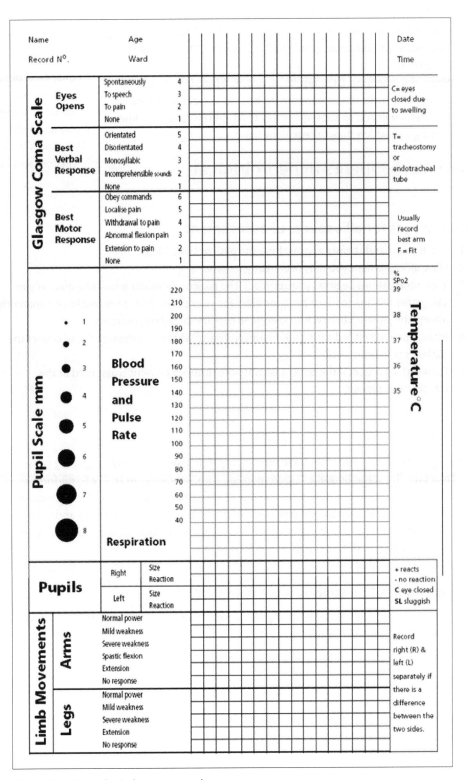

Figure 20.1 Neurological assessment chart

The AVPU and the GCS assessment tools provide a common language to improve communication in reporting neurological findings amongst all healthcare professionals (Aird and McIntosh, 2004; Fischer and Mathieson, 2001).

When documenting GCS results, a dot in black ink should be placed in the middle of the appropriate box on the chart. The dots should then be linked to subsequent observation results with a line to form a graph which shows the patient trend.

Procedures for components of neurological assessment

Core stages for all aspects of assessment

1 Wash your hands before approaching the patient (DH, 2003).
2 Have all equipment you may need ready to hand.
3 Your observations begin as you approach the patient. Consider what information you can gather relating to his or her condition; for example is the patient awake or apparently asleep, the patient's behaviour, position in bed and breathing patterns.
4 Introduce yourself, indicating your name, role and what you intend to do, whatever the patient's conscious level.
5 Gain verbal consent if the patient is conscious. Implied consent is assumed in the unconscious patient.

Assessment of conscious level using AVPU

AVPU is an acronym for the assessing of different levels of consciousness (see Table 20.1) and tends to be documented on existing observation charts or early warning scoring systems as simply A, V, P or U.

Observe your patient to see if they respond spontaneously to your approach, for example saying 'Hello nurse!' If so, than your patient is ALERT, and can be documented as such. If not, then you will need to carry out further assessment. Proceed to talk to your patient, using an agreed name; patients may just be asleep.

You should, from this communication, get an appropriate verbal response. Thus the patient can be documented as responding to

Table 20.1 AVPU

A – Alert	Responds spontaneously
V – Verbal	Responds to voice
P – Pain	Responds to pain
U - Unresponsive	No response to verbal or painful stimuli

verbal stimuli. If no verbal response is obtained, you will need to proceed to apply an appropriate pain stimulus. The patient should at this point respond with a verbal or motor response such as moving limbs. The patient can be documented as responding to pain stimuli. If no verbal or motor response is obtained then the patient is classed and documented as unresponsive.

Procedure for the GCS

The GCS score is obtained by adding together the scores for each component. A minimum score is three (3/15) and a maximum score is 15 (15/15).

Best eye opening

As you approach the patient, note whether the eyes are open or closed. If open, this is classed as open spontaneously and this scores 4.

If the eyes are not open, speak to the patient in a normal tone, raising your voice if necessary. If the eyes open in response to voice, this scores 3.

If the eyes have still not opened, touch your patient on the arm/shoulder with a gentle shake, whilst speaking: for example calling the patient by name, or asking 'can you open your eyes?' If there is no response to this you will then proceed to apply a pain stimulus such as a trapezius muscle squeeze. If the patient responds the score is 2. If there is no eye opening despite all of the above, the patient scores 1.

⚠ Professional alert!

Escalation of assessment from AVPU to GCS should be considered if the patient is only responsive to pain (P) or unresponsive (U). A senior member of the MDT should be informed immediately as this may indicate a serious neurological deterioration (NICE, 2007; Palmer and Knight, 2006).

Table 20.2 Glasgow Coma Scale (GCS): 15 point GCS

Best eye opening	4 Spontaneously 3 To speech 2 To pain 1 None
Best verbal response	5 Orientated 4 Confused conversation 3 Inappropriate words 2 Incomprehensible sounds 1 None
Best motor response	6 Obeys 5 Localises 4 Withdraws 3 Abnormal flexion 2 Extends 1 None

Source: Jennett and Teasdale (1977).

Ⓒ Professional conversation

Mari asks Lena, the staff nurse, 'Do you have any tips on what to do when there's no response from a patient?'

Lena says, 'Some patients respond to better to a familiar family or friend's voice, or the lower pitch of a male voice. It's worth asking someone else to have a try if you get no response yourself. If a patient has severe orbital swelling, it's normal to document closed eyes and not score this component.'

Best verbal

Talk to your patient. Start by asking them to tell you their name. If they can answer correctly, this establishes that they are orientated to person. To establish whether they are orientated to time, ask if they know the date or the day. Some patients may only be aware of the month, season or year. The final component is to assess orientation to place, so ask the patient to identify where they are, for instance the ward name, hospital or city. If they can answer all these components correctly – that is, they are orientated to time, place and person – they score 5.

If they have one or more of these elements wrong, they are classed as disorientated/confused and will score 4.

If they can only answer in monosyllables or words, as opposed to sentences, which are out of context with the questions, they will score 3.

Patients will score 2 if they are unable to format words and are only able to produce incomprehensible sounds such as moans or groans. This may be in response to verbal or pain/ noxious stimuli.

If there is no verbal response despite trying all the above, the patient scores 1.

(C) Professional conversation

Lena the staff nurse offers some key advice to student Mari, 'Remember this is a test of best verbal response. Even if they can write or communicate via other methods, they would still score 1 if there are no verbal sounds.'

(a) Learning activity

Take the opportunity to practise asking a range of different people across the age continuum questions which test their orientation. Reflect on the range of different responses and how you had to alter your questions for different individuals. In paediatrics you may need to assess using an appropriate developmental milestone question such as 'How old are you?' or 'What is your favourite toy's name?'

Best motor response

The best motor response is to be able to obey simple commands convincingly. This is a test of the best response in a single limb as opposed to all limbs. Ask the patient to squeeze and release hands, and/ or place their finger on their nose. Ensure that what you ask the patient to do is within that person's range of movements and physical ability. The patient will score 6 if they are able to obey commands.

If patients localise to pain they will score 5. To identify localisation you must observe them moving their hand to the stimulus and attempting to remove it. This is a purposeful movement.

Patients will score 4 if they withdraw (normal flexion) from pain/noxious stimuli. The limbs will flex (bend at the elbows or knees).

Patients will score 3 if they demonstrate abnormal flexion. Abnormal flexion is easiest to recognise in the arms. The arm will flex at the elbow, wrist and fingers, hands adducted into the body. The thumbs may be pushed through the curled fingers. This is also known as decorticate posturing.

Patients will score 2 if they exhibit extension. In extension the arms and legs are stretched (stiffly) downwards. The forearm pronates (turns away from the body) and the upper arm is held close to the body (adduction). The toes point down (planter flex) and foot may be rolled outwards.

If there is no motor response despite trying all the above, the patient scores 1.

(C) Professional conversation

Lena the staff nurse explains to her student Mari, 'Withdrawal (normal flexion) is often mistaken for localisation. In withdrawal the patient will fail to locate the stimuli being applied; for instance they will not be able to reach and brush the hand away from the area of the body where the stimulus is being applied. To successfully localise they must be able to reach and attempt to remove the stimulus, otherwise it should be documented as withdrawal.'

Procedure for pain/noxious stimuli

A noxious or painful stimulus will need to be applied if the patient does not respond to other auditory (voice) or tactile (touch) stimuli. Initially use a central stimulus (Woodward, 1997; Addison and Crawford, 1999; Shah, 1999; McLeod, 2004) as it can produce an overall body response, and is considered more reliable (Bader and Littlejohn, 2004). A peripheral stimulus is useful in assessing individual limbs.

Start by completing core components as noted above.

Table 20.3 Procedure for pain/noxious stimuli

Central stimuli	
Trapezius muscle squeeze	Pinch/squeeze the trapezius muscle (Figure 20.2). Generally considered best practice in the literature. May be difficult to perform on obese patients (Barker, 2002). **Figure 20.2 Squeezing the trapezius muscle**
Supra-orbital pressure	Do not use in suspected or proven facial trauma. Contradicted in the presence of glaucoma (Barker 2002). Grimacing and eye closure may be the natural response. (Teasdale, 1974), so not always useful to test for best eye opening.
Jaw angle pressure	Do not use in suspected or proven facial trauma. Grimacing and eye closure may be the natural response (Teasdale, 1975), so not always useful to test for best eye opening.
Sternal rub	Sternal rub is *not advocated* in the literature, as it commonly results in bruising of the soft tissue area above. Trauma can be lessened by using a flat open palm (Barker, 2002).
Peripheral stimuli	
Finger pressure	Apply pressure to the side of the finger distal to the last interphalangel joint. Do not apply pressure directly over the nail bed as this can cause damage to the fine capillary network below, resulting in bruising and possible loss of nail. **Figure 20.3 Correct procedure for finger pressure** **Figure 20.4 Incorrect procedure for finger pressure**

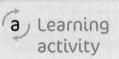

Learning activity

Practise different types of painful stimuli on a consenting volunteer. The above techniques should not cause any marking to the skin.

Vital signs

Assessment of the vital signs is the next section on the neurological assessment chart shown earlier in this chapter. Vital signs give a lot of information about the functioning of the central nervous system. Respiratory rate, rhythm and depth, and pulse and blood pressure are regulated by control centres located within the brain stem, and temperature is controlled by the hypothalamus. These parameters may become altered, indicating neurological deficit; for example, where there is raised intracranial pressure, BP increases, pulse falls and abnormal respiratory patterns may be observed in very late stages. The procedure for vital signs is discussed in Chapter 16.

Procedure for pupil assessment

Pupil assessment is composed of two aspects: pupil size and response to light.

Start by completing core components as described above.

1 Ask the patient to open both eyes (if able).
2 Assess the size of both pupils before testing light reflex. Compare this to size charts commonly included on the neurological assessment chart. The diameter across is measured in mm. Document the size of the pupils, both right and left, before testing for light reaction.

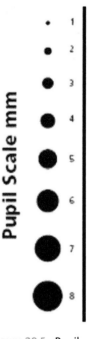

Pupil Scale mm

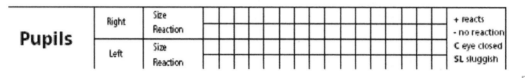

Pupils	Right	Size														+ reacts
		Reaction														− no reaction
	Left	Size														C eye closed
		Reaction														SL sluggish

Figure 20.6 Pupil scale chart

Figure 20.5 Pupil scale measurement

3 The pen torch should be shone onto the eye from the side, rather than directly. Observe for a pupil reaction, that is, pupil constriction.

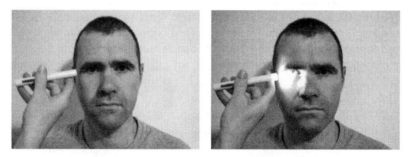

Figure 20.7 Use of pen torch to test pupil reaction

4 If a reaction isn't seen immediately, the light should be held in position to check for a sluggish reaction or establish no response.
5 Document the reaction to light on the observation chart. It is common practice to document a positive reaction using a + sign, no response using a − sign, and sluggish response as SL.

Pupils	Right	Size	4	4	5	6										+ react
		Reaction	+	+	SL	−										− no reaction
	Left	Size	4	4	4	4										C eye closed
		Reaction	+	+	+	+										SL sluggish

Figure 20.8 Pupil scale record

Learning activity

Practise assessing the size and light reaction on a variety of friends and family after gaining their consent. Did you find a particular eye colour more difficult than others?

Practice tip

Unequal pupils, sluggish reaction or no response can be an indicator of raised intracranial pressure (ICP). Photophobia, irritability to light, is another. Pupil size can also be affected by some medications; for example constricted and pinpoint pupils can be caused by the use of opiates, or pupils may be dilated following administration of mydriatic eye drops used in examination of the eye.

Procedure for limb strength (power)/movements

Altered limb strength may be a sign of neurological deficit or dysfunction in some patients. All limbs should be assessed; it may be possible to assess either arms or legs simultaneously in some tests. This facilitates comparison of right and left limbs, which can aid the assessment process.

Limb Movements	Arms	Normal power		Record right (R) & left (L) separately if there is a difference between the two sides.
		Mild weakness		
		Severe weakness		
		Spastic flexion		
		Extension		
		No response		
	Legs	Normal power		
		Mild weakness		
		Severe weakness		
		Extension		
		No response		

Figure 20.9 Limb movements measurement chart

When explaining the assessment to patients, ask if they have any pain or problems that might impair their ability to perform aspects of the test. Ask patients to hold both arms out in front of them and to grip your hands. You can also ask them to pull/push against you if they can, to make your assessment more objective. Arm strength is commonly graded as:

- normal power
- mild weakness
- severe weakness
- spastic flexion
- extension
- no response.

Leg strength can be tested whilst patients are in bed by placing your hands on top of the foot and asking them to pull their toes upwards, and by moving hands to the sole of the foot and asking the patient to push their toes away. If patients are sitting, you can place your hand on their thighs and ask them to lift their legs up, one leg at a time. Leg strength is commonly graded as:

- normal power
- mild weakness
- severe weakness
- extension
- no response.

> **a Learning activity**
>
> Practice assessing limb power on a variety of friends and family after gaining their consent. Reflect on the differences that you find.
>
> As you develop your practice, under supervision you may need to apply a peripheral pain stimulus to limbs that have not been observed to move.

Procedure for sensation

Altered sensation may be a sign of neurological deficit or dysfunction in some patients, especially those with spinal pathology or parietal lobe lesions.

Ask patients if they have any altered sensation over their body. They may describe this in a variety of different ways: numbness, pins and needles, burning, a heavy feeling or woolly sensation (as if being touched through cotton wool). This can be documented in various ways. You may describe the area and altered sensation in the patient notes, or highlight the areas involved on a specific chart such as a dermatone chart. Altered sensation can be assessed in more depth by using fine touch, sharp and dull instruments, temperature or vibration.

Conclusion

Now that you have read through the chapter, it is essential that you go back and complete the learning activities suggested in the text and practise the skills described with your peers and under supervision in the clinical environment.

You should now explore the wider literature around this area. Through discussion with peers, colleagues, mentors and academic advisors, your knowledge base can be further expanded and developed. As you apply the knowledge, the evidence base can be embedded in clinical practice, promoting safe, quality patient care.

References

Addison, C. and Crawford, B. (1999) 'Not bad, just misunderstood', *Nursing Times* **95**(43), 52–3.

Aird, T. and McIntosh, M. (2004) 'Nursing tools and strategies to assess cognition and confusion', *British Journal of Nursing* **13**(10), 621–6.

Bader, M.K. and Littlejohn, L.R. (eds) (2004) *AANN Core Curriculum for Neuroscience Nursing*, 4th edn, St Louis, Saunders.

Barker, E. (2002) *Neuroscience Nursing: A spectrum of care*, 2nd edn, St Louis, Mosby.

Department of Health (DH) (2003) *Winning ways: Working together to reduce healthcare associated infection in England*, Report from the Chief Medical Officer, London, DH.

Evans, R. W. (2007) UpToDate: Concussion and Mild Traumatic Brain Injury (version 15.2) [online] **http://**utdol.com/utd/content/topic. do?topicKey=medneuro/5455&view=print (accessed 9 July 2007).

Fischer, J. and Mathieson, C. (2001) 'The history of the Glasgow coma scale: implications for practice', *Critical Care Nursing Quarterly* **23**(4), 52–8.

Jennett, B. and Teasdale, G. (1977) 'Aspects of coma after severe head injury', *The Lancet* 23, April, 878–81.

McLeod, A. (2004) 'Intra and extracranial causes of alteration in level of consciousness', *British Journal of Nursing* **13**(7), 354–61.

National Institute for Health and Clinical Excellence (NICE) (2007) *NICE Clinical Guideline 56; Head injury: triage, assessment, investigation and early management of head injury in infants, children and adults* (partial update of Clinical Guideline 4), London, NICE.

Palmer, R. and Knight, J. (2006) 'Assessment of altered conscious level in clinical practice', *British Journal of Nursing* **15**(22), 1255–9.

Shah, S. (1999) 'Neurological assessment', *Nursing Standard* **13**(22), 49–56.

Teasdale, G. (1975) 'Acute impairment of brain function – 1: assessing "conscious level"', *Nursing Times*, 12 June, 914–17.

Teasdale, G. M. (2004) 'The Glasgow Coma Scale – 30 years on', Leeds, Neurotrauma Symposium.

Teasdale, G. M. and Jennett, B. (1974) 'Assessment of the coma and impaired consciousness: a practical scale', *The Lancet* 2 (7872), 81–4.

Woodward, S. (1997) 'Practical procedures for nurses No 5.1: Neurological observations 1, Glasgow coma scale', *Nursing Times* **93**(45) supplement, 1–2.

Chapter

21

Pain assessment: child

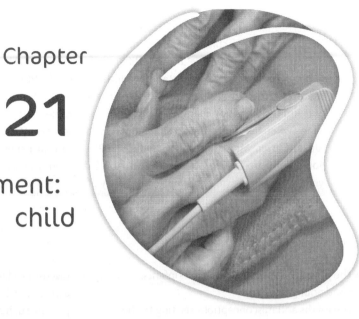

Alyson Davies

 Links to other chapters in *Foundation Skills for Caring*

 Links to other chapters in *Foundation Studies for Caring*

W   Don't forget to visit www.palgrave.com/glasper for additional online resources relating to this chapter.

Introduction

The assessment of children and young people's pain is a complex and challenging issue as children and young people are very different from adults both developmentally and in their cognitive perspective (Simons and Mcdonald, 2006; RCPCH, 2001). This leads to a specific interpretation and perspective of the pain experience. The infant/child/young person may have limited verbal or cognitive skills, making it problematic for them to express themselves clearly when describing the quality and nature of their pain (Carter, Lambrenos and Thursfield, 2002a; Carter, McArthur and Cunliffe, 2002b). Cultural issues also need to be considered (Jongudomkarn, 2006; Gharaibeh and Abu-Saad, 2002) as they can determine the way in which pain is expressed and the acceptability of the method and delivery of analgesia.

Learning outcomes

This chapter will enable you to:

- discuss the purpose of pain assessment in infants, children and young people
- discuss the myths and misconceptions relating to the infant, child and young person's experience of pain
- consider when pain should be assessed and by whom
- describe the ways in which pain can be assessed in infant, child and young person respectively
- discuss the pain assessment tools available to assess the infant, child and young person's pain

- discuss key factors that need to be considered when assessing pain in the infant, the child and the young person, such as development, vocabulary and culture
- identify the coping strategies used by infants, children and young people when they experience pain
- describe the steps involved in assessing the infant's, child's and young person's pain
- describe how the infant, child, young person and family may be supported during the pain experience
- discuss how pain assessment influences pain management.

Concepts

- Infants
- Children
- Young people
- Acute pain
- Chronic pain

- Cognitive development
- Pain myths
- Assessment of pain
- Pain assessment tools
- Pain vocabulary

- Coping strategies
- Family-centred care
- Pain management
- Nursing skills

Children's experience of pain

Children experience physical pain (acute and chronic) as well as psychological pain. Physical pain can be the result of infection, trauma or surgery. Psychological pain can present in relation to the psychosocial influences at home or in the community; effects of hospitalisation where the child or young person becomes distressed by procedures, or by being in hospital and away from home, friends or school; fear of pain or of being injured or hurt in some way; or change in body image (Kortesluoma and Nikkonen, 2004, 2006; RCN, 2001; Twycross, 1998). Unresolved pain profoundly affects the infant, child and young person, leading to withdrawal, regression, non-achievement of milestones, negative recall of hospital and treatment, low self-esteem, poor body image, isolation and depression (Kortesluoma and Nikkonen, 2004, 2006; Carter et al, 2002a; RCN, 2001).

Knowing how much pain a child is experiencing is the first step towards offering appropriate treatment. Pain is a dynamic and complex experience which should be measured and assessed using a multidimensional approach (DH, 2003, 2004; Franck, 2003; RCN, 2001). Effective and accurate pain assessment is a critical step in the process of successfully managing acute pain in the child (Kortesluoma and Nikkonen, 2006; Treadwell, Franck and Vichinsky, 2002) and is an integral part of the care delivered to the child (McArthur and Cunliffe, 1998). Without a good-quality pain assessment, subsequent pain management strategies cannot be based on good information and the care delivered will be flawed. Therefore it is essential that an appropriate, reliable, valid and measurable assessment is performed on a regular basis. Such assessments can be achieved through the use of a validated pain assessment tool (PAT) as a part of the process (RCN, 2001) as well as by observing physiological and behavioural indicators. Healthcare practitioners (HCPs) have a duty of care: a moral, legal and ethical obligation to ensure that children in their care are relieved from pain and suffering (DH, 2003, 2004; Simons, Franck and Roberson, 2001; Simons and McDonald, 2004, 2006; WAG, 2005).

a **Learning activity**

Have you heard any comments about how infants, children, young people experience pain (e.g. 'Babies don't feel pain')?

What did you think of what was said?

Do you think such comments can influence the care given? Give reasons.

Imagine Amy, a 3-year-old who has never experienced pain before. How would you describe the concept of pain to her?

Myths and misconceptions

Despite advances in research into children's pain experiences and the need for evidence-based practice, some common myths and misconceptions still persist about the pain experiences of infants, children and young people (Table 21.1). These are insidious as they influence the practitioner's thinking and view of the child, and can lead to a child's pain being prolonged, debilitating and untreated (Twycross, 1997, 1998, 2007; RCN, 2001; Twycross, Moriarty and Betts, 1998; Collier, 1997).

⚠ **Professional alert!**

Be aware of the many myths and misconceptions that surround the child's experience of pain, its assessment and management (Twycross, 1997, 1998; Twycross et al, 1998; Collier, 1997).

Table 21.1 Twelve pain myths

Myth	Fact
Active children cannot be in pain.	Playing and being active or being distracted is one of the most effective ways in which infants, children and young people cope with pain. Some children and young people spontaneously use this method to focus away from their pain.
Children will always tell you when they are in pain.	Children may not report pain due to fear or a desire to please those around them. A child who conceals pain may do so in an attempt to avoid a further painful experience, such as a needle. Older children may not wish to appear weak by showing their pain, especially in front of their peers.
Children feel less pain than adults.	Younger children experience higher levels of pain than do older ones. For some, pain sensitivity seems to decrease with age. This may be due to cognitive development and the increasing ability to use coping strategies and to rationalise the pain.
Children forget pain quicker than adults.	Children can be traumatised by the pain episode and become fearful of further procedures or admissions. Children and young people's coping skills are not as well honed as an adult's and so they may be unable to rationalise what is happening.
It is unsafe to administer narcotics to children because they become addicted.	Addiction is rare. When used over a short period for pain narcotics are beneficial in resolving pain.
Narcotics always cause respiratory depression in children.	This is very rare. Children tolerate narcotic analgesia well. As long as it is given at the correct dosage and via the correct route it is safe.
Children cannot accurately tell you where it hurts.	Children can describe the intensity, location and meaning of their pain very clearly.

Myth	Fact
The best way to administer analgesia is by injection.	This method is unacceptable to children and young people. It is often the thing they fear most about hospital and pain relief.
Parents always know the best way to manage their children's pain.	Parents may not have seen their child in pain and can feel lost and vulnerable. They will need advice and support to care for their child in this situation.
Generally there is a usual amount of pain associated with any given procedure.	This is untrue and unacceptable as it can lead to children and young people not receiving adequate medication.
The less analgesia administered to children the better it is for them.	Unresolved pain leads to increased stress, delayed wound healing and a child who is fearful.
It is often being restrained during procedures rather than pain that children find distressing.	Restraint can be frightening but should not be assumed to be the cause of the child's distress as pain is heightened during fear-inducing procedures.

Source: Hospital for Sick Children (2008), McDonald and Simons, 2002; RCN (2001), Twycross (1998), Collier (1997).

When is pain assessed?

Pain assessment should be continuous and form part of the HCP's ongoing observations and nursing activities. Formal assessment may occur on a regular basis if analgesia is required or has been administered. It should be an individual, child-centred, holistic process dictated by the needs of the infant, child or young person and not by the routines of the care situation or by people's own preferences or prejudices (Twycross, 2002, 2007). Specific points at which pain can be assessed are:

- As part of the admission process (Twycross, 2002, 2007; RCN, 2001). The infant/child/young person and family will be able to discuss how the infant/child/young person reacts to pain, their pain behaviour, pain vocabulary, previous experiences and management of pain.
- At regular intervals, using a validated PAT (Twycross, 2002; RCN, 2001) to assess the pain and record pain scores and descriptors. The time between assessments will depend on the individual patient.
- When undertaking routine procedures if the child is experiencing or has experienced pain.
- When unexpected intense pain occurs, as indicated by altered vital signs, behaviour or verbal communication.

Who should assess the child in pain?

- *Child*: self-report is the gold standard as only the child/young person can accurately describe their pain experience (Kortesluoma and Nikkonen, 2004; Franck, 2003; RCN, 2001; Polkki, Pietila and Rissanen, 1999; McGrath, 1990). Children as young as 3 years old are able to accurately describe the nature, location and intensity of their pain (RCN, 2001). Children with special needs or undeveloped or limited verbal skills may be unable to communicate about their pain verbally but may be able to do so by signing, pointing or using a picture/letter board (Carter 1993).
- *Parents*: are the experts on their child's behaviour (Casey et al, 2002b). Parents can be a valuable source of information (DH, 2003, 2004; Franck, 2003; RCN, 2001; Twycross, 2002; Simons, Franck and Roberson, 2001; McGrath, 1990; WAG, 2005). They know their child best and may have had previous valuable experience in managing their child's pain (Zisk et al, 2007; Kankkunen et al, 2003; Carter et al, 2002b; 2002; Polkki, Vehilainen-Julkunen and Pietila, 2002 et al, 2002b; Morgan et al, 2001).
- *Healthcare practitioner*: the HCP is able to assess using a multi-faceted approach, gathering information from child and parents, observations and through using a PAT (Twycross, 2002, 2007; RCN, 2001).

> **Learning activity**
>
> What would you observe or notice in a patient who was in pain? What might you look for?

How is pain assessed?

Pain may be assessed by several methods – behaviourally, physiologically and cognitively.

Behavioural indicators focus on the child's behaviour and may include:

- crying
- screaming
- shouting
- pulling knees up to chest
- hitting out
- refusal to be comforted
- withdrawal
- putting on a brave face.

Older children may discuss how they feel but may need encouragement to do so. Young people may become withdrawn and silent, and expect the HCP to 'know' they are in pain (Carter et al, 2002a; RCN, 2001; Twycross, 1997, 1998).

Physiological indicators are initially a guide to the infant/child/young person's status. The patient may have a tachycardia, tachypnoea, raised blood pressure and may be pallid. However these signs cannot be relied on for a prolonged period of time as the autonomic nervous system (ANS) will stabilise the physiological signs.

Cognitive appraisal is particularly useful as it provides the child's perspective on what is happening, giving the HCP insight into the child's experience and which PAT is most appropriate. PATs can be used to assess this dimension and as an adjunct to assess the child's thoughts, experience and vocabulary.

Family-centred care must be given at all times. The family holds valuable information about their child and can provide insight into how their child responds to and manages pain. Family members can play a pivotal role by being involved in the assessment and ongoing management of the pain experience. Roles will need to be negotiated according to the degree of involvement they wish to have (Zisk et al, 2007; Twycross, 2007; Kankkunnen et al, 2003; Polkki et al, 2002; RCN, 2001; Simons et al, 2001).

t ☆ Practice tips

- Be eclectic; use a multidimensional approach to assessing pain in such a wide client group.
- Teach the child/young person and family how to use the PAT.
- Assess the child/young person's ability to use the tool independently; consider for instance how sick children are, and their willingness to participate.

Pain assessment tools

A wide variety of PATs are now available (see examples below). The PAT enables the practitioner to assess with a high degree of accuracy the nature, intensity and effects of the pain. However other variables must be considered too, such as the development of the child and the psychological impact of being sick and in pain. Choose a PAT which is suited to the child's age, cognitive development, verbal ability and cultural background (Simons and McDonald, 2006, 2004; Gharaibeh and Abu-Saad, 2002; Peden and Vater, 2003; RCN, 2001). The PAT will require the patient or parent to make a judgement using faces (Oucher scale, Wong Baker scale), numbers or words (numeric scale/word scale) or to mark on a body diagram the location and intensity of their pain. This will require the HCP to think analytically about the choice of tool as not all PATs are suitable for all infants, children and young people. The HCP must be discerning and choose the appropriate tool to ensure its successful use with the patient and family members who may wish to be involved (Chambers, Giesbrecht and Craig, 1999).

PATs available suitable for different groups of children include:

- neonates and infants – CRIES (Krechel and Bildner, 1995) and NIPS
- nonverbal, cognitively impaired and anxious children – FLACC scale (Merkel et al, 1997)
- children over age of 4 years – Wong-Baker scale (FACES scale)
- older children – visual analogue scales
- body outlines can help establish the location of the child's pain
- behavioural observational scales, the main method of assessment used in infants and children under 3 years, and can also be used in children who are cognitively impaired.

Part

III

CRIES

CRIES is a behavioural assessment tool that assesses crying, oxygen requirement, increased vital signs, facial expression and sleep. The assessor provides a score of 0–2 for each parameter based on changes from a baseline. For example, a grimace, the facial expression most often associated with pain, gains a score of 1 but if associated with a grunt will be scored at 2. The scale is very useful for neonatal postoperative pain.

Wong-Baker scale (FACES scale)

For a child over 3–4 years the faces scale is the most effective. Numerous faces scales have been developed; the most well known is possibly the Wong and Baker (1988). This self-report scale is thought to be easily understood by children as they point directly at the faces and do not need to translate their pain into a numerical value.

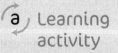

Learning activity

Compare these pain assessment tools and decide which you think would be the most appropriate tool to use to assess the pain experienced by a baby.

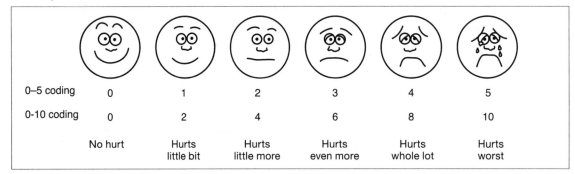

0–5 coding	0	1	2	3	4	5
0-10 coding	0	2	4	6	8	10
	No hurt	Hurts little bit	Hurts little more	Hurts even more	Hurts whole lot	Hurts worst

Figure 21.1 Wong-Baker FACES pain rating scale

Source: Hockenberry, M. J., Wilson, D.: *Wong's Essentials of Pediatric Nursing*, ed.8, St. Louis, 2009, Mosby. Used with permission, copyright Mosby.

Learning activity

Ali is 6 years old and had his appendix removed yesterday. His mother is not present when you assess his pain. He tells you that he is not as sore as yesterday. He scores 4 on the faces scale.
   Do you think that is an accurate score for pain? What may influence his scoring?

Visual analogue scale

For older children the visual analogue scale can be used. This takes the form of a vertical or horizontal line which is numbered 1–10 along its axis. The child then rates where his or her pain is on the scale. Zero at one end indicates no pain and 10 at the other end represents the worst pain imaginable.

Eland colour scale

This scales encourages the child to use different colours to indicate the severity of pain in different body parts.
   After discussing several things that have hurt the child in the past:
1   Present eight crayons or markers to the child. Suggested colours are yellow, orange, red, green, blue, purple, brown and black.
2   Ask the following questions, and after the child has answered, mark the appropriate square on the tool (e.g., severe pain, worst hurt), and put that colour away from the others. For convenience, the word hurt is used here, but whatever term the child uses should be substituted. Ask the child these questions:

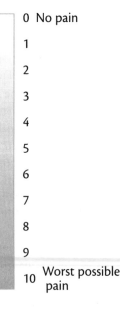

Figure 21.2 Visual analogue scale

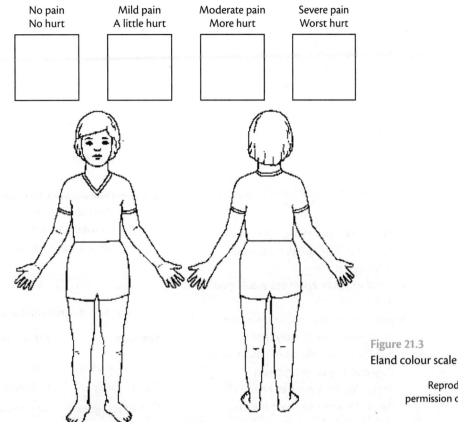

No pain
No hurt

Mild pain
A little hurt

Moderate pain
More hurt

Severe pain
Worst hurt

Figure 21.3

Eland colour scale

Reproduced with
permission of Jo Eland.

- 'Of these colours, which colour is most like the worst hurt you have ever had (using whatever example the child has given), or the worst hurt anybody could ever have?' The phrase that is chosen will depend on the child's experience and what the child is able to understand. Some children may be able to imagine much worse pain than they have ever had, while others can only understand what they have experienced. Of course, some children may have experienced the worst pain they can imagine.
- 'Which colour is almost as much hurt as the worst hurt (or use another phrase, as discussed above), but not quite as bad?'
- 'Which colour is like something that hurts just a little?'
- 'Which colour is like no hurt at all?'

3   Show the four colours (marked boxes, crayons, or markers) to the child in the order s/he has chosen them, from the colour chosen for the worst hurt to the colour chosen for no hurt.

4   Ask the child to colour the body outlines where s/he hurts, using the colours s/he has chosen to show how much it hurts.

5   When the child finishes, ask if this is a picture of how s/he feels now or was feeling earlier. Be specific about what earlier means by relating the time to an event (e.g. at lunch or in the playroom).

W   To download a version of the Eland colour scale visit: http://www.painresearch.utah.edu/cancerpain/attachb6.html.

Word-graphic rating scale

Figure 21.4 shows a simple word rating scale.

No pain	Little pain	Medium pain	Large pain	Worst pain possible

Figure 21.4 Word graphic rating scale

a Learning activity

Can you remember a painful event in your childhood? Thinking back over the experience, how would you have rated that pain on the faces or visual analogue scale?

a Learning activity

- How would you explain pain to a 2-year-old, 5-year-old, 9-year-old, 15-year-old?
- What words or analogies would you use?
- How might they explain their pain? What words might they use?
- Ask friends or colleagues what words they know of or use for pain.
- Keep a log for a week to record all the words you hear from friends, colleagues and patients.

Pain vocabulary

Children and young people have a colourful and varied vocabulary to describe their pain and are able to provide excellent descriptors of it (Kortesluoma and Nikkonen, 2004, 2006; LaFleur and Raway, 1999). An understanding of the child's vocabulary will enable HCPs to interpret the child's experience of pain and tailor their communication and delivery of care appropriately.

t Practice tip

Assess the child's level of cognitive development and use the appropriate level of language to meet his/her level of understanding. Use play or toys to facilitate this assessment and build a trusting relationship with the child or young person.

t Practice tip

The choice of the most suitable tool in each situation should be based on:

- the child's age
- cognitive ability
- time available to educate the child about the scale
- knowledge nurses have about the scale (Twycross, 1998).

Table 21.2 **Pain descriptions used by children**

Sensory	Affective	Evaluative
Lots of banging	Sad	Bad
Get it mostly	Unhappy	Ugly
Comes and goes	Drive you nuts	Awful
Buzzing	Bugged you	No good
Painful	Attacking	Different
Grabbing	Mean	Funny
Fall off	No strength	Terrible
Hitting	Scared	Not nice
Snow	Upset	Yucky
Ouch	Disappointed	Nagging
Sausage	Not well	Weird
Once and a while	Crying	Not good
Needle through	Hard	Like headache
Warm	Dizzy	A lot
Knife hit	Banging	Worst
Cymbals clapping	Falling	Really bad
Bullet	Chilling	Mild
Tickled	Sounds funny	Very sore
Off and on	Mosquitoes buzzing	Little bad
	Wee bit	Feel worse
	Sometimes	

Source: Jerret and Evans (1986).

Coping skills

Children have the ability to cope with pain and have particular strategies which they use. It is important for practitioners to know about these coping strategies so that they can facilitate their use and indeed use them as a nursing intervention when pain is experienced. Also the practitioner must be able to recognise the coping behaviour when it occurs.

Table 21.3 Cognitive and behavioural coping strategies

Cognitive strategies	Behavioural strategies
Distraction – play, singing, reading, watching television. Relaxation – rocking, singing, talking to oneself. Guided imagery. Positive self talk. Thought stopping.	Hiding away – withdrawing physically or psychologically. Fighting it – resisting, pulling away, crying. Making it good – moving position, patting, rubbing, holding comforter.

Sources: Kankkunen et al (2003), Polkki et al (2002), Woodgate and Kristjanson (1995).

> **Learning activity**
>
> What factors would you need to take into account when assessing a child who might be or is going to be in pain?

Assessment skills

You will need:
- a sphygmomanometer
- a thermometer for taking vital signs
- a PAT suitable for the age and cognitive development of the infant, child or young person
- documentation for recording information.

> **t**
> **Practice tip**
>
> When you ask children/young people to give you their own names for their pain, try to do so at a time when they are pain-free/comfortable as they will be more communicative at this stage.

Procedure

Immediate care

1 Observe the child for signs of distress, agitation, crying, restlessness, undue quietness, closed eyes (RCN, 2001),
2 Assess vital signs for tachycardia, tachypnoea, elevated blood pressure.

⚠ Professional alert!

Do not rely totally on physiological indicators as these will return to within normal parameters even if the child is in pain.

3 Ask the child/young person and the parents directly about the pain.
4 Ask the child/young person to describe the pain – location, intensity, duration (use a toy/picture board/letter board as appropriate to communicate).
5 Allow the child/young person time to indicate the pain intensity and describe it using the tool, and his or her own language and interpretation.
6 Record the time of the episode, pain score and descriptors of the pain in the nursing notes, and inform senior staff.
7 Carry out the appropriate nursing interventions to minimise or eradicate the pain, such as positioning the child differently or using non-pharmacological techniques (Table 21.3).
8 Give analgesia as prescribed and as per hospital policy.
9 Document the interventions in the nursing notes.

Part
III

10 Reassess the pain at 15-minute intervals using self-report and PAT, to evaluate whether the nursing interventions/analgesia are effective and make a decision to continue, reassess or alter the nursing care.

11 Once the infant/child/young person is comfortable, continue to reassess the child/young person's pain at frequent intervals (2–4 hourly) to identify whether the pain episode is recurring and the analgesia is remaining effective.

12 Leave a PAT with the family so that they can monitor and report pain if it occurs.

⚠ Professional alert!

If the method of administering analgesia is unacceptable to the child/young person, they might not be wholly truthful about levels of pain.

Admission and ongoing care

Table 21.4 Child and parent report forms

Child form	Parent form
Tell me what pain is.	What word(s) does your child use in regard to pain?
Tell me about the hurt you have had before.	Describe the pain experiences your child has had before.
Do you tell others when you hurt? If yes, who?	Does your child tell you or others when he or she is hurting?
What do you do for yourself when you are hurting?	How do you know when your child is in pain?
What do you want others to do for you when you hurt?	How does your child usually react to pain?
What don't you want others to do for you when you hurt?	What do you do for your child when he or she is hurting?
What helps the most to take your hurt away?	What does your child do for him- or herself when he or she is hurting?
Is there anything special that you want me to know about you when you hurt? (If yes, have child describe.)	What works best to decrease or take away your child's pain?
	Is there anything special that you would like me to know about your child and pain? (If yes, describe.)

Adapted from Hester and Barcus, 1986.

1 Involve the parents in the assessment of the child's pain to gain a holistic view of the experience (DH, 2003, 2004; Zisk et al, 2007; WAG, 2005; Franck, 2003; Carter et al, 2002b, 2002; RCN, 2001; Twycross, 2002).

2 Obtain a detailed pain history from the child and parents on admission if feasible (i.e. if the child is pain free) (Twycross, 2002, 2007; RCN, 2001; Hester and Barcus, 1986 Table 21.4).

3 Assess the child's cognitive level and pain vocabulary on admission (Twycross, 2007, 2002; RCN, 2001; Twycross et al, 1998; LaFleur and Raway, 1999; Hester, Foster and Beyer, 1992; Jerret and Evans, 1986).

4 If the child is admitted as an emergency or is in considerable pain, ask parents for the words the child uses to express their pain.

5 Assess the child's coping strategies on admission or when pain free (WAG, 2005; DH, 2003, 2004; Woodgate and Kristjanson, 1995).

6 Assess the cultural factors which may affect the expression of pain and the assessment process (Gharaibeh and Abu-Saad, 2002; Knott et al, 1994).

7 Give a self-report PAT to the child/young person and parents with instructions on its use, preferably before the pain occurs/recurs (Twycross, 2002; RCN, 2001; Twycross et al, 1998).

> ⚠ Professional alert!
>
> Children who are sleeping, playing or appear quiet may still be in some pain. They may be
> using these activities as a means of distraction, so assess their pain levels regardless.

Conclusion

The infant/child/young person's experience of pain is challenging, complex and debilitating. Unresolved pain leads to long-lasting consequences for the ongoing care, recovery, development and psychological progress of the infant, child or young person. The pain experience is modulated by many factors, including development, vocabulary, family setting, culture and temperament. It is a highly individual experience which must be valued and acknowledged fully by the HCP. It is essential that all HCPs are knowledgeable about the fundamentally important differences that underpin the infant/child/young person's experience of pain. It is vital they understand that children and young people have very different perspectives on pain and expectations of how their pain is managed.

This chapter has provided an insight into the key issues that should be considered and that should inform the delivery of good-quality care. By completing the learning activities in this chapter, HCPs should develop their knowledge of infants', children's and young people's pain and pain assessment. This knowledge must be evidence based and should underpin good-quality practice to ensure that, following a holistic assessment of the infant's, child's and young person's pain experience, prompt, effective management occurs within the context of family-centred care.

References

Agency for Healthcare Policy and Research (AHPR) (1992) *Clinical Practice Guideline: Acute pain management operative and medical procedures and trauma, management of post operative and procedural pain in children*, Washington DC, AHPR.

Carter, B., Lambrenos, K. and Thursfield, J. (2002a) 'A pain workshop: an approach to eliciting the views of young people with chronic pain,' *Journal of Clinical Nursing* 11, 753–62.

Carter, B., McArthur, E. and Cunliffe, M. (2002b) 'Dealing with uncertainty: parental assessment of pain in their children with profound special needs', *Journal of Advanced Nursing* 38(5), 449–57.

Casey, A. (1993) 'Development and use of the partnership model of care,' pp. 183–93 in Glasper, E.A. and Tucker, A. (eds) *Advances in Child Health Nursing*, London, Scutari Press.

Chambers, C. T., Giesbrecht, K. and Craig, K. D. (1999) 'A comparison of faces scales for the measurement of paediatric pain: children's and parent's ratings', *Pain* 83(1), 25–35.

Collier, J. (1997) 'Attitudes to children's pain: exploding the pain myth', *Paediatric Nursing* 9(10), 15–18.

Department of Health (DH) (2003) pp. 27–8 in *Getting the Right Start: The National Services Framework for Children, Young People and Maternity Services, standards for hospital service*, London, DH [online] www.doh.gov.uk/nsf/children/standardhospserviceindex.htm (accessed 14 October 2008).

DH (2004) pp. 32–3 in *The NSF for Children, Young People and Maternity Services: Children and young people who are ill*, London, DH [online] http://www.doh.gov.uk/nsf/children (accessed 14 October 2008).

Franck, L S. (2003) 'Nursing management of children's pain: current evidence and future directions for research', *Nursing Times Research* 8(5), 330–53.

Gharaibeh, M. and Abu-Saad, H. (2002) 'Cultural validation of paediatric pain assessment tools: a Jordanian perspective', *Journal of Transcultural Nursing* 13(1), 12–18.

Hester, N. O. and Barcus, C. S. (1986) 'Assessment and management of pain in children', *Pediatric Nursing Update* 1, 1–8.

Hester, N. O., Foster, R. L. and Beyer, J. E. (1992) 'Clinical judgment in assessing children's pain', pp 236–94 in Watt-Watson, J. H. and Donovan, M. I. (eds), *Pain Management: Nursing perspective*, St. Louis, Mosby-Yearbook.

Hospital for Sick Children (2008) 'About Kid's Health', Hospital for Sick Children [online] http://www.aboutkidshealth.ca/pain/myths-aboutpain (accessed on 14 October 2008).

Jerret, M. D. and Evans, K. (1986) 'Children's pain vocabulary', *Journal of Advanced Nursing* 11, 403–8.

Jongudomkarn, D. (2006) 'The meanings of pain: a qualitative study of the perspectives of children living with pain in North Eastern Thailand', *Nursing and health Sciences* 8, 156–63.

Kankkunen, P., Vehilainen-Julkunen, K., Pietial, A. and Halonen, P. (2003) 'Parents' use of non pharmacological methods to alleviate children's postoperative pain at home', *Journal of Advanced Nursing* 41(4), 367–75.

Knott, C., Beyer, J., Villarruch, A., Denyer, M., Erickson, V. and Willard, G. (1994) 'Using the Oucher developmental approach to pain assessment in children', *MCN American Journal of Maternal and Child Nursing* 19(6), 314–20.

Kortesluoma, R. L. and Nikkonen, M. (2004) '"I had this horrible pain": the sources of and causes of pain experiences in 4–11 year old hospitalised children', *Journal of Child Healthcare* 8(3), 210–31.

Kortesluoma, R. L. and Nikkonen, M. (2006) '"The most disgusting ever": children's pain descriptions and views of the properties of

Part
III

pain', *Journal of Child Healthcare* **10**(3), 213–27.

Krechel, S. W. and Bildner, J. (1995) 'CRIES: a new neonatal postoperative pain measurement score; initial testing of validation and reliability', *Paediatric Anaesthesia* 5, 53–61.

LaFleur, C.J. and Raway, B. (1999) 'School age child and adolescent perception of the pain intensity associated with three word descriptors', *Pediatric Nursing* **25**(1), 45–55.

McArthur, E. and Cunliffe, M. (1998) 'Pain assessment and documentation: making a difference', *Journal of Child Healthcare* 2(4), 164–9.

McDonald, L. and Simons, J. (2002) *Pain Assessment in Children (Surgical and Non Surgical Patients): Information and resource pack for nurses*, London, Pain Control Service, Great Ormond Street Hospital for Children Trust [online] http://www.ich.ucl.ac.uk/website/gosh/clinicalservices/pain_control_services/custom (accessed 8 October 2008).

McGrath, P.A. (1990) 'Pain assessment in children: practical approach', pp. 66–7, 312–13, 354, 364, New York, Raven Press.

McGrath, P.A., Finley, G.A. and Richie, J. (1994) Parents' roles in pain assessment and management, *IASP Newsletter* March/April, 3–4.

Merkel, S., Vopel-Lewis, T., Shayevitz, J. and Malviya, S. (1997) 'The FLACC; a behavioural scale for scoring postoperative pain in young children', *Pediatric Nursing* **23**(3), 293–7.

Morgan, J., Peden, V., Bhaskar, K., Vater, M. and Choonara, I. (2001) 'Assessment of pain by parents in young children following surgery', *Paediatric Anaesthesia* 11, 449–52.

Peden, V. and Vater, M. (2003) 'Validating the Derbyshire Children's Hospital pain tool: a pilot study', *Paediatric Anaesthesia* 13, 109–13.

Polkki, T., Pietila, A. and Rissanen, L. (1999) 'Pain in children: qualitative research of Finnish school aged children's experiences of pain in hospital', *International Journal of Nursing Practice* 5, 21–8.

Polkki, T., Vehilainen-Julkunen, K. and Pietila, A. (2002) 'Parents' roles in using non pharmacological methods in their child's postoperative pain alleviation', *Journal of Clinical Nursing* **11**(4), 526–536.

Royal College of Nursing (RCN) (2001) *Clinical Practice Guidelines: The recognition and assessment of acute pain in children, technical report, guidelines objectives and methods of guideline development*, London, RCN.

Royal College of Paediatrics and Child Health (RCPCH) (2001) *Guidelines for Good Practice: Recognition and assessment of acute pain in children*, London, RCPCH.

Simons, J., Franck, L. S. and Roberson, E. (2001) 'Parent involvement in children's pain care: views of parents and nurses', *Journal of Advanced Nursing* **36**(4), 591–9.

Simons, J. and McDonald, L. M. (2006) 'Changing practice: implementing validated paediatric pain assessment tools', *Journal of Child Healthcare* **10**(2), 160–76.

Simons, M. and McDonald, L. H. (2004) 'Pain assessment tools: children's nurses' views', *Journal of Child healthcare* **8**(4), 264–278.

Treadwell, M.J., Franck, L.S. and Vichinsky, E. (2002) 'Using quality improvement strategies to enhance pediatric pain assessment', *International Journal for Quality in Healthcare* **14**(1), 39–47.

Twycross, A. (1997) 'Nurses' perceptions of pain in children', *Paediatric Nursing* **9**(1), 16.

Twycross, A. (1998) 'Perceptions about children's pain experience', *Professional Nurse* **13**(12), 822–6.

Twycross, A. (2002) 'Managing pain in children: an observational study', *Nursing Times Research* **7**(3), 164–78.

Twycross, A. (2007) 'Children's nurses' post operative pain management practices: an observational study', *International Journal of Nursing Studies* 44, 869–81.

Twycross, A., Moriarty, A. and Betts, T. (1998) *Paediatric Pain Management* (Chapter 1), Oxford, Radcliffe Medical Press.

Welsh Assembly Government (WAG) (2005) 'The NSF for children, young people and maternity services in Wales', Cardiff, WAG [online] http://www.wales.nhs.uk/sites3/documents/441/EnglishNSF%5Famended%5Ffinal%2Epdf (accessed 14 October 2008).

Woodgate, R. and Kristjanson, L.J. (1995) 'Young children's behavioural responses to acute pain: strategies for getting better', *Journal of Advanced Nursing* 22, 243–9.

Zisk, R. Y., Grey, M., Medoff-Cooper, B. and Kain, Z. N. (2007) 'Accuracy of parental-global-impression of children's acute pain', *Pain Management Nursing* **8**(2), 72–6.

Websites

www.rcn.org.uk for clinical practice guidelines. The recognition and assessment of acute pain in children. Implementation guide.

www.ppprofile.org.uk for paediatric pain profile.

Chapter

22

Pain assessment: adult

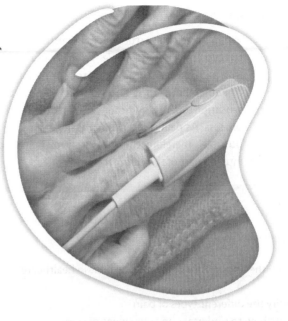

Chris Hanks and Tim Jenkinson

 Links to other chapters in *Foundation Skills for Caring*

 Links to other chapters in *Foundation Studies for Caring*

 Don't forget to visit www.palgrave.com/glasper for additional online resources relating to this chapter.

Introduction

When asked, many students say that they came into the health profession because they want to help and care for people. Whether in the community or on a hospital ward, you will find that pain is a very common reason for people needing help and care.

Remember pain is an important diagnostic sign; the site, intensity and duration of the sensation offers significant information to the doctor and nurse concerning the disease process. As pain is often a distressing symptom it is necessary to alleviate the suffering where possible. Therefore the measuring of pain and instigating interventions to relieve it is an integral part of the caring role.

Learning outcomes

This chapter will enable you to:

- explain the importance of pain assessment in healthcare practice
- identify the different types of pain
- discuss how to undertake an assessment of someone's pain
- debate the use of various pain tools

- identify the various myths and misconceptions relating to the experience of pain
- understand the extent of pain experience in healthcare
- reflect on their own experience of pain
- outline the prevalence of pain in the community
- explore the attitudes of HCPs to patients expressing pain.

Concepts

- Pain as an everyday occurrence
- Pain in older adults
- Communication and body language
- The meaning of pain

- The challenging patient
- Acute and chronic pain
- Stereotyping and labelling
- Assessment skills

(a) Learning activity

Think about the last time you were in pain. How did it feel? What did you think about and how did it affect your behaviour?

In the learning activity it is likely that you will have identified a number of words to describe your feelings, such as 'agony', 'sharp', 'aching', 'hurt', 'burning', 'discomfort' or 'sore'. No doubt you wanted the pain to go away and it might have affected your behaviour in some way; perhaps you started crying, or rubbing the area or just went to bed to get over it. You might have also taken some painkillers to help. It is important to remember that just as you feel pain and it means something to you, so too will the patients you will be nursing. People have their own individual responses to the pain sensation and this will help you understand how behaviour may alter in order to try and cope. In addition there are numerous cultural differences that may affect the expression of pain (see for example Davidhizar and Giger, 2004).

Pain is an everyday occurrence

In a recent survey (NOP, 2005) in the UK, one in four (26 per cent) of almost 1000 people surveyed were in pain on the day they were questioned, and one in five people (21 per cent) experienced pain most days or every day.

In the survey, pain was most commonly caused by back pain (27 per cent), arthritis (24 per cent), headache (16 per cent) or injury (8 per cent). Other reasons were stomach or gastrointestinal pain (4 per cent), migraine (3 per cent), cancer (3 per cent) and heart disease (2 per cent).

Of course, these findings were for people in the community who answered the telephone. The people that nurses may come into contact with may be in hospital undergoing treatment or following surgery, or perhaps in a nursing/residential home.

S   Scenario: pain after an operation for appendicitis

Paul James, aged 37, is a local businessman. For some time he has been troubled by an aching pain on the right side of his abdomen. One afternoon, whilst playing a game of football for his local team, he collapses to the ground holding his right side complaining of pain and then vomits a small amount of clear fluid. An ambulance is called and Paul is taken to hospital. Upon examination, the doctor at A&E suspects acute appendicitis. A blood test reveals an elevated leucocyte (white cell) count which confirms the diagnosis. He requires surgery to remove the appendix. After obtaining his consent the operation takes place under a general anaesthetic. Paul is returning to your ward following an appendectomy. He has regained consciousness but is feeling nauseous and is complaining of pain at the wound site. He looks pale, is perspiring and seems quite anxious.

Even though Paul has had his inflamed appendix removed and that was the primary source of his pain, he is now experiencing a different pain from the wound site. This is most likely to be an acute type of pain that after rest and healing will gradually subside, but until that happens Paul will require prompt and effective pain management in the postoperative period. First, you will need to conduct a pain assessment to ascertain the type of pain he is feeling, its location and intensity. If the wound is visible and can be checked, then this provides a most useful observation to ensure that there is no redness, swelling or discharge. The use of an appropriate pain scale to record the assessment with a numerical rating, the patient's score, is recommended, followed by the appropriate course of action such as the administration of an analgesic and then periodic assessment of its effectiveness.

---

a   Learning activity

Explain the priorities of your postoperative assessment of Paul's pain and indicate how this would be treated.

a   Learning activity

What would you consider to be the most appropriate route for administering this drug to Paul?

In the scenario, given that this is the immediate postoperative period and that Paul is probably feeling nauseous, combined with the fact that he has had a general anaesthetic, the most appropriate route would be an intramuscular injection. Any other route such as oral or intravenous would be ill advised and unnecessary. The analgesia will of course be prescribed by the doctor or specialist nurse depending upon its properties.

Pain in older adults

As people get older, the likelihood of suffering pain increases; nearly one in three (32 per cent) of the over-65s were found to be in pain at least most days. Indeed, National UK statistics in 1997 showed that pain was reported by 65 per cent of women and 56 per cent of men who were over 75 years of age, and this rose even higher among those in residential care. So pain is very common in the community, particularly in the population over 65 years, and these are the people whom you will care for most commonly. It may be surprising, therefore, to find that older people do not always receive adequate pain control. Part of the reason for this may be the following misconceptions:

- Pain is a normal part of ageing.
- Strong analgesics cannot be used for older people.
- If a person does not admit to pain, then they do not have pain.

A well-known and much quoted definition of pain is that offered by McCaffery (1979): 'Pain is whatever the experiencing person says is existing whenever the person says it does.' What do you understand by this definition and what does it tell us about the pain experience? Do you see any difficulties with the definition? First, the quote tells us that pain is unique to the individual. If people complain of pain then they are to be believed and steps should be taken to intervene and relieve the pain where possible. This is a very important perception from a nursing perspective because it implies that patients are the experts on their own pain as Portenoy (1999: 1695) suggests: 'Pain is inherently subjective ... a patient's self-report is the gold standard for assessment.'

All too often healthcare professionals (HCPs) impose their own values on someone else's pain and this can lead to delays in action. However, the McCaffrey definition implies that the person needs to verbalise the pain, speak to someone and complain. It is important to remember that nurses care for a great number of patients who are unable to verbalise their feelings and therefore may show their pain through various non-verbal signs.

> **(a) Learning activity**
>
> Make a list of conditions that might affect a person's ability to communicate verbally. In what way might someone non-verbally (without speech) communicate that they are in pain?

There are many conditions that can affect verbal communication. Many of these affect the central nervous system, so in the learning activity you may have included conditions such as stroke, dementia, multiple sclerosis, learning disabilities, cerebral palsy and Parkinson's disease in your list. For patients who cannot communicate verbally the successful interpretation of non-verbal cues is essential to effective pain control.

You may have identified:

- restlessness
- moaning or crying
- frowning or grimacing
- rocking back and forth
- rubbing the affected area
- tearfulness
- pallor and/or sweating.

(S) Scenario: surgery in an elderly patient

Having retired from a distinguished 30-year career in the police force, Albert Finch has spent the last ten years living with his wife and daughter in their detached cottage in the countryside. He is now approaching his 70th birthday, and Mrs Finch has become increasingly concerned about her husband's forgetfulness. This culminated in her finding him outside on two occasions at night, unsure of where he was. After being referred to a specialist by his GP and after a series of investigations that involved extensive memory tests, Albert is diagnosed with early Alzheimer's disease and is prescribed a course of Aricept. However, since his diagnosis 12 months ago Albert's memory for events has got progressively worse and he now has difficulty expressing himself verbally. Understandably the family are very concerned for him. One evening he is found in his drive by his daughter having fallen and unable to move his right leg or stand. He is admitted as an emergency to the local A&E department.

An X-ray reveals that Albert has fractured the neck of his right femur and he requires surgery under general anaesthetic to stabilise the fracture. The surgeon carefully explains the procedure to both Mr and Mrs Finch, and Albert is able to give his consent for the operation. He returns to your ward two hours later having regained consciousness but is quite restless.

> **(a) Learning activity**
>
> Explain what issues there will be arising from your initial assessment of Albert's pain in the immediate postoperative period.

Surgery of the type that arises in the scenario involves a prolonged period of time on the operating table. Given the nature of the operation it is classed as major surgery; it will have involved a considerable loss of blood that would have necessitated a transfusion in the operating department. As Albert is restless, it is likely that he is in pain or dehydrated or both. The pain will be emanating from the bone and the wound site but may also be a result of lying on the operating table for some considerable time. It is important to talk to Albert about his pain even if he struggles to explain how he is feeling and where the pain is. The priority of care here is for the registered nurse to administer prescribed analgesia as directed so that Albert's pain is managed as soon as possible. As he is restless following surgery, there is a risk that he may hurt himself or damage the wound site, so it is very important to relieve the pain. Given his history, Albert may need to have things explained to him regularly so that he can appreciate what is happening, and the use of bedrails could assist with his ongoing safety as long as these are carefully explained to him and why they are being used. One of the common pitfalls of nursing people with memory problems in orthopaedic surgery is that their postoperative restlessness can be wrongly attributed to the confusion of old age. Unfortunately where this stereotypical error occurs, it is less likely that the person's pain will be managed effectively.

> **Learning activity**
>
> Think of elderly patients you have come across in your own practice. Have any appeared disorientated? How did you handle the situation?

Understanding that not all people can or will express their pain verbally is an important part of the ongoing assessment process. From this particular scenario we learn that Albert is experiencing problems expressing himself with words, so he might find it difficult to actually say when he is in pain and where the pain is coming from. This makes him very vulnerable, and he is largely reliant on an observant nurse or doctor to interpret his non-verbal cues. When people are in pain they often become restless and perspire. They may start to grimace, grind their teeth or frown. They may also start to hold or rub the affected area. All of these non-verbal behaviours may be accompanied by groaning. In the case of Albert, he has come back to the ward in a restless state which is indicative of something being wrong. Therefore it is very important that the nurse correctly assesses this and is able to act on that information, accurately recording in the patient's nursing record the sequence of events. Following the administration of the prescribed analgesia Albert will require ongoing assessment to ascertain the effectiveness of the drug and the need for subsequent doses.

These important non-verbal signs may also accompany the verbal expression of pain. It is perhaps easier to respond to someone who actively complains of pain, so nurses need to develop keen observational skills to help with the assessment of pain in patients who suffer communication difficulties. You also need to be aware that some patients may not complain of pain for the following reasons:

- *Some patients do not want to be perceived as complaining or doubt that carers will believe them.* First, believe the patients. They are the authority on their pain. Patients rarely lie about or exaggerate their pain (Clarke, 2008).
- *Patients may not want to have any further tests, or may want to go home and are concerned that an admission of pain may delay their discharge.* You need to have a good rapport with the patients, and keep them informed about their progress.
- *The patient has a stoic manner and feels that admitting to pain shows weakness.* You could explain the benefits of having the pain treated. Perhaps the patient does not realise that having pain can be detrimental to his or her recovery. McCaffery and Pasero (1999) noted that poorly controlled acute pain can lead to debilitating chronic pain syndromes in some patients.
- *The patient may worry about taking analgesics.* Both patients and HCPs may have misconceptions about strong analgesics such as opiates (for example, morphine). In general these are very effective and safe drugs if used properly: that is, beginning with low doses and slowly increasing them so that the pain is controlled. Many patients think that using opiates will leave them addicted; however this is a very rare occurrence. The patient who has chronic cancer pain may be worried that s/he will 'get used to' the morphine, and then have nothing left to turn to if the pain gets 'really bad'. Of course the patient's pain may not

Part

III

get worse, and many patients do not need to increase their dose significantly, but if there is a need, other types of opiates can be used (McQuay, 1999).

In the course of their work HCPs encounter many people who are in pain. Although the essence of good care is to believe people when they say they are in pain, sometimes nurses and other HCPs such as doctors may come to doubt patients' complaints, viewing them as disingenuous.

ⓐ Learning activity

Why would some HCPs suspect the validity of patients' accounts of their own pain? Make a list of the type of patients who might fall into this category.

In the learning activity it is likely that you have identified those people who are viewed as 'unpopular' (Stockwell, 1972; Johnson and Webb, 1995) or 'difficult' (Kelly and May, 1982). This group of patients may include those who:

- overly complain
- are viewed as attention seekers
- have no definite diagnosis or physical cause for their pain, for example where there is abdominal pain of unknown cause
- are aggressive, rude, demanding or ungrateful
- seem fixated by or exaggerating their pain (Blomqvist, 2003)
- might be addicted to painkillers.

As you can see these are quite negative views to hold of another person, especially someone who is ill, but they are generally born out of a sense of dissatisfaction or frustration with not being able to achieve the reward of successful pain relief. As most HCPs are driven by a motive to care for people who are ill and suffering, the inability to relieve pain with analgesia can leave them unsure on how to proceed, particularly in cases of chronic illness where pain can be ever present.

However, the labelling of patients as 'difficult' is problematic and can lead to the risk of so-called 'non-caring' (Carveth, 1995) where the HCP actually limits the time spent with such patients or avoids them altogether. Although there might be a minority of people who will use their pain to their own advantage, the vast majority do not. It is not for the nurse or doctor to decide, but rather to attempt to understand the behaviour and resolve the difficulties.

The medical diagnosis of illness can depend upon the successful interpretation of a patient's pain, where it is, how long it lasts, what it feels like and what relieves it. If after investigation, there is no obvious reason for the person's pain – that is, a definite physical cause such as an inflamed appendix or renal calculi – then the medical model reaches its limit. If the experience of pain is ongoing without an identifiable cause, this could be a time when the patient's account is brought into question. Again this is not good practice, as the failure to reach a diagnosis might lead to punitive labelling of the person as a 'malingerer' or 'time waster'. Labels such as this, when they are shared between HCPs, can seriously damage the quality of the healthcare experience for the patient. Labelling something as 'trivial' or 'exaggerated', or comparing patient with patient or between genders, completely negates the individual experience of pain.

It is important for the HCP to appreciate that in all cases of complaint of pain the patient is to be believed, and even in the absence of an identifiable cause for the pain the nurse in particular must work at resolving the discomfort through exhibiting professional behaviour, undertaking appropriate assessments and administering prescribed analgesia.

A patient who continually complains of pain even though analgesia has been given can indeed be challenging but still requires attention from the nurse; in some instances there may be scope for an exploration of alternative methods of pain relief to work alongside the medical model.

Patients who are in pain may be grouped into those with acute pain and those with chronic pain.

Acute pain

People who have had surgery, or who attend the A&E department with injuries often have what is termed acute pain. This is the pain that you may have experienced when you stab your finger with a sewing needle, or if you have sprained your ankle. It is the result of injury, surgery (postoperative), a medical illness or childbirth. Acute pain lasts only a short time, a few seconds to a few weeks, and goes away as healing occurs. Acute pain is protective; in addition to providing a warning of injury or tissue damage, pain encourages you to hold the injured part of the body still (immobilising it), which often prevents further injury. Imagine what would happen if you fractured your ankle and did not feel the pain!

Chronic pain

Chronic pain, on the other hand, continues for longer. Reasons for chronic pain may include rheumatoid arthritis or osteoarthritis, cancer or heart disease. Sometimes it is not clear what is causing the pain. Chronic pain has been defined as a pain that lasts three months or longer, and it may come and go over a period of years. It may not be possible to completely alleviate the problem, and some patients have to be helped to 'live with' chronic pain.

Chronic pain may make it difficult to live life as one did previously. It is likely that chronic pain would affect the patient's mood and relationships with family and friends, causing irritability, anger and often depression. This, in turn, may affect the way in which other people respond to the patient, as they become resentful of the situation that is also affecting their lives, and then may feel guilty because they are no longer as sympathetic as they once were.

Chronic pain may affect people's appetite, sleep and movement. Patients may begin to see themselves as disabled, and have a lowered self-esteem. They may no longer be able to work, and be worried about the financial problems.

Unlike acute pain, chronic pain is not a protective mechanism; it serves no function.

As you can see the experience and expression of pain is a complex phenomenon, but it is nonetheless the duty of the nurse to undertake appropriate assessments and implement actions to relieve or lessen pain in patients.

(S) Scenario: rheumatoid arthritis

In 1984, at the age of 33 years Elizabeth Carr was diagnosed with rheumatoid arthritis. She had started to suffer with inflamed joints of the fingers and wrists of both hands and developed similar problems in her right shoulder. During the worst times the inflammation interfered with her mobility, especially her ability to maintain independence and dress herself, which in turn affected her work as a primary school teacher. In addition to this the joints often became very painful and swollen. As the illness progressed other joints in the body were affected, including her knees and ankles, and this further reduced Elizabeth's mobility. Such were the difficulties she faced that at the age of just 40 years Elizabeth was forced to retire from her job on the grounds of ill health.

Throughout the duration of the illness there have been many attempts to try and combat its progression and reduce the inflammation through the prescription of various analgesics and steroids. Now, some 25 years later, Elizabeth's mobility is greatly reduced. She has developed deformities within the small joints of her fingers and feet and is reliant to some extent on others to help her with activities of living. Although her husband does what he can, he still needs to work and has a part-time job as a security officer at a local warehouse. Elizabeth makes use of aids for daily living such as adapted cutlery and kitchen utensils but does require help with washing and dressing. To help her husband to continue with his work, the community nursing team have arranged for Elizabeth to visit a local day centre three times a week. Here she can have her mobility and pain assessed and the nursing staff help her to have a bath. The day centre also gives her the opportunity to meet and talk with other people. Pain is an everyday experience for Elizabeth. It is chronic in nature having lasted many years and is some days visibly upsetting to her. Attempts to control her pain through conventional means have been variable to say the least, and particularly in these later years have been of limited use.

a Learning activity

Explain how you would make an assessment of Elizabeth's pain during her visits to the day centre.

Chronic pain of the nature discussed in the scenario is often difficult to assess. The best person to advise you on how it feels and where it is located is Elizabeth herself as she has an extensive knowledge of the pain. Therefore you will need to enter into a dialogue with her, asking her about her pain and what it is like. Can she describe it? Note the words that she uses, such as aching, stabbing or grinding, and whether there is anything that eases the pain. Given that Elizabeth has been prescribed various analgesics for many years with limited success, it might be that she has adopted different strategies for coping with her pain. Indeed there may be things that actually aggravate the situation, and clearly these need to be avoided; these might include a particular body posture or sitting in an uncomfortable position. With chronic pain it is very important to take time to listen to the patient's perspective as you will gain important insights into to what it is like to suffer with this chronic discomfort, and from this different ways of coping can be discussed.

All too often people with chronic pain complain that nobody listens or understands their predicament and they feel isolated and alone with a pain that never seems to go away. Just imagine how this must be. Think how this type of pain, ever present, might affect your concentration and limit your quality of life. It might also interfere with your sleep and make you tired and irritable, thereby putting a strain on relationships. A thorough, detailed assessment that takes into consideration the patient's point of view and description of their own feelings is an essential component of effective chronic pain assessment.

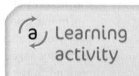

What other approaches to pain management might be available to Elizabeth?

There are many challenges to chronic pain management. Sometimes managing the pain is very difficult and the traditional conventional ways of working, such as prescribing and administering analgesia, can fail or achieve only limited results. This is what Potter (1998) describes as the 'confines of biomedicine' which, he goes on to say, has 'so manifestly failed to address the problem of chronic pain'. People with long-term conditions (LTCs) such as rheumatoid arthritis often experience pain, and the older people with LTCs become, the more likely it is that pain will become a feature of their lives. This is very problematic for the patients and also for the HCPs who work with them, especially if analgesia is viewed as the only solution to the problem. That is why nurses need to have a good knowledge not only of analgesic properties but also how patients deal with their pain at the times when they are alone. This may well reveal other ways of managing and coping that are not so reliant on the biomedical approach.

People who have endured chronic pain for many years can sometimes be challenging to nurse because they may be frustrated and angry about their predicament, or even depressed and despairing that nothing can be done. This can be difficult to deal with, especially if the healthcare system is being blamed for the individual's problems. Sometimes people with chronic pain can become unpopular and difficult to nurse because of their occasional angry outbursts or defeatist talk or their general tired and withdrawn behaviour. But this is what chronic unresolved pain can do.

a Learning activity

Discuss the challenges that nurses face when attempting to manage chronic pain in people with long-term conditions.

As analgesia is known to have numerous limitations in the management of chronic pain, it is often necessary to consider other approaches. Some of these are relatively simple and may involve little more than helping patients to reposition themselves or perhaps apply heat to an affected area. Other therapies (termed complementary therapies because they complement the biomedical approach) such as massage, aromatherapy and reflexology can be offered, and they have been found to achieve results for some people. However it is important to remember that complementary therapies need to be carried out by appropriately qualified individuals who have received training and are fully cognisant with the various contraindications of using these approaches. The use of these therapies can be discussed with Elizabeth in consultation with her GP and can be offered either in the home or during her time at the day centre.

Assessment skills

In order to be effective in your role of pain assessment and thereby inform successful pain management, you need to develop a number of observational, listening and responding skills. In addition you will require knowledge and a good attitude to this part of your work. These are summarised under the following headings.

Knowledge:
- of pain tools and their limitations
- of analgesic properties, doses and side effects
- of alternative approaches to pain control
- of pain and its meaning to people, its emotional significance and pain-related behaviours.

Skills:
- communication: listening and responding
- assessment
- record keeping
- observational: looking, watching, interpreting
- administering prescribed analgesia under supervision
- monitoring effects of analgesia
- problem solving.

Attitudes:
- positive and helping
- motivated to relieve pain
- positive attitude to passing information on to other HCPs (qualified nurses and doctors) so that appropriate analgesia can be prescribed
- empathy with the patient
- evaluating effectiveness of analgesia
- challenging stereotypical views and myths about pain experience that may delay action.

From your own perspective the assessment of pain is largely sense dependent, especially the use of sight and sound to provide you with the information you will need to develop a plan of action. So you will need to carefully *observe* the patient and interpret the various non-verbal cues that you will see. You will also need to converse with the patient and *listen* carefully to their responses to your questions and the descriptions that they give for the pain they are feeling, its location and type. It is useful to practise your opening statement to the patient to elicit information.

(C) Professional conversation

Dev, a staff nurse, comments, 'The use of the word "pain", such as in the questions "Are you in any pain?" or "How is your pain today?" may not always be the correct approach, as some people are reluctant to admit that they are in pain, not wishing to be a burden or showing signs, as they see it, of weakness or dependence. This again shows how complex the meaning and expression of pain can be. Sometimes you need to find a different phrasing to get the answer you are looking for. You might for example ask, "How are you feeling today?" or "Are you in any discomfort?" or "How are you feeling after your operation?" This way the patient might feel more able to complain about their pain without feeling under pressure to do so or admit to it.'

Having made the assessment you will also need to *record* your findings accurately under the supervision of a qualified nurse on the appropriate documentation, such as a pain chart, care pathway or nursing record sheet. In addition, if you have noted anything untoward or unusual about the patient during your assessment you must act accordingly by passing this information on to a qualified nurse.

The purpose of assessment is to build a plan of action that will result in the effective management of the patient's pain. In the hospital setting this most often involves the use

Part
III

of analgesia but must also include an evaluation of the drug's effectiveness with an ongoing review and repeated assessment in order to maintain effective pain control.

In order to assist with the assessment of pain a number of measurement tools have been devised to provide the nurse with information from patients, concerning their individual perceptions of pain.

Pain rating scales

It is helpful to use some form of pain rating scale or measuring tool to assist with the assessment of pain (Williamson, 2005). This gives patients the opportunity to rate their own pain and provides over time a record of how effective the various pain control methods have been. A pain-rating scale can show evidence of the lessening of pain but can also demonstrate unresolved pain or even its escalation. It is very important that the person undertaking the assessment with the patient knows how to use the tool and interpret the findings, for without this knowledge the tool has little relevance. The clinical effectiveness of the tool is dependent on the self-reporting of pain experience from the patient that is facilitated by the skilled questioning of the nurse.

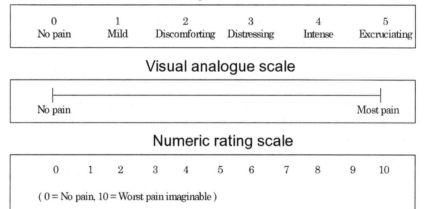

Categorical scale

0	1	2	3	4	5
No pain	Mild	Discomforting	Distressing	Intense	Excruciating

Visual analogue scale

No pain   Most pain

Numeric rating scale

0   1   2   3   4   5   6   7   8   9   10

(0 = No pain, 10 = Worst pain imaginable)

Figure 22.1 **Pain rating scales**

The three types of pain scale shown in Figure 22.1 require the patient to indicate the intensity of pain they are feeling.

The *categorical scale* gives an opportunity to describe the pain, ranging from 0 (= no pain) to 5 (= excruciating). Although easy to use, this type of rating does depend on an understanding of the terms used; for example the interpretation of words such as 'distressing' and 'discomfort' may well vary from person to person and they may use other words to describe their pain such as 'hurting' 'aching', 'dull' or 'sharp'. The differentiation between something that is 'intense' as opposed to 'excruciating' might be difficult to ascertain. A categorical scale such as this is useful if it encapsulates the true meaning of the pain sensation in the patient's own words.

The *visual analogue scale* on the other hand offers the patient an opportunity to rate the pain according to its position along a line that ranges from 'no pain' on the left to 'most pain' on the right. Again this is a convenient method for assessing pain but nonetheless requires the patient to conceptualise the line as a gradient of increasing pain. It is not clear how effectively a very poorly patient would respond to such a diagrammatic representation of pain sensation. Clearly the use of a scale such as this would require a thorough explanation if it is to serve its purpose.

Alternatively the *numeric rating scale* encourages the patient to rate the pain according to a numerical scale where the higher the number recorded the greater the pain. This gives the nurse an indication of how effective pain-relieving methods have been and the results would seem easier to measure than the visual analogue scale.

Another rating scale that is in common usage is the FACES scale, which we also discussed in Chapter 21. This is a more visual assessment that shows a series of faces that are synonymous with the pain sensation. Patients are asked to look at the faces and compare them with their own feelings. They then rate their pain accordingly, once again in numerical fashion depending upon the match they make. Whilst this is particularly successful when assessing the pain of children, it remains to be seen how useful this type of scale is with adults. In particular it could be used with those individuals who have communication difficulties or who have difficulty conversing in English; however, this tool must be used with tact as it may cause offence to some adults who see it as childish and embarrassing to have to point to a picture.

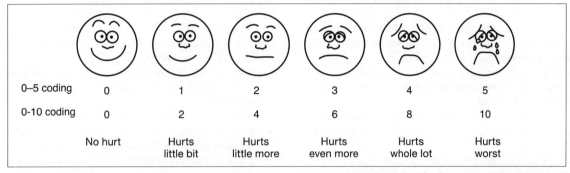

Figure 22.2 Wong-Baker FACES pain rating scale

Source: Hockenberry, M. J., Wilson, D.: *Wong's Essentials of Pediatric Nursing*, ed.8, St. Louis, 2009, Mosby). Used with permission, copyright Mosby.

All of the scales described here need to be tailored to meet the individual patient's needs. The suitability of each scale and the way it will be used need to be carefully discussed with the patients so that they fully understand their role in the assessment process. Therefore the nurse administering the scale needs to be knowledgeable about the tool and supportive of the patient during the assessment.

So, you are faced with a patient who tells you that they are in pain: what do you do?

- Pay attention to the patient, to what they are saying and how it is making them feel. Reassure them that you will report their pain quickly, and then do it.
- A student nurse will need to report the patient's pain to a registered nurse who will administer the prescribed analgesia.
- There may be additional ways, however, to make the patient more comfortable. The patient may require help to reposition themself to make the pain easier. Pillows may be used to support their position or a painful limb for example. The application of a warm blanket may also ease them. Lighting and noise levels may be modified for the patient's comfort. Some patients may want to be left alone in privacy, while others prefer the presence of the nurse.
- Other non-pharmacological approaches may be suggested to the patient. For example, the application of heat or cold may be used to relieve pain (Herr and Kwekkeboom, 2003); however care must be taken to protect the patient from injury. Or relaxation may be encouraged with focused breathing, or with restful music of the patient's choice. The physiological changes that accompany relaxation may reduce the patient's perception of pain.

Conclusion

The experience of pain is commonplace in healthcare practice. Many patients will complain that they are in pain for a variety of reasons. Whilst pain is an important diagnostic symptom, it can also be a most distressing and uncomfortable sensation that requires relief. It is the role of the nurse to effectively assess the patient's pain with the intention to lessen and where possible relieve it by the administration of appropriate analgesia and/or other methods. The skills of assessment are central to effective pain management. This chapter has given you an opportunity to examine the necessary knowledge, skills and attitudes required to succeed in this important aspect of your work.

References

Blomqvist, K. (2003) 'Older people in persistent pain: nursing and paramedical staff perceptions and pain management', *Journal of Advanced Nursing* **41**(6) 575–84.

Carveth, J. A. (1995) 'Perceived patient deviance and avoidance by nurses: what should nurses do to reduce difficulties?', *Nursing Research* 44, 173–7.

Clarke, K. (2008) 'Effects of failing to believe patients' experiences of pain', *Nursing Times* **104**(8), 30–1.

Davidhizar, R. and Giger, J. N. (2004) 'A review of the literature on care of clients in pain who are culturally diverse', *International Nursing Review* **51**(1), 47–55.

Herr, K. A. and Kwekkeboom, K. L (2003) 'Assisting older clients with pain management in the home', *Home Health Care Management and Practice* **15**(3), 237–50.

Johnson, M. and Webb, C. (1995) 'Rediscovering unpopular patients: the concept of social judgement', *Journal of Advanced Nursing* 21, 466–75.

Kelly, M. P. and May, D. (1982) 'Good and bad patients: a review of the literature and a theoretical critique', *Journal of Advanced Nursing* 7, 147–56.

McCaffery, M. (1979) *Nursing Management of Patients in Pain*, 2nd edn, Philadelphia, J.B. Lippincott.

McCaffery, M. and Pasero, C. (1999) *Pain: Clinical manual*, St Louis, C.V. Mosby.

McQuay, H. (1999) 'Opioids in pain management', *The Lancet* 353, 26 June, 2229–32.

NOP (2005) 'Pain survey conducted by the British Pain Society' NOP [online] http://www.britishpainsociety.org/Pain%20Survey%20 NOP%20Report%202005.pdf (accessed 28 April 2008).

Portenoy, R. K. and Lesage, P. (1999) 'Management of cancer pain', *The Lancet* 353, 15 May, 1695–1700.

Potter, R. G. (1998) 'The prevention of chronic pain', in Carter, B. (ed.), *Perspectives on Pain: Mapping the territory*, New York, Oxford University Press.

Stockwell, F. (1972) *The Unpopular Patient*, London, RCN.

Williamson, A. (2005) 'Pain: a review of three commonly used pain rating scales', *Journal of Clinical Nursing* 14, 798–804.

Wong, D. and Whaley, L. (1986) *Clinical Handbook of Pediatric Nursing*, 2nd edn, St. Louis, C.V. Mosby.

Chapter

23

Diabetic foot assessment

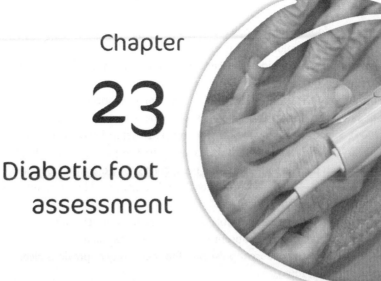

Anita Stuart and Emma Toms

Links to other chapters in *Foundation Skills for Caring*

9   Patient hygiene
14 Basic foot care and managing common nail pathologies
19 Blood glucose measurement
30 Universal precautions
31 Wound assessment
32 Aseptic technique and wound management

Links to other chapters in *Foundation Studies for Caring*

2   Interprofessional learning
7   Public health and health promotion
10 Nutritional assessment and needs
13 Infection prevention and control
25 Care of the older adult – community
34 Primary care

W   Don't forget to visit www.palgrave.com/glasper for additional
online resources relating to this chapter.

Part
III

Introduction

Diabetes mellitus foot-related problems are the single main cause of lower extremity amputations and are a major global health problem (Apelqvist, 2007). It has been shown that almost half of all diabetic amputees had not had an adequate vascular assessment (van Houtum et al, 2001). This is very alarming as around 5 per cent of people with diabetes will develop a foot ulcer in any year, but the risk of ulceration can be reduced through appropriate patient education and timely involvement of a podiatrist (Edmonds, Foster and Sanders, 2004). Effective care involves a working partnership between the patient and the multidisciplinary team where all decisions relating to the patient's care should be shared (Katzen, 2002). Each patient's annual review must consist of a diabetic foot check (Jarvis and Rubin, 2003). As a part of this check both feet should be examined by a trained clinician and a risk factor should be stated:

- *At low risk* – normal sensations, palpable pedal pulses, no foot deformity.
- *At increased risk* – neuropathy or absent pulse plus other risk factor.
- *At high risk* – neuropathy or absent pulse plus foot deformity or previous ulcer.
- *Ulcerated* foot (NICE, 2004).

After the assessment a care plan including foot care education should be agreed with each individual patient (NICE, 2004).

Learning outcomes

This chapter will enable you to:

- discuss the importance of a diabetic foot assessment
- discuss the procedure involved in the vascular assessment of the foot
- discuss the procedure involved in the neurological assessment of the foot
- present basic footcare and footwear advice to patients with diabetes.

Concepts

- Diabetes
- Multidisciplinary team working
- Health promotion
- Health education
- Importance of assessment
- Safety
- Infection control
- Communication

The aim of this chapter is to teach you how to carry out a diabetic foot assessment appropriately. Each assessment must be preceded with a full history taking: diabetic history; complications of diabetes such as retinopathy, nephropathy, cardiovascular problems, cerebrovascular problems; medical history; drug history; family history; psychosocial circumstances; and a past foot history (Mousley, 2006). To conduct the foot assessment the clinician should be in possession of a hand-held Doppler, ultrasonic/coupling gel, 128 MHz tuning fork or neurothesiometer if possible, and a 10 g monofilament (Edmonds and Foster, 2000). The assessment should also include a visual foot check, and any skin breakdown, swelling, change of colour or pain should be investigated further (Edmonds et al, 2004). Before the assessment the clinician should explain to the patient what is going to happen and why. The patient should also be informed of the findings, and the consequences of the outcomes of the tests should be explained (Edmonds and Foster, 2000).

Vascular assessment

This part of the chapter will help you to use terminology correctly, locate and palpate pedal/foot pulses, use a hand-held Doppler device (and distinguish between different sounds), employ the ABPI test (see page 223) and evaluate findings, assess risk status and then proceed with an appropriate care plan.

To start with though, some key terminology is given below (*Oxford Concise Medical Dictionary*, 2000; Kumar and Clark, 2002):

- *ABPI test*: the ankle brachial pressure index test – a test to determine the quality of the blood flow in the lower limb.
- *Brachial pressure*: blood pressure measured in the arm.
- *Cutaneous microcirculation*: blood flow in the skin.
- *Doppler*: an ultrasound device used to detect the arterial and/or venous blood flow.
- *Intermittent claudication*: pains at the back of the legs experienced by patients with poor blood supply during exercise.
- *Ischaemia*: an inadequate flow of blood to a part of the body caused by constriction blockage of the artery supplying it (see examples in the photographs below).
- *Monophasic, biphasic and triphasic wave sound*: the quality of the blood flow sound heard whilst using the Doppler device.
- *NICE*: National Institute of Clinical Excellence.
- *Oedema*: swelling of tissues.
- *Pedal pulses*: pulses found in the foot – dorsalis pedis and the posterior tibial pulse.
- *PVD/POAD*: peripheral vascular disease/peripheral obstructive arterial disease – disease of the arteries resulting in poor quality of blood flow.
- *Palpation*: examining and detection of the pulses using finger tips and hands.
- *Rest pain*: pains in feet due to severe ischaemia that results in patients experiencing pains in feet and legs at rest.
- *SCRT*: subcapilliary plexus refill time – the time allowed for the blood to fully come back to the tissues.
- *Ultrasonic or coupling gel*: water-based gel used with the Doppler.

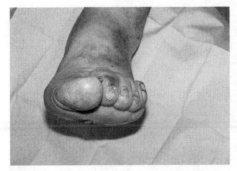

Figure 23.1 Ischaemic foot

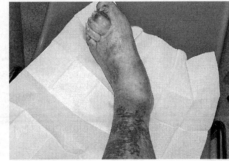

Figure 23.2 Ischaemic limb

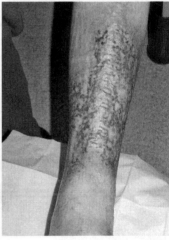

Figure 23.3 Telangiectasis

It is not appropriate to suggest that peripheral vascular disease/peripheral obstructive arterial disease (PVD/POAD) is present on the basis of one examination, so different tests should be used to determine the patient's full vascular status (Davies, 2001).

The easiest test is the palpation of the dorsalis pedis and the posterior tibial pulses. However, clinicians should be aware that in 10–18 per cent of the population the dorsalis pedis may be absent and the posterior tibial artery is absent in approximately 0.2 per cent of people tested. Failing to locate pedal pulses may also be caused by pedal oedema, poor technique, anatomic abnormalities or low cardiac output. In these circumstances the vascular assessment can be extended to the examination of the peroneal, popliteal and the femoral arteries (Cohen and Ratner, 1986).

The dorsalis pedis pulse is palpated on the dorsum of the foot lateral to the extensor hallucis longus tendon, and the posterior tibial pulse is palpable below and behind the medial malleolus. If these pulses are easily palpable it is very unlikely that a POAD is present (Edmonds et al, 2004).

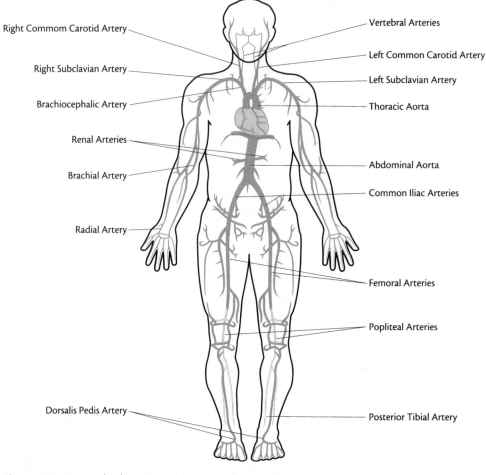

Figure 23.4 Human body: main arteries

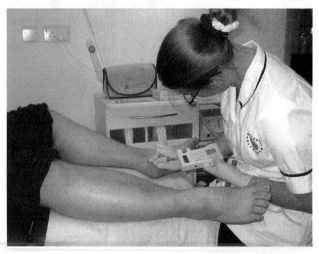

Figure 23.5 Location of the posterior tibial artery of the left foot

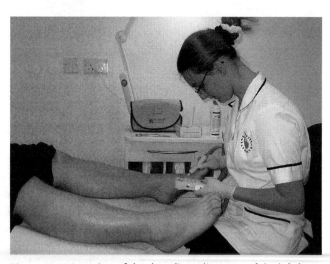

Figure 23.6 Location of the dorsalis pedis artery of the left foot

To fully determine the quality of the arterial flow a Doppler ultrasound should be used (Phillips, 2000). A hand-held Doppler device is widely used in clinical practice by podiatrists as well as nurses and other health professionals to provide an easy, non-invasive assessment of the blood flow to the lower limb (Baker and Rayman, 1999). Doppler probes are available in two different frequencies: 5 MHz used for locating the deep arteries/veins and 8 MHz used for shallow arteries/veins. The probe should be held between forefinger and thumb at an angle of +/– 45° towards the blood flow, firmly against the skin. An ultrasonic/coupling gel must be used to allow correct wave penetration through the skin (Davies, 2001). Three different wave forms can be found: triphasic, biphasic and monophasic.

The triphasic wave form has systolic and diastolic components as well as an elastic vessel wall rebound. In the biphasic wave form some of the elasticity is lost; however the vessels are still working adequately. The monophasic wave form has dramatically reduced systolic peaks and no wall vessel elasticity will be noted (Cohen and Ratner, 1986).

If monophasic pulses are noted an ankle brachial pressure index (ABPI) test can be performed to determine extend of the arterial disease (Austin, Jelinek and McDonald, 2006). Before starting this test the patient should lie flat in a warm room with the limb positioned at the height the heart; if the limb is higher or lower than the heart, the reading might be over/under estimated (Vowden, 1999). The ABPI test provides a good indication of the presence of ischaemia in the lower limb and closely correlates with patient symptoms such as intermittent claudication and rest pain (Grasty, 1999).

This test requires measurements of the systolic blood pressure in both arms (brachial) and of the blood pressure in the posterior tibial arteries (ankle) and the dorsalis pedis arteries of both limbs. The pressure index is the ratio of the ankle: brachial systolic blood pressures (Thomson and Gibson, 2002).

Separate readings should be calculated for each limb and the results recorded:

- ABPI >1.2 indicates calcified arteries which cannot be compressed.
- ABPI 0.9–1.2 indicates normal range.
- ABPI 0.5–0.9 indicates significant peripheral disease.
- ABPI <0.5 indicates severe arterial disease requiring urgent vascular intervention (Jude and Gibbons, 2005).

During the diabetic foot assessment, the subcapillary plexus refill time (SCRT) may also be measured to establish the tone of cutaneous microcirculation, which in turn shows the healing ability of a potential wound. This is done by applying firm digital pressure to the skin

t ⭐
Practice tip

Always remember about infection control and wash your hands before and after handling a patient. Clean the Doppler probe with disinfectant wipes after each patient. Do not use KY-type jelly with the Doppler as it contains air bubbles and the quality of the sound may be affected. The probe may also become damaged as there will not be enough contact with the skin.

t ⭐
Practice tip

If a patient has leg/foot ulcers, consider using cling film before applying the cuff for the ABPI test to prevent the cuff being soiled with bodily fluids. You may use ABPI flow charts instead of calculating the ABPI ratio yourself.

Part

III

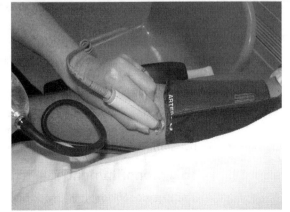

Figure 23.7 ABPI test, ankle pressure   Figure 23.8 ABPI test, brachial pressure

on the apex of the hallux for a few seconds and observing colour changes after removal of pressure. Normal colour should return within three seconds, while a delay of over four seconds indicates impaired microcirculation (Adamson, 1985). During the assessment the clinician must ensure that there are no 'outside' contributory factors such as cold weather, as this would affect the reading.

Other tests which may determine the vascular status include the Buerger's test of elevation and dependency, toe pressure tests or transcutaneous oximetry (Adamson, 1985). However the practitioner must be always aware of his/her scope of practice limitations, and where the adequacy of the peripheral circulation is in doubt referral to a vascular surgeon for further assessment is strongly indicated (Flower and Mitchell, 1998).

Summary of the basic step-by-step vascular foot assessment:

1   Locate and palpate both dorsalis pedis and the posterior tibial pulses.
2   Apply ultrasonic gel to the areas where the pulses were palpable.
3   Use the Doppler holding the probe at +/− 45°; try to locate the loudest and the clearest sound.
4   Record your findings, i.e. triphasic, biphasic or monophasic wave sound.
5   Make sure that the findings 'sound' correct; note that it is very unlikely that the foot will have one monophasic and one triphasic wave sound on the same limb.
6   Now check the SCRT: apply pressure to the apex of the hallux, hold for a few seconds and then release the pressure.
7   Observe the time in which the toe goes back to its normal colour.
8   Record the patient's SCRT.
9   Explain you findings to the patient and refer further if necessary.

Neurological assessment of the foot

A complication of diabetes mellitus that can manifest in the feet is neuropathy. We will now look at testing for sensory neuropathy, which is damage to the nerves that give information about pain and feeling. Sensory neuropathy can lead to parasthesia (burning, tingling, painful or numb sensation) in the feet. There are two other types of neuropathy that may present in diabetes: motor and automonic neuropathy. Motor neuropathy may lead to a weakness in the muscles, possibly leading to foot deformities (a pes cavus or highly arched foot and clawed toes), or loss of proprioception (knowing where the body is in space) that can lead to falls. Autonomic neuropathy is caused by damage to the nerves that work without us being aware of them. It presents in the foot as dry skin, as the sweat glands fail to function normally. The pulses may be bounding when palpated, as the control over the blood vessels is impaired. Veins in the foot may appear distended (more prominent).

The sensation of the diabetic foot should be tested at least annually according to the NICE guidelines (NICE, 2004) on prevention and management of foot problems in diabetes. Failure of the sensory system does not allow a person to respond to the environment adequately. Patients may not be aware that sensory loss has occurred, so it is essential for the practitioner to assess the function of the sensory system (Merriman and Tollafield, 1995). Sensory deficits can lead to patients injuring the foot and not being aware of it, possibly causing a wound and a risk of infection.

A neurological assessment of the foot assesses the function of the small and large afferent nerve fibres. The large afferent nerve fibres transmit proprioception (spatial limb location), cold and vibration sensation, while small nerve fibres are responsible for conducting nociceptive stimuli: sensations of touch and warmth (Vinik et al, 2000).

10 g monofilament

The 10 g monofilament is a nylon fibre calibrated to exert 10 g of pressure on the area to which it is being applied. The 10 g monofilament tests the light touch response and tests the large nerve fibres, which sense anything touching the skin (Jarvis and Rubin, 2003). The test enables the clinician to map an area of reduced pressure perception by exerting a specific repeatable force on the test site. If a patient is unable to feel the 10 g of force they are likely to damage the foot without feeling it; studies have shown patients with an inability to detect pressure have a five-fold increased risk of foot ulceration (Litzelman, Marriott and Vinikor, 1997).

Using the 10g monofilament

- The monofilament should be bent a couple of times before use to remove any residual stiffness.
- Explain to patients what you are going to do and what they should expect to feel. Apply the monofilament to a sensitive area of skin, e.g. inside of the forearm.
- Ask patients to close their eyes and to say 'yes' every time they feel you touch their feet no matter how lightly they perceive the touch.
- Place the 10 g monofilament at 90° to the skin surface and push the monofilament until it bends.
- Hold the monofilament in position for 1–2 seconds – do not jab the skin. Slowly release the pressure on the monofilament until it is straight and remove from contact with the skin.
- The monofilament should be tested on the tip of the hallux, third and fifth toes, three of the metatarsophalangeal joints, the medial and lateral longitudinal arch, the plantar central aspect of the heel and dorsally between the first and second metatarsals.
- Record the responses: if patients say 'yes' this is a positive response. Often patients will say 'No', but on questioning they usually report that they can feel something!

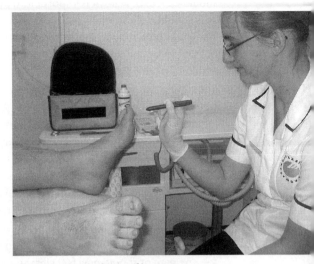

Figure 23.9 Use of monofilament

⚠ Professional alert!

A score of below 8/10 indicates a lack of sensation and patients will need to be given advice on protecting their feet from damage.

t ☆
Practice tips

- The monofilament should be replaced if it has become buckled.
- It should not be used more than ten times in one day and should be left to rest after use.
- The monofilament should not be used over areas of heavy callous and scar tissue due to the altered properties of this type of skin.

Part

III

Vibration sensation testing

The vibration sensation test can detect abnormalities of the large nerve fibres (Jarvis and Rubin, 2003). Vibration is one of the first sensations to be affected in sensory neuropathy, so the tests described below are a useful tool in predicting reduction in sensation (Merriman et al, 1997). Vibration sensation can be tested using a 128 Hz tuning fork or a neurothesiometer. The tuning fork is calibrated and gives us a good guide to the patient's large nerve fibre function. The neurothesiometer gives quantitative data, so changes over time can be monitored.

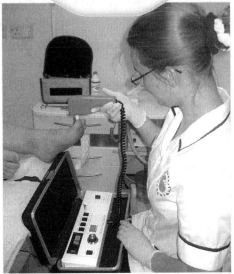

Figure 23.10 Vibration sensation testing

Using the 128 Hz tuning fork

1 Explain to patients what you are going to do and what they should expect to feel – it is important to make it clear that they should feel vibration and not pressure or cold.

2 The vibration sensation should be tested at the apex of the hallux, the lateral aspect of the fifth metatarsophalangeal joint and the medial malleolus.

3 The tuning fork should be held between the thumb and forefinger on the ridged area at the base. With the other hand, using the thumb and forefinger press the two arms at the top of the tuning fork together; sharply pull fingers away from the arms of the tuning fork so it is now vibrating (there should be very little noise).

4 Apply the flat surface of the tuning fork to a sensitive bony area such as the elbow, to demonstrate what the patient should feel.

5 Apply the flat surface of the tuning fork to the tip of the big toe; the patient should now feel vibration. Ask patients to close their eyes and tell you when the vibration or 'buzzing' sensation stops. Record the patients' response.

6 Apply to the outside of the fifth metatarsophalangeal joint and the inside of the ankle joint.

7 Repeat on the other foot.

8 Record all the findings.

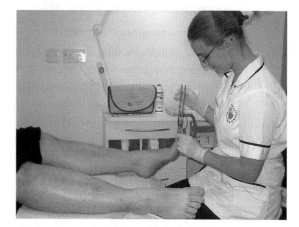

Figure 23.11   Using the tuning fork

Using the neurothesiometer

1 Make sure the settings are correct: *Range* switches should be on 'volts' and 'normal', *Memory* on store and *Power* on.

2 Explain to patients what they should expect to feel and ask them to say 'yes' when they feel a vibration or 'buzzing' sensation.

3 The probe should be held in place with one hand; using your other hand turn the dial slowly and gradually from 0 until the patient reports feeling it – at the point the patient indicates that sensation, press the memory button to record the data (up to 12 results can be stored).

4 Place the probe on a bony area such as the elbow, to demonstrate the sensation to the patient.

5 The neurothesiometer is tested on the same sites as the tuning fork.

6 Record the readings for both feet.

7 A recording of over 25 volts indicates neuropathy.

Sharp and blunt discrimination test

The sharp and blunt discrimination test is carried out using a neurotip: a sterile single-use neurological examination tool. It has a pin end and a blunt end. This test assesses damage to the small nerve fibres. The neurotip should be used at the eponychium (the skin at the base of the toenail) of the big toe as it is the only area sensitive enough to discriminate sharp (or pain) from blunt:

1 Patients should be shown the neurotip and it should be demonstrated on the forearm.

2 Patients should be asked to close their eyes while you conduct the test, as seeing the pin on the foot can lead to false positive testing.

3 The neurotip should be placed in the neuropen with either the sharp or blunt end protruding. The neuropen delivers 40 g of pressure to the area it is applied. The neurotip should be applied to the area of skin at the base of the big toenail and the patient should be asked if it feels sharp or blunt.

4 Repeat this test three times alternating the neurotip in the neuropen between sharp and blunt. Record out of three the number of correct responses.

Temperature testing

Using a warm or cold item on the foot can test for damage to the small nerve fibres. If the small fibres are damaged patients will be at risk of damaging their feet, especially of scalding the feet if they are unaware they are getting into a scalding-hot bath for example or sitting with feet too close to a fire.

Light touch testing

Testing the light touch gives an indication of the large fibre function. The large nerve fibres transmit proprioception of cold and vibration. The large fibres are sensitive to anything touching the skin. Light touch can be tested using cotton wool or a tissue, but these tests have been superseded by the monofilament.

Proprioception

Proprioception is the body's positional sense, knowing where the body is in space. Proprioception is tested by holding the most distal joint of a digit by its side and moving the toe up or down slightly. The patient should be able to detect two to three degrees of movement in the toe.

1   Demonstrate the test with the patient's eyes open, to ensure they understand what is expected of them.
2   Ask the patients to close the eyes. Holding the distal phalanx of the hallux (the end of the big toe) at the sides, move the toe up or down slightly.
3   Ask the patient to inform you whether the toe is going up or down.
4   If the patient cannot accurately detect the movement, then progressively test a more proximal joint (such as the big toe joint) until the patient can identify the movement correctly (Larsen and Stensaas, 2007).

Deep reflex testing

Deep reflexes at the patellar and achilles tendons can be tested with a reflex hammer. When a muscle tendon is tapped briskly, in a healthy person the muscle immediately contracts due to a two-neuron reflex arc. Hyporeflexia is an absent or diminished response to tapping. It usually indicates a disease that involves one or more of the components of the two-neuron reflex arc itself. Hyperreflexia is shown by hyperactive or repeated (clonic) reflexes, and indicates a lesion above the spinal reflex pathways.

Deep tendon reflexes are graded:

- 0 = no response
- 1+ = a slight but definitely present response
- 2+ = a brisk response
- 3+ = a very brisk response
- 4+ = a tap elicits a repeating reflex (clonus).

Whether 1+ and 3+ indicate normal responses depends on what the responses were previously. If a change is noted it should be assessed in conjunction with the muscle tone, muscle strength and any evidence of other disease. Asymmetry of reflexes suggests abnormality. 2+ is a normal response. 0 and 4+ are abnormal responses (Walker, Hall and Hurst, 1990).

Knee jerk (patellar reflex) can be tested in the following way:

1   Allow the patient to swing one leg off the side of the patient couch.
2   Place one hand on the quadriceps muscle to feel it contract.
3   Palpate the patellar tendon, just below the kneecap and gently tap the tendon. Feel for a contraction in the quadriceps muscle and grade the response using the system outlined earlier.

Ankle jerk (Achilles reflex) can be tested in the following way:

1   With the patient sitting, place one hand under the sole of the foot and dorsiflex the foot slightly.

Part
III

2 Tap the Achilles tendon just above its insertion into the calcaneus (heel) and feel for movement in the foot.

3 Grade response using the grading system.

Abnormal responses may indicate peripheral neuropathy and it may be appropriate to refer patients back to their GP with this information, so they can be referred on for further investigation.

Treatment of diabetic peripheral neuropathy

The first-line treatment in diabetic peripheral sensory neuropathy is rigid blood glucose control and patient education regarding the risks and hazards associated with nerve damage. Neuropathy can often be very painful. Superficial nerve pain can sometimes be managed with Capsicum cream. Deeper nerve pain can sometimes be managed with tricyclic antidepressant medications like amitirptylene or gabapentin (Lorimer et al, 2006). The patient would need to be referred back to their GP in order to receive these prescription only medicines.

> **a Learning activity**
>
> Use an internet search engine to look at the mode of action of drugs to treat peripheral sensory neuropathy, including capsicum cream, gabapentin and amitriptylene.

Advice for the patient

It should be clearly explained to the patient that they are at risk of injuring the foot and not realising it. This education could be in the form of demonstration (i.e. using the neurotip to show the sharp sensation on the patient's forearm and then the contrast in sensation on the foot). The demonstration can be reinforced with verbal advice and written information leaflets. The patient should be given advice on the correct type of footwear to support the foot and avoid injury; if patients with evidence of neuropathy have difficulty in finding suitable footwear (due to oedema/swelling or deformity), they may be referred to an orthotist for specialist footwear.

General foot care and footwear advice

Good foot care increases your comfort, mobility and independence. Many people, especially when they get older, have difficulty in managing their own basic foot care. Reaching toenails to cut them, for example, can prove difficult, but there are easy to do alternatives that usually get around the problem. This information is intended to help you advise patients. If they follow these simple steps, it will help them retain their independence and avoid the need to rely on others for help.

Hygiene

Following these simple rules will help prevent basic foot problems:

- Wash feet daily with soap and water.
- Dry carefully, especially between the toes where moisture may become trapped.
- Use moisturising cream daily on dry skin to keep skin supple and prevent cracks but avoid putting it between your toes.
- Do not use talc or medicated powders; instead use surgical spirit for 'sweaty feet' – avoiding broken skin.
- Change socks or tights daily.
- Avoid socks that are too tight around the ankle and foot. Ensure seams are smooth to prevent rubbing toes.
- Be careful to avoid overheated baths. The water temperature must not exceed 43 °C or 110 °F measured by using a bath thermometer.

Cutting and filing nails

When tending to nails:

- Always ensure you are in a safe position; for example, don't balance on the edge of the bath where you could slip and fall.
- When the toenails need cutting, do this after bathing.
- Cut nails to follow the natural line of the end of the toe – essentially straight.
- Do not cut down the sides of the nail grooves but allow them to grow forward free from the groove.
- Ensure some of the free white edge is still showing.
- Don't try to cut the whole nail in one go; use a gradual 'nipping' action.

If patients cannot reach their feet well enough to cut them safely, suggest they try filing them once a week instead or ask a carer or relative to help. The patient should use a sturdy emery board or a long-handled file (these can be purchased at most pharmacies). This will make reaching the nails easier and safer. Nails should always be filed when they are hard and dry.

Follow these simple steps:

- Always file from the top of the nail in a downward direction using single strokes.
- File the edge of the nail to remove sharp corners but do not file down into the sides.
- Help reduce nail thickness by gently filing the top of the nail down.

Callouses and corns

Callouses (plaques of hard, thick, yellowish skin) form to protect our feet from stress and strain. If your patient has callouses which aren't painful, they are not a cause for concern – the callous is simply doing its job! It has probably been caused by poor fitting footwear, especially if found around the toes. However, if patients are experiencing pain or discomfort, suggest they use a pumice or foot file to thin down the callous, being careful not to overdo it – they should not aim to remove it all. They should do this on a regular basis to prevent the callous building up again. Also recommend the daily use of an emollient (not to be put between the toes), specifically E45 or aqueous cream for dry skin or an oil-based product such as vaseline or baby oil for hard skin.

First-aid measures

Minor injuries can be treated quite adequately by patients, provided they seek help if the injury does not respond quickly to their first aid.

⚠ Professional alert!

When cutting toenails never:

- cut nails too short
- use a sharp instrument to clean the free edge or the nail grooves
- leave sharp corners
- cut a 'v' in nails to 'cure ingrowing toenails' – it does not work and can cause problems.

⚠ Professional alert!

Tell your patients to seek advice if they notice:

- any colour change in the leg or foot
- any discharge from a break or crack in the skin or from a corn or from beneath a toenail
- any swelling or throbbing in any part of the foot, which does not resolve in two to three days.

Part

III

t☆ Practice tips

Advise your patient on some basic first aid:

- Clean wounds with some tepid salty water (ordinary table salt is suitable).
- Cover minor cuts and abrasions with a clean, sterile, non-adherent dressing.
- Never use cotton wool to clean or dress wounds.

- Do not encircle toes with adhesive tape or tight bandages.
- If blisters occur do not prick them. If they burst dress them as for a minor cut.
- Never place adhesive strapping directly over a wound.

- If a wound gets worse or doesn't start to heal in a couple of days, seek professional help immediately. Remind patients to be vigilant. Even mild infections may spread quickly, and cause problems for diabetics.

Footwear

Badly fitting footwear can be very damaging to feet. In fact, many simple foot problems occur because of poorly fitting shoes. To help prevent damage to feet, recommend that patients apply the following rules (similar rules will help for buying children's shoes or shoes for specialist conditions such as diabetes):

- Avoid wearing slippers. It is an easy habit to wear them but they often do more harm than shoes. Instead, consider buying a pair of shoes to wear at home. Do not walk around barefoot or wear a pair of socks with rubber grips on the soles.
- Choose the right shoes for the right occasion. If patients need to be on their feet for a long time or have to walk a long way, remind them to wear something that fits well and will support the foot. Good fitting footwear will also help prevent falls. Save dress shoes for special occasions.

> ⚠ **Professional alert!**
>
> Some patients, such as diabetics, should never go barefooted. Patients should be encouraged to speak to a qualified podiatrist if they are unsure whether this rule will apply to them.

To find a well-fitting shoe, the patient should consider the following:

- *Length*: Fit to the longest toe, leaving a small gap between the tip of it and the end of the shoe. As we get older our feet often become longer and wider as the ligaments stretch.
- *Width*: This is not measured across the toe of the shoe and so you need to ensure that, whilst you have the correct width fitting across the middle of the foot, the toe box is equally wide and rounded.
- *Fastenings*: These hold the foot in the shoe. Shoes should have laces, straps with buckles, or velcro to keep them in place. 'Slip-on' shoes are kept in place either because they are too small for the foot, or by curling the toes. They should therefore be avoided for everyday use.
- *Toe box*: The toe of the shoe should be rounded, deep and wide. It should match the shape of the toes so they do not become squashed. Make sure the width of the shoe is correct and that the toe box does not taper too much as this will squash the toes.
- *Heel*: This takes a large proportion of a person's weight. Unfortunately, the height of the heel is often determined by fashion, not by the needs of the feet. Ideally, the heel should have a broad base and the heel height should be no greater than 4 cm/1.5".
- *Heel counter*: The portion of the shoe that grasps the heel of the foot at the sides and back, preventing the heel from sliding up and down while walking. Most importantly, it stabilises or helps maintain the position of the heel when the shoe contacts the ground. As the heel counter softens or breaks down and loses its shape, the shoe becomes less supportive – when shoes become old and worn, replace them.
- *Sole*: The entire bottom of the shoe. It should be flat, except for a gentle slope upwards under the toes. Try to buy something that will cushion the foot. Leather soles tend to be very slippery and hard so they are best avoided.
- *Upper*: The material that forms the main part of the shoe covering the top of the foot. Ideally, it should be composed of a natural material such as leather, and should be soft without hard seams or stitching.
- *Lining*: Found inside the shoe, it should be smooth and without seams.

Shoe buying tips

- 'They'll feel more comfortable when I've worn them in ...'. Don't accept the need to 'break in' new shoes. Shoes that fit well will feel comfortable straight away!
- Take the socks or insoles likely to be worn most often when going to buy shoes.
- Shop at stores with well-trained staff and a large selection of styles, sizes and fittings.
- Always try on both shoes and fit the larger foot.
- For maximum comfort, buy a shoe with adjustable fastening, such as laces or a strap with a buckle.

- It is not the cost but the fit that is important when buying shoes. Paying a lot for shoes will not make them fit better if they are not right for your feet. It is all about shape and fit.
- Buy shoes late in the day, as feet tend to swell as the day goes on. This is especially true if you suffer from swollen feet and legs.

Conclusion

In summary, diabetic foot screening is important to allow health professionals to assess the risk of a diabetic patient developing foot ulceration as diabetic foot complications can have a very detrimental effect on a person's quality of life. Ischaemia and neuropathy can be painful conditions to live with, and increase the individuals risk of developing ulcerations. Ulcerations need to be tended by a health professional several times per week and can take many weeks to resolve; they can be malodorous and cause immobility, often causing affected individuals to feel depressed as their quality of life is reduced. It is therefore better to prevent these complications in the first place by offering good multidisciplinary care to ensure tight control of blood glucose levels and promoting a healthy life style. It is important to offer patients advice, in a format that they can understand, about how to prevent foot injury and promote good health to minimise the risk of developing ulcerations and in turn reduce the amputation rate.

References

Adamson, D. I. (1985) *Circulatory Problems in Podiatry*, Switzerland, Karger.

Apelqvist, J. (2007) 'Diabetic foot ulcers: evidence, cost and management', *The Diabetic Foot Journal* **10**(1).

Austin, M. Jelinek, H. C. and McDonald, K. (2006) 'Age and gender do not affect the ankle-brachial index', *The Diabetic Foot*, **9**(2), 93–101.

Baker, N. and Rayman, G. (1999) 'Clinical evaluation of Doppler signals', *The Diabetic Foot – Supplement* **2**(1), 22–5.

Cohen, S. and Ratner, S. (1986) 'Peripheral arterial disease: a complete review', *Cardiology Product News* July–August.

Davies, C. (2001) 'Use of Doppler ultrasound in leg ulcer assessment', *Nursing Standard* July, 18–24.

Edmonds, M. and Foster, A. (2000) *Managing the Diabetic Foot*, Oxford, Blackwell Publishing.

Edmonds, M., Foster, A. and Sanders, L. (2004) *A Practical Manual of Diabetic Footcare*, Oxford, Blackwell Publishing.

Flower A. and Mitchell, D. (1998) 'Assessment of the vascular status of the diabetic foot', *The Diabetic Foot* **1**(3), 105–7.

Grasty, M. S. (1999) 'Use of the hand-held Doppler to detect peripheral vascular disease', *The Diabetic Foot – Supplement* **2**(1), 18–21.

Jarvis, S. and Rubin, A. (2003) *Diabetes for Dummies*, Chichester, Wiley.

Jude, E. and Gibbons, J. (2005) 'Identifying and treating intermittent claudication in people with diabetes', *The Diabetic Foot* **8**(2), 84–92.

Katzen, B. T. (2002) 'Clinical diagnosis and progress of acute limb ischaemia', *Cardiovascular Medicine (USA)* **3**, supplement 2.

Kumar, P. and Clark, M. (2002) *Clinical Medicine*, 5th edn, Edinburgh, W. B. Saunders.

Larsen, P. D. and Stensaas, S. S. (2007) *NeuroLogic Exam: An anatomical approach*, University of Utah [online] http://library.med.utah.edu/neurologicexam/html/home_exam.html (accessed 9 February 2009).

Litzelman, D. K., Marriott, D. J. and Vinikor, F. (1997) 'Independent physiological predictors of foot lesions in patients with NIDM', *Diabetes Care* 20, 1273.

Lorimer, D., French, G., O'Donnell, M, Burrow, G. and Wall, B. (2006) *Neal's Disorders of the Foot*, Edinburgh, Churchill Livingstone.

Merriman, L. M. and Tollafield, D. R. (1995) *Assessment of the Lower Limb*, Edinburgh, Churchill Livingstone.

Mousley, M. (2006) 'Diabetic foot screening: why it is not assessment', *The Diabetic Foot* **9**(4).

National Institute for Clinical Excellence (NICE) (2004) Type 2 Diabetes Prevention and Management of Foot Problems, Clinical Guideline 10, London, NICE.

NICE (2004) 'Type 2 Diabetes: prevention and management of foot problems', *Clinical Guideline* 10.

Oxford Concise Medical Dictionary 2000, Oxford, Oxford University Press.

Phillips, G. W. (2000) 'Review of arterial vascular ultrasound', *World Journal of Surgery* **24**(2), 232–40.

Thomson, C. and Gibson, J. N. (2002) *50 Foot Challenges: Assessment and management*, Livingstone, Churchill.

van Houtum, W., Bakker, K., Rauwerda, J. A. and Heine R. J. (2001) 'Vascular assessment before lower extremity amputation', *The Diabetic Foot* **4**(4), 165–72.

Vinik, A. L., Park, T. S., Stansberry, K. B. Park T. S. and Erbas, T. (2000) 'Diabetic neuropathies', *Diabetologia* 43, 957–73.

Vowden, P. (1999) 'Doppler ultrasound in the management of the diabetic foot', *The Diabetic Foot – Supplement* **2**(1), 15–17.

Walker, H. K., Hall, W. D. and Hurst, J. W. (1990) *Clinical Methods; The history, physical and laboratory examinations*, Oxford, Butterworth.

Part

III

Part IV

Skills for care management

Chapters

Chapter

24

Assessing and managing hydration

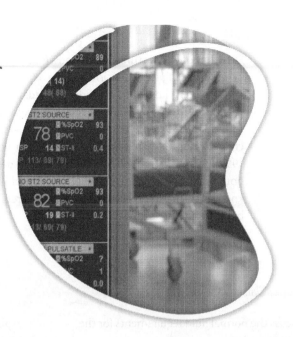

Veronica Lambert and Doris O'Toole

Links to other chapters in *Foundation Skills for Caring*

9 Patient hygiene
10 Pressure area care
12 Mouth care
16 Vital signs
17 Blood pressure
25 Intravenous therapy
26 Enteral feeding

Links to other chapters in *Foundation Studies for Caring*

10 Nutritional assessment and needs
11 Fluid balance in children
12 Fluid balance in adults
19 Care of the neonate
21 Care of the acutely ill child
23 Care of the adult – surgical
24 Care of the adult – medical
25 Care of the older adult – community
34 Primary care

W Don't forget to visit www.palgrave.com/glasper for additional
online resources relating to this chapter.

Part

IV

Introduction

Dehydration is a disturbance in body fluid that occurs as a result of inadequate fluid intake or abnormal fluid losses, irrespective of the underlying cause, which can vary in adults and children. In adults, underlying medical conditions, including neurological disorders, respiratory infections, urinary infections and cardiac failure, may alter the person's ability to drink adequate fluids. Gastroenteritis is a common cause of dehydration in infants and children due to increased fluid losses from vomiting and diarrhoea (McVerry and Collin, 1999). Early recognition and management of dehydration are key in preventing and reducing both adult and child susceptibility to critical illness. This chapter aims to provide you with knowledge and understanding of the skills required in assessing and managing hydration in both the adult and child.

Learning outcomes

This chapter will enable you to:

- discuss the normal fluid requirements for the child and adult
- discuss the risk factors for developing dehydration for the child and adult
- describe the signs and symptoms of dehydration for the child and adult
- explain the assessment you would undertake for a child and an adult presenting with dehydration
- outline the procedure for measuring and recording fluid intake and output
- discuss the procedure you would undertake for restoring fluid balance in a child and adult presenting with dehydration.

Concepts

- Assessing fluid status
- Hydration
- Dehydration
- Fluid balance
- Fluid requirements
- Fluid intake, fluid output
- Measuring and recording
- Restoring fluid balance

To achieve the above learning outcomes, two patient scenarios are presented. The first scenario introduces Mary, 70 years of age. The second scenario introduces Lata, 2 months old. Read through the two scenarios, presented below, and we will then explore how you would assess and manage both Lata's and Mary's hydration.

[S] Scenario: introducing Mary

Mary, a 70-year-old woman, presents with a history of increased confusion over the last two days, dizzy spells, dry skin and mucous membranes. She is living alone and has a history of mild dementia. Mary's daughter decided to bring her to the emergency department for assessment because she was less responsive than usual and she had an episode of urinary incontinence.

[S] Scenario: introducing Lata

Lata, a 2-month-old girl, is admitted to the infant ward, with a two-day history of vomiting and diarrhoea. Lata has a history of vomiting a number of feeds over the previous 48 hours, has loose stools, is very lethargic and sleepy, and has not had as many wet nappies as she usually does.

a Learning activity

In your learning group reflect on Mary and Lata's history as illustrated above and think about what skills and knowledge you would use to develop an assessment. Some points are included below to help you with this.

Assessment

It is necessary to obtain accurate information about Lata and Mary's food and fluid intake and output. Mary, like other older people, may experience greater difficulty with providing detailed information due to slower functioning, reduced energy, memory deficits, confusion, dementia or illness. It is therefore important not only to gather information firstly from Mary but also to involve her family. Information about Lata can be obtained from her parents.

The percentage of body water depends on age, gender and amount of body fat (Heath, 1995; Kanneh, 2006). Infants have the highest amount of water in relation to body weight, that is 75–80 per cent, as compared with approx 60–70 per cent in adolescents and 50–60 per cent in adults (Hazinski, 1988). Body fluids are distributed in two compartments, one containing intracellular (within body cells) and the other extracellular (outside body cells) fluid (Heath, 1995). Although the percentage of fluid that comprises each compartment varies with age, in a healthy person and under normal conditions fluid within the compartments remains relatively balanced (Gobbi, Cowen and Ugboma, 2006).

a Learning activity

Make a list of questions you would ask Mary and her family, and Lata's parents to find out about Lata and Mary's fluid/food intake and output.

a Learning activity

Fluid intake

In your learning group discuss the sources of fluid intake.

Consider the average daily amount of fluid intake for Mary and then for Lata.

What factors might prevent Mary and Lata from taking in the recommended amount of fluid?

a Learning activity

Fluid output

Now consider sources of fluid output.

Consider the average daily amount of fluid output for Mary and then for Lata.

What factors might affect Mary's and Lata's fluid output?

W   Refer to the companion webpages for this chapter to help you with your estimations of normal fluid requirements.

a Learning activity

In your learning group reflect on the signs and symptoms of dehydration in the child and adult; refer to Willock and Jewkes (2000), Suhayda and Walton (2002), Gobbi et al (2006), Berman et al (2008) and the accompanying website presentation to help develop your assessment.

To assess Lata's and Mary's fluid state you will need to focus on their skin, mouth, mucous membranes and eyes, as well as their cardiovascular, respiratory, neurological and muscular systems.

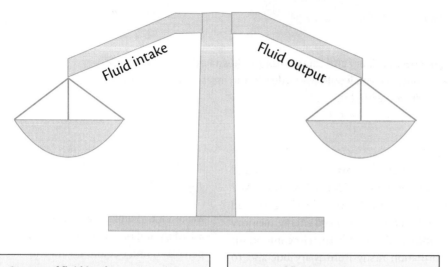

Sources of fluid intake

◆ Fluid (drinks) taken orally with and between meals
◆ Liquid foods e.g. soup, gelatine/jelly
◆ Tube feedings
◆ Water to flush tube feeds
◆ Liquid medications
◆ Intravenous (IV) infusion of fluids/medications

Sources of fluid output

◆ Urine (urinary catheter, bedpan, urinal, nappy)
◆ Stool/diarrhoea
◆ Vomit
◆ Nasogastric (NG) tube aspirations
◆ Stomal fistulas
◆ Wound drainage e.g. chest, closed wound drainage

Figure 24.1 Balancing fluid intake and output

a) Learning activity

What signs/symptoms did you identify that Mary and Lata might present with, and why?

Did you consider any of the questions in Table 24.1?

Table 24.1 Questions to consider when assessing Mary's and Lata's hydration status

Physical assessment	Clinical measurements
How do Mary/Lata look physically?	What are Lata's/Mary's vital signs?
Are Mary/Lata quiet, lethargic, irritable, sleepy, drowsy, confused?	Do Mary/Lata appear to be breathing faster than normal?
What is Lata's muscle tone like?	What is Mary's/Lata's temperature?
Is Lata floppy to hold? Has she poor head control?	What is Mary's/Lata's heart rate?
What is the appearance of Mary's/Lata's mouth?	What is Mary's/Lata's blood pressure?
Are Mary's/Lata's eyes sunken?	What is Mary's/Lata's capillary refill time?
Are Mary's/Lata's mucous membranes dry?	What is Mary's/Lata's blood glucose?
Does Mary's/Lata's skin look inelastic?	What is Mary's/Lata's weight?
Is Lata's fontanel sunken?	

t☆ Practice tips

The 'pinch test' is a guide to establishing the extent of dehydration by assessing skin turgor.

Child: gently lift the skin folds over the abdomen. Recoil within one to two seconds indicates mild to moderate dehydration, whereas a pause of greater than two seconds represents severe dehydration (Armon et al, 2001).

Elderly: due to the gradual loss of skin elasticity with age inspect the skin over the forehead, sternum or inner aspect of the thigh as the skin maintains its elasticity in these areas (Heath, 1995; Berman et al, 2008).

t☆ Practice tips

As an older adult Mary may have decreased salivation; therefore mucous membrane moistness is best assessed by inspecting the area underneath the tongue for a pool of saliva (Heath, 1995).

In Lata's case examine the infant's anterior fontanel which may be sunken (a small soft 'dip' may be observed or palpated) due to fluid volume deficit (Willock and Jewkes, 2000; Wong and Hockenberry, 2003).

⚠ Professional alert!

If a child has a history of a reduced fluid intake or an excessive fluid loss, as in Lata's case, and appears very lethargic and drowsy, it is vital to measure the blood glucose level immediately. Glucose levels may drop significantly and lead to an unconscious state if not treated promptly. The frequency of blood glucose monitoring will depend on the condition of the patient.

The frequency of recording vital signs (temperature, pulse, respiration and blood pressure) will also depend on each patient's clinical condition. Temperature and heart rate may be raised due to underlying infection, fever or low circulating blood volume (hypovolaemia). Breathing may be faster than normal (tachypnoea) as the body compensates for the fluid loss. Low blood pressure is a late sign of dehydration and is often related to hypovolaemia. Oxygen saturation may also need to be recorded at intervals or continuously depending on the condition of the patient. Capillary refill time should also be regularly assessed with the vital signs recording.

ⓐ Learning activity

Think about the significance of the outcome of the vital signs such as temperature, pulse, respirations and blood pressure.

t☆ Practice tip

Capillary refill time indicates circulatory return. It can be assessed by pressing gently on the nail bed, then releasing the pressure, and observing the time taken for the colour to return to pink. Delayed capillary return is a sign of the body 'shutting down' because of a fluid volume deficit. Normal capillary refill is less than two seconds (APLS, 1997).

Measuring and recording intake and output

Maintaining an accurate intake and output is critical to assessing the patient's fluid balance and maintaining hydration. A comparison of intake and output is necessary to prevent dehydration.

Procedure

- Obtain an accurate patient history and identify risk factors that might affect the patient's ability to maintain an adequate fluid balance, such as current illness, pre-existing disease, surgery, medications and mental status. Refer to the companion website for more information on potential risk factors.
- In Mary's (70 years) case, her semi-dependency places her at high risk of dehydration because she is reliant on others to assist her with maintaining adequate hydration (Hodgkinson, Evans and Wood, 2003).
- Lata (2 months) is also reliant on others for help and a disturbance in her digestion, with vomiting and diarrhoea, enhances her risk of becoming dehydrated quickly (Holman, Roberts and Nicol, 2005).

⚠ Professional alert!

- Use caution when handling an infant because as a result of severe dehydration they might be 'floppy' to hold, with poor head control.
- Elderly patients may become particularly confused, restless or dizzy because of dehydration, as in Mary's case, so ensure the environment is safe, for example, bed sides up.

W

Part
IV

- Instruct the patient and family of the need to accurately measure all intake and output.
- Involve the patient and family in accurately measuring and recording fluid intake and output. However, first assess the patient and family's ability to measure and record intake and output.
- Tell the patient and family exactly what is to be measured, how it is to be measured, and where and how to record these measurements.
- Adhere to standard universal infection control procedures (for example, use of gloves, aprons), following local policy and guidelines relating to body fluids, when measuring sources of intake and output. Refer to Chapter 30 on universal precautions.
- Measure and record all measurable sources of fluid intake and fluid output, including the amount, type, source and route of fluid gain or loss (McConnell, 2002; Holman et al, 2005). Measurement of fluids should be recorded in millilitres (mls). Refer to the accompanying website PowerPoint presentation for practical exercises on measuring different fluid sources.
- To accurately measure fluid losses, for example urinary output, use a clean graduated measuring container. Observe the fluid volume in the gradient container at eye level and read the measurement from the bottom of the meniscus, which is the curvature of the liquid surface (McConnell, 2002). Use a separate gradient container for each patient.
- Some patients may have a urinary catheter in place; if so it may be necessary to record urinary output every hour (via an attached drainage receptacle) or at various intervals throughout the day, depending on the individual patient's condition.
- In infants/young children, urine can be measured by weighing nappies or by the use of urine collecting bags. The amount of wet nappies will provide an indication of the severity of dehydration. Most infants will have six to eight wet nappies in 24 hours. Refer to the accompanying webpages to learn about weighing wet nappies.
- If the infant has a bowel movement with every nappy change it will be difficult to differentiate one type of fluid loss from another (urine and stool), and this must be documented on the fluid balance chart. The number of wet/soiled nappies may be recorded as opposed to the volume of urine (Gobbi et al, 2006; Berman et al, 2008).
- Some fluid outputs, such as incontinence and vomit, can be difficult to measure accurately. Where you cannot measure exact amounts, record an estimated volume on the fluid balance chart.
- Be aware that outputs entered on the fluid balance chart will in some situations underestimate body fluid loss due to the immeasurability of insensible losses such as fluid lost through respiration, perspiration and faeces (Holman et al, 2005; Chapelhow and Crouch, 2007).
- All measurements (time, amount and description) of intake and output should be documented on a bedside fluid balance chart. This provides a record of all fluid taken in and excreted over a 24-hour period, Measurements should be recorded as soon as possible

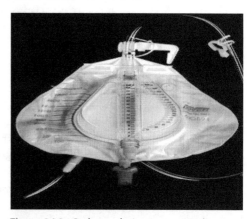

Figure 24.2 Catheter drainage receptacle

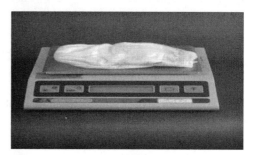

Figure 24.3 Weighing a nappy

⚠ Professional alert!

Report urinary output of less than 25–30 ml per hour or 500 ml in 24 hours for an adult, or less than 2 ml/kg/hour for an infant and 1 ml/kg/hr for a child (Willock and Jewkes, 2000; Berman et al, 2008).

Measuring daily weight is extremely important in both Mary's and Lata's case because weight helps you to evaluate fluid balance changes and also provides a guide for fluid replacement. Refer to the companion website for key points in relation to recording patient weights.

after they have been taken (Holman et al, 2005). This will help to maintain accuracy, minimising recall errors.

- Fluid balance is the difference between total fluid intake and total fluid output. This should be calculated at the same time each day, for example at 08.00 am, 08.00 pm, 12 midnight or 12 midday (Holman et al, 2005).
- It is vital to estimate on an ongoing basis, throughout the day, patterns and volumes that might fall outside the normal range, bearing in mind the average 24 hour intake and output values (McConnell, 2002).

Practical calculation: Lata weighs 6.0 kg. She is feeding orally and normally takes approximately 120 ml/kg daily. She feeds usually every four hours.

a Learning activity

Complete the fluid balance chart (Table 24.3) by referring to the practical calculation, which relates to Lata:

- How many millilitres (ml)/kilogram(kg) did Lata take in orally?
- Is Lata's urinary output normal?
- What would Lata's fluid balance be at 14.00 hours?
- What is Lata's overall fluid balance at 24.00 hours?

Table 24.2 Lata's fluid intake and output

Intake: Lata takes the following volumes orally:	**Output:** Lata voids urine (wet nappy) at the following times:
06.00 hours: 120 ml	06.00 hours: 42 ml
10.00 hours: 110 ml	10.00 hours: 40 ml (with small soft bowel motion)
14.00 hours: 120 ml	14.00 hours: 48 ml Episode of vomiting (approximately 20 ml of milk)
18.00 hours: 120 ml	18.00 hours: 46 ml
22.00 hours: 120 ml	22.00 hours: 50 ml (with small soft bowel motion)
02.00 hours: 100 ml	02.00 hours: 49 ml

Table 24.3 Fluid balance chart

Name					Weight				
ID No					Date				
Intake	(mls)				Output	(mls)			
Time	Oral	Tube	I.V.	Total	Vomit	Urine	Stool	Drain	Total
01.00									
02.00	100					49			
03.00									
04.00									
05.00									
06.00									
07.00									
08.00									
09.00									
10.00									
11.00									
12.00									
13.00									
14.00									
15.00									
16.00									
17.00									
18.00									

Name					Weight				
ID No					Date				
Intake	(mls)				Output	(mls)			
Time	Oral	Tube	I.V.	Total	Vomit	Urine	Stool	Drain	Total
19.00									
20.00									
21.00									
22.00									
23.00									
24.00									
Total Intake					Total Output				
Fluid Balance									

⚠ Professional alert!

There are ways that error can occur when recording fluid balance, such as variations in measurements, estimations, omissions, mathematical and shift change errors. Refer to the accompanying website for more information.

Ⓒ Professional conversation

Rose, a first-year nursing student, says, 'I approached Tamali, my mentor, about calculating and administering intravenous fluids to dehydrated children. Although we had discussed elements of this in one of our lectures I was still shocked to be reminded that babies only have a circulating blood volume of 80 millilitres per kilogram of body weight. This made me realise why it is so important to monitor carefully intravenous intake and why infusion pumps are so invaluable'.

Restoring fluid balance

If patients are dehydrated, there is an urgent need to re-establish normal hydration in order to restore metabolism, circulation, and renal function. Interventions in relation to restoring fluid balance may range from encouraging patients to drink more fluids orally to managing intravenous fluid infusions. 'Push fluids', record intake and output and daily weights are instructions commonly encountered (Gobbi et al, 2006).

Procedure

- In mild to moderate cases of dehydration patients should be encouraged and assisted in restoring and maintaining their own hydration by increasing their intake of fluids orally (Woodrow, 2003).
- Assess whether the patient is able to drink independently or whether assistance is required. Consider, for example, ability to open drink cartons or bottles, and handle glasses/cups/jugs (Holman et al, 2005). Liaise with the occupational therapist for additional supportive aids, if needed.
- Inform the patient of the specific amount of oral fluid to be taken and the importance of taking this amount (Berman et al, 2008). This promotes patient cooperation.
- Determine the patient's fluid preferences and ensure a variety of the preferred fluids are available (Berman et al, 2008; Holman et al, 2005). This will assist with encouraging fluid intake. Avoid soft drinks, tea and coffee as these have dehydrating effects (Bennett, 2000).
- Ensure fluids are available at regular intervals for elderly patients. This will enhance the likelihood that the elderly will drink an increased volume of fluids (Hodgkinson et al, 2003).

- Offer small amounts of fluids at regular intervals and offer drinks between set meal times (Woodrow, 2003).
- Regular hourly prompts are helpful, particularly if the patient is confused or has dementia, as in Mary's case (Holman et al, 2005).
- Ensure that the fluids are kept fresh and served at a correct temperature. Water should be available, with or without ice as preferred.
- Ensure fluids are accessible to the patient. Drinks must be placed within easy reach for patients with limited mobility because the inability to reach drinks often accounts for patients consuming insufficient fluids (Woodrow, 2003). Open containers, pour liquids into cups and provide straws as appropriate to each individual patient need (Bennett, 2000).
- Young children may need encouragement so use creative tactics to increase oral fluid intake. For example, try freezer pops made from juice, jelly in fun shapes, small medicine cups, a tea party, a crazy straw or sticker rewards for drinking a certain amount (Wong and Hockenberry, 2003).
- Older children can be involved as active participants in planning and developing their own intake schedule (Wong and Hockenberry, 2003).
- Oral hygiene should be provided at two to four-hour intervals to keep lips moist, promote patient comfort and maintain integrity of the oral membranes. Refer to Chapter 12.
- Mild to moderate cases of dehydration may be corrected with the administration of commercially available oral re-hydration solutions. These solutions contain a mixture of water, glucose and electrolytes that help to re-hydrate by replacing fluid losses and providing maintenance fluid requirements (Dale, 2004).
- In cases of severe dehydration, or if the patient is unable to take in sufficient amounts of fluids orally for any reason, intravenous fluids will need to be considered. Refer to Chapter 25.

Conclusion

Through the use of two patient scenarios and a number of practical activities, this chapter has provided an outline of factors to consider when assessing, measuring, recording and restoring fluid balance in both an adult and a child presenting with dehydration. It is advised that you draw upon the accompanying website to supplement the theoretical and practical information presented in this chapter. It is imperative that you become familiar with the normal fluid requirements of both adult and child patients in your care, as early recognition and management of dehydration are crucial to prevent and minimise both adult and child susceptibility to critical illness.

References

Advanced Paediatric Life Support (APLS) (1997) *Advanced Paediatric Life Support: The practical approach.* 2nd edn, London, BMJ Publishing Group.

Armon, K., Stephenson, T., MacFaul, R., Eccleston, P., Werneke, U. and Baumer, H. (2001) 'An evidence and consensus based guideline for acute diarrhoea management', *Archives of Disease in Childhood* **85**(2), 132–42.

Bennett, J. A. (2000) 'Dehydration: hazards and benefits', *Geriatric Nursing* **21**(2), 84–8.

Berman, A., Snyder, S. J., Kozier, B. and Erb, G. (2008) *Kozier and Erb's Fundamentals of Nursing: Concepts, process and practice.* 8th edn, New Jersey, Pearson/Prentice Hall.

Chapelhow, C. and Crouch, S. (2007) 'Applying numeracy skills in clinical practice: fluid balance', *Nursing Standard* **21**(27), 49–56.

Dale, J. (2004) 'Oral rehydration solutions in the management of acute gastroenteritis among children', *Journal of Pediatric Health Care* **18**(4), 211–12.

Gobbi, M., Cowen, M. and Ugboma, D. (2006) 'Fluid and electrolyte balance', Chapter 20 in Alexander, M.F., Fawcett, J.N. and Runciman, P.J. (eds), *Nursing Practice: Hospital and home: The adult*, Edinburgh, Elsevier.

Hazinski, M. F. (1988) 'Understanding fluid balance in the seriously ill child', *Pediatric Nursing* **14**(3), 231–6.

Heath, H. B. M. (1995) *Potter and Perry's Foundations in Nursing Theory and Practice*, London, Mosby Elsevier.

Hodgkinson, B., Evans, D. and Wood, J. (2003) 'Maintaining oral hydration in older adults: a systematic review', *International Journal of Nursing Practice* 9, S19–S28.

Holman, C., Roberts, S. and Nicol, M. (2005) 'Promoting adequate hydration in older people', *Nursing Older People* **11**(4), 31–2.

Part

IV

Kanneh, A. B. (2006) 'Caring for children with body fluid and electrolyte imbalance', Chapter 26 in Glasper, A. and Richardson, J.A. (eds), *Textbook of Children's and Young People's Nursing*, Edinburgh, Churchill Livingstone.

McConnell, E. A. (2002) 'Measuring intake and output', Nursing **32**(7), 17.

McVerry, M. and Collin, J. (1999) 'Managing the child with gastroenteritis', *Nursing Standard* **13**(37), 49–53.

Suhayda, R. and Walton, J. C. (2002) 'Preventing and managing dehydration', *MedSurg Nursing* **11**(6), 267–78.

Willock, J. and Jewkes, F. (2000) 'Making sense of fluid balance in children', *Paediatric Nursing* **12**(7), 37–42.

Woodrow, P. (2003) 'Assessing fluid balance in older people: fluid replacement', *Nursing Older People* **14**(10), 29–30.

Wong, D. L. and Hockenberry, M. J. (2003) *Wong's Nursing Care of Infants and Children*, 7th edn, St Louis, Mosby.

Chapter

25

Intravenous therapy

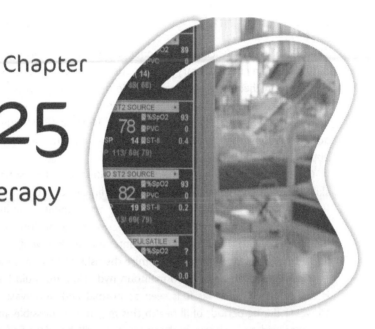

Carol Chamley and Michelle Wilson

 Links to other chapters in *Foundation Skills for Caring*

 Links to other chapters in *Foundation Studies for Caring*

W Don't forget to visit www.palgrave.com/glasper for additional online resources relating to this chapter.

Part

IV

Introduction

The role of the healthcare practitioner is continually evolving to meet the diverse needs of patients within contemporary society. Therefore increasingly procedures such as intravenous (IV) infusion therapy, which may include drug administration have become a fundamental aspect of care rather than being considered as an extension of an existing role (Shawyer et al, 2007). Indeed, the Royal College of Nursing (RCN) identified the preparation and administration of IV drugs as 'a core skill for general nursing practice, allowing a holistic approach to patient care' (RCN, 2005).

Caring involves the integration and coordination of personal, technical and professional skills based upon a sound knowledge base, clinical competence, and evidence-based practice. Intravenous infusion (IV) therapy may be an element of individual patient care which is integral to the patient's well-being and recovery. The healthcare practitioner (HCP) needs to be equipped with the underpinning contemporary knowledge and skills for competent, safe and ethical practice, which will minimise the risks and complications to the patient.

Most individuals are able to maintain hydration and fluid balance with oral fluids which is the preferred route, as it is seen as normal and noninvasive with fewer complications. However during periods of ill health this may not be possible and alternative methods must be employed to maintain hydration which will be identified through patient assessment (Brooker, 2007).

This chapter aims to identify key concepts associated with the safe administration of IV fluids:

- principles of normal fluid balance and body compartments, identification and location of common routes, and the classification of IV fluids commonly used in clinical practice
- principles of safe administration of fluids and caring for the patient who is receiving IV fluids, whilst observing and assessing the patient for side effects and complications such as anaphylaxis, speedshock infection, phlebitis and extravasation
- record keeping, documenting and monitoring fluid balance as endorsed by the Nursing and Midwifery Council (2002).

Learning outcomes

This chapter will enable you to:

- define the term 'IV infusion therapy'
- explain the principles of normal fluid balance and differentiate between body fluid compartments
- outline the different types and classifications of IV fluids commonly administered in practice
- describe the common routes for the infusion of fluids

- discuss the principles of IV infusion therapy
- describe the care of a patient who is receiving IV infusion therapy
- explain the common site effects and complications of IV infusion therapy.

Concepts

- Historical context
- Applied anatomy and physiology
- Classification of IV fluids
- Principles of safe administration

- Caring for the patient receiving IV therapy
- Professional responsibilities
- Record keeping and documentation

- Monitoring fluid balance
- Side-effects and complications

Intravenous infusion therapy

Modern IV infusion therapy is less than 100 years old yet it was recognised that medication could be injected into a vein as early as the 1600s. The history of cannulation of a central venous structure can be traced back to 1929, when Forssmann described how he advanced a plastic tube near to the heart by puncturing his own arm, and in the 1950s Aubaniac used the subclavian vein to insert a central venous catheter. However, initially IV therapy was reserved for the critically ill, but it was following the First and Second World Wars that an era of modern IV therapy emerged. Most notably the greatest advances in drugs, equipment and procedures have occurred during the last 25 years (Millam, 1996). Refer to the companion webpages for this chapter to read an outline of the history of IV infusion therapy.

W

The term IV is defined as 'inside or within a vein' (Macpherson, 2002), and is commonly referred to as IV therapy.

The infusion of sterile fluid can be:

- blood or blood products
- medication
- sterile fluid.

Intravenous fluid therapy is of benefit when oral or enteral routes, which include nasogastric, nasoenteric and gastrostomy routes, are inappropriate, therefore IV therapy can deliver fluid to the patient quickly and safely. According to Brooker (2007) IV infusion therapy may be used to:

- replace fluids and correct imbalances
- maintain fluid, electrolyte and acid-base balance
- administer blood and blood products
- administer medication
- provide parenteral nutrition
- monitor cardiac function.

Physiology: fluid compartments, movement of body fluids and acid-base balance

Fluid compartments

Water is the major constituent of the human body, and body tissue fluids have an important role in maintaining homeostasis. Functionally total body water in a lean adult can range from between 45–75 per cent of body weight. Differences would occur because of age, fat content of the body and sex (Thibodeau and Patton, 2007). Because of several important characteristics, infants and children have a greater need for water and are subsequently vulnerable to alterations in fluid and electrolyte balance. The fluid compartments in the infant will vary significantly from those of an adult, primarily due to an expanded extracellular compartment which constitutes more than half of the infant's body weight (Hockenberry, Winkelstein and Kline, 2003).

Functionally total body water can be subdivided into two major compartments; outside cells and inside cells known as:

- *Extracellular fluid* (ECF) (extra = outside) 80 per cent of extracellular fluid is interstitial which occupies the microscopic spaces between the cells, and 20 per cent of extracellular fluid is plasma which is the liquid portion of blood.
- *Intracellular fluid* (ICF) (intra = within) also known as cytosol is the fluid within the cells.

However, it is important to note that the composition of extracellular and intracellular fluids are strikingly different (Clancy and McVicar, 2002; Costanzo, 2006).

Extracellular fluid

Extracellular fluid consists of plasma, blood, lymph, cerebrospinal fluid and the intercellular or interstitial fluid which bathes all the cells in the body, except for the outer layer of the skin. It is the medium through which substances pass from the blood to body cells, and from the cells into the blood.

Part

IV

Intracellular fluid

The composition of intracellular fluid is largely controlled by the cell itself, because there is selective uptake and discharge mechanisms present in the cell membrane. The composition of intracellular fluid is very different from that of extracellular fluid. Sodium levels are approximately ten times higher in extracellular fluid than intracellular fluid (Waugh and Grant, 2003).This differential is due to the fact that although sodium diffuses into the cell down its concentration gradient there is a pump in the cell membrane which selectively pumps it back out again. This concentration gradient is essential for the normal functioning of some cells particularly nerve and muscle cells.

The body is in fluid balance when the required amounts of water and solutes are correctly proportioned and present in the various compartments. Various physiological processes, including osmosis and diffusion ensure the continual exchange of water and solutes among body fluid compartments. Most solutes in the body are known as electrolytes, which are inorganic compounds that dissociate with ions which are atoms that have a positive (+ve) or negative (-ve) charge (Tortora and Grabowski, 2003).

Movement of substances within the body

Within the body it is essential that substances such as molecules, or electrolytes can move around the body. Water, which is the principle constituent of the body, has to move in order to be distributed throughout the body fluids and keep solutes at appropriate physiological concentrations, thereby maintaining homeostasis (Waugh and Grant, 2003). Substances will always travel from an area of high concentration to a low concentration. A concentration gradient exists between two such areas.

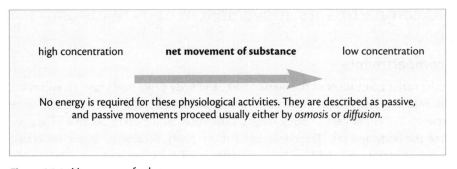

Figure 25.1 Movement of substances

Osmosis

This is the movement of water in the cell, which goes down the concentration gradient across a semipermeable membrane, when equilibrium cannot be achieved by diffusion of solute molecules. This can occur when the solute molecules are too large to pass through the pores in the cell membrane. The force with which this occurs is referred to as osmotic pressure. The process of osmosis continues until equilibrium is reached, at which point the solution on each side of the membrane are of the same concentration and are said to be isotonic.

Diffusion

Diffusion is the physiological process whereby chemical substances move from an area of high concentration to an area of low concentration, and occurs mainly in liquids, gases and solutions. The process of diffusion enables the transfer of oxygen from the alveoli of the lungs (high concentration) into the blood (low concentration). The process of diffusion is accelerated under conditions such as when the temperature increases and/or the concentration of the diffusing substance is increased.

Acid- base balance and pH values

Body fluids have pH values that must be maintained within relatively narrow limits for normal cell activities (acid-base balance). A pH reading below 7 indicates an acid solution while a reading above 7 indicates alkalinity. It is important to note that a change of one whole number on the pH scale indicates a tenfold change in the acid-base balance of the body. However pH values are not the same in all parts of the body . The normal pH value for blood has a value between 7.35–7.45 whereas bile has a pH range between 6–8.5. Refer to the companion webpages for background physiology of fluid compartments, movement of body fluids and acid-base balance and pH values.

Intravenous fluids

There are three main types of fluid:

- isotonic fluids
- hypotonic fluids
- hypertonic fluids.

Isotonic fluids

Isotonic fluids closely resemble the osmolarity of serum and remain inside the intravascular compartment and expand it: for example, in a patient who is hypotensive.

Hypotonic fluids

These fluids have less osmolarity than serum and act by diluting serum, which in turn reduces serum osmolarity. Hypotonic fluids are useful when the cells are dehydrated: for example, when a patient is on diuretic therapy or kidney dialysis.

Hypertonic fluids

These fluids have a higher osmolarity than serum. They act by pulling fluid and electrolytes from the intracellular and interstitial compartments into the intravascular compartment. Hypertonic fluids can be useful to help stabilise blood pressure, increase urine output and reduce oedema.

Crystalloid and colloid solutions

Intravenous fluids are sterile and commonly divided into:
- crystalloids
- colloids.

   Crystalloid solutions are composed of a clear aqueous solution of mineral salts and other water-soluble molecules, which move between tissue fluids and the blood stream. Most commonly they are used intravenously to support and maintain hydration and electrolyte balance.

   The most commonly used crystalloid fluid is normal saline which is a solution of sodium chloride 0.9 per cent which is isotonic and close to the physiological concentration in the blood. A solution of 5 per cent dextrose in water may be used if a patient is at risk of having elevated sodium (salt) and a low blood sugar.

t☆
Practice tip

Examples of crystalloid solutions include:
- 5 per cent dextrose solution (sodium chloride 0.9 per cent)
- Sodium chloride 0.18 per cent with glucose 4 per cent.

⚠ Professional alert!

Hospitals are currently being advised to remove sodium chloride 0.18 per cent with glucose 4 per cent IV infusions, from areas that treat children to minimise the risk of hypontraemia. The National Patient Safety Agency (NPSA) also recommends that the NHS and independent sector organisations in England and Wales restrict availability of these infusions to critical care and specialist units www.npsa.nhs.uk.

Part

IV

W

Colloid solutions contain large insoluble molecules or particles which are referred to as solutes. These particles can stay in the blood because they are unable to pass through the capillary membranes. Examples of colloid solutions include:

- blood or blood products
- synthetic solutions containing gelatine (for example Gelofusine) or starch (for example Hepsan)
- human albumen.

W   See the companion website for more information on the classification of solutions.

Intravenous access

An IV drip is the continuous infusion of fluids. This may be with or without medication, and the fluid is delivered through an IV access device, also known as an administration set or drip. The device is designed to deliver a measured amount of fluids and or drugs over a period of time via a number of different routes, which may be IV, subcutaneous or epidural. The method of IV drug administration depends upon the patient's condition, and the drug(s) which has been prescribed. In the main there are three methods for delivering IV drugs (Dougherty, 2002; Figure 25.2).The infusion devise is set at an appropriate rate to achieve the desired therapeutic response and prevent complications, and the use of infusion devices both mechanical and electrical have increased the level of safety in IV therapy (see image right). Furthermore the frequency of human error highlights the need for nurses to be competent working with both simple and complex infusion devises (Medical Devices Agency, 2003; Dougherty and Lister, 2006).

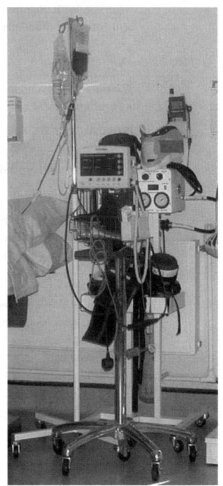

Figure 25.3 Mechanical intravenous device

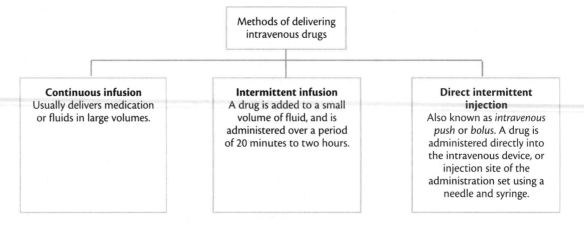

Methods of delivering intravenous drugs		
Continuous infusion Usually delivers medication or fluids in large volumes.	**Intermittent infusion** A drug is added to a small volume of fluid, and is administered over a period of 20 minutes to two hours.	**Direct intermittent injection** Also known as *intravenous push* or *bolus*. A drug is administered directly into the intravenous device, or injection site of the administration set using a needle and syringe.

Figure 25.2 Main methods of administering intravenous drugs

Needle and syringe

The simplest from of IV access is using a needle and syringe which will deliver a single dose of medication. A tourniquet is normally applied in the first instance and then the needle is inserted directly into a vein and the contents of the syringe are injected directly into the bloodstream. The tourniquet is then removed.

Peripheral IV lines

This is the most common form of IV access. A peripheral IV line consists of a short catheter (cannula) which is inserted into a peripheral vein (Figure 25.4), most commonly on the back of the hand or the arm in adults (see photograph below), although leg and foot veins are occasionally used.

Ideally vein selection should be based upon the one with the straightest appearance and should feel firm and round when palpated. Veins that cross over joints should be avoided to ensure patient comfort.

Intravenous cannulation and venepuncture are the most commonly performed clinical procedures carried out on young children, and may increase psychological and emotional distress (Melhuish and Payne, 2006). Intravenous access is more difficult to obtain in infants and children owing to the size of their veins, and their ability to understand and cooperate (Willcock et al, 2004; Trigg and Mohammed, 2006). A variety of sites are commonly accessible in infants and children (see Figure 25.6), however venous anatomy varies with each individual

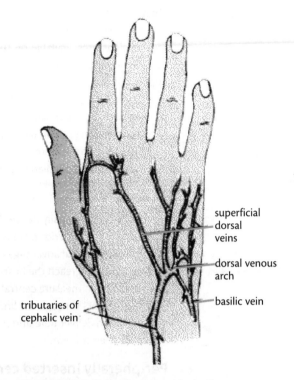

superficial dorsal veins
dorsal venous arch
basilic vein
tributaries of cephalic vein

Figure 25.4 Peripheral veins on the back of the hand

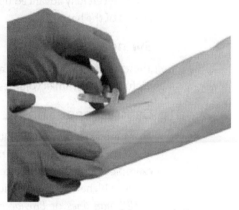

Figure 25.5 Insertion of the cannula into a peripheral vein

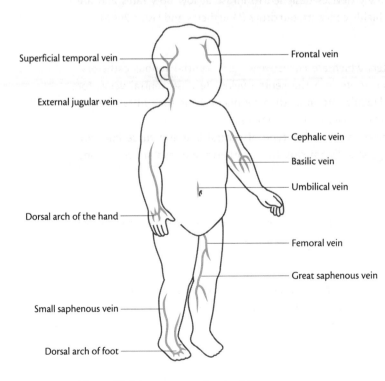

Superficial temporal vein
Frontal vein
External jugular vein
Cephalic vein
Basilic vein
Umbilical vein
Dorsal arch of the hand
Femoral vein
Great saphenous vein
Small saphenous vein
Dorsal arch of foot

Figure 25.6 Intravenous sites in children

Part IV

child and care must be taken not to damage adjacent structures such as nerves and arteries (Trigg and Mohammed, 2006). Most infants have two possible sites on each arm and foot and four to eight sites available on the scalp. Parenteral fluids may be given to high-risk neonates via several routes including umbilical venous and arterial routes (Hockenberry et al, 2003). Superficial veins on the infant's scalp have no valves and can therefore be infused from either direction (Wong, 1999), and arteries should be avoided for peripheral IV therapy. Infusion therapy within the paediatric setting requires very specific skills particularly in relation to:

- competency in relation to calculation of paediatric drug dosages
- maintaining an accurate fluid balance chart
- use of dedicated paediatric devices.

Central IV lines

Central IV lines normally deliver fluids through a catheter which has its tip situated in a large vein, usually the superior or inferior vena cava, or the right atrium of the heart. Furthermore this route has several advantages over peripherally sited infusions including:

- Medication can reach the heart immediately and be distributed to the rest of the body.
- Caregivers can measure central venous pressure (CVP) and other physiological measurements through the line.
- The line can deliver fluid and medications safely that would be irritating to peripheral veins, such as chemotherapy.

Peripherally inserted central catheter (PICC)

Peripherally inserted lines are used when IV access may be required over a prolonged period of time, such as patients who may require extended periods of antibiotic treatment, chemotherapy or parenteral nutrition. The line is inserted into a peripheral vein, usually in the arm and carefully advanced upward until the catheter is in the superior vena cava, or the right atrium of the heart.

Syringe pumps

These are low volume, high accuracy devices designed to infuse at low flow rates and are useful to deliver small volumes of highly concentrated drugs (Dougherty and Lister, 2006).

Central venous lines

There are several types of catheters which are collectively called 'central venous catheters/ lines' and there is more than one route into the central veins. Because central veins, for example the subclavian or internal jugular, are larger than peripheral veins, the central line can deliver a higher volume of fluid and can have multiple lumens.

Hickman lines or Broviac catheters are another type of central line and these lines are tunnelled under the skin to emerge at a distant site. These catheters are resistant to clotting and infection.

Implantable ports

A port such as Port-a Cath or Mediport is a central venous line that does not have an external connector. Instead it has a small reservoir under the skin.

Epidural pump

These pumps deliver analgesia through a fine catheter which has been inserted into the epidural space. This is a space between the spinal dura mater and the vertebral canal, containing areolar connective tissue and a plexus of veins.

Ambulatory pump

Ambulatory devices are small and allow patients more freedom thereby enabling patients to move more widely and continue with their activities of living. They are used to deliver small volumes of a variety of drugs.

Subcutaneous infusion (hyperdermolysis)

According to Brooker (2007) this route is utilised increasingly for older adults or those who are receiving palliative care. This method is less invasive than other methods, is convenient and more cost effective. Sites include:

- thighs
- abdomen
- chest wall
- area over the scapula.

Intraosseous infusion

The rapid establishment of systematic access may be vital in some situations and venous access may be seriously compromised by venous circulatory collapse. Intraosseous infusion provides a rapid, safe and alternative route for the administration of fluids and medication until intravascular access is re-established. Intraosseous cannulation can be secured rapidly with either a large bore needle or intraosseous needle inserted into the medullary cavity of a long bone. The most common site is the anteromedial aspect of the tibia (Figure 25.7). However, the dorsal tibia is an alternative site and the distal one third of the femur may be used in newborn infants.

In the main, IV fluid therapy is short term. However, should fluid replacement be required to be delivered for the long term, fluids may be infused into the superior vena cava. This is particularly important for the infusion of hypertonic fluids which may be physiologically irritant, however the vena cava is a large central vein and the blood flow is such that it is sufficient to dilute the fluid (Brooker, 2007). Refer to the companion webpages for an overview of methods of cannulation and fluid delivery.

W

Intravenous equipment

IV fluid is normally administered through bags or bottles of fluid which are delivered through a sterile single-use administration set (also referred to as a 'giving set') composed of several parts. This is attached to a cannula which has been normally inserted into a vein and collectively this will form a closed system of delivery. A variety of administration sets are available, and their selection and use will be based upon the type of fluids to be infused and safety issues.

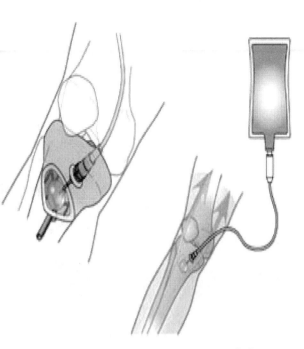

Figure 25.7   Intraosseous cannulation

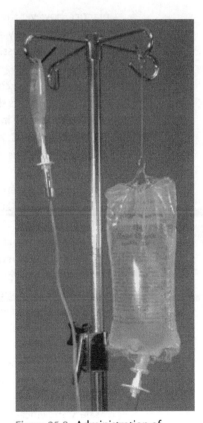

Figure 25.8   Administration of intravenous fluids through a bag

Procedure

All fluids and medication for IV use are prescribed by the doctor but checked by the registered nurse (RN), to ensure that the correct fluid is administered to the correct patient at the correct time. Infusion therapy is now an integral part of the majority of nurses' professional

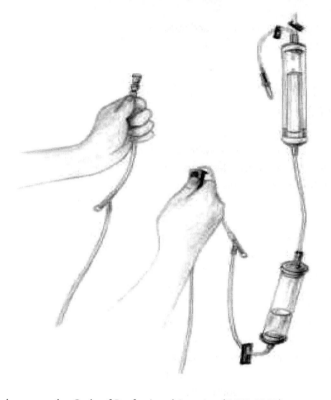

Figure 25.9 Component parts of an intravenous set

Reprinted with permission
© Kathy Mak.

practice; however the Code of Professional Practice (RCN, 2003) encourages nurses to expand their practice. They need to accept responsibility for their actions and undertake the necessary training (RCN, 2003).

- Nurses must:
    - seek informed consent before initiating any procedure; this should be obtained by explaining the procedure in an honest and age appropriate manner (NMC, 2004a; Dimond, 2005)
    - pay meticulous attention to hand washing (Winn, 2005)
    - adequately prepare patient for procedure and ensure dignity at all times (Crow and Keenan, 2007)
    - administer Emla cream or Ametop gel local anaesthetic if required and prescribed, and follow manufactures guidelines (Pedlar, 2001)
    - prepare equipment (collect everything prior to beginning procedure) including identification of suitable sized IV cannula
    - wear gloves.
- Use aseptic technique throughout (NICE, 2003).
- Position the patient correctly ensuring dignity and prepare the immediate environment to ensure safety and efficacy, for example making sure there is adequate lighting.
- The doctor or an appropriately qualified nurse will select an appropriate insertion site, demonstrating knowledge of anatomy and physiology of veins (palpation and visually) and indications and contraindications of venepuncture/cannula site

t☆ Practice tip

Gloves may be sterile or nonsterile and are available in a variety of materials including: natural rubber latex, synthetic latex and vinyl. The choice of glove will very much depend upon the clinical activity. According to Rennie-Meyer (2007) latex gloves should be used for procedures requiring dexterity such as cannulation or catheterisation and vinyl gloves are more appropriate for cleaning spillages.

a Learning activity

The National Institute of Clinical Excellence (NICE, 2003) has produced guidelines and advice relating to latex allergies and sensitivity. Refer to the NICE website and read the guidelines.

selection (Collins, 2006). This should be done in partnership with the patient (Brooker, 2007).

- The practitioner will undertake the procedure accurately and safely, cleaning the patient's skin with an alcohol-impregnated swab, applying traction, inserting the cannula at a 15–30 degree angle, advancing the catheter and withdrawing the needle (Lilley, 2006) with as little discomfort as possible to the patient (VAN, 2005). A flashback of blood should be observed prior to advancing the catheter.
- The cannula is taped in place securely using a transparent dressing (Tagaderm) to observe for any complications (Günnewicht and Dunford, 2004; Morgan, 2004).
- The cannula is flushed to check potency.
- Immobilise the limb if required.
- Care should be taken to avoid needlestick injuries throughout the procedure and during sharps disposal as per local policy (DH, 2001; NICE, 2003; EPINet, 2004).
- Clear the area, disposing of equipment following the trust policy.
- Ensure the comfort and dignity of the patient.
- Complete patient documentation (NMC, 2002).

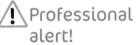

⚠ Professional alert!

According to NHS Scotland (2005) and Rennie-Meyer (2007), it is estimated that 100,000 needlestick injuries occur annually to healthcare workers. These involve:

- 48 per cent nursing staff
- 7 per cent medical and dental staff
- 20 per cent ancillary staff.

⟳a⟲ Learning activity   W

Investigate needlestick injuries further by looking at the information available through EPINet (2004) 'Exposure prevention network (EPINet)' on www.needlestickforum.net/3epinet/latestresults.htm

Caring for the patient with IV therapy

IV infusion therapy is a relatively common procedure, and for various medications it is the only effective route of administration (Campbell and Glasper, 1995). The procedure, however, continues to be associated with various high-risk complications (Higgins, 2004), varying from local irritation and venous oedema to rapid life-threatening systemic reactions (Ingram and Lavery, 2005; Morris, 2006). Therefore, to assist with the recognition and prevention of IV-related complications and to facilitate the safe and effective care for the patient undergoing IV therapy, it is essential that nurses demonstrate an in-depth awareness of:

- The advantages and disadvantages of the IV route for drug administration.
- The anatomy and physiology involved with the procedure.
- The method of delivery (including equipment) will be dependent on the condition of the patient, the drug to be administered and the desired effect of the drug (Dougherty, 2002).
- A sound understanding of normal fluid balance and electrolyte requirements, including the losses experienced by adults and children during the maintenance of homeostasis.
- Types of fluids to be used: crystalloids (water soluble molecules) and colloids (insoluble molecules).
- The duty of care and accountability they have in relation to drug administration, which incorporates safe drug calculation, checking, selecting, dispensing, preparing and administering. These are fundamental to safe practice (NMC, 2004b; Depledge and Gracie, 2006).
- Documentation should also involve complete information regarding infusion therapy and vascular access (Infection Control Nurses Association, 2000; INS, 2000).
- Additional information should include the date and time of insertion, number and location of attempts, identification of the site, type of dressing, patient's tolerance of the insertion and the name of the practitioner inserting the device (Randle and Clarke, 2007).

Part

IV

- Infection control, including the use of universal precautions, and intrinsic and extrinsic sources of infection.
- The risk of anaphylaxis, phlebitis, infiltration, extravasation and speedshock occurring, their diagnosis and management, and those at greatest risk of experiencing them.
- Trust policy in relation to the replacement of peripheral IV cannulas.
- The maintenance of accurate patient records (NMC, 2002).

Medicines must be administered in accordance with the NMC guidelines (NMC, 2004b). These incorporate the legal and professional requirements that must be adhered to when preparing and administering any medication, ensuring patient safety. Additionally, nurses should demonstrate an awareness of any contraindications or incompatibilities that may occur between the drugs they are administering. This is essential for safe practice (Depledge and Gracie, 2006). They should also be familiar with the local policy and procedures for reporting medication errors. Prior to administering the IV drugs the nurse should assess the patient's baseline observations, including pulse, temperature, blood pressure and respiratory rate. Following drug administration, in addition to routinely monitoring the insertion site, observations should be checked regularly and recorded to aid in the detection of any complications at the earliest stage possible (Dougherty and Lister, 2006). Before drug administration check that you have the right patient, the right drug, the right dose, the right route and the right time (Dougherty and Lister, 2006).

> **a) Learning activity**
>
> Detailed information relating to the care of IV infusions, can be found in Jamieson, McCall and White (2002); Nicol, Bavin and Bedford-Turner (2004) and Brooker (2007).

Calculating flow rates

It is the responsibility of the nurse to determine the correct rate of flow of the IV infusion.

The infusion rate may be calculated in one of two ways (Dougherty and Lister, 2006; Brooker, 2007):

Drops per minute: used for infusions regulated by gravity. The administration set (giving set) has a specific drop factor.

For example:

$$\text{Flow rate (drops per minute)} = \frac{\text{volume of fluid (ml) x drop factor (number of drops/ml)}}{\text{Time (min)}}$$

Millilitres per hour: the method used when the flow rate is regulated by volumetric infusion pump or syringe driver.

For example:

$$\text{Flow rate (ml/hour)} = \frac{\text{Volume of fluid (mls)}}{\text{Time/hour}}$$

> **⚠ Professional alert!**
>
> In addition to meeting the needs of high-risk neonates, infusion pumps must be accurate to within ± 5 per cent of the set rate when measured over a period of 60 minutes (Springhouse Corporation, 2002).

> **a) Learning activity**
>
> Richard has been prescribed 1000 mls of sodium chloride 0.9 per cent in eight hours. A standard administration set will be used. Calculate the drops per minute.

> **t☆ Practice tip**
>
> When deciding which administration set to use, remember the following (Brooker, 2007):
> - Standard administration set delivers 20 drops/ml for crystalloids.
> - Standard administration set delivers 15 drops/ml for colloids.
> - Blood administration set delivers 15 drops/ml.
> - Burette administration set delivers 60 drops/ml to children.

Adjusting the infusion rate

It does not matter how carefully you calculate the drip rate, and adjust the flow rate of the IV infusion, it is possible for the rate to still change. It may be that the patient has changed position, the IV tubing has become kinked, or the fluid has infiltrated the skin (extravasation). Such factors may cause the infusion to slow down or speed up ahead of schedule. When these problems occur recalculate the drip rate taking into account the remaining time and volume (Scott and McGrath, 2009).

Changing the infusion bag/bottle

Ensure that:
- There is a meticulous washing of hands.
- The dignity of the patient is certain.
- The empty bag/bottle is changed before the fluid level falls below the spike of the administration set. This will prevent the formation of air bubbles in the tubing leading to the cannula (Brooker, 2007).
- The expiry and patent date is checked by the RN, also that the solution is not contaminated by particles, or appears discoloured.
- The fluid type and volume is checked against the patient's prescription sheet and identity band.
- The information is recorded in the nursing records including batch number.
- The bag change is documented on the fluid balance chart.
- The patient is left comfortable.

> ## ⚠ Professional alert!
>
> It is important to note that in some areas of practice it may require two nurses, one of whom is registered, to check IV fluid administration. You will need to check Trust policy in your area of practice.

W   Refer to the companion webpages for an overview of the principles of caring for a patient with an IV infusion.

Complications associated with IV therapy

Infection

Although IV insertion is carried out using a strict aseptic technique, and requires a sound knowledge of the principles of infection control, the procedure causes trauma to the skin, and can facilitate the introduction of organisms such as *coagulase-negative staphylococcus* or *Candida albicans* (bacteria, fungi, yeast and viruses) into the site. Therefore, prevention is the key. This incorporates being aware of the potential sites for organisms to enter the IV infusion system (see Figure 25.10). These can be *intrinsic* occurring before the start of the IV, or *extrinsic* occurring during infusion. Infection can also be classed as *local* to the device site, or *systemic*, which can include organ failure and septicaemia. Nurses should encourage patients to inform them if they begin to experience any of the signs and symptoms of infection as this will aid early detection and management. Equally, nurses should be encouraged to utilise their observation and assessment skills and not rely solely on electronic infusion devices to detect problems such as infiltration and extravasation.

Anaphylaxis is the systemic immediate hypersensitive reaction, caused by an immunoglobulin (Ig)-E- mediated immunological release of mediators from

> ## ⚠ Professional alert!
>
> A peripheral IV line cannot be left in place for a long time because of the risk of insertion-site infection. This may include cellulites, phlebitis or bacteremia. You must adhere to the policy of your trust which will give you evidence-based guidelines, indicating how often the IV site must be relocated to a different site and the cannula changed. However, Randle and Clarke (2007) suggest that peripheral IV cannulas should be removed every 72–96 hours depending upon the type of therapy, or removed sooner if complications develop.

Part

IV

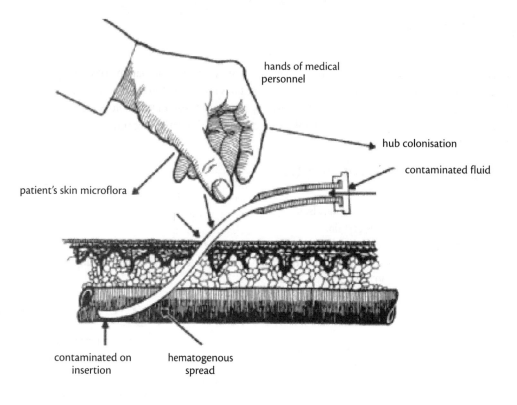

hands of medical
personnel

hub colonisation

contaminated fluid

patient's skin microflora

contaminated on
insertion

hematogenous
spread

Figure 25.10 Intravenous therapy sources of cross-infection

mast cells and basophils (Drain and Volcheck, 2001). Reactions from patients experiencing anaphylaxis vary diversely and can range from a mild skin irritations and urticaria to cardiovascular collapse. Nursing actions therefore will depend on the severity of the reaction.

Speedshock occurs when a foreign substance is introduced rapidly into the circulation. This can cause organs such as the brain and heart to become flooded by toxins. This is due to medication concentrating within the plasma and reaching toxic levels (Dougherty, 2002), resulting in syncope, shock and cardiac arrest. Plumer and Weinstein (2001) suggest that this is common during the rapid delivery of bolus injections. However, it can also be instigated by rapid flushing, the guidance of which is often overlooked even though this is a vital component of IV care, and therefore it is essential that guidance such as that provided by the Royal College of Nursing in *Standards for Infusion Therapy* (2005) is strictly adhered to.

Phlebitis is inflammation of the vein. This is linked directly to vascular access devices (Jackson, 1998). The condition is very painful and is typically treated with analgesia and heat (Philpot and Griffiths, 2003). Phlebitis can be further classified as mechanical, chemical or infective in origin, and many clinical areas now use a phlebitis scale such as the one adapted from Jackson (1998).

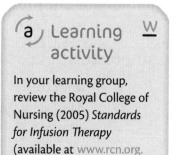

Learning activity

In your learning group, review the Royal College of Nursing (2005) *Standards for Infusion Therapy* (available at www.rcn.org. uk).

Table 25.1 Phlebitis scale

Healthy IV site	0	No signs of phlebitis
One of the following evident: Pain near IV site. Redness near site.	1	Possible first signs of phlebitis: regular observation required.
Two of the following experienced: Pain at IV site. Erythema. Swelling.	2	Early stages of phlebitis: resite cannula.
All of the following evident: Pain. Erythema. Induration.	3	Medium phlebitis: resite cannula. Consider treatment.
All of the following evident and extensive: Pain. Erythema. Induration. Palpable venous cord.	4	Advanced stage of phlebitis: possible thrombophlebitis. Resite cannula.
All of the following evident and extensive: Pain. Erythema. Induration. Palpable venous cord. Pyrexia.	5	Advanced phlebitis. Initiate treatment. Resite cannula.

Source: adapted from Jackson (1998).

Infiltration occurs when a non-vesicant drug such as 0.9 per cent sodium chloride or blood/ products are delivered into the surrounding tissues (Weinstein, 2001). *Extravasation* is the unintentional administration of vesicant drugs such as cytotoxic drugs (phenytoin and doxorubicin) into surrounding tissues. The following list of clinical characteristics of infiltration and extravasation is adapted from Dougherty (2000).

Table 25.2 Clinical features of infiltration and extravasation

Venous irritation	**Infiltration**	**Extravasation**
Erthema/discolouration. Aching and tightness along the vein. Absence of swelling or leaking at site.	Coolness at site. Blanching. Discomfort. Inability to obtain blood return. Quality of infusion altered. Swelling. Leakage. Taut skin.	Burning. Stinging. Swelling. Possible redness. Possible blistering. Potential tissue necrosis and ulceration. Inability to obtain blood return. Quality of infusion altered. Leakage at site.

Source: adapted from Dougherty (2000).

W

Refer to the companion webpages for an overview of complications associated with IV therapy.

Nurses should remain alert to the possibility of complications arising during IV therapy and act accordingly if the need arises. It is also vital that they are knowledgeable about the medicines in use within their clinical area and that they attend any training relevant to maintaining their professional competence. Equally, all care should be appropriately documented (NMC, 2002).

Monitoring fluid balance

Accurate record keeping and careful documentation are an essential part of nursing practice, which is endorsed by the NMC (2002). The fluid balance chart, which may also be referred to as the 'intake and output chart' or 'fluid chart', records fluid intake and output over a 24-hour period. This includes all intakes of fluids and outputs, and documentation should include the commencement or discontinuation of intravenous therapy, and changes of bags or bottles of fluid.

Patients who are receiving IV therapy may also be taking fluids orally, and in some cases the patient may be catheterised. Therefore careful monitoring and recording of all inputs and outputs is an essential part of total patient care.

Conclusion

The role of the nurse in the safe administration of IV fluids is an essential component of holistic care of the patient. Contemporary nursing practice requires the application of evidence-based practice, and the practitioner working from an informed position, in order to assess, plan and deliver care and make informed decisions, thus ensuring the safe administration of IV therapy. This awareness will enable the practitioner to deliver a high standard of care whilst also recognising professional roles and responsibilities and adhering to the Code of Conduct (NMC, 2002, 2004a, 2007). By maintaining a safe environment with respect to infection control and being alert to complications and side effects, the nurse will further ensure the patient's safety, which is paramount during IV therapy. Careful monitoring of observations and fluid balance will alert the practitioner to any impending problems which can be addressed early, thus preventing further complications. By applying professional knowledge and skills which are relevant to the safe administration of IV therapy, and reflecting upon your own learning needs and achievements, it is possible to make a real difference to the patient's experience during IV therapy.

> **ⓐ Learning activity**
>
> Compare your calculation for Richard's 'drops per minute' to the worked example. If your answer is different, go back and review this section.
>
> $$\frac{100 \times 20}{480} = \frac{20,000}{480} = 41.7 \text{ drops per minute (42 rounded off)}$$
>
> (Adapted from Brooker and Waugh, 2007)
>
> Then, using a model of structured reflection, think about your learning in this chapter. You can refer to the companion website for more information on reflective practice.

References

Brooker, C. (2007) 'Promoting hydration and nutrition', pp. 531–68 in Brooker, C. and Waugh, A. (eds), *Foundations of Nursing Practice: Fundamentals of holistic care*, London, Mosby.

Brooker, C. and Waugh, A. (eds) (2007) *Foundations of Nursing Practice: Fundamentals of holistic care*, London, Mosby.

Campbell, S. and Glasper, A. E. (eds) (1995) *Whaley and Wong's Children's Nursing*, Edinburgh, Mosby.

Clancy, J. and McVicar, A. (2002) *Physiology and Anatomy: A homeostatic approach*, London, Hodder Headline Group.

Collins, M. (2006) 'A structured learning programme for venepuncture and cannulation', *Nursing Standard* **20**(26), 34–40.

Costanzo, L. S. (2006) *Physiology*, 3rd edn, Philadelphia, Saunders.

Crow, J. and Keenan, I. (2007) 'Changing staff behaviour to encourage dignity and respect', *Nursing Times* **103**(13), 36–7.

Department of Health (DH) (2001) 'Standard principles for preventing hospital-acquired infections', *Journal of Hospital Infection* Supplement S21–S37, 47.

DH (2004) *Toward Cleaner Hospitals and Lower Rates of Infection: A summary of action*, London, DH. [online] www.dh.gov.uk (accessed 18 February 2009).

Depledge, J. and Gracie, F. (2006) 'Providing IV therapy education to community nurses', *British Journal of Community Nursing* **11**(10), 428–32.

Dimond, B. (2005) *Legal Aspects of Nursing*, 4th edn, London, Pearson Longman.

Dougherty, L. (2000) 'Drug administration', pp. 211–54 in Mallett, J. and Dougherty, L. (eds), Royal Marsden Manual of Clinical Nursing Procedures, 5th edn, Oxford, Blackwell Science.

Dougherty, L. (2002) 'Delivery of intravenous therapy', *Nursing Standard* **16**(16), 45–52.

Dougherty, L. and Lister, S. (2006) *The Royal Marsden Hospital Manual of Clinical Nursing*, 6th edn, Oxford, Blackwell Science.

Drain, K.L. and Volcheck, G. W. (2001) 'Preventing and managing drug-induced anaphylaxis', *Drug Safety* **24**(11), 843–53.

EPINet (2004) Exposure Prevention Network (EPINet) [online] www.needlestickforum.net/3epinet/latestresults.htm (accessed 20 February 2008).

Günnewicht, J. and Dunford, C. (2004) *Fundamental Aspects of Tissue Viability Nursing*, London, Quay Books.

Higgins, D. (2004) 'Priming an IV infusion set', *Nursing Times* **100**(47), 32–3.

Hockenberry, M. J., Winkelstein, M. and Kline, N. (2003) *Wong's Nursing Care of Infants and Children*, London, Mosby.

Infection Control Nurses Association (2000) *Guidelines for Preventing Intravascular Catheter-related Infections*, Bathgate, Fitwise Publications.

Infusion Nurses Society (INS) (2000) *Standards for Infusion Therapy*, Plymouth, Becton Dickenson.

Ingram, P. and Lavery, I. (2005) 'Peripheral intravenous therapy: key risks and implications for practice', *Nursing Standard* **19**(46), 55–64.

Jackson, A. (1998) 'Infection control: a battle in vein; infusion phlebitis', *Nursing Times* **94**(4), 68–71.

Jamieson, E. M. McCall, J. M. and Whyte, L. A. (2002) *Clinical Nursing Practice*, 4th edn, Edinburgh, Churchill Livingstone.

Jones, E. (2004) *A Matron's Charter: An action plan for cleaner hospitals*, London, Department of Health. [online] www.nhsestates.gov.uk (accessed 30 March 2008).

Lilley, M. (2006) 'Venepuncture and cannulation', pp. 433–9 in Trigg, E. and Mohammed, T.A. (eds) *Practices in Children's Nursing : Guidelines for hospital and community*, 2nd edn, London, Churchill Livingstone.

Macpherson, G. (2002) *Black's Student Medical Dictionary*, London, A. and C. Black.

Medical Devices Agency (2003) *Infusion System Devices Bulletin DB 9503*, London, Medical Devices Agency.

Melhuish, S. and Payne, H. (2006) 'Nurses' attitudes to pain management during routine venepuncture in young children', *Paediatric Nursing* **18**(2), 20–3.

Millam, D. (1996) 'The history of intravenous therapy', *Intravenous Nurse* **19**(1), 5–14.

Morgan, D. (2004) *Formulary of Wound Management Products*, 9th edn, Haslemere, Euromed Communications.

Morris, R. (2006) 'Intravenous drug administration: a skill for student nurses?', *Paediatric Nursing* **18**(3), 35–8.

NHS Scotland (2005) Needlestick Injuries: *Sharpen your awareness*, Report of the Short Life Working Group on Needlestick Injuries [online] http://needlestickforumnet.securepod.com/saferneedles/downloads/nursingsafetysurvey2005.doc (accessed 30 January 2009).

National Institute for Clinical Excellence (NICE) (2001) *Standard Principles for Preventing Hospital Acquired Infections*, London, NICE.

NICE (2003) *Infection Control: Prevention of healthcare-associated infection in primary and community care*, London, NICE [online] www.nice.org.uk/pdf infection_ control_full (accessed 25 January 2008).

Nicol, M., Bavin, C. and Bedford-Turner, S. (2004) *Essential Nursing Skills*, 2nd edn, Edinburgh, Mosby.

Nursing and Midwifery Council (NMC) (2002) *Guidelines for Records and Record Keeping*, London, NMC.

NMC (2004a) *Code of Professional Conduct*, London, NMC.

NMC (2004b) *Guidelines for the Administration of Medicines*, London, NMC.

NMC (2007) *Code of Professional Conduct*, London, NMC.

Pedlar, J. (2001) 'A study of topical skin analgesics', *British Medical Journal* **190**(8), 437.

Philpot, P. and Griffiths, V. (2003) 'The peripherally inserted central catheter', *Nursing Standard* **17**(44), 39–46.

Plumer, A. L. and Weinstein, S. M. (2001) *Plumer's Principles and Practice of Intravenous Therapy*, 7th edn, Philadelphia, Lippincott.

Randle, J. and Clarke, M. (2007) 'Maintenance of peripheral intravenous catheters', *Nursing Times* **103**(12), 30–1.

Rennie-Meyer, K. (2007) 'Preventing the spread of infection', pp. 391–423 in Brooker, C. and Waugh, A. (eds), *Foundations of Nursing Practice: Fundamentals of holistic care*, London, Mosby.

Royal College of Nursing (RCN) (2003) *Standards for Infusion Therapy*, London, RCN.

RCN (2005) *Standards for Infusion Therapy*, 2nd edn, London, RCN.

Scott, W. N. and McGrath, D. (2009) *Dosage Calculations Made Incredibly Easy*, London, Lippincott Williams and Wilkins.

Shawyer, V., Copp, A., Dobrojevic, J. and Goding, L. (2007) 'Nursing student and the administration of IV drugs', *Nursing Times* **103**(4), 32–3.

Springhouse Corporation (2002) *Intravenous Therapy Made Incredibly Easy*, Pennsylvania, Springhouse Corporation.

Thibodeau, G. and Patton, K. (2007) *Anatomy and Physiology*, 6th edn, London, Mosby.

Tortora, G. J. and Grabowski, S. (2003) *Principles of Anatomy and Physiology*, 10th edn, London, John Wiley.

Trigg, E. and Mohammed, T. A. (2006) *Practices in Children's Nursing: Guidelines for hospital and community*, London, Churchill Livingstone.

Vascular Access Network (VAN) (2005) *Venepuncture and Cannulation Structured Learning Programme*, London, VAN.

Waugh, A. and Grant, A. (2003) *Ross and Wilson Anatomy and Physiology in Health and Illness*, 9th edn, London, Churchill Livingstone.

Weinstein, S. (2001) *Plumers Principles and Practice of Intravenous Therapy*, 7th edn, Philadelphia, PA, Lippincott.

Willcock, J., Richardson, J., Brazier, A., Powell, C. and Mitchell, E. (2004) 'Peripheral venepuncture in infants and children', *Nursing Standard* **18**(27), 43–50.

Winn, C. (2005) *NHS Professionals Special Health Authority: Infection control guideline*, London, NHS Professionals.

Wong, D. L. (1999) *Whaley and Wong's Nursing Care of Infants and Children*, 6th edn, London, Mosby.

Useful websites

www.accessabilitybard.co.uk
www.bapen.org.uk
www.dh.gov.uk
www.go-needlefree.com

www.icna.co.uk
www.IVteam.com
www.nurseminerva.co.uk
www.nice.org.uk

www.nmc-uk.org
www.npsa.nhs.uk
www.rcn.org.uk
www.saferhealthcare.com

Part

IV

Chapter

26

Enteral feeding

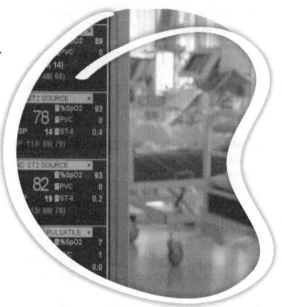

Chris Hanks and Gill McEwing

Links to other chapters in *Foundation Skills for Caring*

Links to other chapters in *Foundation Studies for Caring*

W Don't forget to visit www.palgrave.com/glasper for additional online resources relating to this chapter.

Introduction

One of the pleasurable experiences of life is eating. From the baby at the breast to the adult in the restaurant, feeding is an enjoyable experience. However, when individuals are unable to eat in the normal way it is crucial that nutrition is still provided by the enteral route. Although some nutrition can be provided parenterally (nutritional fluid administered through a tube directly into a vein) it is more beneficial physiologically for the individual to have nutrition via the gastro-intestinal route (enteral nutrition) even if the mouth and oesophagus are bypassed.

For most individuals this may be a short-term event, and in this instance, a small tube is inserted through the nose and passed into the stomach. If longer-term nutritional support is required, this is usually achieved by surgically inserting a small tube through the abdominal wall into the stomach.

This chapter introduces and discusses the notion of malnutrition and the ways in which health professionals may manage this.

Learning outcomes

This chapter will enable you to:

- explain the reasons why a person may require enteral feeding
- describe the possible complications, risks and side-effects
- identify the equipment necessary for enteral tube insertion and feeding.

Concepts

- Malnutrition
- Enteral feeding
- Safety
- Routes of enteral feeding
- Patients' experience

Rationale for enteral feeding

Malnutrition usually implies that the individual is getting too few nutrients but could also mean that the individual is getting enough of some nutrients, say sugar, but too little of other nutrients, such as particular vitamins or minerals. The term undernutrition is more specific, and indicates a deficiency of calories or of one or more essential nutrients. This deficiency, if it persists for more than a few days, will affect a patient's health by impairing immunity, delaying wound healing and reducing muscle strength. Psychosocial function can also be affected, leading to anxiety and depression (Stroud, Duncan and Nightingale, 2003). Schenker (2003) notes that about 40 per cent of all patients admitted to hospitals are undernourished, half of them severely so. She suggests that one factor in this situation is the inadequacy of current catering and feeding practices. Extra education and training for staff should emphasise the importance of nutrition for the patient, and how practitioners can ensure that appropriate food and snacks are easily available. Improving nutritional intake has been shown to reduce morbidity, mortality and hospital stay in undernourished or critically ill patients (Dobson and Scott, 2007; Stroud et al, 2003).

When a patient is at risk of, or is suffering from, undernutrition then enteral nutrition can be considered, providing the patient has a functioning gastrointestinal tract. Screening for malnutrition should be carried out by specifically skilled health professionals; the National Institute for Health and Clinical Excellence (NICE) guidelines (2006) suggest that all acute hospital trusts should employ at least one specialist nutrition support nurse. Nutritional support should be considered when patients are malnourished, such as when adult patients have a body mass index of less than 18.5 kg/m^2 or the patient has unintentionally lost 10 per cent of body weight in the past three to six months. Other patients who may be at risk of malnutrition are those who have not eaten or are likely to not eat anything for five days or have high nutritional losses, for example from ileostomies or poor absorption.

Part

IV

'Enteral feeding' refers to the delivery of a nutritionally complete feed containing protein, carbohydrate, fat, water, minerals and vitamins directly into the stomach, duodenum or jejunum (NICE, 2006). This can be by an orogastric route (usually used in neonates), a nasogastric or gastrostomy route.

In adults the groups of patients that may benefit from enteral feeding are:

- critically ill patients, for example, patients who are being ventilated
- post operative patients who are unable to maintain adequate oral intake
- acutely ill patients, such patients who have had a stroke
- patients with some long-term conditions
- patients approaching the end of life.

Enteral feeding is provided for children and young people when their growth and development is faltering, their recovery from illness will be delayed without nutritional assistance or they have a life-limiting condition that requires respite care (Corkin, Price and Gillespie, 2006). The lack of desire to eat can be due to many things, such as nausea, vomiting, dysphagia, pain on swallowing, altered taste due to medications and psychological factors. The ability to eat can be affected by impaired sucking, chewing and swallowing mechanisms and respiratory or cardiac conditions leading to breathlessness when feeding (Corkin and Chambers, 2008).

Other groups of children who benefit from enteral feeding are those with:

- short-term feeding problems, for example, prematurity, severe burns, cancer treatment (Huband and Trigg, 2000)
- neurological disorders, for example, cerebral palsy (Samson-Fang, Butler and O'Donnell, 2003)
- chronic conditions, for example, cystic fibrosis, renal failure, inflammatory bowel disease
- some psychological problems such as anorexia nervosa.

To provide best practice, the patient and carers/parents should be fully informed about the treatment. All information should be given verbally, and when appropriate supported by written information to meet the patient's and the family's needs (NICE, 2006). Only by being fully informed can a patient give informed consent. A fully informed patient can participate in choices about their healthcare, including the decision to proceed with the procedure, realistic alternatives to the proposed intervention and the relevant risks, benefits and uncertainties related to each choice.

When giving information, the individual's ability to understand must be taken into consideration. This may be affected by cognitive ability, in young children and also some adults. Language may interfere with understanding and cultural perspectives may influence the acceptability of the procedure. Physical, sensory or learning disabilities may make it difficult for the patient to understand what is involved and, later, to live with the effects of the procedure. It is important to gain patients' consent if they are competent, or act in their best interest, if they are not competent (Mental Capacity Act, 2005). The General Medical Council provides guidance on withholding and withdrawing treatment (www.gmc-uk.org).

W

National Patient Safety Agency (NPSA) and the administration of medications

Babies, young children and adults who have impaired ability to swallow tablets are often given their medications in a liquid form. These medications can be measured using a graduated spoon, medicine cup or an oral/enteral syringe. If standard injection/intravenous syringes are used, there is a risk of mistakes being made and oral medications being given into the intravenous or parenteral line if the patient has one in situ. The incorrect administration of oral medication by the intravenous route resulted in three deaths between 2001 and 2004 (NPSA, 2004). The NPSA has given advice to healthcare organisations to improve patient safety. This advice includes:

- Syringes used to measure oral medications are designed not to be compatible with intravenous catheters, systems or ports.
- Intravenous syringes should never be used to measure oral medications.
- The design of the feeding tubes/systems should include only ports that cannot be connected to intravenous syringes; no three-way taps should be included in the system and the tubes should be labelled.
- Organisations should have clear policies identifying and managing the risk of administering oral medications by the wrong route. Training in this procedure should be part of the organisation's programme.
- Careful use of colour and design should be used to help healthcare staff identify oral/ enteral syringes to prevent mistakes being made. The NPSA recommends that there should be a standard for colour design and labelling. Some manufacturers have started to use purple to help recognition of the correct syringes, and they will have male luer lock tips or catheter tips (NPSA, 2007).

W   **Further information can be found at** www.info.doh.gov.uk/sar2/cmopatie.nsf.

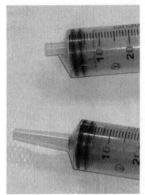
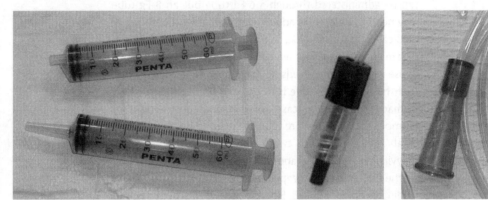

Figure 26.1 Enteral syringes

In adults, guidance regarding the route of enteral feeding is outlined in the NICE guidelines on *Nutrition Support in Adults*, which states:

> Nasogastric feeding can be used for patients unless there is upper gastrointestinal dysfunction. If the patient does have upper gastrointestinal dysfunction then a duodenal or jejunal tube should be used. If the need for enteral feeding will continue for more than four weeks then a gastrostomy should be considered.
>
> (NICE, 2006:13)

Nasogastric feeding

A nasogastric tube is passed though the nostril, down the back of the throat, into the oesophagus and then into the stomach. Nasogastric feeding is the most common route for enteral feeding and can be used for up to four to six weeks (Bowling, 2004).

> **(a) Learning activity**
>
> Think about how it might feel to have a nasogastric tube passed into your stomach. If you have the opportunity, ask your patient to tell you how it felt to have a nasogastric tube passed into his or her stomach.

Part
IV

⚠ Professional alert!

The nasogastric route is contraindicated in patients with following conditions:

- base of skull fractures
- nasal injuries
- when they have a high risk of aspiration

- gastric stasis
- gastro-oesophageal reflux
- upper gastro-intestinal stricture (Best, 2005).

Selecting a nasogastric tube

When choosing a nasogastric feeding tube, the principle considerations should be its size and material. Tubes are sized according to their internal lumen, for example 6, 8, and 10 French gauge (Fg). Fine-bore tubes, less than 9 Fg, are more comfortable for the patient and reduce the risk of inflammation of the nose (rhinitis), throat (pharyngitis) or oesophageal erosion (Bowling, 2004). Standard feeds can be administered through a 6 Fg tube but an 8 Fg tube may need to be used in adults receiving a high-fibre feed or medications (Stroud et al, 2003). It has also been reported that in children small lumen tubes (6 Fg) may be too narrow to use with thickened feeds (Huband and Trigg, 2000).

If the nasogastric tube is to be used for aspiration of the stomach contents, in cases of intestinal obstruction for example, then a wide-bore tube will need to be used (Stroud et al, 2003). There are two main types commonly used, polyvinylchloride (PVC) and polyurethane tubes.

The PVC tubes are cheaper and are suitable for short-term feeding of up to ten days. However, the chemical plasticisers in the PVC tubes, which keep the tube flexible, leach out when in contact with gastric secretions, and therefore after a short time the tube becomes brittle and cracks. The leaching plasticisers can also cause nasal and oesophageal erosion (Best, 2005). PVC tubes are therefore primarily used for short-term feeding, as they need changing frequently according to the manufacturer's guidance (Hockenberry et al, 2003). Large-bore PVC tubes should be avoided as they can cause irritation of the nose, oesophagus and increase the risk of aspiration and gastric reflux (Stroud et al, 2003). The polyurethane tubes are more suitable for longer-term feeding as they are softer and more flexible and can remain in situ for up to one month. These tubes usually have a guide wire to assist with passing the tube; the wire is removed when the tube has been passed but should be labelled with the patient's name and hospital number and kept by the bedside in case the tube needs to be re-passed. Never re-introduce the guidewire while the tube is in the patient (Nursing and Midwifery Practice Development Unit, 2003).

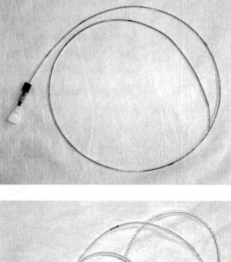

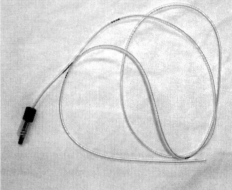

Figure 26.2 Nasogastric tubes

© Professional conversation

Margoscha, a registered nurse, says, 'I needed to decide which type of nasogastric tube would be best to use for Mrs Randolf. She was 78 years old and suffered a stroke three days ago, and due to her paralysis she had difficulty swallowing and was unable to maintain her nutritional requirements orally. I had to take into consideration that Mrs Randolf would require nutritional support for several weeks and therefore the tube should be made from polyurethane. Mrs Randolf would require normal feeds and therefore, to cause the least irritation, I decided to use a fine-bore tube such as a 6 Fg. However, as it would be likely that Mrs Randolf would be prescribed oral medications, I took the decision to use the bigger 8 Fg. Because the tube would be in situ for a longer period and there was a risk that Mrs Randolf might dislodge the tube, I felt it important that the tube should be radio-opaque, so that if necessary the tube's position could be checked using x-ray. To gain a more accurate estimate of the length of tube to be inserted I selected a tube with clear centimetre markings; once it was inserted, the measurement at the tip of the nose was recorded. This can be used to check the tube remains in the same place. I remembered that some tubes have multiple ports to aid aspiration, but in the case of Mrs Randolf I didn't think this would be necessary.'

a Learning activity

What type and size of nasogastric tube would you select for an adult patient who has had extensive abdominal surgery and has paralytic ileus requiring regular gastric aspiration for several days?

Procedure for passing a nasogastric tube

1   Explain the procedure and gain consent.

Child/infant: Explain the procedure to the parent and gain consent. Depending on the age of the child, explain in age-appropriate terms, or delay explanation until ready to perform procedure. Passing a nasogastric tube is a distressing experience (Penrod, Morse and Wilson, 1999) and children should be prepared for this procedure in a manner sensitive to both their and their family's needs. A risk assessment should be completed, including an enquiry into the patient's medical history to identify whether there had been any previous nasal fractures, nasal surgery, polyps or any other causes of potential blockage (Best, 2005).

2   Collect the required equipment.

- nasogastric tube
- syringe 50 ml (polyurethane tubes) OR 5–10 ml (PVC tubes)
- pH indication paper
- tape to secure the tube
- hydrocolloid dressing
- glass of oral fluid

- 2 gallipots
- water or water-based lubricant/2 per cent xylocaine
- disposable gloves
- scissors
- plastic apron
- tissues
- child/infant dummy.

⚠ Professional alert!

Syringe size

A negative pressure is created at the tip of the syringe when aspirating; the strength of this is dependent on the size and type of syringe and the force exerted. The manufacturer's guidelines must be followed when aspirating the tube in order to prevent damage (Viasys, 2000). Bunford (2006) recommends that 5–10 ml syringes should be used with PVC tubes and 50 ml syringes with polyurethane tubes (Kelsey and McEwing, 2008).

pH indication paper

Blue litmus paper should not be used to check the acidity of the aspirate as it is not sensitive enough to accurately determine the level of acidity.

3   Wash and dry hands and put on plastic apron to prevent cross-infection.
4   Decide on a signal the patient can use to stop the procedure if necessary.

Part

IV

Child/infant: Explain to the child and parent that you are going to pass the nasogastric tube; explain what the child should do if he or she wishes you to stop.

5   Clean work surface/trolley prior to placement of equipment as this is a clean procedure Prepare a hydrocolloid dressing; to prevent epidermal damage this should be three times the width of the tube and cover two-thirds of the cheek between the side of the nostril and the ear.

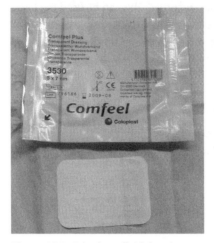

Figure 26.3   A hydrocolloid dressing

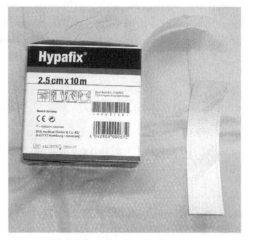

Figure 26.4   Adhesive tape

6   Cut adhesive tape. This should be wide enough to cover the nasogastric tube and overlap the sides sufficiently to hold it securely in place; however it should not overlap the hydrocolloid dressing. Place this within easy reach.

7   Wash and dry hands to avoid bacterial contamination of the tube.

8   Have water/lubricant in the galipot, to be used to lubricate the tip of the tube. Place a strip of pH paper in the second galipot.

9   Open syringe and place it within easy reach.

10   Put on disposable gloves to prevent bacterial contamination of the tube. Remove nasogastric

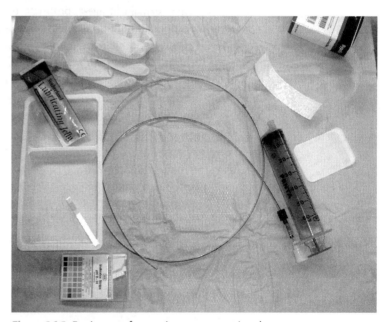

Figure 26.5   Equipment for passing a nasogastric tube

tube from packaging, checking that it is not damaged or beyond its expiry date. Measure

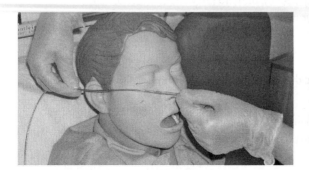

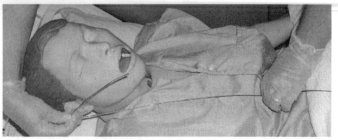

Figure 26.6   Passing a nasogastric tube

length of tube, using the measurement from nostril to the earlobe (NEX) and then from ear to stomach, just past the xiphoid process. Note/mark the point on the tube or hold the tube at the calculated point and keep it between the fingers of your less dominant hand. Ensure the end cap of the tube is in place to prevent leakage of gastric contents.

Child/infant: Klasner, Luke and Scalzo (2002) suggest that for paediatric gastric tube insertion, a graphic method based on height is more accurate than the standard NEX method for determining depth of tube insertion.

11   Sit the patient in an almost upright position with the head in a central position supported with pillows. This aids insertion of the tube and helps avoid the tube entering the respiratory tract. Do not tip the head backwards or forwards (Best, 2005).

Child/infant: Ask an assistant (parent) to supportively hold the child as appropriate to age and level of understanding. Older children should sit up with their head supported. Babies can be wrapped in a blanket and encouraged to suck a dummy throughout the procedure.

12   When selecting which nostril to use for insertion of the tube, it is sometimes helpful if the patient blows his or her nose to clear the nasal passages. Observe the nose for deviation of nasal septum, any inflammation, tenderness or visible obstruction.

Ask patients to remove any dentures in case they vomit during the procedure (Nicol et al, 2004).

13   Examine the nostrils for any obstruction or deformity, which may prevent easy insertion of the tube.

Child/infant: Older children may prefer to choose which nostril is to be used. Airway maintenance must be considered in infants as they are obligatory nose breathers.

14   Lubricate the tip of the tube using a water-based solution; this reduces the risk of friction and tissue damage. Follow the manufacturer's guidelines regarding type of lubrication. Encourage the patient to breathe steadily and try to relax if possible (Nicol et al, 2004).

15   Insert the tip of the tube into nostril; angle the tube slightly upwards and slide it backwards along the floor of the nose into the pharynx, following the normal contour of the nasal passage.

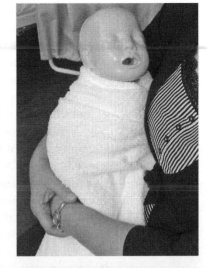
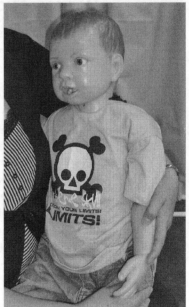

Figure 26.7 Gastric tube insertion for a child or infant

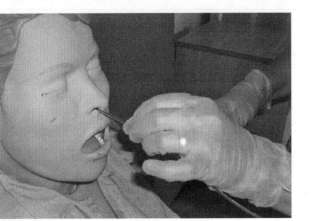

Figure 26.8 Inserting the tip of tube into the nostril

⚠ Professional alert!

If at any time during this procedure the adult or child starts to cough or gasp, or their colour deteriorates (becoming cyanosed), the procedure should be stopped immediately and the tube removed.

The tube should also be withdrawn if it coils in the mouth.

Part

IV

16 Continue to gently feed the tube downwards. In the case of obstruction, pull the tube back and turn it slightly and advance again. If the obstruction is felt again, try the other nostril. Do not force the tube down.

The tube should be gently inserted as the child/adult swallows as this will assist with the movement of the tube and reduce any discomfort.

A short pause may be necessary for the tube to pass through the cardiac sphincter into the stomach

Child/infant: As the tube passes to the back of the nose, advise child to take sips of water (if appropriate) to help the tube go down, or in the case of a baby offer a dummy. Continue until the point marked on the tube reaches the outer edge of the patient's nostril.

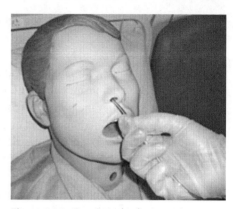

Figure 26.9 Continued tube insertion

⚠ Professional alert!

Only three attempts should be made at intubation. If intubation appears technically impossible then the advice of senior members of the healthcare team should be sought (Best, 2005).

17 Ask the person assisting to hold the tube in position. It is important to check that the nasogastric tube is in the stomach. Remove the end cap. Using the syringe, aspirate a small amount of gastric contents (0.5–1 ml) by gently pulling back on the plunger. Detach the syringe, and replace the end cap. Test the pH of the fluid using pH indicator paper; readings should be less than 4. NB: if the patient is taking acid-inhibiting drugs such as antacids, proton pump inhibitors or H_2 receptor antagonists, then a pH of 4–6 is acceptable.

Replace aspirate in infants at risk of electrolyte imbalance. There is no totally reliable bedside test of nasogastric tube placement, but measuring pH is the recommended method for determining tube position in infants and children. If bilirubin testing can be shown to be accurate in children then the two could be used jointly to discriminate among gastric, intestinal and respiratory placements (Kelsey and McEwing, 2008).

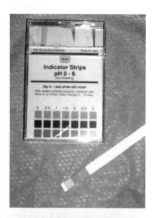

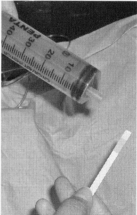

Figure 26.10 Testing the pH of fluid

⊝ Evidence-based practice

Assessment of aspirate acidity

Blue litmus paper should not be used to test the aspirate as it only identifies the presence of acid, not the level of acidity (Khair, 2005).

Following a fatality due to the misplacement of a nasogastric tube in a child (DH, 2004), the Medicines and Healthcare Products Regulatory Agency (MHRA) advised health professionals on methods used to check the correct placement of nasogastric tubes (MDA/2004/026, 14 June 2004).

If the tube is in the stomach the pH should be less than 4. If the tube is in the intestine then a pH of 4–6 will be obtained. If the tube is in the respiratory tract the patient will usually show signs of distress and the pH will be 6–8.

The National Patient Safety Agency (NPSA, 2005b) recommends that feeding can commence if aspirate is below pH 5.5.

Difficulty in obtaining aspirate

When there is difficulty obtaining aspirate try the following:

- If possible encourage patients to swallow a small amount of oral fluid if allowed (Stroud et al, 2003).
- Attempt to push the tube away from the stomach wall by inserting 5–10 ml of air down the tube using a 20 or 50 ml syringe.
- Inject 10 ml of air into the tube; if the patient belches then the tube is probably in the oesophagus, advance the tube a little.
- Try advancing or retracting the tube slightly to alter the position in the stomach (Stroud et al, 2003).
- Lay the patient on his or her left side for ten minutes (NPSA, 2005a).
- For infants and children: Inability to aspirate fluid is more likely to occur in children because the tubes used have a smaller diameter and are therefore more likely to collapse; however Ellet and Beckstrand (1999) showed that injecting air (1 ml in infants and 5 ml in adolescents) into the tube enabled aspirate to be obtained in 88.2 per cent of nasogastric tubes. Guidance from the NPSA (2005b) supports injecting 1–5 ml of air using a 20 or 50 ml syringe, waiting for 15–30 minutes and then attempting to re-aspirate.

Checking the tube position

If there is any doubt regarding the position of the nasogastric tube in the stomach, then consider re-passing the tube or checking its position by x-ray. X-ray, however, can only confirm the position of the tube at the time of the x-ray and the position may have altered by the time the patient is returned to the ward. There is also evidence that x-rays have been misinterpreted. The NPSA (2005b) cites cases of misinterpretation of x-rays by physicians who were not trained in radiography.

X-ray of tube position also presents problems, including the time taken to get and read the x-ray resulting in lost feeding time, radiation exposure in patients who frequently pull out tubes, inconvenience and discomfort for patients, cost, and the possible displacement of the tube after x-ray and prior to feeding (Kelsey and McEwing, 2008).

Methods of checking the tube position that are not recommended:

- Injecting air through the tube whilst listening for a bubbling sound over the epigastrium (the 'whoosh' test) is considered unsafe and is not recommended (Metheny et al, 1998; Stroud et al, 2003).
- Absence of respiratory distress does not necessarily mean the tube is not in the lungs (Best, 2005).
- Trying to confirm the tube is in the lungs by placing the proximal end under water and observing for bubbles is dangerous as there is a risk of water being sucked into the lungs on inspiration and can give false results as there may be bubbles from air in the stomach (Metheny and Meert, 2004).

(e) Evidence-based practice

Metheny et al (1994) examined the colour of gastric aspirate in 880 patients. The colour ranged from green, tan to off-white, bloody or brown and on some occasions clear and colourless. Aspirate from the bronchial tree was found to be off-white, yellow or green, and contained mucus which may be bright red or rusty coloured from blood. Therefore examining the colour of aspirate is not a safe method of determining the position of the tube.

Part

IV

⚠ Professional alert!

Difficulties with neonates

Two main problems exist with neonates: obtaining an aspirate and the use of the aspirate pH to confirm position of the tube. The NPSA (2005b) acknowledges that gaining aspirate from fine-bore feeding tubes can be difficult and that factors which may affect results from pH indicator strips or paper include:

- gestation
- postnatal age
- small volumes of aspirate
- the effect of medications on gastric pH
- continuous and frequent feeding.

The NSPA (2005b) recommends that a risk assessment is carried out to consider factors that may contribute to a high gastric pH particularly:

- the presence of amniotic fluid in a baby under 48 hours old
- milk in the baby's stomach if they are on one to two hourly feeds
- the use of medication to reduce stomach acid.

The detection of bilirubin in the aspirate is considered to be one of the determining factors for tube position in neonates (Kelsey and McEwing, 2008). Absence of bilirubin could suggest that the tube is in the lungs, but there may be occasions where no bilirubin will be detected in the stomach. Metheny and Stewart (2002) suggest a bilirubin concentration of <5 mg/dL as a good predictor of gastric tube placement in adults irrespective of fasting, while a bilirubin level of >5 mg/dlL is an indication of intestinal placement. These studies have been carried out on adults; only one study has investigated this in children, Metheny et al (1999) noted that comparable bilirubin is found in the gastric fluid of neonates. Metheny, Smith and Stewart (2000) suggest a combination of pH test, colour and bilirubin concentration is useful in assessing tube position.

> ### t☆ Practice tip
>
> When securing a nasogastric tube, a barrier such as a hydrocolloid dressing should be used to protect the skin and prevent epidermal stripping under the adhesive tape (Nursing and Midwifery Practice Development Unit, 2003).
>
> If it is necessary to continue with nasogastric feeding for an extended period, alternate nostrils should be used. If nasogastric tube feeding is initiated in infancy, areas around the face may become hypersensitive to touch and taste (Holden, 1997).

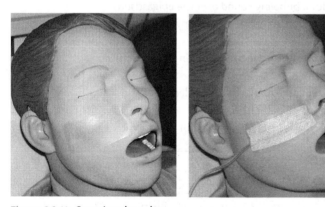

Figure 26.11 Securing the tube

> ### t☆ Practice tip
>
> PVC tubes lose their flexibility when in contact with gastric secretions and need changing frequently according to the manufacturer's guidance.

18   Apply hydrocolloid dressing to patient's cheek and secure tube using adhesive tape. Most patients benefit from using a barrier product such as hydrocolloid dressings and transparent films to protect the skin under strong adhesive tapes.

19   Document nostril used, size of tube, date and time of insertion. It is useful to make a note of the length of the tube extending from the nostril as this may help determine whether the tube has been displaced (Best, 2005).

Care required for a patient with a nasogastric tube in situ

- Ensure the tube is fixed securely.
- Avoid damage to or infection of the skin around the entry site.
- Maintain the patency of tube by regular flushing.
- Check the tube is positioned in the stomach before infusing anything down the tube.
- Always stop infusion immediately if the patient shows any signs of distress.
- Follow precautions to prevent bacterial contamination of feed.
- Record and act on signs of nausea, vomiting, abdominal pain or distention.
- Record and act on conditions of diarrhoea or constipation.
- Provide oral and dental care.
- Provide psychological support.

How the patient might feel

Having a nasogastric tube inserted can be uncomfortable and distressing, particularly if it takes more than one attempt to complete the procedure. Once it is in place and attached to the side of the face, the patient may feel embarrassed.

(e) Evidence-based practice

Displacement of the tube

There is a relatively high risk of displacement of the nasogastric tube after insertion, due to the patient coughing, retching, vomiting or knocking or pulling the tube up (Best, 2005). Safe and accurate checking of the tube's position is therefore essential. Errors can include initial mistaken positioning as well as displacement over time. If a tube is located in the airway or the oesophagus, feeding through the tube will result in pulmonary aspiration with subsequent morbidity and mortality. If a tube is placed in the duodenum, this can result in malabsorption due to a lack of gastric enzymes required for digestion (Kelsey and McEwing, 2008).

Metheny, Spies and Eisenberg (1986) found that 15 per cent of tubes were displaced without the nurses being aware that this had occurred. Ellett and Beckstrand (1999) found error rates in tube placement to be between 20.9 per cent and 43.5 per cent in a study of 39 hospitalised children. Children with swallowing difficulty or reduced levels of consciousness were found to have an increased risk of tube placement error.

Maintaining patency

Obstruction of the tube can occur, particularly with the smaller tubes used in children and babies. The most likely causes of blockage are the build-up of material from large molecule feeds, partially digested gastric residue, or the instilling of crushed or hydrophilic medications (Wiggins, 2007a). To prevent this happening the tube should be flushed regularly. A flush of 30–50 ml of tap water should be used before and after each feed and 10–15ml between and after each medication to ensure all medication is delivered to the stomach. If the patient is immuno-compromised, sterile water should be used. If a patient is on restricted intake then smaller flushes can be used providing the tube remains patent (Best, 2005). If continuous feeding is in progress then the tube should be flushed every four hours. Only use a 30–50 ml syringe (or follow the tube manufacturer's instructions) as smaller syringes can exert too high a pressure, which can cause the tube to split (Rollins, 1997).

t☆ Practice tip

Management of tube blockage

In the first instance roll the tube gently between the thumb and forefinger from the tip of the nose to the end of the tube; this can sometimes break up the blockage. Then try and aspirate the tube using a 50 ml syringe. If this is unsuccessful, then attempt to flush the tube, taking care to avoid excessive pressure.

A variety of solutions are suggested for removing blockages of enteral tubes including:
- use warm water, leave for 30 minutes, flush again (Bunford, 2006)
- carbonated drinks (Bunford, 2006)
- pineapple juice
- pancreatic enzyme solution (Green, 2005).

⚠ Professional alert!

Some of the disadvantages of using a nasogastric tube are:
- It can cause irritation to both the nose and oesophagus.
- It may increase mucus secretion and partially block the nasal airways.
- In some babies it may decrease their sucking reflex.
- It is possible for the tube to be passed into the trachea, delivering fluid into the lungs; this could be fatal.

⟲ Learning activity

Think about how it might feel to have a nasogastric feed. If you have the opportunity, ask your patient to tell you how it feels.

Feeding via nasogastric tube

A dietician will be involved to plan a feeding regime to ensure that the patient has the correct calorific and nutritional intake.

When possible, plan to feed patients at normal meal times. If they are able to take any food or fluid orally this should be given at the same time as the feed. With babies and young children, when progression onto oral feeding is intended they should be given finger food or soft food that they can touch and taste to help with the transition to oral feeding (Wiggins, 2007b).

Feeds can be given by gravity as a bolus, or by a pump as a bolus, or continuously. Feeds given continuously reduce the risk of gastrointestinal symptoms but this does mean that the patient needs to be connected to the pump most of the time, which limits mobility.

t☆ Practice tip

If a dietician is not available, in adults use the criteria for assessment of feed requirements as 30 ml/kg/day of standard 1 kcal/ml prepared feed. Inadequate or excessive feeding can be harmful to the patient, so the involvement of dietetic advice is imperative (Stroud et al, 2003).

Equipment required to administer a nasogastric tube feed

- pH paper
- disposable latex gloves
- boiled cooled water for flushing tube
- two sterile galipots
- plastic apron
- two syringes 5–10 ml for PVC tube or 50 ml for polyurethane tube
- feed prepared and heated to room temperature
- fluid balance chart (Wiggins, 2007b).

Method

1 This is a clean procedure; wash your hands and put on the gloves.
2 Reassure patient, explain what you are going to do and gain consent.
3 Make sure the patient is in a comfortable position; the head should be at a higher level than the stomach, with the patient preferably sitting or at 30°. A baby can be prone or on its right side.

4   Using the appropriate syringe aspirate fluid from the stomach and test using pH paper. The paper should read below 4. Remember that some medications can alter the pH of the aspirate.

5   Flush the tube to ensure it is patent and to prime tube.

6   Clamp the tube.

7   Attach the recommended syringe with the plunger removed and fill the barrel with feed.

8   Release the clamp allowing the feed to slowly enter the stomach.

9   The feed flows by hydrostatic pressure; therefore the higher the syringe is held above the stomach the faster the feed will flow down the tube. Administer the feed at a rate similar to the time taken to have a meal or feed orally, approximately 15–30 minutes. If the feed is administered too quickly, the patient may feel nauseated.

10   Top up the barrel of the syringe as it empties to prevent air entering the system.

11   When the feed is complete, flush tube with water.

12   Cap off the feeding tube.

13   Make sure the patient is comfortable; observe for signs of nausea, gastric reflux or dyspnoea.

14   Complete the fluid balance chart.

15   Provide oral hygiene and care to lips and nostril.

Administering medicines via a nasogastric tube

The pharmacist should be consulted for advice when administering medications through a nasogastric tube as most medication is not licensed for administration by this route. For some medications an empty stomach may be required to aid absorption, and therefore continuous feeding may need to be interrupted for a period before and after the medication is administered.

Medicines should be in liquid or dispersible form and must be measured by using amber-coloured oral syringes which have been designed with a wider neck, in order to promote safety. 'Press-in-bungs' are also available for medicine bottles to allow easy removal of doses (Corkin and Chambers, 2008). The position of the tube in the stomach must be confirmed before administration of any medication. As previously stated the tube must be flushed between and at the end of administration of medications to ensure they are not mixed and have reached the stomach.

Remember to accurately record the volume of medication administered and the flushing volumes when calculating the 24-hour total fluid volume; this is very important when caring for patients with fluid restriction.

t ☆
Practice tip

Medicines should always be given separately from the feed and not mixed together (Stroud et al, 2003). When possible, syrups or solutions should be given. If tablets are used then they should be crushed into a fine powder and dissolved into a small amount of sterile water. Enteric-coated or sustained-release tablets or capsules should not be crushed, and therefore should be avoided. Oil-based medicines should be avoided as they cling to the lumen of the tube.

Gastrostomy insertion and feeding

Gastrostomy

A gastrostomy is when an artificial opening is made surgically into the stomach via the abdomen through which a tube is inserted into the stomach (Samson-Fang et al, 2003). Gastrostomy tubes are feeding tubes used to provide nutritional support for patients with long-term problems such as neurological disorders of swallowing, depressed consciousness or mechanical obstruction to swallowing, including cerebral palsy, head injury, multiple sclerosis and motor neuron disease. The tube is made of very soft plastic and needs to be changed every two to three months. When changing the tube it is important to replace the tube quickly before the stoma closes.

The position of the gastrostomy tube is confirmed by testing the gastric aspirate with pH indicator paper to ensure safe administration of feeds, fluids or medications (Corkin and Chambers, 2008).

Types of gastrostomy tubes available include percutaneous endoscopic gastrostomy (PEG), balloon gastrostomy tube and a skin-level 'button' device.

Percutaneous endoscopic gastrostomy (PEG)

'Percutaneous' means through the skin, and in this case the flexible polyurethane tube is surgically inserted through the skin into the stomach (gastrostomy means an opening into the stomach). The endoscope (a flexible tube with a light) is introduced into the patient's mouth and down into the stomach, and the light is pushed against the abdominal wall, guiding the surgeon to make a well-placed incision (Cancer Backup, 2008).

A small incision is made in the abdomen and the tube is brought to the surface and secured in position inside the stomach and held against the skin using a fixation device. The procedure is performed under sedation and local anaesthetic in adults, and general anaesthetic in children. A tract will form over the following two weeks, and the fixation device should be kept in position to allow this to take place. It is important to avoid the device being too tight, which may lead to necrosis, or too loose, which could lead to leakage and peritonitis (Corkin and Chambers, 2008).

After insertion the stoma site should be cleaned daily with gauze swabs and sterile water for about a week. Then for the next two weeks cooled boiled water can be used. When the stoma has completely healed it can be cleaned in the bath. Follow the manufacturer's instructions as to when the fixation device can be opened; opening too early can lead to peritonitis.

There is a danger of the fixation device becoming buried under the skin after about six weeks (buried bumper syndrome). Once the tract has healed, the fixation device should be opened daily, the tube completely rotated and moved in and out of the stoma site 1–2 cm, then cleaned; this will prevent the tube adhering to the surrounding skin. A PEG can usually stay in position for 18–24 months (always check the manufacturer's instructions). When required the tube is removed endoscopically (Deaves, 2007).

A *balloon gastrostomy tube* is a wider-diameter flexible tube that is inserted surgically through an incision in the abdomen. The section of the tube in the stomach is held in position by an inflated silicone balloon. The portion of the tube extending from the skin may be initially held in place with sutures. After about six to eight weeks this tube may be replaced with a skin-level button device (Corkin and Chambers, 2008). Further surgery is not required when changing or removing the tube, but the procedure must be undertaken by a healthcare practitioner who is competent to carry it out.

A *balloon retention low-profile gastrostomy tube* (skin-level 'button' device) is a shorter tube with the external part of the device situated close to the skin. A silicone balloon or mushroom-shaped end is positioned inside the stomach to keep it in place. This device is less conspicuous and is preferred by many patients. The patient needs to be measured for the appropriate size tube prior to fitting by an experienced healthcare professional. Attachments are used when feeding the patient. The water in the balloon will require changing every week. The device will need to be changed every three to six months according to the manufacturer's advice.

Patients with respiratory conditions may require a shaft length of 0.5 cm longer than measured; this will aid movement when the patient is coughing and prevent the balloon splitting (Deaves, 2007).

Complications of gastrostomy insertion and maintenance

Early complications include haemorrhage, bowel perforation, gastrocolic fistula, bowel obstruction, peritonitis, local or septicaemia (Corkin and Chambers, 2008; Stroud et al, 2003).

Other problems that can occur include: Leakage at the stoma site can cause skin irritation, local skin infection, formation of granulation tissue at the stoma site, accidental removal of the tube, migration of the tube, tube blockage or diarrhoea.

Leakage at the stoma site may be due to the patient being fed too large a volume at one time. It may be necessary to reduce the volume of the feed and feed more frequently. Feeds may have to be given continuously using a pump. The other cause of leakage may be deflation of the balloon that secures the tube in the stomach (check 5–7 ml of water is in the balloon) or the tube moving out of position.

Granulation tissue may form at the gastrostomy site; this is a normal body healing response. Granulation tissue is bright red and moist, and leakage of fluid from the tissue can cause irritation of the surrounding skin. This may need to be reduced to improve patient comfort. If the area appears generally sore Cavillon spray or sticks can be used, which act as a barrier enabling the skin to heal. Candida infection should be treated with a course of Nystatin both orally and topically. A sample of stomach aspirate should be sent for analysis. Once treatment is completed, if possible change the gastrostomy tube as this may contain residual infection (Deaves, 2007). Excessive moisture can be contained around the site by using an absorptive dressing such as Mepilex or Lyofoam (Bunford, 2006). A steroid-based ointment or antifungal cream may be prescribed for irritated skin (Bunford, 2006).

Over granulation can be managed with the application of silver nitrate, using prescribed sticks applied daily. Take care to protect the skin around the site with petroleum jelly.

Diarrhoea related to enteral feeding can sometimes be resolved by the use of fibre-containing feeds or a break in feeding of four to eight hours (Stroud et al, 2003).

Care of stoma site

When the gastrostomy tube is surgically inserted, the stoma at this stage is a wound. Aseptic technique is therefore required for the first five days. When initial healing has taken place, cleaning of the stoma becomes a clean procedure. The patient should shower and wash with mild soap daily. The healthcare professional should then examine the stoma.

To perform this procedure, wash hands thoroughly with soap and water and dry with a clean towel. The site should be checked for any sign of leakage, inflammation, excoriation, swelling, soreness, infection or movement of the tube. The gastrostomy device should be rotated daily to help reduce peristomal infections and to prevent mucosal overgrowth that can lead to blockage of the tube (Stroud et al, 2003). The gastrostomy tube should be taped securely to the abdomen as this will prevent unnecessary traction on the tube, which may cause the stoma site to enlarge and allow leakage of gastric fluid which can damage the skin.

After two to three weeks the stoma will have healed and the patient can bath or shower normally; care should be taken to dry the site thoroughly.

> **ⓐ Learning activity**
>
> Think about how it might feel to have a gastrostomy. If you have the opportunity, ask your patients to tell you how it feels and whether they miss the experience of eating. Do they prefer continuous or bolus feeding?

Feeding via a gastrostomy tube

Feeding is usually possible approximately 6–12 hours after insertion of the gastrostomy tube providing bowel sounds are present; check trust policy and medical guidelines (Nicol et al, 2004). Feeds can be given as bolus feeds at meal times, or continuous or overnight feeds using a feeding pump. In some cases the patients benefit from bolus feeds throughout the day and then an overnight feed to complete their nutritional requirements.

Practice tip

Continuous pump feeds can provide maximum nutritional support for the patient and reduce gastrointestinal discomfort. However a return to intermittent feeding should be made as soon as possible to avoid gastric acid suppression; enabling the stomach pH to fall will help prevent bacterial growth (Stroud et al, 2003).

Procedure

1 Equipment required: prescription chart and prescribed feed, enteral feed administration set, enteral feed pump, infusion stand, syringe and sterile water (Nicol et al, 2004).
2 Explain the procedure to the patient and gain consent.
3 To minimise the risk of aspiration the patient should be sat up or propped at a 30° angle during the feed and for 30 minutes after it (Stroud et al, 2003).
4 Bowel sounds should be present.
5 Feeds should be administered at room temperature; if possible use sterile specifically prepared feeds which may have a giving set directly attached.
6 Wash and dry hands thoroughly.
7 Put on apron.
8 Remove the end cap from the feed bottle.
9 Maintain asepsis whilst opening the feed administration set, attach the bottle and close the flow-control clamp.
10 Attach the hanger to the feed container and hang onto the infusion stand.
11 Prime the tube by slowly opening the roller clam and allowing feed to run through the tube expelling the air; when priming is completed close the clamp and replace the end cap to maintain sterility.
12 Flush the tube with sterile water following local policy guidelines.
13 Following the manufacturer's instructions, insert the administration set into the pump apparatus.
14 Remove the end cap and attach to the PEG tube.
15 Open the clamp, turn on the pump and set to the desired flow rate; start the pump.
16 Check that the feed is running into the tube and that there are no blockages or kinks in the tube.
17 Check the patient is comfortable.
18 Regularly check the feed is running correctly and document the time the feed commenced, type of feed, flow rate and volume of water used to flush the tube.
19 When the feed is completed, disconnect the administration set and flush the tube with sterile water.

Care of the patient with a gastrostomy tube

- Check for tube displacement.
- Avoid damage to skin around the stoma site.
- Observe gastric aspirate confirming the tube position in the stomach.
- Maintain patency of the tube by regular flushing.

- Record and act on signs of nausea, vomiting, abdominal pain or distention.
- Record and act on conditions of diarrhoea or constipation.
- Provide oral and dental care.
- Provide psychological support.

Conclusion

Healthcare practitioners tending to patients requiring enteral feeding need to be skilled in the procedures of inserting nasogastric tubes, feeding and care of stoma sites. Without this skilled care, patients will be in danger not only of poor nutrition, but of infection, inflammation or death from asphyxiation. It is also important that all healthcare professionals involve the patient in care, listening to them and taking account of their experiences.

References

Best, C. (2005) 'Caring for the patient with a nasogastric tube', *Nursing Standard* **20**(3), 59–65.

Bowling, T. (2004) *Nutritional Support for Adults and Children*, Abingdon, Radcliffe Medical Press.

Bunford, C. (2006) 'Part 2: enteral feeding', Chapter 10, p. 173, in Trigg, E. and Mohammed, T.A. (eds), *Practices in Children's Nursing: Guidelines for hospital and community*, 2nd edn, Edinburgh, Churchill Livingstone.

Cancer Backup (2008) Cancer Backup [online] http://www. cancerbackup.org.uk/Resourcessupport/Eatingwell/ Nutritionalsupport (accessed 31 January 2009).

Corkin, D. and Chambers, J. (2008) 'Nutrition via enteral feeding devices', pp. 137–56 in Kelsey, J. and McEwing, G. *Clinical Skills in Child Health Practice*, Edinburgh, Elsevier.

Corkin, D.A.P., Price, J. and Gillespie, E. (2006) 'Respite care for children, young people and families: are their needs addressed?' *International Journal of Palliative Nursing* **12**(9), 422–7.

Deaves, J. (2007) 'Gastrostomy care', in Glasper, A., McEwing, G. and Richardson, J. *Oxford Handbook of Children's And Young People's Nursing*, Oxford, Oxford University Press.

Department of Health (DH) (2004) *Chief Medical Officer Update*, Issue 39 (August), London, DH.

Dobson, K. and Scott, A. (2007) 'Review of ICU nutrition support practices: implementing the nurse-led enteral feeding algorithm', *British Association Of Critical Care Nurses, Nursing In Critical Care* **12**(3), 114–23.

Ellett, M. L. and Beckstrand, J. (1999) 'Examination of gavage tube placement in children', *Journal of the Society of Pediatric Nurses* **4**(2), 51–60.

General Medical Council (2008) 'With and withdrawing life prolonging treatments: good practice in decision making', General Medical Council [online] www.gmc-uk.org (accessed 31 January 2009).

Green, S. (2005) 'Options and techniques in enteral tube feeding', *Clinical Nutritional Update* **9**(2), 6–9.

Hockenberry, M. J., Wilson, D., Winkelstein, M. L. and Kline, N. E. (2003) *Nursing Care of Infants and Children*, 7th edn, Philadelphia, Pa., Mosby.

Holden, C. E., MacDonald, A., Ward, M., Ford, K and Patchell, C. (1997) 'Psychological preparation for nasogastric tube feeding in children', *British Journal of Nursing* **6**, 376–85.

Huband, S. and Trigg, E. (2000) *Practices in Children's Nursing: Guidelines for hospital and community*, Edinburgh, Churchill Livingstone.

Kelsey, J. and McEwing, G. (2008) 'Nasogastric tube insertion and feeding', pp. 139–47 in Kelsey, J. and McEwing, G. *Clinical Skills In Child Health Practice*, Edinburgh, Elsevier.

Khair, J. (2005) 'Guidelines for testing the placing of nasogastric tubes', *Nursing Times* **101**(20), 26–7.

Klasner, A.E., Luke, D.A. and Scalzo, A.J. (2002) 'Pediatric orogastric and nasogastric tubes: a new formula evaluated', *Annual Emergency Medicine* **39**, 268–72.

McClave, S., Sexton, L., David, A., Adams, J., Owens, N., Sullins, M., Blandford, B. and Snider, H. (1999) 'Enteral tube feeding in the intensive care unit: factors impeding adequate delivery' *Critical Care Medicine* **27**(7), 1252–6.

Mental Capacity Act 2005 for England and Wales, [online] http:// www.opsi.gov.uk/acts/acts2005/ukpga_20050009_en_1 (accessed 31 January 2009).

Metheny, N.A., Eikov, R., Rountree, V. and Lengettie, E. (1999) 'Indicators feeding-tube placement in neonates', *Nutrition in Clinical Practice* **14**(5), 307–14.

Metheny, N.A and Meert, K. L. (2004) 'Monitoring feeding tube placement', *Nutrtion in Clinical Practice* **19**(5), 487–95.

Metheny, N. A., Reed, L., Berglund, B. and Wehrle, M. A. (1994) 'Visual characteristics of aspirates from feeding tubes as a method for predicting feeding tube placement', *Nursing Research* **43**(5), 282–7.

Metheny, N.A., Smith, L. and Stewart, B.J. (2000) 'Development of a reliable and valid bedside test for bilirubin and its utility for improving prediction of feeding tube location', *Nursing Research* **49**(6), 302–9.

Metheny, N.A., Spies, M. and Eisenberg, P. (1986) 'Frequency of nasoenteral tube dispalcment and associated risk factors', *Research in Nursing and Health* **9**(3), 241–7.

Metheny, N.A. and Stewart, B.J. (2002) 'Testing feeding tibe placement during continuous tube feedings', *Applied Nursing Research* **15**(4), 254–8.

Metheny, N .A., Whrie, M. A., Wiersama, L. and Clark, J. (1998) 'Testing feeding tube placement:auscultatation vs pH method', *American Journal of Nursing* **98**(5), 37–43.

Mohammed, T. A. and Trigg, E, (eds) (2006) *Practices in Children's Nursing: Guidelines for hospital and community*, 2nd edn, Edinburgh, Churchill Livingstone.

National Institute for Health and Clinical Excellence (NICE) (2006) *Nutrition Support in Adults*, London, NICE.

National Patient Safety Agency (NPSA) (2004) 'Fatal report of wrong route errors with oral liquid medicines', Personal communication from the MHRA to the NPSA.

NPSA (2005a) *How to Confirm the Correct Position of Nasogastric*

Feeding Tubes in Infants Children and Adults, London, NPSA.

NPSA (2005b) 'Reducing the harm caused by misplaced nasogastric feeding tubes', *Patient Safety Alert,* February 21, London, NPSA.

NPSA (2007) 'Promoting safer measurement and administration of liquid medicines via oral and other enteral routes' NPSA/2007/19.

Nicol, M., Bavin, C., Bedford-Turner, S., Cronin, P. and Rawlings-Anderson, K. (2004) *Essential Nursing Skills,* 2nd edn, Edinburgh, Mosby.

Nursing and Midwifery Practice Development Unit (2003) *Nasogastric and Gastrostomy Tube Feeding for Children Being Cared for in the Community: Best practice statement,* Edinburgh, NHS Quality Improvement Scotland.

Ozer, S. and Benumof, J. (1999) 'Oro- and nasogastric tube passage in intubated patients: fiberoptic description of where they go at the laryngeal level and how to make them enter the esophagus', *Anesthesiology* **91**(1), 137–43.

Penrod, J. Morse, J. M. and Wilson, S. (1999) 'Comforting strategies used during nasogastric tube insertion', *Journal of Clinical Nursing* **8**(1), 31–8.

Rollins, H. (1997) 'A nose for trouble', *Nursing Times* **93**(8), 68–70.

Rollins, H. (2000) 'Hypergranulation tissue at gastrostomy sites', *Journal of Wound Care* **9**(3), 127–9.

Samson-Fang, L., Butler, C. and O'Donnell, M. (2003) 'Effects of gastrostomy feeding in children with cerebral palsy: an AACPDM evidence report', *Developmental Medicine and Child Neurology* 45, 415–26.

Schenker, S. (2003) 'Undernutrition in the UK', *Nutrition Bulletin* **28**(1), 87–120.

Stroud, M., Duncan, H. and Nightingale, J. (2003) 'Guidelines for enteral feeding in adult hospital patients', *Gut: An international journal of gastroenterology and hepatology* **52**(7), 1.

Viasys (2000) 'Effect of syringe pressure on Viasys feeding tubes', *Protocol 170,* August.

Wiggins, S. (2007a) 'Enteral feeding tubes', pp. 396–7 in Glasper, A., McEwing, G. and Richardson, J. *Oxford Handbook Of Children's And Young People's Nursing,* Oxford, Oxford University Press.

Wiggins, S. (2007b) 'Feeding via a nasogstric tube', pp. 398–9 in Glasper, A., McEwing, G. and Richardson, J. *Oxford Handbook Of Children's And Young People's Nursing,* Oxford, Oxford University Press.

Chapter

27

Preparation of infant feeds

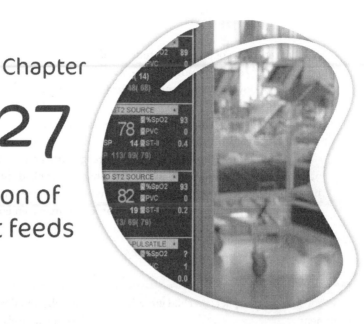

Doris Corkin and
Andrea McDougall

Links to other chapters in *Foundation Skills for Caring*

Links to other chapters in *Foundation Studies for Caring*

W   Don't forget to visit www.palgrave.com/glasper for additional
online resources relating to this chapter.

Part

IV

Introduction

This chapter will be of interest to students of both nursing and allied health professions when undertaking child health modules. The overall aim is to promote understanding, knowledge, skills and a positive learning attitude towards providing safe and effective infant bottle-feeding practice, thus enabling children's nurses and other healthcare professionals to know how to select and prepare age-appropriate infant feeds and be able to give clear, consistent evidence-based advice to mothers and those caring for infants, in the hospital and community.

Good nutrition is fundamental to ensure growth and development. Infancy is a time characterised by rapid growth which can only be supplied by an adequate dietary intake. Those children considered to be at risk, however, will need a comprehensive assessment by a dietician, ideally with experience in paediatrics, for management of any feeding difficulties.

Learning outcomes

This chapter will enable you to:

- explain how bottle feeding impacts on child growth and development
- appreciate that good nutrition is fundamental
- discuss the differences between the various infant formulae
- describe with theory how to calculate an infant's feed requirements

- describe and demonstrate the safe preparation of bottle-feeding, utensils and the making-up of an infant milk formula feed
- discuss the weaning process
- explain how to bottle feed an infant
- recognise the importance of keeping up to date with advances in infant formulae and evidence-based practice.

Concepts

- Nutrition
- Infant formulae
- Calculation of requirements
- Safety issues

- Growth and development
- Education and support; risks identified
- Infection control

- How to bottle feed
- Weaning process

[S] Scenario: feed intake of a 12-month-old infant

Jamie, who is 12 months old, lives with his mum on the third floor of rented accommodation. His mum has reported to the consultant paediatrician that Jamie looks pale and will not eat much solid food, but enjoys his bottle feeds. Jamie remains on five SMA White formula bottle feeds of about 240 ml per day and weighs 10 kg.

Jamie's dietary intake is as follows:

7.00 am:	240 ml SMA White via bottle
9.30 am:	240 ml SMA White via bottle Jamie sleeps from 10 am to 12 midday.
12.30–1.00 pm:	Slice of toast cut into fingers and small spoonful of beans; 1 Petit Filous; 240 ml SMA White via bottle
3.00 pm	1 digestive biscuit; SMA White via bottle.
5–6 pm:	2 tablespoons mashed potato with soup
9.00 pm:	240 ml SMA White via bottle

[a] Learning activity

Calculate Jamie's nutritional requirements, then estimate his current nutritional intake and consider:

- What advice should be given to Jamie's mum?
- Are there any other nutritional risks you would consider?
- Who are the healthcare professionals that should be involved and what would their role be in Jamie's care?

> **C** **Professional conversation**
>
> Andrea, paediatric dietician, says, 'I visited Jamie and his mum soon after admission to the children's ward. After looking through his medical notes I talked to the nurse caring for Jamie and was asked for advice on the most appropriate diet for him. Following a detailed assessment of Jamie's likes and dislikes, I was able to give his mum some practical guidance relating to his nutritional needs.'

Bottle feeding

Bottle feeding is an acceptable method of feeding an infant and refers to the preparation of artificial feeds, using a bottle and teat to feed an infant milk formula instead of using the breast (Hockenberry et al, 2003; Corkin, 2006). Although breast feeding is universally endorsed as the best way of feeding infants, human milk may not be nutritionally complete for every infant. Neonates <1500 g may require the addition of breast-milk fortifiers such as Nutriprem (Cow & Gate) or SMA (SMA Nutrition), as suggested by Wheeler and Chapman (2000). The composition of infant formulae is however similar to human milk and when it is prepared correctly, it is a safe alternative for mothers who decide not to breast feed (Lawson, 2007). All new mothers should be given accurate and consistent information regarding the preparation of milk formulae, which are derived from cow's milk protein and the only alternative to human milk (DH, 2006).

During the early days, weeks and months of a child's life, milk is the main source of nutrition. Infant formulae can be continued until 1 year of age (DH, 2003). It is essential to ensure infants receive optimum nutrition, which is a basic human requirement in order to allow for normal growth and development (Holden and MacDonald, 2000; WHO, 2003; Trigg and Mohammed, 2006). Even though there is a wide range of written information on bottle feeding (Ellis and Kanneh, 2000; DH, 2006) much of this literature may become a source of tension for new mothers and a negative experience for healthcare professionals (Hehir, 2005). Mothers need education and support in relation to specific information about formulae and how to make up infant formula feeds safely (Corkin, 2008).

t☆ Practice tips

- Recommend that infant milk formulae are made-up as required and only changed following advice from an identified health professional such as a midwife, health visitor or paediatric dietician.
- New mothers should be informed that infants will demand frequent feeds, usually every three to four hours over a 24-hour period, averaging six to eight feeds daily.
- Infants generally double their weight between birth and 6 months old. Furthermore, an infant may triple in weight and increase in length by 50 per cent in the first 12 months of life (Coleman, 2007).
- Milk from cows and goats is unsuitable for infant consumption as it is too high in some nutrients and too low in others, for example iron (Ellis and Kanneh, 2000).

Infant formulae

According to Barness (1991), milk-based infant formulae first became available in the late nineteenth century, and since the early 1970s whey-based formulae have been nutritionally modified to closely resemble the content of human milk.

Whey and casein-based milks are the two main types of infant formulae:

- Whey-based or 'first milk' is recommended from birth as it is easy to digest; it has a 60:40 whey:casein ratio, protein composition with essential amino acids and low renal solute load, and closely resembles breast milk (RCN, 2007).
- Casein-based or 'second milks' are similar to cow's milk, with a 20:80 whey:casein ratio. They are often given to hungrier infants although there is no scientific evidence to support this practice, and therefore it should not be encouraged.

Formulae are available in:

- ready-to-feed liquid, which is often used in hospitals – remember to check seal and 'use by date'
- dry powder for reconstitution with freshly boiled, cooled water (70 °C–80 °C); bottle should be labelled after reconstitution if made-up in hospital.

Table 27.1 Main types of infant formulae

Whey-based	Casein-based
Aptamil First	Aptamil Extra
Farleys First Milk	Farleys Second Milk
Cow & Gate Premium	Cow & Gate Plus
SMA Gold	SMA White

⚠ Professional alert!

Infant formulae must be prepared according to the manufacturer's instructions, using the measuring scoop provided in the tin of powder; avoid exchanging scoops between brands.

Preterm/low-birthweight formulae

Although preterm infants should be encouraged to breastfeed or be fed expressed breast-milk via a bottle, this practice may not always be possible. Infants who are born prematurely have greater nutritional requirements than infants born at term. Medical staff may recommend low-birthweight formulae while these infants are in hospital, such as Nutriprem 1 (Cow & Gate) or SMA Goldprem (SMA Nutrition). These provide preterm infants with more calories and protein which can help with weight gain/growth, and are mainly introduced while the infant is in the neonatal unit. Once an infant is ready for discharge, and should preterm formulae still be required, Nutriprem 2 (Cow & Gate) is available on prescription and can be continued at home until 6 months corrected age, providing growth and development are under regular clinical review of a consultant paediatrician and/or paediatric dietician.

Other high-energy infant formulae are available, for example SMA High Energy (SMA Nutrition) or Infatrini (Nutricia), which are both nutritionally complete and should be considered for infants with a history of faltering growth.

Follow-on milk formulae

These milk formulae should only be used from 6 months of age. They are beneficial for infants where intake of dietary iron may be of concern (Ellis and Kanneh, 2000; Lawson, 2007).

Examples of follow-on milks are:

- Aptamil Forward (Milupa)
- Cow & Gate Step-up (Cow & Gate)
- SMA Progress (SMA Nutrition)
- Farleys Follow-on milk (Farleys).

Follow-on formulae can be given as the main milk drink between 6 and 12 months and, should the child's weaning diet be inadequate, may be continued until 18 months of age.

Soya protein-based formula

Soya formula is based on whole-soy protein isolate. Soya formula however is no longer considered an appropriate treatment for the intolerance of lactose or cow's milk protein for infants under the age of 6 months (More, 2003). This is because infants who are at risk of allergy may also be sensitive to soya protein (Fiocchi et al, 2003). Lactose-free formulae are available and should be used if lactose intolerance is suspected. Extensively hydrolysed formulae are first line treatment options for cow's milk protein intolerance/allergy such as Nutrimagen, Pregestimil (Mead Johnston) or Pepti-junior or Pepti (Cow & Gate).

Examples of soya formulae are:

- Farley's Soya (Farleys)
- Cow & Gate Infasoy (Cow & Gate)
- SMA Wysoy (SMA Nutrition).

In 2003, the Chief Medical Officer advised against the use of soya-based formulae in infants under the age of 6 months unless there is a specific indication because of their high phytoestrogen content. This is supported by the Paediatric Group of the British Dietetic Association (2004), which highlighted the need to protect infant organ systems which are immature and vulnerable. Soya-based formulae should only be used for infants with galactosaemia or infants born to vegan parents (DH, 2004).

Elemental formulae

Neocate (SHS) is a special formula available on prescription. It is a nutritionally complete amino acid/hypoallergenic milk and may be required if the infant has multiple food allergies or malabsorption problems, and should be used if symptoms have not resolved using a protein hydrolysate infant formula. Neocate is free of cow's milk protein, soya and lactose and is only available in powder form (Hockenberry et al, 2003). Neocate can provide relief of gastrointestinal cow's milk allergy symptoms and can be used until 1 year of age. Neocate Advance (SHS) is available for children over 1 year of age.

Anti-reflux formulae

Enfamil AR (Mead Johnston) and SMA Stay-down (SMA Nutrition) are examples of gastric-thickening feeds which thicken when in contact with stomach acid. They may be used for reflux management when the addition of a thickener such as Carobel to infant formula is not appropriate. However these formulae should not be used with an anti-reflux medication (for example, Infant Gaviscon) because they will not thicken when the stomach acids have been neutralised. Therefore specialist medical advice must be sought when dealing with gastric reflux.

Goats' milk

Healthcare professionals do not recommend goats' milk as it is totally unsuitable for infants under 1 year of age because it is not always pasteurised, is a poor source of iron and vitamins and has an excessively high protein and salt content. Goats' milk may have been perceived by some parents as less allergenic, but this claim has not been substantiated (Hockenberry et al, 2003).

Calculating an infant's feed requirements

The children's nurse should be able to calculate the appropriate amount of feed an infant is expected to take to ensure adequate nutrition and hydration. Infants can differ greatly in their feed requirements as all infants are individual and will demand feeds frequently. A newborn infant will gradually increase feed intake from 30 ml/kg on the first day of life to 120 ml/kg on the fourth day and 150 ml/kg by the seventh day (Shaw and Lawson, 2001; Corkin, 2006).

Example: A 4-day-old infant weighing 3.0 kg should receive: 3.0 x 120 = 360 ml in 24 hours.

The formulae containers show tables based on the age and weight of the infant and these are useful guidelines when making up feeds. There may however be exceptional medical and dietetic reasons for adjusting calculations. This most often occurs when an infant has a history of faltering growth and requires extra calories (for example, 200 ml/kg/day) or indeed needs restricted fluids (for example, 75 ml/kg/day) if suffering from cerebral oedema, renal or cardiac problems (Trigg and Mohammed, 2006).

Preparation procedure

1 Preparation

Wash and dry hands, then collect the equipment for bottle feeding:
- plastic disposable apron to prevent cross-infection
- steam sterilising unit and instructions
- feeding bottle, disc, screw-ring, teat and cap
- kettle with cooled, freshly boiled water from tap
- container of infant milk formulae with scoop
- plastic knife with straight-edged back – plastic to allow for sterilisation and straight-edged to ensure correct measurement of milk powder
- bottle brush for washing utensils.

2 Prepare bottle-feeding utensils

All the utensils used for bottle feeding need to be thoroughly washed with the aid of an appropriate bottle brush which is only used for this cleaning purpose, in warm soapy water. Rinse with running water from tap and then place brush in sterilising unit with teats, discs, screw-rings, bottles and caps to protect against infections such as gastroenteritis and oral thrush, until infant is at least 6 months old.

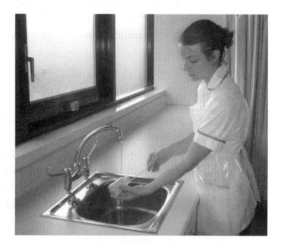

Figure 27.1 Washing utensils

3 Ensure safety of feeding teats

Clean teats carefully by squeezing the water through the hole of the teat with the aid of the bottle brush to ensure removal of milk residues and liquid soap (Ellis and Kanneh, 2000).

⚠ Professional alert!

Salt is no longer recommended for cleaning teats as this can damage silicone teats (DH, 2006). Cracked or split teats must be discarded.

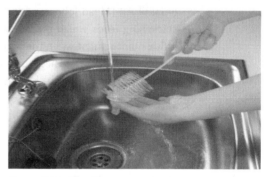

Figure 27.2 Cleaning teats

4 Sterilise

Steam sterilising is done either by electric or microwave; both are quick and efficient. Follow the manufacturer's instructions and add the recommended amount of water to sterilising unit. Cold-water sterilising requires a tank and either chemical solution or tablets. Ensure the manufacturer's guidelines are followed to protect against infections.

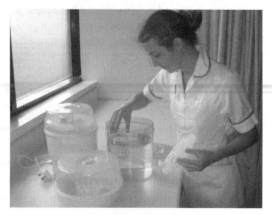

Figure 27.3 Sterilising feeding equipment

5   Prepare the feed

Before making up a bottle feed, wipe the work surface with a damp clean cloth and then dry it with a hygienic paper towel to cleanse the surface working area. Ensure effective hand hygiene to protect against infection. Wet hands with warm running water, then apply liquid soap and wash hands, ensuring fingers have been interlaced. Rinse and dry hands before touching the sterilised utensils (NICE, 2003; Trigg and Mohammed, 2006).

6   Make up a bottle feed

Boil fresh cold water supplied from the mains tap in a kettle. Leave the water to cool for no more than 30 minutes; meanwhile read the instructions on the formulae container. Freshly boiled water should not be used for making up feeds as it may destroy or significantly reduce the vitamin C content of milk. Evidence has supported safe practice to reduce the risk of E sakazakii and salmonella proliferation by making up infant formulae with boiled water cooled to between 70 °C and 80 °C. Cool the prepared feed and store it in a fridge at between 2 °C and 4 °C, unless the feed is being given within two hours after preparation (Foods Standards Agency, 2007).

Place the empty bottle on a flat clean surface. Always pour the cooled boiled water into the bottle first, then check the water level to ensure accurate measurement of water before adding milk powder.

7   Safe preparation of milk formulae

- Remember to check the expiry date on the infant formulae container and use within four weeks of opening; powder is not sterile (RCN, 2007).
- Follow the manufacturer's instructions regarding the number of scoops to amount of water.
- Loosely fill the scoop supplied with the milk powder and level it with the sterilised straight-edged back of the plastic knife, to ensure accurate measurement (Trigg and Mohammed, 2006).
- Add scoops of powder to the bottle of cooled boiled water (for example, one scoop to 30 ml of water).
- Seal the bottle with the supplied disc, screw-ring and cap, then gently shake it to dissolve the milk powder.

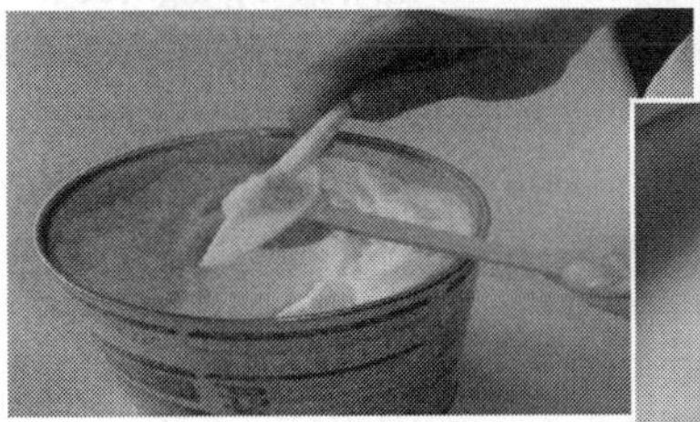

8   Before bottle feeding the infant

- Remove the disc and secure the sterilised teat with screw-ring provided.
- Ensure the teat has a hole that lets the milk out in regular drops, rather than a stream.
- Check the temperature of the milk feed by squirting a few drops onto the inside of your wrist.
- Cool the bottle of milk formulae under cold running water if necessary.

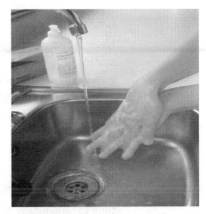

Figure 27.4 Washing hands before preparing the feed

> ⚠ Professional alert!
>
> Bottled mineral water, filtered water and repeatedly boiled water are not recommended as they may contain high concentrations of salts (Ellis and Kanneh, 2000; DH, 2006).

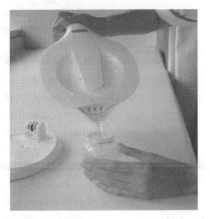

Figure 27.5 Pouring water into the bottle

Figure 27.6 Filling the scoop

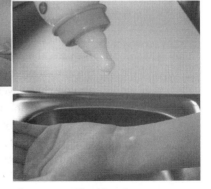

Figure 27.7 Checking the temperature of infant feed

Part

IV

⚠ Professional alert!

Never reheat a bottle feed in the microwave because the heat is not equally distributed and milk could scald the infant's mouth (Hockenberry et al, 2003); warming a bottle feed with warm water is sufficient. It is unsafe practice to reheat a bottle feed more than once as bacteria can multiply rapidly. Discard any remaining milk formula after bottle feeding (European Food Safety Authority, 2004).

Weaning process

When a child makes progress from drinking to eating solid food this is the process of weaning, which should not be encouraged before the age of 6 months. This is to allow the infant gut time to functionally mature, and only then should the diet be developed to include foods and drinks other than human milk or infant formulae (DH, 2003; WHO, 2003). Furthermore, solid food should never be added to an infant's bottle. Infants who find sucking difficult, however, may find the eating of soft pureed foods easier. Drinking from a lidded free-flow cup should be encouraged from 6 months and bottle feeding discontinued by 1 year of age, as spoon feeds should be well established and finger feeding introduced by this stage. Cow's milk must only be used to mix solid foods from 6 months and should not be given as a main drink until after 12 months of age (DH, 2006).

Stages in the development of feeding

- Milk first by breast or bottle.
- Then weaning from 6 months.
- Offer soft pureed foods and drinking from cup.
- Gradually introduce textured food to help develop muscles in the mouth.
- Introduce finger foods.

How to bottle feed an infant

Prior to bottle feeding, ensure the infant's nose is clean and clear of mucous and that he/she has a dry nappy in order to promote comfort.

1 Wash and dry hands thoroughly as highlighted in Point 5 of preparation procedure. A plastic disposable apron may be worn to prevent cross-infection, but be careful as plastic can be slippery on the knee of the carer.
2 Feeding bottles and teats are available in various shapes and sizes. Please choose and sterilise appropriately prior to use.
3 Calculate and prepare the bottle feed as recommended by manufacturer of infant formulae, ensuring the milk scoop is used correctly – see Point 7.
4 Test the temperature of the milk as highlighted in Point 8. Should the milk feel hot it can be cooled under cold running water from the tap before it is offered to infant, to avoid scalding (Hockenberry et al, 2003).
5 In order to protect clothing, it is best for infant to wear a bib; keep tissues within easy reach in case the infant should possset a mouthful.
6 The carer should sit down in a comfortable chair with the infant's head supported in the upright position. Relax and enjoy the experience, as bottle feeding is an ideal time to observe child development, whilst promoting eye contact and verbal stimulation.
7 Ensure the infant does not lie flat when feeding as there is a danger of choking and possible aspiration of stomach contents into lungs.
8 Offer the bottle feed by gently placing it to the lips of the infant. Never force a bottle feed into an infant's mouth.
9 Hold the bottle feed at an angle/tilted so that the teat is always full of milk, to prevent the infant swallowing air (Corkin, 2006).

10 Should the teat flatten while feeding, gently ease the bottle to release the vacuum in the teat.

11 Swallowed air will cause the infant to cry due to discomfort, so with the head supported, position the infant upright two or three times during bottle feed and gently rub the infant's back to release the trapped air, expect either a burp or passing of flatus.

12 Clear away the bottle-feeding equipment and wash the bottle and teat thoroughly before sterilising as explained in Points 2, 3 and 4 of the reparation procedure.

> **Learning activity**
>
> Reflect upon the identified risks and discuss how to prepare bottle-feeding utensils and infant milk formulae safely.

Conclusion

The purpose of this chapter has been to provide evidence-based practical guidance regarding safe care of infants when preparing bottle feeds. All infants and children go through different stages in their feeding behaviours and it is important to remember that different formulae may work at different times.

References

Barness, L. A. (1991) 'Brief history of infant nutrition and view to the future', *Pediatrics* 88, 1054–6.

Coleman, V. (2007) 'Promoting child health', pp. 60–115 in Coleman, V., Smith, L. and Bradshaw, M. (eds), *Children's and Young People's Nursing in Practice*, Basingstoke, Palgrave Macmillan.

Corkin, D. (2006) 'Bottle feeding', pp. 692–3 in Glasper, E.A., McEwing, G. and Richardson, J. (eds), *Handbook of Children's and Young People's Nursing*, Oxford, Oxford University Press.

Corkin, D. (2008) 'Artifical feeding', Chapter 14 in Kelsey, J. and McEwing, G. (eds), *Clinical Skills in Child Health Practice*, Edinburgh, Churchill Livingstone, Elsevier.

Department of Health (DH) (2003) *Infant Feeding Recommendations*, London, DH.

DH (2004) *Chief Medical Officer Update 37*, London, DH.

DH (2006) *Birth to Five: Your complete guide to parenthood and the first five years of your child's life*, London, DH, [online] www.dh.gov.uk (accessed 10 February 2009).

Ellis, M. and Kanneh, A. (2000) 'Infant nutrition: part two' *Paediatric Nursing* 12(1), 38–43.

European Food Safety Authority (2004) 'Opinion adopted by the BIOHAZ Panel related to the microbiological risks in formulae and follow-on formulae', *The European Food Safety Authority Journal* 113, 1–34.

Fiocchi, A., Restani, P., Gualtiero, L. and Martelli, A. (2003) 'Clinical tolerance to lactose in children with cow's milk allergy', *Pediatrics* 112(2), 359.

Food Standards Agency (2007) 'Guidelines for making up special feeds for infants and children in hospital', Food Standards Agency [online] www.food.gov.uk (accessed 10 February 2009).

Glasper, E. A., McEwing, G. and Richardson, J. (eds) *Oxford Handbook of Children's and Young People's Nursing*, Oxford, Oxford. University Press.

Hehir, B. (2005) 'Stop hitting the bottle', *Nursing Standard* 19(52), 28–9.

Hockenberry, M.J., Wilson, D., Winkelstein, M.L. and Kilne, N.E. (2003) *Nursing Care of Infants and Children*, 7th edn, Philadelphia, Mosby.

Holden, C. and MacDonald, A. (2000) *Nutrition and Child Health*, London, Bailiere Tindall.

Lawson, M. (2007) 'Contemporary aspects of infant feeding', *Paediatric Nursing* 19(2), 39–44.

More, J. (2003) 'New guidelines on infant feeding in the first 12 months of life', *Journal of Family Health Care* 13(4), 89–90.

National Institute for Health and Clinical Excellence (NICE) (2003) *Infection control: Prevention of healthcare-associated infection in primary and community care*, London, NICE.

Paediatric Group of the British Dietetic Association (2004) *Position Statement on the Use of Soya Protein for Infants*, Birmingham, British Dietetic Association.

Royal College of Nursing (2007) 'Formula feeds: RCN guidance for nurses caring for infants and mothers', London, RCN [online] www.rcn.org.uk (accessed 10 February 2009).

Shaw, V. and Lawson, M. (2001) *Paediatric Dietetics*, 2nd edn, Oxford, Blackwell Science.

Trigg, E. and Mohammed, T. A. (2006) *Practices in Children's Nursing: Guidelines for hospital and community*, 2nd edn, Edinburgh, Churchill Livingstone.

Wheeler, J. and Chapman, C. (2000) 'Feeding outcomes and influences within the neonatal unit', *International Journal of Nursing Practice* 6(4), 196–206.

World Health Organisation (WHO) (2003) 'Global strategy for infant and child feeding', Geneva, WHO [online] www.who.int/nutrition/publications/infantfeeding/en/ (accessed 10 February 2009).

Chapter

28

Routes of medication administration

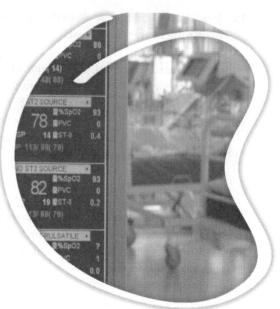

Tracey Harrington and Carol Barron

Links to other chapters in *Foundation Skills for Caring*

Links to other chapters in *Foundation Studies for Caring*

W Don't forget to visit www.palgrave.com/glasper for additional
online resources relating to this chapter.

Introduction

This chapter aims to give you the foundations required to safely administer medications to patients, focusing specifically on:

- relevant anatomical and physiological knowledge
- the understanding and application of the relevant mathematical formulations required in the calculations of medication dosages
- the theoretical knowledge underpinning the clinical skills required for the safe administration of medications via the numerous routes available founded on current evidence-based practice
- the importance of aseptic technique in the prevention of infection and sharps injuries which underpins all nursing care and practice.

Learning outcomes

This chapter will enable you to:

- discuss the role of the nurse in the preparation, administration and recording of medication administration to patients
- recognise the importance of the most common route of medication administration to all patient groups – orally administered medicines
- explain the relevant medication calculation formulae required in the calculation of accurate medication dosages for clients/patients
- demonstrate knowledge and understanding of the theoretical and clinical skills required in the administration of injections to clients/patients utilising current evidence-based practice
- recognise the importance of differing routes for the administration of medications such as rectal, ear, eye, nasal and topical

- appreciate the differing methods of medication administration, for example nebulisers and metered dose inhalers
- recognise the essential requirements of safe practice in the administration of medicines to patients
- demonstrate knowledge of the standard precautions involved in drug administration
- appreciate the importance of preparing the patients and gaining their consent for medication administration
- discuss the possible advantages and disadvantages associated with the different routes of medication administration.

Concepts

- Medication calculations
- Clinical skills
- Safe nursing practice
- Routes of medication administration
- Nurse's role
- Standard precautions

Drug calculations

To administer medications it is necessary to first calculate how much medicine you will be giving, so a good place to start is the mathematical formulation for medicine dosages.

Drug calculations are an important aspect of the nurses' responsibility in relation to the safe administration of medications. Two of the main mathematical formulations required are:

- ability to convert metric units
- multiplication and division.

Weight

The basic unit of weight is the gram (g). We also use the milligram (mg) and the microgram (mcg) for the (sometimes tiny) amounts involved in drug dosages. Larger weights sometimes use the kilogram (kg).

Part

IV

Weight unit conversions and terminology

1 kilogram (kg) = 1000 grams (g)
1 gram (g) = 1000 milligrams (mg)
1 milligram (mg) = 1000 micrograms (mcg)
1 microgram (mcg) = 1000 nanograms (ng)

Table 28.1 Weight conversion

1 kg = 1000 g
1 g = 1000 mg
1 mg = 1000 mcg

Look at the conversion table and unit terminology above. To convert g to mg, we multiply by 1000. To convert g to mg, we divide by 1000. When calculating medication dosages, all weights and volumes in any equation must be in the same units prior to the drug calculation.

In this case, in order to convert a larger unit to a smaller unit you must multiply by 1000. The decimal point moves three places to the right:

0.250 mg = 250 mcg

In order to convert a smaller unit to a larger unit you divide by 1000. The decimal point moves three places to the left:

125 mcg = 0.125 mg

a) Learning activity

Try the following exercises yourself (see the end of this chapter for the answers):

1. Convert 68735 milligrams to grams.
2. Convert 92763 millilitres to litres.
3. Convert 93074 milligrams to grams.
4. Convert 44343 millilitres to litres.

Multiplication and division

There is no single right way to calculate drug dosages; however there is one formula, in the form of an equation that always works:

$$\text{Dose} = \frac{\text{What you want}}{\text{What you've got}} \times \text{What it's in}$$

a) Learning activity

Try following the worked examples below.

S Scenario: medication for Sanjeev

A child, Sanjeev, is prescribed oral chloral hydrate 250 mg. The drug is available as an elixir containing 200 mg in 5 ml.

You need to estimate a sensible dose. If 5 ml contains 200 mg, then you will need more than 5ml for a dose of 250mg. You *want* 250 mg. You *have* 200mg in 5 mls.

Therefore: 250 mg divided by 200 mg x 5 = 6.25 mls

$$\text{Dose} = \frac{250}{200} \times \frac{5}{1} = \frac{1250}{200} = 6.25 \text{ ml}$$

OR

$$= \frac{\overset{50}{\cancel{250}}}{\underset{40}{\cancel{200}}} \times \frac{5}{1} = \frac{250}{40} = 6.25 \text{ ml}$$

(S) Scenario: medication for Joe

Joe King requires analgesia. He has severe difficulties swallowing tablets so all medications are given in a liquid form. He can have paracetamol elixir 500 mg every six hours. The elixir contains 250 mg in 10 ml.

How much should you pour out for Joe?

$$\text{Dose} = \frac{\text{What you want}}{\text{What you've got}}$$

$$\frac{500 \text{ mg}}{250 \text{ mg}} \times \frac{10}{1} = 20 \text{ ml}$$

You *want* 500 mg. You *have* 250 mg in 10 ml.
Therefore: 500 mg divided by 250 mg x 10 = 20 ml.

(a) Learning activity   W

Why is it important to be able to accurately calculate drug dosages? Using the following website complete the tablet dosage drugs quiz: http://www. testandcalc.com/quiz/index.asp

(S) Scenario: medication for Paul

Paul is prescribed 0.5 milligrams of Digoxin; 250 microgram tablets are available.
How many tablets will you give Paul? First ensure all weights are in the same unit.

250 mcg = 0.25 mg

$$\frac{0.5 \text{ mg}}{0.25 \text{ mg}} = 2 \text{ tablets}$$

You *want* 0.5 mg. You *have* 0.25mg (same as 250 microgram) tablets.
Therefore; 0.5mg divided by 0.25 mg = 2 tablets.

(a) Learning activity

Try the following exercises.
- Clare is ordered 500 mg of Amoxicillin orally. It is available in suspension form as 125 milligrams per 5 millilitres. How many millilitres of Amoxicillin will you administer?
- Tony is ordered 30 milligrams of Codeine phosphate. 60 milligram tablets are available. How many tablets will you give?
- Catherine requires 85 mg of cortisone; there is 100 mg in 5 ml. How many ml will you administer?

⚠ Professional alert!

When calculating medication dosages, all weights and volumes in any equation must be in the same units prior to the drug calculation.

If the dose of drug prescribed is greater than the safe dosage limit recommended in the British National Formulary (BNF), always check with the person who prescribed the medication, as there may have been an error.

(S) Scenario: medication for John

John is a 27-year-old civil servant who was diagnosed with asthma as a child. Generally he manages his asthma well, with periodic exacerbations normally associated with chest infections. Otherwise John is fit and well and is a non-smoker. At weekends he enjoys clubbing with his mates and does drink in excess of the recommended alcohol intake guidelines. John lives in a rented apartment with his Thai girlfriend, aged 25 years. They have been together for three years.

John and Chanakarn Ng are really excited as they are planning to visit Chanakarn's parents in Thailand later this summer. As John has never been to Thailand he has come to the GP surgery to ask you as the nurse about any vaccinations that he will need in preparation for their trip.

While John is talking to you in the surgery/clinic he tells you that he has become more wheezy, breathless and tired over the last few weeks and asks for his current asthma medication to be reviewed.

Part

IV

> ### (a) Learning activity   W
>
> Research the answers to John's questions using the British National Formulary website; http://www.bnf.org/bnf/. You will need to consider:
>
> - The use of bronchodilator in the management of asthma.
> - The rationale for vaccination when travelling to certain geographical locations.
>
> Using a web search engine such as Google, search for the recommended routes of administration. Now look for the British Thoracic Society guidelines for the pharmacological management of asthma in adults. Make a list of things from your search that you may have to consider in the management of John's asthma.

Standard precautions

Standard (or universal) precautions are a list of infection control practices recommended for healthcare workers when engaging in practices that may result in contact with a patient's blood or body fluids (Siegel et al, 2007; NICE, 2003). Standard precautions/principles have to be adhered to for the prevention of healthcare-associated infections and apply to every patient, regardless of actual infection status, in any setting in which healthcare is delivered. The recommendations include hand hygiene, and the use of personal protective equipment such as gloves, gowns, masks, eye protection, or face shields, depending on the potential exposure; and safe injection practices.

When preparing for medication administration it is very important to follow the principles of standard precautions. First on the list as always is wash your hands. Throughout this chapter, we recommend when it is necessary to use protective equipment such as gloves, but hands must also be washed after disposing of gloves, as gloves are not a replacement for good hand hygiene. Medications should be prepared on a clean surface. When drawing up medications for injections, use aseptic technique to avoid contamination of sterile injection equipment (Siegel et al, 2007). Safe disposal of sharps, that is needles and syringes, is fundamental for the prevention of blood-borne infections. Never bend, break or recap needles; both needles and syringes must be disposed of into a sharps container (Siegel et al, 2007; NICE 2003).

> ### (a) Learning activity   W
>
> Take the time to explore the following websites:
> - http://healthcarea2z.org/index.aspx: complete the A to Z quiz on infection control. Use the search window to examine standard precautions.
> - http://www.cdc.gov/ncidod/dhqp/index.html: on this website, locate the resource 'Exposure to blood – what health-care workers need to know' and read to increase your knowledge and understanding.
> - http://www.nice.org.uk/Guidance/CG2/NiceGuidance/pdf/English: read the guidelines in full for infection control in relation to hand hygiene, personal protective equipment and safe injection practices.

Administration of oral medications

Oral medications are any medications the patient swallows. These include pills, tablets, capsules, syrups, elixirs, suspensions and medicines in spray form. Oral administration of medication is the most common route via which medications are administered.

You will need:
- a prescription chart

- a formulary to check drug dosage such as the British National Formulary (BNF)
- a clean work surface.

  You will also need some of the following:
- a medication pot
- medicine spoons
- a variety of sizes of oral syringes
- a tablet crusher, tablet cutter
- a drink such as water for the patient if allowed.

> **t** ☆
> ### Practice tip
> Do not break a tablet unless it is scored, and use the appropriate tablet cutter.

Procedure

1   Hands should be washed (decontaminated) before and after patient contact, to prevent cross-infection (NICE, 2003; DH, 2003).
2   Consult the patient's prescription and ascertain the following:
    - right drug
    - right dose
    - right route
    - right date and time of administration
    - right patient.

    These checks are performed prior to all medication administrations to avoid medication errors.
3   Select the drug in the appropriate volume, dilution or dosage and the check expiry date.
4   Proceed with preparation of the drug according to pharmaceutical and healthcare setting's guidelines.
5   Empty the required dose into the drug container, ensuring your hands do not come into contact with the medication.
6   Take the prescribed dose of medication and prescription chart to the patient.
7   Discuss and explain the procedure to the patient, and gain the patient's consent.
8   Check the patient's identity by asking them to state name and date of birth. If the patient is unable to confirm details then check these details with the patient's identity band (Greenstein and Gould, 2004).
9   Administer the medication following the manufacturer's recommendations and as prescribed. Offer the patient a drink such as water to aid the movement of the medication to the stomach if allowed.
10 Record the medication given in the prescription chart and any other place necessary, as indicated by individual hospital policy (NMC, 2004).
11 Wash hands (NICE, 2003; DH, 2003).

> ⚠ ### Professional alert!
> Certain drugs interact with food and must be given in between meals or on an empty stomach. Other drugs act as irritants on an empty stomach and must be given with meals or snacks (Dougherty and Lister, 2004).
>
> Always ensure you stay with the patient until you are certain that he or she has taken the medication.

Oral medication administration in patients with enteral feeding tubes

Some patients will have enteral tubes in place as a temporary method of feeding.

When medication is administered via an enteral tube, van den Bemt and colleagues, (2006) suggest five golden 'tube rules':

- Stop the enteral feeding prior to drug administration.
- Flush the enteral feeding tube.
- Crush only what can be crushed.
- Use the 'dispersing method' when possible and do not mix different tablets.
- Flush after administration.

Part

IV

The dispersing method refers to dissolving a tablet in an oral syringe containing 10 mls of water. This method is only recommended if the tablet will disperse fully within two minutes (van den Bemt et al, 2006).

Inappropriate crushing of tablets can lead to obstruction of the enteral tube (Belknap, Seifert and Petermann, 1997) or interfere with the efficacy of enteric-coated drugs in relation to the controlled release effect (Schier et al, 2003). Furthermore if the function of the enteric coat is to prevent irritation of gastric mucosa by the medication, then removal of the coat can affect the mucosa as well as leading to loss of efficacy if the drug is destroyed by gastric juices (van den Bemt et al, 2006).

Administration of rectal medications

Rectal medications are administrated mainly in suppository and enema form. Creams or ointments may also be prescribed. Absorption of medication is via the mucous membrane lining.

⚠️ **Professional alert!**

Crush only what can be crushed (van den Bemt et al, 2006). When in doubt, contact the pharmacist and check the BNF.

You will need:

- a prescription chart
- a formulary to check drug dosage such as the BNF
- a clean work surface
- disposable gloves
- a medicine tray
- topical swabs
- lubricating gel
- a disposable incontinence pad
- a bedpan, commode or toilet to hand.

Procedure

1   Hands should be washed (decontaminated) before and after patient contact, to prevent cross-infection and apply gloves (NICE, 2003; DH, 2003).
2   Consult the patient's prescription and ascertain the following:
    - right drug
    - right dose
    - right route
    - right date and time of administration
    - right patient.
3   Select the drug in the appropriate volume, dilution or dosage, and check the expiry date.
4   Proceed with preparation of the drug according to pharmaceutical and healthcare setting's guidelines.
5   Take the prescribed dose of medication and prescription chart to the patient.
6   Discuss and explain the procedure to the patient, and gain the patient's consent.
7   Ensure patient privacy and ensure the bedpan or commode is to hand or the toilet is in close proximity.
8   Position the patient on the left lateral position with the patient's buttocks close to the edge of the bed (Dougherty and Lister, 2005).
9   Place an incontinence pad underneath the patient.

For administration of suppositories

10   Apply lubricating gel to the tip of a topical swab and then use the tip of swab to lubricate the suppository.
11   Separate the patient's buttocks and insert the suppository, rounded end first, 2–4 cm into the anal canal.
12   Advise the patient to try to retain the suppositories for at least 20 minutes.
13   Dispose of gloves and incontinence pad, and wash hands (NICE, 2003; DH, 2003).
14   Record the medication given in the prescription chart and any other place necessary, as indicated by individual hospital policy (NMC, 2004).

For administration of enemas

Follow steps 1–9 then:

10 Apply lubricating gel to a topical swab and use the swab to lubricate the tip of the rectal funnel (neck of enema).

11 Separate the patient's buttocks and insert the funnel gently through the anus 2–4 cm, following the manufacturer's recommendations.

12 Gently and slowly administer the contents of the enema into the rectum.

13 Advise the patient to try and retain the enema for as long as possible.

14 Dispose of gloves and wash hands (NICE, 2003; DH, 2003).

15 Record the medication given in the prescription chart and any other place necessary, as indicated by individual hospital policy (NMC, 2004).

Administration of injections

Intradermal injection (ID)

An intradermal injection is an injection most commonly given into the ventral (volar) forearm, which is the inner aspect of the lower arm. The upper arm, upper chest and shoulder blades may also be used (McConnell, 2000). ID injections can be given to test for hypersensitivity, extrinsic allergens and TB sensitivity.

You will need:

- a prescription chart
- a formulary to check drug dosage such as the BNF
- a clean work surface
- disposable gloves
- an appropriate size syringe and needle
- medication
- a gauze pad or cotton ball and plaster if required, following local healthcare area guidelines
- a medicine tray
- a sharps container.

Procedure

1 Wash hands and put on disposable gloves as there is potential exposure to blood in the administration of ID injections (NICE, 2003; DH, 2003).

2 Consult the patient's prescription and ascertain the following:
- right drug
- right dose
- right route
- right date and time of administration
- right patient.

3 Prepare the syringe by removing the needle cover, inverting the syringe, and expelling any excess air.

4 Select the drug in the appropriate volume, dilution or dosage, and check the expiry date.

5 Proceed with preparation of the drug according to pharmaceutical and healthcare setting's guidelines.

6 Take the prescribed dose of medication and prescription chart to the patient.

7 Discuss and explain the procedure to the patient, and gain consent.

t☆ Practice tip

Medication such as enemas should be at room temperature before administration to reduce discomfort for the patient.

t☆ Practice tip

The inner aspect of the lower arm is the most common site for ID injections.

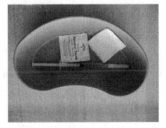

Figure 28.1 Equipment for administration of an intradermal injection

Source: courtesy of Barron and Cocoman (2007).

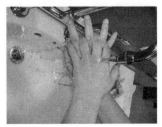

Figure 28.2 Washing hands

Source: courtesy of Barron and Cocoman (2007).

Part

IV

8   Ensure you have identified the correct patient and assist him or her into a position that is comfortable and practical for access to the injection site you have chosen.

9   Follow the individual healthcare setting's policy and procedure with regard to cleansing of the injection site.

10 Locate the correct area for injecting and stretch the skin using the thumb and forefinger of your less dominant hand.

11 Angle the syringe at 15° along the long axis of the arm (parallel).

12 Insert the needle with the bevel facing up, ensuring the entire bevel penetrates the skin about 2 mm.

13 Inject the medication, raising a 'bleb' with injected solution under the skin.

14 Withdraw the needle smoothly; do not apply pressure to site. Draw a ring around the site if allergen testing (McConnell, 2000).

15 Dispose of the syringe and needles in the sharps box (never recap a needle).

16 Dispose of clinical waste and gloves and wash hands (NICE, 2003; DH, 2003).

17 Record the medication given in the prescription chart and any other place necessary, as indicated by individual hospital policy (NMC, 2007).

⚠ Professional alert!

Do not give ID injections in the ventral (volar) forearm if the patient is suffering from dermatitis or cellulites as the injection and/or medication may exacerbate the pre-existing condition.

Sharps injuries and/or needle stick injuries pose a serious occupational hazard to nurses and may result in the transmission of blood-borne viruses such as human immunodeficiency virus (HIV), hepatitis C and hepatitis B (HSE, 2004). The risk of such injuries can be greatly reduced by adhering to procedures for safe handling and disposal of sharps (HPA, 2005).

To reduce the risk of needle stick injuries, it is important to carry out immediate and safe disposal of sharps into appropriate, puncture-proof sharps bins. It is also important not to overfill the sharps container and under no circumstance should you place your hands into it. Never re-sheath needles as research indicates that this practice is particularly likely to result in injury (HPA, 2005). Sharps also should never be carried by hand or in pockets. If an injury should occur it is imperative that the incident be reported and documented according to local policy.

Subcutaneous injection (SC)

Many medications must be injected subcutaneously. A subcutaneous injection is the administration of medication into the adipose tissue just under the skin. You will use a small needle that causes very little discomfort. Traditionally, subcutaneous injections were administered at a 45° angle; however with the introduction of shorter needles (13 mm x 25 gauge) a full-depth perpendicular injection (90°) into a raised skin fold is recommended for subcutaneous injections, in particular of heparin (Newton, Newtown and Fudin, 1992) and insulin. The rationale for the use of the shorter needle is to prevent leakage of the drug to the superficial layers of the skin on withdrawing the needle after injection (Wooldridge and Jackson 1988). However, with very thin patients a 45° angle may be needed to ensure that the end of the needle does not pierce the muscle (Ellis and Bentz, 2007; Cocoman and Barron, 2008).

> **t** ☆
> ### Practice tip
> There are many sites that can be used for subcutaneous injection. Probably the most convenient, easy and comfortable site is the anterior abdomen (belly).

You will need:

- a prescription chart
- a formulary to check drug dosage such as the BNF
- a clean work surface
- disposable gloves

- an appropriate size syringe and needle
- medication
- a gauze pad or cotton ball and plaster if required
- a medicine tray
- a sharps container.

Procedure

1   Wash hands and put on disposable gloves as there is potential exposure to blood in the administration of subcutaneous injections (NICE, 2003; DH, 2003).

2   Consult the patient's prescription and ascertain the following:
- right drug
- right dose
- right route
- right date and time of administration
- right patient.

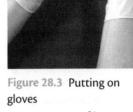

Figure 28.3 Putting on gloves

Source: courtesy of Barron and Cocoman (2007).

3   Prepare the syringe by removing the needle cover, inverting the syringe, and expelling any excess air.

4   Select the drug in the appropriate volume, dilution or dosage and check expiry date.

5   Proceed with preparation of the drug according to pharmaceutical and healthcare setting's guidelines.

6   Take the prescribed dose of medication and prescription chart to the patient.

7   Discuss and explain procedure to the patient and gain the patient's consent.

8   Ensure you have identified the correct patient and assist him or her into a position which is comfortable and practical for access to the injection site you have chosen.

9   Follow the individual healthcare setting's policy and procedure with regard to cleansing of the injection site.

10 Locate the correct area for injecting.

11 With your non-dominant hand pinch a fold of skin and hold it up.

12 Using your dominant hand pick up the syringe, hold like a pencil and insert it in to the skin fold at a 45° angle. Routine aspiration of the syringe is not necessary.

13 Inject the medication and quickly withdraw the needle.

14 Dispose of the syringe and needles in the sharps box (never recap a needle).

15 Dispose of clinical waste and gloves, and wash hands (NICE, 2003; DH, 2003).

16 Record the medication given in the prescription chart and any other place necessary as indicated by individual hospital policy (NMC, 2004).

> ⚠ **Professional alert!**
>
> Do not give injections in scarred areas, in moles, or inflamed or oedematous areas (Barron and Cocoman, 2006, 2007, 2008).

Intramuscular (IM) injection

Intramuscular (IM) injections are given directly into the central area of selected muscles. There are a number of sites on the human body that are suitable for IM injections; the four most commonly used in this procedure are the deltoid, vastus lateralis, ventrogluteal and dorsol gluteal muscles. The intramuscular route offers a faster rate of absorption than the oral or subcutaneous route.

> t☆ **Practice tip**
>
> The technique for the administration of IM injections varies according to the site used (Barron and Cocoman, 2006).
>
> Always use the Z-track technique, which involves displacing the skin and subcutaneous layer in relation to the underlying muscle so that the needle track is sealed off when the needle is withdrawn thus minimising reflux.
>
> Injection into muscle is less painful if the muscle is relaxed.
>
> To relax the muscle:
> - Ask the patient to place their hand on their hip when injecting into deltoid.
> - Internally rotate the femur by flexing the knee to relax the gluteal muscles.

Part

IV

You will need:

- a prescription chart
- a formulary to check drug dosage such as the BNF
- a clean work surface
- disposable gloves
- an appropriate size syringe
- appropriate needles to draw up and then administer medication
- medication
- a gauze pad/cotton ball and plaster if required
- a medicine tray
- a sharps container.

Procedure

1   Wash hands and put on disposable gloves as there is potential exposure to blood in the administration of IM injections (NICE, 2003; DH, 2003).

2   Consult the patient's prescription and ascertain the following:
- right drug
- right dose
- right route
- right date and time of administration
- right patient.

3   Prepare the syringe by removing the needle cover, inverting the syringe, and expelling any excess air.

4   Select the drug in the appropriate volume, dilution or dosage and check the expiry date.

5   Proceed with preparation of the drug according to pharmaceutical and healthcare setting's guidelines.

6   Take the prescribed dose of medication and prescription chart to the patient.

7   Discuss and explain the procedure to the patient and gain the patient's consent.

8   Ensure you have identified the correct patient and assist him or her into a position which is comfortable and practical for access to the injection site you have chosen.

9   Follow the individual healthcare setting's policy and procedure with regard to cleansing of the injection site.

10   Locate the correct area for injection using:

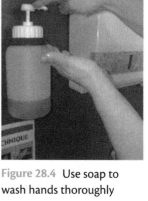

Figure 28.4 Use soap to wash hands thoroughly

Source: courtesy of Barron and Cocoman (2007).

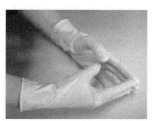

Figure 28.5 Putting on gloves

Source: courtesy of Barron and Cocoman (2007).

Ventrogluteal site

- Patient position – standing or supine.
- Place heel of the left hand on right greater trochanter.
- Index finger touches iliac crest.
- Stretch middle finger as far as possible to form a V.
- Access gluteus medius muscle.
- The ventrogluteal site is the safest site for administering IM injections (Beyea and Nicoll, 1995) as it is furthest away from major blood vessels and nerves.
- Maximum volume: 5 ml adult, 2 ml child and 1 ml infant.

Dorsogluteal site

- Patient position: draw a line horizontally from the centre of the cleft of the buttocks.
- Draw a second line vertically midway along the first line. This is referred to as the upper outer quadrant.
- Maximum volume for injection: 2 ml adult.

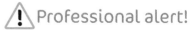 Professional alert!

The dorsogluteal site is contraindicated in children and should never be used, due to the risk of sciatic nerve damage.

Adaptation of the dorsogluteal site

- The 'double cross'.
- Divide the buttock with an imaginary cross.
- *Then* divide the upper outer quadrant by another imaginary cross.
- Inject into the upper outer quadrant of the upper outer quadrant.

11 Aspirate at the injection site by holding the barrel of the syringe with the non-dominant hand and pulling back on the syringe plunger with the dominant hand. If blood appears in the syringe, withdraw the needle and prepare a new injection. If no blood is aspirated, continue by slowly injecting the medication at a constant rate (1 ml every ten seconds) until all medication has been delivered (Soanes, 2000).

12 Withdraw the needle and syringe smoothly to minimize discomfort. Do not massage the site after injection as this reduces the effect of the medication. If there is leakage, apply gentle pressure with a cotton wool ball or gauze swab for 30 seconds.

13 Dispose of the syringe and needles in the sharps box (never recap a needle).

14 Dispose of clinical waste and gloves and wash hands (NICE, 2003; DH, 2003).

15 Record the medication given in the prescription chart and any other place necessary, as indicated by individual hospital policy (NMC, 2007).

⚠ Professional alert!

Never attempt to resheath a needle as this increases the risk of needlestick injuries (DH, 2001).

ⓔ Evidence-based practice

Z-track technique and intramuscular injections

Z-tracking involves displacing the skin and subcutaneous layer in relation to the underlying muscle to be injected so that the needle track is sealed off when the needle is withdrawn, thus minimising reflux of the medication into the subcutaneous tissue. The Z-track technique is endorsed in all literature related to intramuscular injection administration (Keen, 1990; Newton et al, 1992; Beyea and Nicoll, 1995); the exception is in the case of infant vaccination, where the literature advocates compressing the skin between the index finger and thumb (Diggle and Deeks, 2000, 2006; Diggle, 2007). In order to make use of the Z-track technique when administrating intramuscular injections, nurses should use their non-dominant hand to displace the skin and subcutaneous tissue ½ inch or 1 cm laterally to the injection site prior to injecting. The Z-tracking must be kept in place until after the medication is administered and the needle is withdrawn. This manoeuvre seals off the puncture tract and traps the drug in the muscle.

Minimising pain associated with injections

Invasive procedures, particularly those that involve needles, can cause substantial anxiety and pain to patients (Ellis and Bentz, 2004). In the paediatric setting many children view receiving needles as one of the most traumatic aspects of being in the hospital (Cordoni and Cordoni, 2001; Cummings et al, 1996). Parents regard needle procedures as the second most distressing event during their child's hospitalisation (Sharp, 2004). On average, younger children experience more pain and anxiety than older ones (Fowler-Kerry Lander, 1987; Fradet et al, 1990). For some individuals, a fear of needles persists into adulthood and may have lifelong negative repercussions, such as preventing them from donating blood (Sharp, 2004) or precipitating fainting episodes in response to a needle (Pavlin et al, 1993). A patient's distress during intramuscular and subcutaneous injections needs to be acknowledged and every effort should be made to control the pain and minimize the distress. While injections can never be perceived as pain free, some patients are more at risk of trauma and stress due to injections than others.

Part
IV

Research suggests that if painful procedures such as injections are not properly managed, patients may suffer negative short and long-term psychological effects such as nausea, insomnia and treatment non-adherence (Weisman, Bernstein and Schechter, 1998). Therefore it is important for the nurse to minimise injection-induced pain and thus reduce the patient's distress, using both pharmacological and non-pharmacological methods.

Pharmacological management of injection site pain

- Topical anaesthetics: topical anaesthetics provide pain relief at the insertion point of the needle. EMLA, a lidocaine-prilocaine cream, is used predominantly in children beyond neonatal age. It is applied to the skin, then covered with an occlusive dressing and left in place for at least 60 minutes. The peak action for EMLA occurs at two hours and lasts for as long as four to five hours (Sharp, 2004).
- Ametop Gel (tetracaine 4 per cent) provides analgesia similar to EMLA's but has the advantage of a more rapid onset of action. It works in about 30 to 45 minutes, and lasts for four to six hours after a single application (Sharp, 2004).
- The use of topical anaesthetics gives children a sense of control and they are easy to apply. However, they have a slow onset and may cause anxiety in children who identify them with needle sticks, which are soon to follow (Conte et al, 1999).
- Analgesic agents: use of a non-aspirin-containing analgesic may be considered to decrease discomfort and fever following vaccination.

Nonpharmacological management of injection site pain

- Establishing a relationship: establish a rapport with the patient and explain why the procedure is necessary. Answer clearly any questions the patient may have.
- Positioning: ensure the patient is in the most comfortable position possible that allows for full access to the injection site. Children may be cuddled or held depending on their age.
- Privacy: ensure the patient has total privacy and no more of their body than is necessary is exposed.
- Allow for patient choice: allow the patient to choose which site the injection is to be administered to wherever possible.
- Distraction technique: adults may wish to listen to music through headphones or watch TV in the room as the injection is being administered. With children distraction can involve counting, blowing bubbles, music, television or computer games, depending on the child's age.
- Muscle relaxation: progressive muscle relation – deep and rhythmic breathing, cleansing-breaths.
- Guided imagery: used with both adults and children, for example favourite place, most treasured memory.
- Use of ice on the injection site prior to injection may act as a form of local anaesthetic; however it does not affect the pain receptors.

Proper injection technique

One of the most successful methods of minimising site pain and trauma from injections is proper injection technique (Barron and Cocoman, 2008).

- Explain the procedure to patients and gain their consent prior to drug administration to reduce their anxieties.
- Good communication skills are an essential part of the psychological preparation of the patient prior to the injection.
- Positioning of the patient to relax the muscle significantly reduces pain (Roger and King, 2000).
- Administer the injection with a dart-like motion to quickly pierce the skin to reduce the pain experienced (Ellis and Bentz, 2006).

- Pain receptors are concentrated in the dermis layer of the skin and hence the length of needle has no association with pain experienced by the patient.
- Keen (1990) and Roger and King (2000) advocate that an administration rate of 1 ml per ten seconds facilitates absorption of the medication and minimises pain.
- Good Z-track technique ensures that medication is deposited into muscle with no reflux back through the needle track causing seepage into subcutaneous tissue, which can cause irritation and pain (Beyea and Nicoll, 1995).
- The nurse has a responsibility to understand the actions of all medications administered. Thus certain pharmacological preparations are known to be 'irritants'. Analgesics may be offered to the patient prior to the procedure, based on the nurse's individual assessment.
- Insert the needle at a 90° angle using the Z-track technique.
- Spread the skin, using the fingers of the non-dominant hand. Holding the syringe with the thumb and forefinger of the dominant hand at a 90° angle, pierce the skin and enter the muscle.

a Learning activity

Use an internet search engine to find pictures of Z-tracking technique. Also find pictures of the ventrogluteal site, dorsalgluteal site, deltoid site and vastuslateruras site.

Administration of ear drops

Administration of ear drops entails the instillation of a prescribed solution directly into the ear drum. This type of medication may be necessary for relieving discomfort and inflammation, providing an antibacterial role or simply for softening of ear wax. While the procedure is not painful it may cause discomfort and therefore requires the patient's cooperation.

You will need:
- a prescription chart
- medication with dropper or syringe
- a medication tray
- disposable gloves
- tissues or swabs if required
- a towel or protective sheet for the patient's clothes.

t ☆ Practice tip

Medications formulated for the ear have a short shelf life after opening and it is necessary to store them in the refrigerator. As well as checking the expiry dates it is recommended that the medication is allowed to warm to room temperature before inserting into the ear (Trigg and Mohammed, 2006).

Procedure

1 Wash your hands to reduce any risk of cross-infection (NICE, 2003; DH, 2003).
2 Consult the patient's prescription and ascertain the following:
   - right drug
   - right dose
   - right route
   - right date and time of administration
   - right patient.
3 Select the required medication and check the expiry date.
4 Take the prescribed dose of medication and prescription chart to the patient.
5 Explain and discuss the procedure with the patient to gain cooperation and consent.
6 Check the patient's identity by asking his or her name and date of birth. If the patient is unable to confirm details then check these details with the patient's identity band.

Part

IV

7   Place the patient lying on their side or sitting upright with the ear requiring the medication uppermost. Put a towel or a protective cover over the patient's clothing to ensure that these items are kept clean and dry.

8   Gently lift the ear cartilage of the pinna backwards and upwards and allow ear drops to fall in the direction of the external canal for adults (Dougherty and Lister, 2005). For placement of ear drops in a child aged 3 years or less, pull pinna down and back (Trigg and Mohammed, 2006).

9   Hold dropper 6 mm above ear canal, and instil prescribed number of drops.

10 Ensure the patient stays in this position for one to two minutes to ensure medication reaches the eardrum to allow for absorption (Dougherty and Lister, 2004).

11 Remove gloves and wash hands (NICE, 2003; DH, 2003).

12 Record the medication given in the prescription chart and any other place necessary, as indicated by individual hospital policy (NMC, 2007).

> ⚠ **Professional alert!**
>
> Don't use a dry cotton wool ball in the eardrum after insertion of ear drops as it will absorb the medication away from the eardrum (Campbell and Glasper, 1995).

Administration of eye medications

The two main forms of eye medications are eye drops and eye ointments. They are normally administered to treat conditions which directly affect the eye and or eye socket. Medication administered directly onto the eye may cause a significant amount of discomfort, visual blurring and irritation to the patient (Trigg and Mohammed, 2006).

> ⭐ **Practice tip**
>
> Ask the patient to close (but not squeeze) their eyelids and to roll eyes in all directions to ensure even distribution of eye ointment.

You will need:

- a prescription chart
- a formulary to check drug dosage such as the BNF
- a clean work surface
- a towel
- medication
- a medication tray
- tissues or swabs as required
- a waste disposal bag.

Procedure

1   Hands should be washed (decontaminated) before and after patient contact, to prevent cross-infection (NICE, 2003; DH, 2003).

2   Consult the patient's prescription and ascertain the following:
- right drug
- right dose
- right route
- right date and time of administration
- right patient.

3   Select the required medication and check the expiry date.

4   Take the prescribed dose of medication and prescription chart to the patient.

5   Explain and discuss the procedure with the patient to gain cooperation and consent.

6   Check the patient's identity by asking his or her name and date of birth. If the patient is unable to confirm details, then check them with the patient's identity band.

For administration of eye drops

7   Ask the patient to lie in the supine position or to sit with head slightly tilted back and to look up.

8 Pull lower lid down gently to expose the conjunctival sac, creating a pocket.

9 Hold eyedropper 3–6 to mm above the conjunctival sac (pocket).

10 Place the hand holding the dropper on the patient's cheek or forehead to stabilise as needed.

11 Drop the prescribed number of drops into the centre of the pocket (conjunctival sac). Avoid touching the eye or conjunctival sac with the tip of the eyedropper.

12 Instruct the patient to gently close the eye.

13 Apply gentle pressure with finger to the lacrimal duct at the inner canthus for one to two minutes. This is to avoid overflow drainage into nose and throat, thus minimizing risk of absorption into the systemic circulation.

14 With a tissue, remove excess medication around eye.

For administration of ointment

7 Pull the lower lid down gently, and instruct the patient to look up.

8 Apply a thin line of ointment evenly along the inner edge of the lower lid margin, from inner to outer canthus.

9 Avoid touching the tip of applicator to the eyelid or eye.

10 Instruct the patient to close eyelids and to roll eyes in all directions to distribute medication.

11 Dispose of clinical waste and gloves and wash hands (NICE, 2003; DH, 2003).

12 Record the medication given in the prescription chart and any other place necessary, as indicated by individual hospital policy (NMC, 2007).

Administration of nasal medications

Nasal medications are administered into the nose using either drops or sprays. The medication is absorbed via the mucous membrane lining of the nose.

You will need:

- a prescription chart
- a formulary to check drug dosage such as the BNF
- a clean work surface
- medication
- tissues
- disposable gloves
- a towel, to protect the patient's clothes.

Procedure

1 Hands should be washed (decontaminated) before and after patient contact, to prevent cross-infection, and gloves should be worn (NICE, 2003; DH, 2003).

2 Consult the patient's prescription and ascertain the following:
- right drug
- right dose
- right route
- right date and time of administration
- right patient.

3 Select the required medication and check the expiry date.

4 Take the prescribed dose of medication and prescription chart to the patient.

5 Explain and discuss the procedure with the patient to gain cooperation and consent

6 Check the patient's identity by asking his or her name and date of birth. If the patient is unable to confirm details then check them with the patient's identity band.

⚠ **Professional alert!**

Always wear disposable gloves when administering eye drops or ointments to prevent the spread of infections.

t ☆
Practice tip

Ensure patients have clear nostrils by asking them to blow their nose prior to insertion of drops.

Part

IV

7   Ensure the nasal passages are clean and clear prior to administration by getting the patient to blow their nose.

8   Ensure the patient is sitting comfortably and hyperextend the neck unless contraindicated.

9   Avoid touching the external nares with the nasal dropper as it may cause the patient to sneeze (Trigg and Mohammed, 2006).

10 Insert the required number of drops into the nare(s) as prescribed.

11 Clean any secretions or medication with the tissues/swab.

12 Ensure the patient stays in the same position for one to two minutes to allow for absorption of the medication (Dougherty and Lister, 2004).

13 For nasal sprays follow steps 1–7 then insert the tip of the spray inside the nasal passage and administer the correct number of sprays.

14 Remove gloves and wash hands (NICE, 2003; DH, 2003).

15 Record the medication given in the prescription chart and any other place necessary, as indicated by individual hospital policy (NMC, 2007).

> ⚠ **Professional alert!**
>
> Patients should have their own nasal medication to avoid cross-contamination.

Administration of medications via nebuliser

A nebuliser is a device which turns an aqueous solution of a drug into a mist of fine particles for inhalation. The aim of nebuliser therapy is to deliver a therapeutic dose of the desired drug within a short delivery time, usually ten minutes. Nebulised therapy should be delivered by a mouthpiece whenever possible as this provides increased lung drug deposition. Beta agonists, anti-cholinergics, corticosteroids and antibiotics are the main drugs commonly administered by nebuliser. Other medications are used in specialist areas.

> t ☆
> **Practice tip**
>
> Wash the patient's face after using a facemask, especially if you have administered steroids.

You will need:

- a prescription chart
- a formulary to check drug dosage such as the BNF
- a clean work surface
- disposable gloves
- a nebuliser pot, mouthpiece/mask and filter/valve set
- a vial of saline
- medication
- a syringe
- a medicine tray.

Procedure

1   Hands should be washed (decontaminated) before and after patient contact, to prevent cross-infection, and gloves should be worn (NICE, 2003; DOH, 2003).

2   Consult the patient's prescription and ascertain the following:
- right drug
- right dose
- right route
- right date and time of administration
- right patient.

3   Select the required medication and check the expiry date.

4   Proceed with preparation of the drug according to pharmaceutical and healthcare setting's guidelines. If a dilutent is required, unless otherwise stated, only sodium chloride 0.9 per cent for injection should be used as hypotonic solutions can cause bronchospasm.

5   Explain and discuss the procedure with the patient to gain cooperation and consent

6   Check the patient's identity by asking their name and date of birth. If the patient is unable to confirm details then check them with the patient's identity band.

7   Assist the patient into a position which is comfortable, sitting upright and leaning slightly forwards whenever possible.

8   Ensure the mask fits properly and is comfortable, and encourage the patient to breathe steadily through the mouth (not nose) where possible.

9   Ensure the driving gas of air flow rate is set at 8 litres per minute. Note: in acute asthma use oxygen as the gas, at all other times use air.

10 The delivery time should not exceed ten minutes and the nebuliser chamber needs to remains upright at all times

11 Wash the patient's face after using a facemask – especially after steroids.

12 To clean after each use:
- Disconnect the nebuliser chamber from the tubing.
- Wash the nebuliser chamber and mask/mouthpiece in warm water and detergent.
- Rinse thoroughly and dry well.
- Reassemble and then run the nebuliser empty to dry the tubing.

13 Dispose of clinical waste and gloves, and wash hands (DH, 2003).

14 Complete relevant documentation (NMC, 2007).

> ⚠ **Professional alert!**
>
> Oxygen should be the driving gas in acute asthma only. Otherwise it should be air. The gas to be used should be stated by the prescriber.

Administration of topical medications

Topical administration of medication refers to the application of medication directly to the surface where the action is required (Trounce, 2004) such as the skin. This may include patches, creams or ointments applied directly to the skin. The absorption of medication may vary with age due to reduced skin density and integrity (Trigg and Mohammad, 2006). Patches provide a reliable and controllable dose administration.

> t☆
> **Practice tip**
>
> Gloves must always be worn when administrating any form of topical medication.

You will need:
- a prescription chart
- a formulary to check drug dosage such as the BNF
- a clean work surface
- disposable gloves
- topical medication
- sterile topical swabs
- a medication tray
- dressings/bandages if required.

Procedure

1   Hands should be washed (decontaminated) before and after patient contact, to prevent cross-infection, and gloves should be worn (NICE, 2003; DH, 2003).

2   Consult the patient's prescription and ascertain the following:
- right drug
- right dose
- right route
- right date and time of administration
- right patient.

3   Selected the required medication and check the expiry date.

4   Take the prescribed dose of medication and prescription chart to the patient.

5   Explain and discuss the procedure with the patient to gain cooperation and consent

6   Check the patient's identity by asking his or her name and date of birth. If the patient is unable to confirm details, then check them with the patient's identity band.

7   Using a gloved hand remove semi-solid/stiff ointment and apply to the area as prescribed and following the manufacturer's recommendations. In the case of steroid creams, apply specifically to the site required and sparingly.

8   In the case of a transdermal patch, follow manufacturers' guidelines and apply the patch to clean smooth skin. Ensure the plastic protective coating is removed. Ensure the old patch is removed and disposed of and the skin is cleaned.

9 Remove gloves, dispose of clinical waste receptacle, and wash hands (NICE, 2003; DH, 2003).

10 Record the medication given in the prescription chart and any other place necessary, as indicated by individual hospital policy (NMC, 2007).

> **⚠ Professional alert!**
>
> Topical medications should always be single-patient use to avoid cross contamination.

> **ⓐ Learning activity**
>
> Review your calculation questions at the start of the chapter. The correct answers are:
>
> 1 Answer 68.735 grams.
> 2 Answer 92.763.
> 3 Answer 93.074 grams.
> 4 Answer 44.343.
>   Claire: 20 ml.   Tony: 0.5 tabs.   Catherine: 4.25 ml.
> If you made any errors, go back and reread the section.

Conclusion

This chapter aimed to give you the foundations required to safely administer medications to patients. We have investigated both the theory and practice that accompanies a range of medication administration routes, and laid the foundations for future development of your clinical skills in this area.

References

Barron, C. and Cocoman, A. (2006) *Theory and Practice of Intramuscular and Subcutaneous Injections*, Dublin, Campus Print, Dublin City University.

Barron, C. and Cocoman, A. (2007) *Theory and Practice of Intramuscular and Subcutaneous Injections; Perfecting the art of injection techniques for student nurses*, Dublin, Campus Print, Dublin City University.

Barron, C. and Cocoman, A. (2008) 'Administering intramuscular injections to children: what does the evidence say?' *Journal of Children's and Young People's Nursing* 2(3), 138–44.

Belknap, D. C., Seifert, C. F. and Petermann, M. (1997) 'Administration of medications through enteral feeding catheters', *American Journal of Critical Care* 6, 382–92.

Beyea, S. and Nicoll, L. (1995) 'Administration of medications via IM route: an integrative review of literature and research based protocol for the procedure', *Applied Nursing Research* 8, 23–33.

British National Formulary (BNF) (2008) British Medical Journal Publishing Group, London.

Campbell, S. J. and Glasper, E. A. (1995) 'Family centred care', in Campbell, S. J. and Glasper, E. A. (eds), *Whaley and Wong's Children's Nursing*, UK edn, London, Mosby.

Cocoman, A. and Barron, C. (2008) 'Administering subcutaneous injections to children: what does the evidence say?' *Journal of Children's and Young People's Nursing* 2(2), 84–9.

Conte, P., Walco, G., Sterling, C., Engel, R. and Kuppenheimer, W. G. (1999) 'Procedure pain management in pediatric oncology: a review of literature', *Cancer Investigation* 17, 448–59.

Cordoni, A. and Cordoni, L. E. (2001) 'Eutectic mixture of local anaesthetics reduces pain during intravenous catheter insertion in the paediatrics patient', *Clinical Journal of Pain* 17(2), 115–18.

Cummings, E. A., Reid, C. J., Finley, G. A., McGrath P. J. and Ritchie, J. A.

(1996) 'Prevalence and source of pain in paediatric inpatients', *Pain* 68, 25–31.

Department of Health (DH) (2001) *Seeking Consent: Working with children*, London, Stationery Office.

DH (2003) *Winning Ways: Working together to reduce healthcare associated infection in England*, London, DH.

Diggle, L. (2007) 'Injection technique for immunisation', *Practice Nurse* 33(1), 34–7.

Diggle, L. and Deeks, J. (2000) 'Effect of needle length on incidence of local reactions to routine immunisation in infants aged 4 months: randomised controlled trial', *British Medical Journal* 14(321), 931–3.

Diggle, L., Deeks, J. and Pollard, A. (2006) 'Effect of needle size on immunocenicity and reactogenecity of vaccines in infants: randomized controlled trial', *British Medical Journal* 333, 571.

Dougherty, L. and Lister, S. (2004) *The Royal Marsden Hospital Manual of Clinical Nursing Procedures*, 6th edn, Oxford, Blackwell.

Ellis, J. R. and Bentz, P. M. (2004) *Modules for Basic Nursing Skills*, 7th edn, Philadelphia, Pa., Lippincott Williams & Wilkins.

Fowler-Kerry Lander, J. (1987) 'Management of injection pain in children', *Pain* 30, 169–75.

Fradet, C., McGrath, P., Kay, J., Adams, S. and Luke, B. (1990) 'A prospective survey of reactions to blood tests by children and adolescents', *Pain* 40, 53–60.

Greenstein, B. and Gould, D. (2004) *Trounce's Clinical Pharmacology for Nurses*, 17th edn, Edinburgh, Churchill Livingstone.

Health Protection Agency (HPA) (2005) *Eye of the Needle: Surveillance of significant occupational exposure to bloodborne viruses in healthcare workers: seven year report*, London, Health Protection Agency Centre for Infections [online] www.hpa.org.uk (accessed 18 February 2009).

Health and Safety Executive (HSE) (2004) *Blood Borne Viruses in the*

Workplace: Guidance for employers and employees, London, HSE [online] http://www.hse.gov.uk/pubns/indg342.pdf (accessed 10 February 2009).

Keen, M. F. (1990) 'Get on the right track with Z-track injections', *Nursing*, 10, 59.

McConnell, E.A (2000) 'Administering an intradermal injection', *Nursing* 30(3), 17.

National Audit Office (NAO) (2003) *A Safer Place to Work: Improving the management of health and safety risks to staff in NHS trusts*, London, National Audit Office.

National Institute for Clinical Excellence (NICE) (2003) *Prevention of Health-associated Infection in Primary and Community Care*, London, NICE [online] http://www.nice.org.uk/nicemedia/pdf/Infection_control_fullguideline.pdf (accessed 10 February 2009).

Newton, M., Newtown, D. W. and Fudin, J. (1992). 'Reviewing the big three injection routes' *Nursing* 22, 34–42.

Nursing and Midwifery Council (2004) *Medication Policy for Nurses*, London, NMC.

NMC (2007) *Standards for Medicines Management*, London, NMC.

Pavlin, D. J., Links, S., Rapp, S. E., Nessley, M. L. and Keyes, H. J. (1993) Vasovagal reactions in an ambulatory surgical centre, *Anaesthesia and Analgesia* 76, 931–5.

Roger, M. A. and King, L. (2000) 'Drawing up and administering intramuscular injections: a review of literature', *Journal of Advanced Nursing* 31(3), 574–82.

Royal College of Paediatrics and Child Health (RCPCH) (2002) *Position Statement on Injection Technique*, London, RCPCH and RCN.

Schier, J. G., Howland, M. A., Hoffman, R. S. and Nelson, L. S. (2003) 'Fatality from administration of labetalol and crushed extended-release nifedipine', *Ann Pharmacother.* 37, 1420–3.

Sharp, D. (2004) 'Selling comfort: a survey of interventions for needle procedures in a paediatrics hospital', *Pain Management Nursing*, 5(4), 144–52.

Siegel, J. D., Rhinehart, E., Jackson, M., Chiarello, L. and the Healthcare Infection Control Practices Advisory Committee (2007) *Guideline for Isolation Precautions: Preventing transmission of infectious agents in healthcare settings*, Center for Disease Control and Prevention (CDC) [online] http://www.cdc.gov/ncidod/dhqp/pdf/guidelines/Isolation2007.pdf (accessed 5 May 2008).

Soanes, N. (2000) 'Injection site safety', *Nursing Standard* 14(25), 55.

Trigg, E. and Mohammed, T. (2006) *Practices in Children's Nursing Guidelines for Hospital and Community*, 2nd edn, Edinburgh, Churchill Livingstone.

van den Bemt, P., Cusell, M., Overbeeke, P., Trommelen, M., van Dooren, D., Ophorst, W. and Egberts, A. (2006) 'Quality improvement of oral medication administration in patients with enteral feeding tubes', *Quality Safety Health Care* 15, 44–7.

Weisman, S. J., Bernstein, B. and Schechter, N. L. (1998) 'Consequences of inadequate analgesia during painful procedures in children', *Archives of Paediatrics Adolescent Medicine* 152, 147–9.

Wooldridge, J. B. and Jackson, J. G. (1988) 'Evaluation of bruises and areas of induration after two techniques of subcutaneous heparin injection', *Heart and Lung* 17, 476–82.

Chapter

29

Patient-controlled analgesia

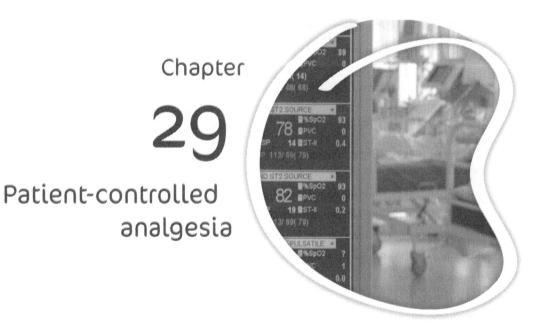

Mark Broom and Gareth Parsons

Links to other chapters in *Foundation Skills for Caring*

Links to other chapters in *Foundation Studies for Caring*

W Don't forget to visit www.palgrave.com/glasper for additional online resources relating to this chapter.

Introduction

When someone is in pain they need a method of managing their pain that is:

- easy to use
- safe
- flexible
- fast.

Patient-controlled analgesia (PCA), when used effectively, achieves this as it enables the patient to access analgesia without needing to ask for assistance – much as if they were taking pain killers for a headache or toothache at home. The patient is therefore in control of when they have analgesia and how frequently they take it. This means that they do not need to rely upon nurses giving them analgesia in a timely manner, a common problem in pain management. However, whilst it relieves nurses of the demands of administering analgesia, it does impose other demands on monitoring, educating and supporting patients.

Learning outcomes

This chapter will enable you to:

- Understand the concept of PCA
- Discuss the rationale behind PCA
- Consider factors that would influence patient selection
- Explore the differing individual types of PCA infusion equipment
- Appreciate the safety issues encountered using PCA
- Describe how to start PCA
- Evaluate the effectiveness of PCA
- Monitor the patient receiving PCA
- Recognise common problems associated with the use of PCA
- Care for the patient following PCA

Concepts

- Self care
- Patient education
- Assessment
- Pain management
- Patient safety
- Pharmacology
- Equipment
- Intravenous infusions
- Management and prevention of complications

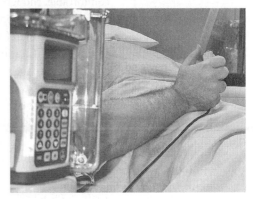

Figure 29.1 PCA infusion device

Basic principles of PCA

PCA is a tried, tested and safe way of administering postoperative opioids for acute pain relief (Fisher et al, 2003). It can be delivered in a number of ways, although the most common is through intravenous administration with a specific type of pump or syringe driver. The PCA infusion device operates by delivering frequent preprogrammed doses of analgesia when the patient presses the device's hand piece (Thomas, 1994).

We shall concentrate upon the intravenous method, but whichever method you use there are a few common basic principles that require consideration.

Patient selection

The patients need to be able to appreciate the concept of PCA. If they cannot grasp that when in pain they must demand a dose (usually by pushing a button) from the PCA device then they should not be using this method. This is facilitated by good preparation of

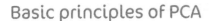

Learning activity

Consider how pain is managed in clinical areas you have worked in. How has the control of access to analgesics affected the quality of pain management in patients you have cared for?

You may want to think about the types of drugs that are available, how patients are communicated with, the legal and organisational constraints and how easy is it for patients to request painkillers.

Part

IV

Learning activity

How are patients in your area prepared for PCA?

patient that includes education in the basic principles of PCA.

Usually patient incapacity can be recognised before the method is selected; for example, a patient may be unable to physically press the button on the device. Occasionally someone who seems suitable may not cope with the method or the effects of medication or anaesthetic and may become incapable. At this point an alternative should be sought.

On-demand analgesia

PCA operates on an 'on-demand' basis; unless the patient demands a dose, they will not receive pain relief. As the drugs used in a PCA are usually analgesics with strong effects, this acts as a safety measure. Several demands for an opioid-like morphine will induce drowsiness and a drowsy patient will be unable to demand another dose. This allows the patient to be comfortable without overdosage, and this is the reason that only the patient should press the button, not the nurse or some other party.

Titration

Another safety feature is the size of the dose. In a typical morphine sulphate PCA, a single dose usually contains 1 mg of morphine. This is not enough to relieve moderate or severe pain on its own; several doses are required, a process known as 'titration'. When the patient is comfortable, enough analgesia has been administered to maintain comfort at rest as well as giving the patient control of pain on movement.

Titration is therefore an important element in PCA and is necessary before a PCA is first commenced. Titration involves getting patients comfortable before giving them manual control of the pain. Failure to do this will render the PCA ineffective. Titration can be achieved through:

- a loading dose of analgesia administered either orally or intravenously
- nurse-controlled intravenous administration following an algorithm (Parsons and Edwards, 1999)
- good pain control before starting the PCA
- using the best drug for PCA.

There is no universal ideal opioid for PCA (Woodhouse, Ward and Mather, 1999) but the characteristics of the ideal drug to choose for PCA are:

- a rapid onset
- moderate duration
- a high margin of safety between effectiveness and troublesome side-effects.

In practice and in the literature, morphine seems to be the most popular drug although pethidine, fentanyl and hydromorphone have been mentioned; diamorphine and tramadol can also be used.

Lockout period

Titration is necessary because of another safety feature: the 'lockout period'. Each delivery of a successful dose is followed by a predetermined 'lockout' period when the PCA remains inactive. A lockout period is normally set at five minutes although in some cases it may need to be lengthened. This prevents overdosing as, no matter how many times patients demand a dose, they will only receive it when the programmed device allows them to. In theory, this

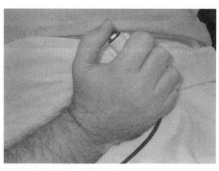

Figure 29.2 Hand-held device

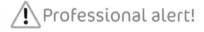

Professional alert!

Phantom hands

Do not press the button for the patient as this removes an essential safety feature. The patient must be aware enough to press the button him/herself. However, it is perfectly acceptable to encourage the patient to press the button.

allows the minimum effective analgesia concentration in plasma to be maintained, and the side-effects associated with the swinging from pain to pain-free states seen with conventional intermittent 'as-required' analgesia can be avoided (Charlton, 1997). The basic principle of PCA is a simple feedback loop (Harmer and MacIntyre, 2003); the patient who experiences pain presses the demand button and the PCA releases a small dose of an opioid into the systemic circulation. The pain is either reduced or stays the same. If pain relief is adequate, the patient makes no further demand, but if the dose is inadequate then a repeat demand is made. (See Figure 29.3.)

Bolus dose

The optimal bolus dose for morphine is 1 milligram (mg) with a five-minute lockout (Owen, Plummer and Armstrong, 1989). Occasionally a 2 mg bolus may be substituted. This may occur if the patient is expected to have difficulty achieving the minimum effective analgesic concentration. This might, for example, be because the patient is opioid tolerant, has a greater body weight or has not had the pain controlled on the lower dose.

Dose limit

It should be recognised that patients using PCA usually titrate their analgesia to a relief point where they are comfortable (Mercadante, 2007); however in certain vulnerable groups at risk of prolonging the effect of the drug, such as the elderly or those with liver or renal disease, a dose limit can be set on infusion pumps. As mentioned previously, another safety measure might be to lengthen the lockout period. These measures cannot be taken with non-programmable or mechanical PCA devices, which should therefore be avoided in these groups.

As with the administration of any medication or mode of drug delivery, caution needs to be exercised with certain patients who are at particular risk of experiencing the side-effects of a particular drug or, for any number of reasons, may be unable to exercise the autonomy necessary to use a PCA.

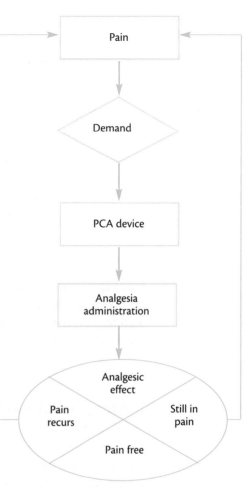

Figure 29.3 The PCA effect

Source: reproduced with permission from Parsons, Jenkins and Comerford (2005).

(a) Learning activity

When caring for a patient receiving PCA, look at the prescription and set up of the equipment. Compare this with other methods of analgesia and consider its effectiveness.

Rationale for PCA

PCA is suitable for:

- the management of acute postoperative pain
- the management of pain in those patients who are unable to tolerate oral medication
- those patients who require frequent intramuscular or intravenous injections of opioids.

Those who benefit most from PCA tend to be younger age groups undergoing major abdomen or orthopaedic surgery (Sherwood, 1996).

PCA is unsuitable for patients who:

- Have a severe respiratory problem or suffer from obstructive sleep apnoea. This is a problem as strong opioids are likely to exacerbate these problems and could be an iatrogenic cause of morbidity. In this group of patients a low-opioid method such as epidural analgesia or intravenous paracetamol is preferred.

- Are reluctant to use the device.
- Feel threatened by personal responsibility for pain control and would prefer some other method.
- Are likely to experience severe pain or are nursed in high-dependency areas with high nurse-to-patient ratios. Myles and colleagues (1994) demonstrated that ITU and HDU areas where nurses gave intermittent IV boluses provided pain relief that was as good as or better than PCA for patients after coronary artery bypass grafts. Patients in these units might also have their pain managed by a continuous intravenous infusion.

> **ⓐ Learning activity**
>
> What seems to be the basis for patient selection in your clinical area?

Types of PCA devices

It would not be practical to explore the different individual types of PCA infusion equipment in this chapter, although most devices can be categorised as:

- programmable PCA devices
- disposable PCA devices
- other PCA methods.

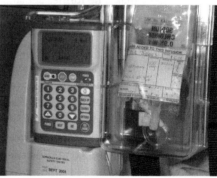

Figure 29.4 A programmable patient-controlled analgesic device

The programmable PCA device

This type of infusion device began its life as an intravenous syringe driver or infusion pump, and had added to its basic design a patient-demand button and a display window to show the number of demands and the total amount of drug in mass concentration and volume the patient had accessed. Its power source is electricity with back-up batteries, and it tends to be bulky and heavy.

The introduction of the microprocessor has led to:

- audible alarms for trouble shooting
- separate protocols configured into the device for different opioids
- electronic records of the entire infusion history.

⚠ Professional alert!

Programming some PCA devices can take time and skill, and requires training and supervision of designated staff if serious errors are not to occur (Vicente et al, 2003). In these devices access to the syringe, bag or cassette containing the drug is restricted by a key or access code in order to prevent tampering or theft of the opioid. The key or pass codes for these devices should be kept secure.

The major advantage of programmable PCA devices is their flexibility, as they have a wide range of variable parameters; however, this can be a disadvantage as programming has to be controlled in order to avoid errors (Lehmann, 2005). These devices tend to be restricted in practice to a limited range of programmes according to organisational protocols. These are designed to limit human error and they have the advantage that a programme can be set prior to commencement of a PCA.

Dedicated PCA equipment is required for these machines and the PCA administration set should incorporate:

- An anti-siphon valve. This is a one-way valve that prevents rapid uncontrolled downloading of the opioid to the patient. Several deaths have been attributed to free flow as a result of siphonage (Elcock, 1994).

- An anti-reflux valve. This prevents backflow up into a secondary infusion that may be piggybacked into the PCA infusion line. If vasoocclusion occurs, for example, as a result of extravasation of the intravenous cannula, this would mean that no analgesia could enter the patient and the resulting pain would cause the patient to make several demands of the PCA device. The pump would administer the dose, and without the presence of an anti-reflux valve the drug would be pushed up into the secondary infusion line. When the occlusion is identified and cleared, or the infusion lines reconnected to a new cannula, the opioid in the secondary infusion would cause an inadvertent bolus with possibly serious consequences. An anti-reflux valve also maintains infusion line pressure and ensures that the pressure-sensitive infusion pump alarms earlier when occlusion occurs.

Disposable PCA devices

These infusion devices have no external power source and depend upon simple mechanical devices such as springs or elastomer technology (usually an inflatable elastic sack) to drive the drug into a patient-activated reservoir chamber.

The advantages of using disposable PCA devices are that:

- if using small volumes they can be safely and easily set up for pain management
- they are light and portable and therefore do not interfere with patient movement
- they are easy to store and move around
- they do not require servicing or maintenance
- they do not require an electric power source.

These advantages have led to their use in areas where patients are ambulant, such as day surgery, in the community and in some specific settings such as field hospitals and battlefield and trauma scenes. However, they are not as flexible in their use, as the only factors that can be varied are:

- choice of drug
- concentration of the drug.

Limitations to using the disposable PCA device are that:

- They are only able to deliver a preset bolus dose volume, usually 1 millilitre (ml) with a preset lockout of five minutes inbuilt in the system.
- It is a relatively expensive way of providing PCA if using large volumes.
- The drug reservoir can be more readily accessed by the public and staff.

⚠ Professional alert!

Standardisation of drug concentration has been a key risk management strategy to avoid drug errors. With disposable devices however, the only way to vary the bolus dose is to increase or decrease the concentration of the drug.

Other PCA methods

Transmucosal PCA devices

There is on the market a range of metered aerosol containers available to allow the administration of a fixed dose of analgesic drug via the nose (intranasal administration). This type of intranasal PCA has been shown to be as effective as intravenous PCA (Borland et al, 2007). At present, fentanyl appears to be the drug of choice administered via this route.

Transdermal PCA devices

This type of administration is based upon the transdermal fentanyl patch, but with the addition of a PCA mode. A process is used that applies a small electrical charge to the agent (usually fentanyl) that accelerates the rate of absorption through the skin. The technical term for this process is 'iontophoretic PCA'.

This technology is still in the development stages but papers are beginning to be published on its efficacy and use. For example, Viscusi and colleagues, (2004) in a randomised controlled trial demonstrated that transdermal fentanyl PCA was as effective as conventional morphine PCA after major surgery.

Part

IV

Identifying and managing potential complications

Opioids, like morphine, act primarily on the body's μ receptors and despite having a desired analgesic effect can also contribute to several unwanted effects such as:

- respiratory depression
- excessive sedation
- nausea and vomiting
- confusion and hallucinations
- pruritis
- hypotension
- constipation.

⚠ Professional alert!

Respiratory depression can be detected by a combination of low respiratory rate (below eight to ten respirations per minute) and increasing sedation. If this occurs, PCA should be stopped and emergency measures should be taken (see Professional alert on use of naloxone).

⚠ Professional alert!

An anti-emetic should always be prescribed. When a patient complains of nausea, give the anti-emetic but continue with the PCA. If the anti-emetic does not work consider trying an alternative anti-emetic.

⚠ Professional alert!

The use of naloxone

One way of dealing with some of these effects, such as respiratory depression, sedation and pruritis is to ensure that naloxone is prescribed alongside the PCA prescription. Naloxone is an opioid antagonist and blocks the action of opioids. These properties mean that naloxone works very quickly and a small dose will produce an effect. However it also means that the effect will not last for long.

Management of a PCA

Patients receiving PCA should be monitored closely to minimise the unwanted side-effects of the opioids used. Nursing observation should include hourly:

- observation of pulse
- observation of respiratory rate
- observation and documentation of the volume delivered
- pain assessment
- sedation scores
- documentation of incidents of nausea and vomiting.

Continuing pain

PCA opioids may not be enough to reduce pain to tolerable levels on their own. In this case a process of 'balanced analgesia' should be adopted. If not contraindicated, patients should also receive regular paracetamol 1 g and a non-steroidal anti-inflammatory drug such as diclofenac. This may have an opiate sparing effect and help in pain relief and weaning from PCA at a later stage. The importance of this should be emphasised, as often these drugs are omitted by the nurses, even when prescribed when a PCA is in situ. They can be given rectally, or in the case of paracetamol intravenously, if the oral route is not available.

ⓢ Scenario: continuing or discontinuing PCA

Harry is two days postoperative following abdominal surgery. He has now started on oral fluids and his intravenous infusion has been discontinued. He is becoming increasingly mobile and is beginning to get frustrated by his attachment to the patient-controlled analgesia pump. What factors need to be considered before the PCA is discontinued?

Discontinuing the PCA

Stopping a PCA early is one of the biggest causes of pain in the postoperative period (Carr, 2007). Before a patient gives up the PCA, a suitable alternative analgesia regime should be prescribed and commenced.

⚠️ **Professional alert!**

Only discontinue a PCA when you are confident that the patient's pain will be adequately managed by any alternative.

Conclusion

In this chapter you have read about and explored the principles of PCA. You should have a sound understanding of how to care for a patient receiving this form of pain management. This chapter should be read alongside the chapters on Vital signs, Intravenous therapy, Pain assessment and Routes of administration.

References

Borland, M., Jacobs, I., King, B. and O'Brien, D. (2007) 'A randomized controlled trial comparing intranasal fentanyl to intravenous morphine for managing acute pain in children in the emergency department', *Annals of Emergency Medicine* **49**(3), 335–40.

Carr, E. (2007) 'Barriers to effective pain management'. *Journal of Perioperative Practice* 17(5), 200–8.

Cashman, J. (2003) 'Routes of administration', Chapter 10 in Rowbotham, D.J. and MacIntyre, P.E. (eds), *Clinical Pain Management: Acute pain*, London, Arnold.

Charlton, E. (1997) 'The management of postoperative pain practical procedures', *Anaesthesia Update* 2, 1–7.

Elcock, D. H. (1994) 'Overdosage during patient-controlled analgesia', *British Medical Journal* 309, 1583.

Fisher, C. G., Bilanger, L., Gofton, E., Umedaly, H. S., Noonan, V. K., Abramon, C., Wing, D. C., Brown, J. and Dvorak, H. F. (2003) 'Prospective randomized clinical trial comparing patient-controlled intravenous analgesia with patient-controlled epidural analgesia after lumber spine fusion', *Spine* **28**(8), 739–43.

Harmer, M. and MacIntyre, P. E. (2003) 'Patient controlled analgesia', Chapter 11 in Rowbotham, D.J. and MacIntyre, P.E. (eds) *Clinical Pain Management: Acute pain*, London, Arnold.

Hawthorn, J. and Redmond, K. (1998) 'Pain: causes and management', *Journal of Psychiatric and Mental Health Nursing* 6(5), 409–10.

Lehmann, K. A. (2005) 'Recent developments in patient-controlled analgesia', *Journal of Pain and Symptom Management* 29(1), 72–89.

Mercadante, S. (2007) 'Opiod titration in cancer pain: A critical review', *European Journal of Pain* **11**(8), 823–30.

Myles, P. S., Buckland, M. R., Cannon, G. B., Bujor, M. A., Langley, M., Breaden, A., Salamonsen, R. F. and Davis, B. B. (1994) 'Comparison of patient-controlled analgesia and nurse-controlled infusion analgesia after cardiac surgery', *Anaesth Intensive Care* 22, 672–8.

Owen, H., Plummer, J. L., Armstrong, I. et al (1989) 'Variables of patient-controlled analgesia: 1 bolus size', *Anaesthesia* 44, 7–10.

Parsons, G. and Edwards, P. (1999) '"Acute pain algorithm",*Prof essinoal Nurse* 15(2), 136 .

Parsons, G., Jenkins, L. and Comerford, D. (2005) 'Patient Controlled Analgesia'. *Therapeutic Approaches to Pain Management*, Unit 2, Pontypridd, University of Glamorgan (unpublished).

Sherwood, K. (1996) *Patient-controlled Analgesia Booklet*, Australia, Ryde Hospital.

Southern, D. A. and Read, M. S. (1994) 'Lesson of the week: overdosage of opiate from patient-controlled analgesia devices', *British Medical Journal* 309, 1002.

Thomas, N. (1994) 'Patient controlled analgesia: how it works', *Elderly Care* **6**(3) 25–7.

Vicente. K. J., Kada-Bekhaled, K., Hillel, G., Cassano, A. and Orser, B. A. (2003) 'Programming errors contribute to death from patient-controlled analgesia: case report and estimate of probability', *Canadian Journal of Anaesthesia* **50**(4), 328–32.

Viscusi, E. R., Reynolds, L., Chung, F., Atkinson, L. and Khanna, S. (2004) 'Patient-controlled transdermal fentanyl hydrochloride vs intravenous morphine pump for postoperative pain: a randomized controlled trial', *Journal of the American Medical Association* **291**(11),1333–41.

Woodhouse, A., Ward, E. M. and Mather, L. E (1999) 'Intra subject variability in post operative patient-controlled analgesia (PCA): is the patient quality equally satisfied with morphine, pethedine and fentanyl?', *Pain* **80**(3), 545–53.

Chapter

30

Universal precautions

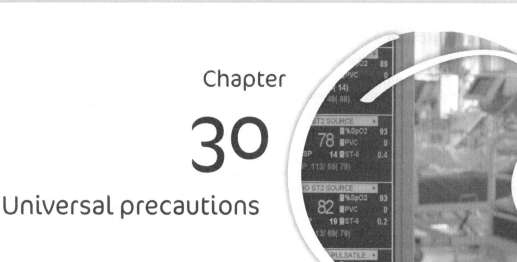

Siobhan MacDermott

 Links to other chapters in *Foundation Skills for Caring*

1 Fundamental concepts for skills
9 Patient hygiene
23 Diabetic foot assessment
31 Wound assessment
32 Aseptic technique and wound management

 Links to other chapters in *Foundation Studies for Caring*

3 Evidence-based practice and research
4 Ethical, legal and professional issues
8 Healthcare governance
13 Infection prevention and control
16 Safeguarding children
17 Safeguarding adults
33 HIV and infectious disease management

W Don't forget to visit www.palgrave.com/glasper for additional online resources relating to this chapter.

Introduction

Infection is considered a significant risk in healthcare settings, to both patients and healthcare staff. The UK National Audit Office (2000) reported that at least 9 per cent of patients in hospitals have acquired a healthcare-associated infection (HAI) at some time.

The implications for patient care, hospital stays and financial costs of such infections are huge. However healthcare workers' knowledge of and compliance with universal precautions is variable.

Universal precautions are set out in guidelines designed to protect healthcare workers from the risk of becoming contaminated with potentially infectious blood or body secretions (Bennett and Mansell, 2004). They involve the routine use of protective measures such as gloves, masks, gowns and handwashing. They were first introduced in the United States in 1985 in response to growing concerns among healthcare workers about the risk of infection from patients with the human immunodeficiency virus (HIV). It is impossible to identify every person who has an infectious disease, so all patients should be considered as a potential hazard in relation to infection, and universal precautions should be applied to all patients irrespective of infectious status (DH, 1998). Use of such precautions should be based on assessment of the risk associated with the procedure about to undertaken and not the antibody status of the patient (Cockcroft and Elford, 1994); for example, gloves are necessary for venepuncture.

In 2003, the UK National Institute of Clinical Excellence (NICE) launched a new clinical guideline on the prevention of HAI in primary and community care. The guidelines outlined ways of avoiding infection which included handwashing, the use of gloves and aprons, safe disposal of sharps, and educating patients and their carers about infection. This chapter explores these issues and aims to highlight the principles of universal precautions as an effective means of protecting patients and staff and controlling infection.

Learning outcomes

This chapter will enable you to:

- understand the principles of universal precautions in controlling the spread of infection
- describe the procedure and indications for the following procedures using evidence-based knowledge:
  - handwashing
  - the use of gloves and aprons
  - disposal of linen
  - environmental cleaning
  - educating patients and their carers about infection.

Concepts

- Hand hygiene
- Improved practice
- Healthcare associated infection
- Protective clothing
- Hygiene promotions

Hand hygiene

Hand hygiene is a term that usually applies to either handwashing, antiseptic handwash, antiseptic hand rub or surgical hand antisepsis.

Handwashing has long been described as the single most effective way of preventing the spread of infection (Gammon and Gould, 2005), as hands are considered the route most commonly responsible for the transmission of such infection in hospitals. However compliance rates among healthcare workers are reported to be unacceptably low, ranging from less than 50

⚠ Professional alert!

The NHS estimated that HAI costs £1 billion a year, and that 15 per cent of this could be prevented by the introduction of good practice.

per cent to just 14 per cent (Hughes, 2006). High workloads, time pressures (Ardle et al, 2006), lack of hygiene promotion and role models (Hughes, 2006), and inadequate equipment/facilities have been blamed for such non-compliance.

When should handwashing be carried out?

Hands should be washed:

- before and after patient contact which includes any contact with the patient's skin, dressing or equipment (NICE, 2003; Pratt et al, 2001)
- between every patient contact when skin-to-skin contact has occurred between the healthcare worker and the patient
- before each clinical procedure that involves patient contact
- after contact with any blood/body fluids or contaminated items
- after removal of gloves
- before and after entering an isolation cubicle
- before all aseptic procedures
- before all invasive procedures.

An effective handwashing technique includes three stages: preparation, washing and rinsing, and drying (NICE, 2003).

Handwashing preparation

- Hand jewellery should be removed before handwashing.
- Cuts and abrasions should be covered with waterproof dressings.
- Fingernails should be kept short, clean and free from nail polish.

Handwashing procedure

Wet hands under tepid running water, apply soap or antimicrobial preparation, rub hands together for a minimum of 10–15 seconds with careful attention to finger tips, thumbs and between fingers (NICE, 2003). Remember to rub all skin areas (five strokes backwards and forwards) using the approach shown in Figure 30.1. The same technique should be used when applying alcohol rubs.

The procedure shown in Figure 30.1 was identified by Ayliffe et al (1978). It is a six-step technique to ensure that all parts of the hands are covered by the handwashing procedure, and consists of five strokes forward and five strokes backwards.

t ☆
Practice tip

- Protective emollients or hand creams should be encouraged to prevent skin damage to healthcare workers (MMWR, 2002).
- Disposable hand towels should be used for drying hands.
- A suitable hand cream should be available for staff.

Table 30.1 Situations requiring hand washing

Risk	Precaution	Function
Routine patient contact (before and after)	Handwashing using liquid soap	Removes transient bacteria
Invasive procedures	Handwashing using antiseptics	Kills resident bacteria, with residual effectiveness
Contact with immuno-compromised patient	Handwashing using antiseptic hand rub	Kills bacteria, with residual effectiveness
Contaminated hands	Handwashing using antiseptics	Cleans physically soiled hand and transient bacteria
Potential heavy hand contamination	Gloves followed by handwashing	Protects hands from potential contamination

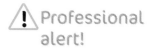

⚠ Professional alert!

Tell hospital management/supervisor if a particular soap or antimicrobial is irritating your skin.

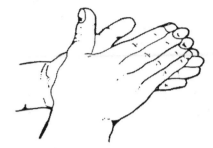

1. Palm to palm

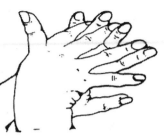

2. Right palm over left dorsum and left palm over right dorsum

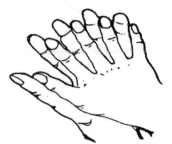

3. Palm to palm fingers interlaced

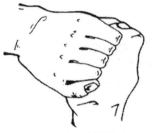

4. Backs of fingers to opposing palms with fingers interlocked

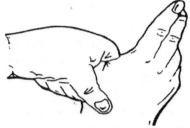

5. Rotational rubbing of right thumb clasped in left palm and vice versa

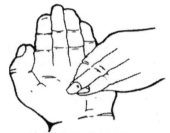

6. Rotational rubbing, backwards and forwards with clasped fingers of right hand in left palm and vice versa

Figure 30.1   Six step handwashing technique devised by Ayliffe et al (1978) ensuring that all parts of the hands are covered

The role of alcohol rubs

Alcohol hand rubs or gels are suitable for use as an adjunct to handwashing provided hands are clean initially. Antiseptic soaps are only slightly more effective at killing residual bacteria on hands than soap and water. However hand rubs that contain 70 per cent alcohol and chlorhexidine can kill bacteria more effectively than many antiseptic hand solutions. In addition they have a cumulative effect that can kill bacteria for several hours afterwards, an effect known as residual effectiveness (Gould et al, 2000). They are better at preventing re-growth of bacteria on hands. Alcohol-based hand rubs also contain added emollients and skin softeners (Fry and Burger, 2005).

Alcohol rubs or gels are particularly useful in:

- areas where frequent handwashing is required, such as intensive care.
- outside isolation cubicles
- areas with an inadequate supply of handwashing facilities (Kaplan and McGuckin, 1986).

(e)   Evidence-based practice

Alcohol hand gels are associated with less skin damage than antiseptic handwash solutions (Fry and Burger, 2005).

The role of gloves

The role of gloves in preventing cross-infection in healthcare has been promoted since the 1970s and 1980s. Several studies at the time recommended the use of gloves for procedures likely to result in heavy hand contamination (Lowbury and Lilley, 1973). The Royal College

Part

IV

of Nursing (1997) recommends that healthcare workers wear gloves for invasive procedures such as venepuncture and when there is any other risk of contact with body fluids or blood.

It is important to distinguish between the appropriate use of sterile disposable gloves and the less costly non-sterile disposable gloves:

- non-sterile gloves – to prevent contamination
- sterile gloves – to prevent cross-infection.

The role of gloves in universal precautions is to reduce the risk of cross-infection to healthcare workers.

⚠ **Professional alert!**

- Gloves should always be single use only and should be changed between contacts with different patients.
- Gloves must be disposed of as clinical waste immediately after the procedure (DH, 2003b).
- Handwashing is considered necessary following the use of gloves because hands can become contaminated on removal of gloves, which can also puncture or leak (Korniewicz et al, 1994).

The role of protective clothing

In hospitals, patients' secretions can often be a major source of infection. The role of protective clothing is to reduce the risk to staff and patients, and it should be worn where there is a risk of splashing and contamination from bodily fluids. Typical potentially infectious bodily fluids include blood, sputum, vomit, saliva, urine and faeces.

The choice of protective clothing should depend on the risk of exposure to bodily fluids. Procedures where the risk of contamination is low, like collecting specimens or assisting patients with bed baths, may require a plastic apron only, whereas operating theatres may require disposable waterproof clothing, masks and eye protection because of the risk of splashing.

Disposal of linen

While hands are typically regarded as the main cause of spreading HAI, decontamination of the clinical environment (Gammon and Gould, 2005) and correct disposal of linen and equipment are pivotal in preventing such infection.

Hospital linen can become contaminated with patients' secretions and bodily fluids and therefore should be treated as potentially infectious.

⚠ **Professional alert!**

Disposal of linen should conform to local hospital policy.

Laundering of contaminated linen must be carried out using industrial washing and drying machines. Laundries that deal with hospital linen must comply with local DH guidelines and statutory regulations (May, 2000).

Guidelines for the safe handling of soiled linen/disposal of hospital linen

- Never shake linen as this will disperse skin scales.
- Wear gloves and plastic apron when changing soiled bed linen, and discard apron afterwards (McCulloch, 1998).
- Use the correct colour-coded system for linen bags as laid down in hospital/local policy (McCulloch, 1998).
- Heavily soiled linen should be placed in a water-soluble or soluble-stitched bag, otherwise known as alginate bag, before being put into a linen bag. These bags are then placed directly into suitable washing machines without opening, thus reducing the risk of contamination.
- Wash hands after contact with soiled linen.
- Bring the linen skip to the bedside and do not carry soiled linen (McCulloch, 1998).
- Display a colour-coded chart indicating the correct disposal of types of linen.
- Double the bag first in an alginate bag and then in a clear plastic or cloth bag.
- Do not over-fill bags or skips.

- Tie each bag securely.
- Label with ward label (May, 2000).

Table 30.2 Colour chart for disposal of linen and waste

Colour	Content	Disposal
Black	Domestic waste (not contaminated)	Landfill
Yellow	Clinical or infected waste	Incinerated
Clear/white plastic	Used linen	Emptied into washing machine
Alginate bag inside clear plastic or cloth bag	Soiled or infected linen	Laundered whole as alginate bag dissolves in washing machine

Environmental cleaning

Healthcare environments can easily become contaminated with dust, debris and bodily fluids with potentially infectious micro-organisms. Since airborne infection can remain suspended in the air for long periods, its risk is much greater than that of droplet infection.

The aim of environmental cleaning or disinfection is to reduce the number of microbes present and remove any substances that might encourage growth or interfere with disinfection or sterilisation processes (Parker, 1999).

- Warm/hot water and detergent are usually sufficient to reduce environmental contamination.
- Disinfectants such as alcohol or chlorine-releasing agents help to reduce the number of pathogens present but should not be used indiscriminately.
- Local/hospital disinfection policies must be adhered to.
- Hospital/ward environments should be kept uncluttered and easy to clean (May, 2000).

Education

Education is considered the cornerstone for improvement with hand-hygiene practices (Boyce and Pittet, 2002) and universal precautions. Healthcare programmes and clinical skills education centres should include handwashing techniques which help improve handwashing, such as the glogerm system.

Topics that should be included in educational programmes

- information about hospital-acquired infection and cross-transmission of micro-organisms
- information about the impact of improved hand hygiene on healthcare-associated infection
- awareness of local guidelines for hand hygiene
- information on hand-hygiene compliance rates by healthcare workers and the implications for infection control
- knowledge about the use, appropriateness and understanding of hand-hygiene protection agents in universal precautions.

Hygiene promotions

There have been a number of campaigns to improve public and patient hygiene, some of the most significant being:

⚠ Professional alert!

Only use alginate bags for contaminated linen as they are expensive and require special laundry.

ⓐ Learning activity

- Identify what precautions are necessary in your working area to minimise risk of infection.
- Check to see if there are any posters displayed in your clinical area advising patients or relatives of the risk of infection.
- Read your local policy regarding universal precautions.

W

- The 'Cleanyourhands' campaign: this is aimed at improving hand-hygiene compliance, using poster and promotional materials to influence healthcare workers in the UK: www.npsa. nhs.uk/cleanyourhands.
- *Winning Ways: Working together to reduce healthcare associated infection in England* (DH, 2003b) outlines strategies to reduce HAI in England.
- *Getting Ahead of the Curve* (DH, 2003a) examines controlling interventions. This is the Chief Medical Officer's Report on Infectious Diseases Strategy for England.
- In 2005 the Royal College of Nursing launched the 'Wipe it out' campaign with support from the Infection Control Nurses' Association in the UK, outlining minimum standards in the prevention and control of HAI.
- *Healthcare Associated Infections* (Welsh Assembly Government, 2004) outlines a strategy developed by the Welsh Healthcare Associated Infection subgroup (WHAISG) of the Committee for the Control of Communicable Disease aimed at reducing HAI in acute hospitals.
- 'Cleanliness Champions' is an NHS Education for Scotland initiative promoting infection control via educational resources in the Scottish NHS: www.space4.me.uk/hai.

W

- 'Clean your hands: say no to infection' (Health Service Executive, Ireland, 2007) lays out a plan to prevent and control of healthcare-associated Infections in Ireland.
- Chief Medical Officer (2005) *Protecting Patients and Staff: A strategy for prevention and control of healthcare associated infections in Northern Ireland 2005–2010.* (Belfast, Department of Health, Social Services and Public Safety) is available online at http://www. dhsspsni.gov.uk/publications/2005/prevention-of-HCAIs.pdf.

W

(a) Learning activity

W

Refresh your learning by asking yourself these commonly asked questions. The answers are below.

- When should you wash your hands?
- Are alcohol-based hand gels accepted in place of washing with soap and water?
- Should disinfectants be used for washing hands?

Answers:

- Hands should be washed before and after contact with patients.
- Alcohol rubs are effective if used on clean hands.

- No; disinfectants are designed for objects and surfaces and may be too harsh for use on skin tissue. Soaps containing antiseptic should be used for proper handwashing.

Now try creating a poster related to the Health Science Education curriculum, such as 'Hand Hygiene – Preventing the Spread of Infection'.

Finally, to test your knowledge, complete the online RCN 'Wipe it out' quiz available at http://www.rcn.org.uk/resources/mrsa/healthcarestaff.

Conclusion

This chapter has introduced you to the main precautions for preventing the spread of infection. It is important that all healthcare professionals take note of these, and follow the guidelines carefully for the safety and well-being of both practitioner and patient. Before commencing any care, take the time to familiarise yourself with the guidelines issued by your local health authority.

References

Ardle, F., Lee, R. J., Gibb, A. P. and Walsh, T. S. (2006) 'How much time is needed for hand hygiene in intensive care? A prospective trained observer study of rates of contact between healthcare workers and intensive care patients', *Journal of Hospital Infection* **62**(3) 306–10.

Ayliffe, G. A. J., Babb, J. R. and Quoraishi, A. H. (1978) 'A test for hygienic hand disinfection', *Journal of Clinical Pathology* 31, 923–8.

Ayliffe, G. A. J., Collins, B. J. and Taylor, L. J. (1990) *Hospital Acquired Infection: Principles and prevention*, 2nd edn, Cambridge, Wright.

Bennett, G. and Mansell, I. (2004) 'Universal precautions: a survey of community nurses' experience and practice', *Journal of Clinical Nursing* 13, 413–21.

Boyce, J. M. and Pittet, D. (2002) 'Guidelines for hand hygiene in health-care settings: MMWR recommendations of the Healthcare Infection Control Practices Advisory Committee and the HICPAC/SHEA/APIC/IDSA Hand Hygiene Task Force', *American Journal of Infection Control* 30(8), S1–S46.

Cockcroft, A. and Elford, J. (1994) 'Clinical practice and the perceived importance of identifying high risk patients', *Journal of Hospital Infection*, **28**(2) 127–36.

Department of Health (DH) (1998) *Guidance for Healthcare Workers: Protection against infection with blood borne viruses, recommendations of the Expert Advisory Group on AIDS and the Advisory Group on Hepatitis*, Wetherby, DH Publications.

DH (2003a) *Getting Ahead of the Curve: A strategy for combating infectious diseases*, London, DH.

DH (2003b) *Winning Ways: Working together to reduce healthcare associated infection in England*, London, Stationery Office.

Fry, D. and Burger, T. L. (2005) 'Hand hygiene compliance: step up reach out', *Nursing Management* 36(11) (suppl.), 12, 14–15.

Gammon, J. and Gould, D. J. (2005) Universal precautions, a review of knowledge, compliance and strategies to improve practice, *Journal of Research in Nursing* **10**(5), 529–47.

Gould, D. J., Gammon, J., Donnelly, M., Batiste, L., Ball, E. Carneiro, De Melos, A. M., Alidad, V., Miles, R. and Halablab, M. (2000) 'Improving hand hygiene in community health settings', *Journal of Clinical Nursing* 9, 95–102.

Health Services Executive (2007) *Say No to Infection: Infection Control Action Plan. The prevention and control of healthcare associated Infections in Ireland*, Dublin, The Stationery Office.

Hughes, N. (2006) 'Handwashing: Going back to basics in infection control', *American Journal of Nursing* 106(7), 96.

Kaplan, L. M. and McGuckin, M. (1986) 'Increasing handwashing compliance with more accessible sinks', *Infection Control*, **7**, 408–9.

Korniewicz, D. M., Kirwin, M., Cresci, K., Sing, T., Choo, T. E., Wool, M. and Larson, E. (1994) 'Barrier protection with examination gloves: double versus single', *American Journal of Infection Control* 22(1),12–15.

Lowbury, E. J. L. and Lilley, H. A. (1973) 'Use of 4% chlorhexidine detergent solution (Hibiscrub) and other methods of skin disinfection in wards', *British Medical Journal* 1, 510–15.

May, D. (2000) 'Infection control', *Nursing Standard* **14**(28), 51–7.

McCulloch, J. (1998) 'Infection control: principles for practice', *Nursing Standard* 13(1), 49–53.

MMWR (2002) Centers for Disease Control and Prevention. *Guideline for Hand Hygiene in Health-Care Settings: Recommendations of the Healthcare Infection Control Practices Advisory Committee and the HICPAC/SHEA/APIC/IDSA Hand Hygiene Task Force*, MMWR Vol. 51, no. RR-16.

National Audit Office (2000) *The Management and Control of Hospital Acquired Infection in NHS Trusts in England*, London: Stationery Office.

National Institute of Clinical Excellence (NICE) (2003) *Infection Control: Prevention of healthcare-associated infection in primary and community care* (NICE guideline), London, NICE, [online] www.nice.org.uk (accessed 10 February 2009).

Parker L. J. (1999) 'Managing and maintaining a safe environment in the hospital setting', *British Journal of Nursing*, 8(16), 1053–66.

Pellowe, C., Pratt, R., Loveday, Harper, P., Robinson, N. and Jones, S. R. (2004) 'The epic project: updating the evidence-base for national evidence-based guidelines for preventing healthcare-associated infections in NHS hospitals in England: a report with recommendations', *British Journal of Infection Control* 5, :10–15.

Pratt, R. A. Pellowe, C. M., Loveday, H. P. et al (2001) 'The epic project: developing national evidence based guidelines for preventing healthcare associated infections', *Journal of Hospital Infection* 47, Supplement A.

Royal College of Nursing (1997) 'Universal precautions', *Nursing Standard* 11, 32.

Scottish Executive Health Department (2004) *The NHS Scotland National Cleaning Services Specification*, Edinburgh: Scottish Executive.

Welsh Assembly Government (2004) *Healthcare Associated Infections: A strategy for hospitals in Wales*, Cardiff, Welsh Assembly Government.

Chapter

31

Wound assessment

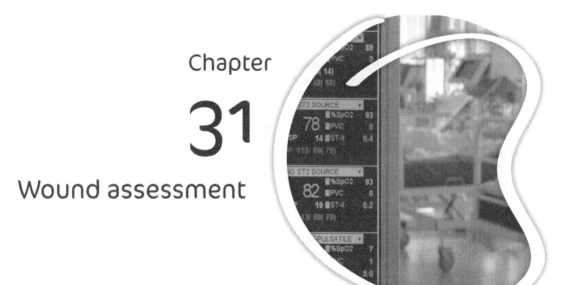

Lesley Wayne

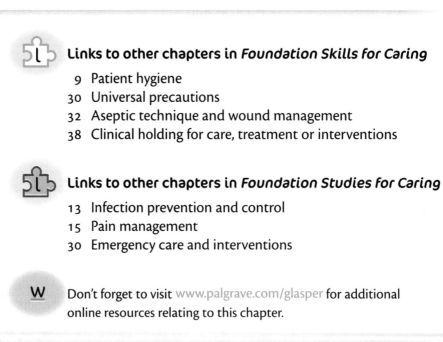

Links to other chapters in *Foundation Skills for Caring*

9 Patient hygiene
30 Universal precautions
32 Aseptic technique and wound management
38 Clinical holding for care, treatment or interventions

Links to other chapters in *Foundation Studies for Caring*

13 Infection prevention and control
15 Pain management
30 Emergency care and interventions

W Don't forget to visit www.palgrave.com/glasper for additional online resources relating to this chapter.

Introduction

Wound evaluation can present many challenges but accurate assessment is essential as it provides the basis on which to formulate treatment and management. The aim of this chapter is to provide an introduction to accurate wound assessment and documentation. The chapter will define and describe wounds and detail how to take a focused history. The assessment and examination procedure is explained (including a short review of wound measurement tools and their uses) and the significance of findings outlined. A brief synopsis of wound healing is given.

Learning outcomes

This chapter will enable you to:

- define a wound
- take a history of the presenting complaint
- identify tetanus prone wounds
- understand the principles of wound assessment

- describe different types of wound
- accurately measure a wound
- understand the basic principles of wound healing
- be able to accurately document your findings.

Concepts

- wound definition
- types of wound
- history taking

- wound assessment and examination procedure
- significance of wound colour and odour

- wound measurement guides
- principles of wound healing
- documentation

A wound can be defined as: 'An injury to the person by which the skin is divided, or its continuity broken; a lesion of the body, involving some solution of continuity' (Biology online, 2007).

Types of wound

Acute wounds
- contusion (bruise)
- abrasion (graze)
- laceration (tear)
- puncture (stab)
- burn (dry heat) or scald (wet heat) (Dougherty and Lister, 2004).

Chronic wounds

Some wounds (a minority) will become chronic and non-healing and will require regular reassessment (Grey, Enoch and Harding, 2006). Examples include:
- *Pressure ulcers*: caused by the compression soft tissue between a bony prominence and an external surface for a lengthy period thereby causing an area of tissue necrosis (James and Bayat, 2007).
- *Venous ulcers*: improper functioning of valves in the veins (usually of the legs) results in venous hypertension. 'The increased pressure in the veins causes extravasation of fibrinogen, which leads to deposition of fibrin around the vessel. This in turn results in poor oxygenation of the surrounding skin' (James and Bayat, 2007).
- *Arterial ulcers*: 'arterial insufficiency ulcers are caused by arteriosclerosis which leads to insufficient oxygenation of the skin and underlying tissues. This kills the affected tissues and causes wounds' (Tyco Health Care, 2007).
- *Diabetic ulcers*: commonly occur on the feet of type 1 and type 2 diabetic patients due to poor circulation and peripheral neuropathy.

Part

IV

Procedure

Prior to assessment and examination, the patient should be informed of your role and consent obtained.

Taking a history

The prime objective of taking a history is to formulate a diagnosis on which to base treatment and management. The history should also include the patient's past medical history of relevant illness or underlying disease. Nutritional status and history of smoking are also important as these factors influence healing rates. Potential complicating factors, which might delay healing, should be sought during the history. These include patients with disease processes such as diabetes, HIV, drug-resistant infections or peripheral vascular disease; patients who are immunosuppressed; patients receiving chemotherapy or steroid treatments; and any patient over the age of 50. Known allergies should be ascertained.

Remember to ask about the patient's occupation and leisure activities as this may influence your management.

⚠ Professional alert!

Remember to ascertain the patient's tetanus status when assessing acute wounds.

Tetanus infection can gain entry through an open wound. The time elapsed since the injury occurred is important in deciding whether to close the wound and the need for tetanus prophylaxis.

⟳ⓐ Learning activity

Search the internet or consult the literature to find out which wounds are considered tetanus prone.

What is the Department of Health's current advice about tetanus vaccination? Consult the Department of Health's 'Green Book' (available online).

Focused history

A focused, detailed history is essential. This involves asking the 'how, what, where, why, when' questions:

- How did the injury occur?
- What exactly happened? For example, did the patient fall, did they cut themselves with a knife, on glass? Have they been stabbed? If so, with what? How long was the blade?
- Where did it happen? – inside/outside?
- Was there any preceding event, for example to cause a fall?
- When did the injury occur?

The mechanism of injury will indicate whether there is likely to be damage to underlying structures or the presence of a foreign body. The place where the injury occurred will similarly indicate whether the wound is clean or dirty and whether there are likely to be any contaminants or foreign bodies in the wound.

It is important to establish whether there was any preceding event, for example cardiac pain or dizziness, that may indicate an underlying illness requiring treatment.

⚠ Professional alert!

You must identify the patient's dominant hand when assessing upper limbs. Injuries to a dominant hand require particular care when assessing and managing an injury.

History of chronic wounds

The history of a chronic wound should include information on the duration of the lesion or ulcer, previous ulceration, history of trauma and family history of ulceration (Grey et al, 2006).

S Scenario: hand injury in A&E

David is a 12-year-old boy who has presented to the accident and emergency (A&E) department with his mother. Half an hour ago, while ice-skating, David fell over and landed on his outstretched right hand. His hand was then run over by another skater. He has sustained wounds to the dorsum of his right ring and middle fingers over the proximal phalanges. He is right-hand dominant.

a Learning activity

Apart from the wounds, what other injuries do you think that David might have sustained?

What concerns do you think David and his mother might have?

Wound assessment and examination

- Before commencing your examination make the patient comfortable and adjust the lighting to allow inspection of the wound.
- Show concern for the patient's privacy and modesty by drawing the curtains in the ward or examining room (Bickley and Szilagyi, 2007).
- Wash your hands in accordance with local protocols.
- Don protective clothing, i.e. plastic apron, gloves, goggles as required.

Procedure for wound assessment

The following practices ensure accuracy of assessment and will aid the review of the wound at a later date.

- Expose patients who have sustained trauma (as appropriate) in order to ensure that further injuries are not missed.
- Note the exact anatomical site of the wound. The location of the wound will affect healing rates and choice of treatment.
- Note the direction and shape of wound: transverse, oblique, longitudinal, stellate, ragged, y shaped or others. Identification of the type and shape of wound, together with the measurements will ensure accuracy and aid the review process (Reynolds and Cole, 2006).
- Note any skin loss and the viability of the surrounding tissue. Viable tissue is healthy undamaged tissue whereas non-viable tissue is damaged and contused and is without an adequate blood supply.
- Note any associated bruising, haematoma, swelling, erythema.
- Note whether the wound is clean or dirty. Contaminants will impair healing and require removal.
- Visualise the base of wound, in order to exclude involvement of underlying structures, such as tendons, nerves, joints and fractures.
- Where appropriate palpate for underlying fractures, x-ray if required.
- For *acute* wounds, identify the type of wound: flap wound, laceration, cut, puncture wound, amputation injury.
- Measure the wound accurately, including the length, depth and breadth.
- Assess limbs for motor function and tendon function where applicable. Delay in identifying tendon injury may result in permanent loss of function.
- Assess neurovascular function distal to wound. Sensory deficit may indicate nerve damage and requires further assessment. Any circulatory deficit will need attention in order to preserve and restore healthy tissue. Control bleeding in order to promote healing and prevent the formation of a haematoma.
- For *chronic* wounds, note ulcer characteristics such as pain or odour. Establish whether there is any exudate or discharge.
- Examine the edge of the wound. The history of the wound together with this examination may give an indication of the aetiology of the wound. For example, venous leg ulcers usually have gently sloping edges while arterial ulcers often appear well demarcated, dry with deep

'cliff edges' and localized oedema. Rolled or everted edges, or non-healing ulcers should raise the suspicion of malignancy' (Wayne and Bunn, 2007, Grey et al, 2006; Smith and Nephew, 2000; Guly, 1996).

Wound colour and odour

Wound colour and odour are very important to wound assessment. Consider the tasks in the 'Learning activity' carefully.

---

a Learning activity

Search the literature and internet or consult your tissue viability professional to answer the following questions:

- Wound appearance by colour:
  - Pink is indicative of ...
  - Red is indicative of ...
  - Dark red bleeds easily: is indicative of ...
  - Creamy yellow adherent to wound surface: is indicative of ...
  - Black/yellowish brown is indicative of ...

- Wound odour:
  - A fruity smell is indicative of ...
  - Foul smells are indicative of ...

Wound measurement guides

A variety of guides and tools are available to assist wound measurement. All methods have advantages and disadvantages and choice is largely a matter of clinical judgment.
   Commonly used methods are outlined below:

- Simple measurements can be made by means of a tape measure; however this can be difficult to use accurately if the wound is an irregular shape.
- A more accurate method may be to use a grid. The outline of the wound is traced onto sterile transparent film marked with a grid, so allowing subsequent grid measurements to be compared with the original. Difficulties can arise in tracing the wound boundaries and may again lead to inaccuracies.
- Scaled photographs, which incorporate a ruler in the margin, are also available for use. Photographs also enable comparisons to be made, but these can be subject to errors in magnification.
- Moulds of the wound can be created by taking a cast of the cavity using saline or alginate fillings. These have the advantage of being three-dimensional (Fette, 2006).

---

t Practice tip

The wound assessment tool selected for use should be:

- User friendly: to ensure continuity of use, consistency and reliability. 'Differences in the manual skill and/or experience of the measuring clinician can result in considerable variations.'

- A valid tool: 'the validity of any wound assessment tool must be based on its ability to measure accurately what it is intended to measure' (Fette, 2006).
- Able to provide an accurate basis for the formulation of management and treatment.

(Fette, 2006)

Wound healing

In order to assess a wound's progress, a basic knowledge of the process of wound healing is essential. Normal wound healing comprises three distinct phases. For healing to take place, each phase needs to occur.

1 The inflammatory phase: this primary phase is characterized by inflammation and haemostasis of the wound. The body's defences are activated to protect against bacterial infection and clotting factors are initiated (platelet aggregation occurs).

2 The proliferative phase: granulation, contraction, and epithelialisation take place.

3 Maturation: vascularisation is reduced. Collagen is synthesised, thereby increasing the tensile strength of the wound. Scar contraction and remodelling occur (Dougherty and Lister, 2004).

In a chronic wound, the order of the stages of wound healing has become disrupted. This can occur when there is defective remodelling, failure to re-epithelialise or prolonged inflammation.

> **a Learning activity**
>
> Wound healing can be affected by intrinsic factors and extrinsic factors. Search the internet or consult the literature to find out the meaning of these terms. How many intrinsic and extrinsic factors can you identify?

Documentation

Accurate and timely documentation of your assessment is essential. It is a legal record of your intervention and, should a complaint be made or a malpractice suit result, you will be glad that you have a definitive record to refer to. Remember, if it's not documented you didn't do it (Guly, 1996)! Additionally, you may recall (possibly) what the wound looked like the last time you saw it, but fellow clinicians will have no idea.

Your documentation should:

• record the patient's medical history
• identify aetiological factors
• identify intrinsic and extrinsic factors that may affect wound healing
• obtain a baseline for future comparison
• provide a legal and systematic record (Templeton, 2004).

It should be legible, concise and comprehensive. A labelled diagram can be invaluable in conveying an accurate record of your findings. Use of abbreviations should be restricted to those universally recognised and approved. It must be signed and printed with your name and designation, timed and dated.

Good documentation will aid communication and ensure consistency and continuity of care with the team, thereby providing quality patient care.

> **a Learning activity W**
>
> Look up the advice given by your professional body regarding documentation.
>
> See the companion webpages for this chapter for an example of a wound assessment tool.

Summary

• A detailed focused history is essential.
• The type of wound should be clearly defined.
• Wounds may be acute or chronic.
• Regular reassessment of wounds to evaluate treatment and progress of the wound is essential.
• Use of a 'user-friendly' standardised wound assessment tool is advised in order to ensure that valid, reliable and consistent information is gained.
• Accurate and timely documentation is essential.

a) Learning activity

Check your answers to the chapter Learning activities against those given below. Where you have made an error, return to the relevant section and revise the material:

Tetanus-prone wounds

The following wounds are considered to be tetanus prone:

- puncture wounds
- wounds with a significant degree of devitalised tissue
- wounds contaminated with soil or manure
- wounds containing foreign bodies
- compound fractures
- wounds with clinical signs of sepsis
- wounds or burns sustained more than six hours before surgical treatment (PRODIGY, 2004).

David

David might have sustained a tendon injury to his finger. He may also have sustained a fracture to his arm (anywhere from the shoulder downwards) and/or finger. David may be concerned about pain and the treatment and management of his injury. He and his mother may be worried about complications in the healing process, for example scarring or impaired function.

Significance of wound colour and odour

Wound appearance by colour:

- Pink is indicative of epithelialising tissue.
- Red is indicative of healthy granulation tissue.
- Dark red bleeds easily; it is indicative of unhealthy granulation tissue, may indicate infection.
- Creamy yellow adherent to wound surface is indicative of slough, dead tissue, which will impede healing.
- Black/yellowish brown is indicative of necrotic, non-viable tissue due to loss of blood supply.

Wound odour

- A fruity smell is indicative of staphylococcus organisms.
- Foul smells are indicative of gram-negative bacteria.

Intrinsic/extrinsic factors

Intrinsic factors are those which originate from within the patient, for example, diseases such a diabetes, nutritional status. Extrinsic factors are external to the patient, for example, wound dressings.

Conclusion

Wound assessment helps in identifying the cause and extent of the wound; it also enables evaluation of the progress of wound healing, and from this decisions can be made regarding the management of care to treat the wound. Assessment is essential for the early identification of any factors that might cause a delay in the natural healing process so that these can be considered in the treatment plan. Wound assessment is essentially subjective but using a standardised approach can make the process more objective, and management can be based on accurate evidence.

References

Bickley, L. S. and Szilagyi, P. G. (2007) *Bates' Guide to Physical Examination and History Taking*, 9th edn, Philadelphia, Lippincott, Williams & Wilkins.

Biology online (2007) http://www.biology-online.org/ (accessed 10 January 2007).

Department of Health (DH) (2007) *The Green Book*, DH [online] www.dh.gov.uk/en/Policyandguidance/HealthandSocial caretopics/Greenbook/index.htm (accessed 30 December 2008).

Dougherty, S. and Lister, S. (eds) (2004). 'Wound management', in *The Royal Marsden Manual of Clinical Nursing procedures*, 6th edn, Oxford, Blackwell Publishing.

Fette, A. M. (2006) 'A clinimetric analysis of wound measurement tools', [online] http://www.worldwidewounds.com/2006/january/Fette/Clinimetric-Analysis-Wound-Measurement-Tools.html (accessed 16 February 2009).

Grey, J. E., Enoch, S. and Harding, K. G. (2006) 'ABC of wound healing: wound assessment', *British Medical Journal* 332, 285–8.

Guly, H. (1996) *History Taking, Examination and Record Keeping in Emergency Medicine*, Oxford, Oxford Handbooks in Emergency Medicine, Oxford University Press.

James, A. L. and Bayat, A. (2007) 'Basic plastic surgery techniques and principles', [online] www.studentbmj.com/back_issues/1103/education/406.html–50k (accessed 30 January 2007).

Miller, M. (1995) 'Principles of wound assessment', *Emergency Nurse* **3**(1), 16–18.

Prescribing Nurse Bulletin (1999) 'Modern wound management dressings', *Prescribing Nurse Bulletin* **1**(2) [online] www.npc.co.uk/nurse_prescribing/pdfs/modWoundvol1no2.pdf (accessed 12 February 2009).

PRODIGY (2004) www.prodigy.nhs.uk/Lacerations 'Clinical knowledge summaries. prodigy guidance lacerations', PRODIGY [online] http://www.prodigy.nhs.uk/lacerations/extended_information/

management_issues (accessed 2 February 2007).

Reynolds, T. and Cole, E. (2006) 'Techniques for acute wound closure', *Nursing Standard* **20**(21), 55–64.

Smith and Nephew Ltd (2000) *Leg Ulcers The Facts. Formulary support service*, Hull, Smith and Nephew Ltd.

Templeton, S. (2004) 'Nursing documentation and legal considerations in wound management' [online] www.sawma.org.au/newsletters/2004/sawma_documentation_and_legalities_wound_management.pps (accessed 10 March 2007).

Tyco Health Care (2007) 'Arterial ulcers', Tyco Health Care [online] www.kendallhq.com/catalog/ClinicalInformation/Arterial%20Ulcers.pdf (accessed 30 January 2007).

Wayne, L. E. and Bunn, L. (2007) pp. 74–83 in Cleaver, K. and Webb, J. (eds), *Emergency Care of Children and People* Oxford, Blackwell Science.

Chapter

32

Aseptic technique and wound management

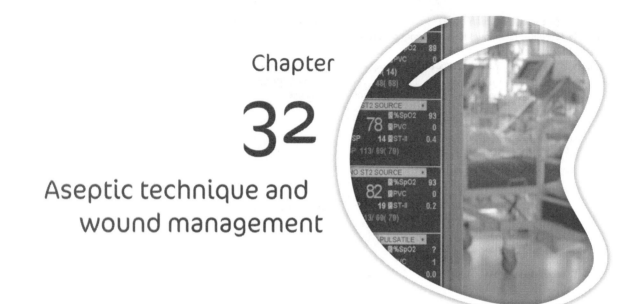

Pauline Cardwell

Links to other chapters in *Foundation Skills for Caring*

Links to other chapters in *Foundation Studies for Caring*

W Don't forget to visit www.palgrave.com/glasper for additional online resources relating to this chapter.

Introduction

Wound care is an essential aspect of nursing and as such all professional practitioners must ensure their knowledge and skills are up to date so that the care they provide is evidence-based and effective. With increasing evidence and insights into wound healing processes, this area of nursing care is developing into a diverse and challenging area of practice. This aspect of care is supported by the development of roles such as that of the tissue viability nurse, who possesses expert knowledge and skills relating to the management of wounds, and as such is a valuable resource. The nurse must understand the wound healing process and the principles of wound management so as to accurately assess wounds and their progress, with the appropriate use of dressings and nursing care to support healing.

Initially, it is pertinent to define the term wound to ensure that a common view of the concept is shared at the beginning of this chapter. *The Oxford Mini-dictionary for Nurses* (1998: 677) defines a wound as 'a break in the structure of an organ or tissue caused by an external agent; for example a bruise, cut or burn'. Wounds can be further classified according to the nature of the injury, the stage of the healing process and any underlying associated illnesses.

Learning outcomes

This chapter will enable you to:

- review the wound healing process
- discuss the principles which underpin asepsis
- describe the procedure with evidence-based rationale for:
  - using aseptic technique
  - preparation of equipment
  - wound assessment and cleansing
  - choice of wound dressings
  - wound drains
  - wound closure – sutures and staples
  - care planning and documentation
- discuss possible hazards and problems associated with wound management, including standard precautions of infection control, nutritional intake and nursing care.

Concepts

- Wound healing
- Principles of asepsis
- Wound dressing equipment
- Wound assessment
- Problems associated with wound management
- Wound dressings
- Pain assessment and management
- Wound closure and drains
- Care planning

The wound healing process

Wound healing is a highly complex process which is not yet fully appreciated; however it is known that the process consists of three phases:

- the inflammatory/destructive phase
- the proliferation stage
- the maturation stage.

Whilst children experience the same stages in the wound healing process as adults, it is worth noting that several factors influence wound healing in children, including increased metabolic rate and efficient circulation which contribute to a dynamic healing response (Bastin and Newton, 2007).

After an injury occurs or a wound is sustained, the initial *inflammatory phase* of the healing process is initiated. This stage involves increased cell activity that causes redness and heat at the site. The damaged tissues release various enzymes and histamine, which triggers a vasodilation reaction and increases the cell permeability, leading to the leakage of inflammatory exudates which includes plasma, antibodies and white cells that cause swelling and oedema of the surrounding tissue. Macrophages arrive at the site of injury and provide a defence against bacteria (Tortora and Reynolds Grabowski, 2000). This phase may last up to six days after the injury.

Some texts (Taylor, 2001; Bastin and Newton, 2007) discuss the discrete *destruction phase*, which occurs concurrently, from two to five days following injury, and relates to the role of macrophages in wound healing. The macrophages continue alongside polymorphs in clearing devitalised tissue whilst also continuing to attack bacteria. Fibroblasts begin to develop which initiate the creation of collagen fibres, during which time it is essential not to disturb the wound in order to support tissue regeneration (Collier, 2003).

The second main phase of the wound healing process occurs usually from the third day to day 24 after the injury, and is known as the *proliferation phase*. Collagen fibres support the healing of the wound edges, whilst cells start to migrate across the wound supported by the growth of new blood vessels and hair follicles; epithelialisation takes place during this phase. The presence of moisture is essential in supporting the healing process throughout the whole process and is known to accelerate repair of the wound (Bryan, 2004). The growth of new blood vessels around the framework provided by the collagen structure is referred to as angiogenesis. Whilst the wound edges appear strong, the healing is at a delicate stage and requires care to prevent further damage or any interruptions to the healing processes (Kingsley, 2002).

The final phase of wound healing is the *maturation phase*, which involves the re-epithelialisation and reorganisation of the collagen fibres. This phase of the process usually starts from around 24 days after the injury and can continue for up to one year. After epithelialisation has occurred the vascularity of the wound reduces, thus causing the wound to appear less red; with the reorganisation of the collagen fibres the size of the scar reduces during this maturation phase.

Principles of asepsis

Asepsis is the practice of reducing or eliminating the entry of contaminants into the operative wound in order to prevent infection. Ideally, a wound is 'sterile' or free of contaminants, a situation that is difficult to attain. However, the goal is elimination of infection, not sterility. Aseptic technique, or aseptic non-touch technique (ANTT) as it is sometimes referred to, has several aims which include:

- promoting healing through the creation of an optimal environment in which healing can occur
- ensuring the reduction of any risk of cross-infection through the appropriate use of personal protective equipment and good hand hygiene
- preventing the introduction of infection due to poor wound management technique, and the use of appropriate dressing and wound care products.

In order to heal effectively, the wound has several requirements that must be met; these include moisture, warmth, and a good blood and nutrient supply. Nursing care and wound management practices should aim to support and meet these requirements. The use of an aseptic technique during the assessment and dressing of wounds will reduce the risk of introducing infection to the wound site. Simultaneously, it is important to recognise and use effective personal protective equipment (PPE) such as aprons and gloves, whilst also ensuring effective hand hygiene practices before providing wound care to the infant, child, young person or adult. The World Health Organization (2005) in the 'Clean Hospital, Clean Healthcare' programme identifies the key role of good hand hygiene by practitioners as an undervalued activity in the realisation of this initiative.

Handwashing technique

Figure 32.1 demonstrates how to wash your hands in a socially clean technique, as supported by NICE (2003). There is more information on handwashing in Chapter 30.

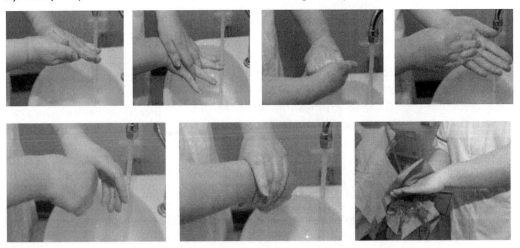

Figure 32.1
How to wash your hands

Using aseptic technique

In attempting to achieve an aseptic technique (ANTT) the nurse aims not to contaminate the wound and to prevent the introduction of infection where possible (Gould, 2001). This can be very challenging, especially if you are working with an infant, child or young person who is frightened, upset and unwilling for the nurse to 'touch' the injury or wound. The importance of good hand hygiene cannot be overestimated as the key to achieving an aseptic technique. With an increasing focus on infection control by both healthcare organisations and the general public, practitioners must update their knowledge and skills regularly in infection control management.

The use of sterile equipment and dressing products when delivering wound care is another key aspect in achieving aseptic technique. It is important to choose equipment or dressing products which will support effective, evidence-informed wound care whilst preventing disruption to the healing process, for example by the over-zealous cleaning of a wound bed with cotton wool swabs or use dressing products which are easily dislodged.

Preparation of equipment

In preparing to perform aseptic technique, it is essential the practitioner prepares all equipment required or potentially required for the activity prior to performing the wound care, as interruptions can increase the risk of introducing infection, cause distress to the patient and delay the completion of the procedure. Equipment such as dressing packs and wound care products should be examined for undamaged packaging and expiry dates during this preparation stage of the activity, to ensure sterility of equipment prior to usage. Essential equipment required includes:

- trolley or appropriately clean surface, washed with detergent and water and disinfected with 70 per cent ethyl alcohol hard surface wipe
- a sterile dressing pack containing a gallipot, disposable clinical waste bag, swabs, forceps, non-woven balls, sterile gloves and additional sterile field
- normal saline (0.9 per cent sodium chloride), warmed
- appropriate dressing – refer to patient's care plan or dependent on wound assessment recommendations
- surgical tape and bandaging if required to secure dressing
- sterile scissors: to modify dressing to wound contours and to cut tape

Part

IV

- PPE: plastic apron, clean disposable gloves for removal of old dressing, and hand disinfectant.

In children's nursing it is important to note the vital role of the practitioner in preparing the child and parent for the procedure, giving age-appropriate information and using distraction techniques (Taylor, 2001). Infants, children or young people and their parents may be distressed if they have just sustained the wound, are in pain or fearful of the procedure, or have previously experienced a painful dressing change. The children's nurse must help the child and parent to discuss their concerns by explaining the procedure and answering any questions posed, appropriately and honestly.

Wound assessment and cleansing

Initially it is important to perform an accurate assessment of the wound, taking account of the holistic needs of the patient. In order to perform such an assessment a sound knowledge of the wound healing process and familiarity with the wound assessment tool may assist the nurse in effectively managing the wound. Vuolo (2006) advocates timely and effective care as being integral to the healing process, which is further supported by accurate, structured assessment of the wound and its healing. Factors that should be considered in the assessment of wounds include:

- wound site and appearance
- nature of injury
- size and depth of wound
- condition of surrounding skin
- appearance of wound including stage of healing
- presence and level of exudate
- signs of infection including odour
- associated pain
- the patient's response to the wound
- environment
- mobility
- nutritional status
- underlying conditions which may effect the healing process
- medications.

Wound cleansing is an area of care around which there is a lot of debate regarding the type of cleansing and suitable solutions for this procedure. Bastin and Newton (2007) suggest wound cleansing should only be performed if there is obvious debris in the wound bed, by the use of gentle irrigation with a syringe and warmed sterile saline. The use of steripods and gentle swabbing around the wound is sufficient to cleanse the area without disrupting the healing process. Vuolo (2006) also highlights the need to avoid cleansing wounds that are clean and have minimal exudate as this may cause pain and has no purpose. In her article on the use of tap water for wound cleansing, Platt (2005) identifies it as cost effective, safe and a more convenient means of wound cleansing; however she emphasises the need to base this on an individual assessment of the patient. Briggs (2006) in a systematic review identifies tap water as being effective in cleaning simple lacerations in children. The most commonly used solutions for wound cleansing are sterile saline and tap water; the choice should be based on individual assessment of the wound and the holistic assessment of the patient.

Choice of wound dressing

Careful reflection on the type of dressing required is vital in supporting wound healing, and requires the nurse to be familiar with the types of dressings available and their individual properties. In choosing wound dressings there are certain criteria that the product must meet in relation to the needs of the individual; these include:

- supporting high humidity, so providing an optimal wound-healing environment
- removal of excess exudate and debris
- impermeability to micro-organisms

Table 32.1 Choice of wound dressing

Dressing	Action	Indications for use	Guidelines for use
Thin hydrocolloid: Activheal Hydrocolloid®	Encourages autolysis to debride wounds that are sloughy or necrotic. Waterproof. Provides an optimal moist wound healing environment.	Low to moderate exudating wounds (e.g. extravasation injury). Protect vulnerable skin (e.g. bony pressure sites).	Choose a dressing which allows for 1–2 cm overlap onto healthy skin. Do not replace unless clinically indicated.
No-sting barrier film and cream: Cavilon®	Provides a waterproof barrier. Provides a protective interface between the skin and bodily fluids, adhesive products and friction.	As a primary barrier against irritation from bodily fluids (e.g. faeces, urine). A protective barrier against adhesives from wound dressings and surgical tapes. Skin protection around stoma sites. Peri-wound protection from exudate damage. Protection from damage caused by friction and shear. Can be used on broken skin.	Clean and dry skin. Apply coat of film; allow drying for 30 seconds. Ensure skin contact areas are separated and allowed to dry before returning to normal position (e.g. cleft of buttocks). Reapply every 24 hours (nappy area). Reapply following removal of stoma bag, surgical tape, wound dressing. Do *not* use on infected skin.
Nonadherent dressing: Mepitel®	Mepitel is a nonadherent soft silicone wound dressing. It minimises trauma/pain at wound dressing as it only adheres to dry healthy skin, and not a moist wound bed. It minimises maceration and does not compromise fragile surrounding skin.	Skin tears, abrasions. Surgical incisions. Second degree burns. Blisters. Lacerations. Partial and full thickness grafts. If in doubt use Mepitel.	Mepitel should overlap the surrounding skin by 2 cm, if necessary cut to size. Moisten gloves with sterile saline to avoid gloves adhering to Mepitel. In large area, dressings may be overlapped but ensure the pores are not blocked. Mepitel is *not* absorbent so a wound will need to be covered with an absorbent secondary dressing. Mepitel can be left in place on a wound bed for up to *seven* days. The wound must still be *inspected* on a regular basis. The wound can be cleaned by irrigating through the Mepitel and then a new secondary dressing applied. Hydrogel can also be applied to the wound through the Mepitel. Mepitel should only be left in place if it is still effective and the wound bed can still be visualised after irrigation. Change Mepitel *before* seven days if the wound is infected or the Mepitel is compromised. If used for fixation of skin grafts and protection of blisters, Mepitel should not be changed for five days. *Wounds must still be monitored regularly for signs of infection and/or deterioration.*

Dressing	Action	Indications for use	Guidelines for use
Hydrogel: Askina Gel® Actiform Cool®	Facilitates the autolytic debridement of sloughy and necrotic tissue.	Can be used on flat or cavity wounds where there is no exudate (e.g. dry, sloughy and necrotic wounds).	Apply directly to area of wound that requires to be rehydrated. Can be kept in place with a film dressing, hydrocolloid or foam.
Foam dressing: Mepilex®	Absorbs exudate. Low adherence, Adhesive and nonadhesive versions available.	Wounds with moderate exudate. As a secondary dressing when Hydrogel is required.	Mepilex can be left in place on a wound bed for up to *seven* days. The wound must still be *inspected* on a regular basis.
Film dressings: Opsite® Tegaderm®	Helps prevent bacterial contamination. Is waterproof.	To secure non adhesive dressings. To protect friction sites.	Use on prepared dry skin. For removal: alternatively stretch and release the film section to break the adhesive bond.
Alginate: Kaltostat®	Wounds with moderate to high exudate level		Use Mepitel at base of all wounds prior to applying Kaltostat to prevent adherence to wound bed. Can be kept in place with a film dressing or foam.

- being age appropriate
- easily removed: atraumatic for children (although this may also be a disadvantage if the child can remove the dressing easily)
- conformable to wound site
- cosmetically pleasing, particularly for the young person if wound dressings are visible to others
- hypoallergenic
- protecting and providing additional padding for wound to prevent further trauma
- cost-effective
- available both in the hospital and community setting.

Please note that other products such as silver dressings, honey, topical negative pressure and larvae treatment may also be of benefit to the patient under the direction of an experienced wound care practitioner.

⚠ Professional alert!

It is not possible to include all types of dressings available in Table 32.1. Additionally, it is worth noting that wound care is a dynamic area of care provision and new products are constantly being produced and marketed. Therefore it is prudent to recommend that manufacturer's guidelines and literature are consulted prior to using any product with which you are not familiar.

Securing dressings and dressing removal

Equally important is the securing of dressings, as excessive movement or disturbance can reduce healing or increase the incidence of infection. Most dressing products come with an adhesive option and it is important to discuss with the patient, child or parent the importance of not tampering with the dressing product whilst it is in place. Adhesive dressings are an obvious choice to promote the security of the dressing, but on occasions the use of supplementary, secondary dressings is required. Additional securing may be in the form of vapour-permeable film borders if compatible with the primary dressing, bandaging or the use of tubular conforming stockinette to support the security of the primary dressing.

Dressing removal can cause a lot of distress and anxiety particularly to the child, young person or parent and this requires careful consideration when selecting a dressing. Moffatt

(2002) and Moffatt, Franks and Hollinworth (2002) identify pain associated with dressing removal as the most important factor to consider when changing a dressing. Strategies to manage pain and prevent trauma, including the choice of dressings which possess pain-free removal characteristics, are major considerations for the children's nurse. The use of adhesive removal wipes or of sterile solutions to aid pain-free removal can be effective in reducing the pain associated with the dressing change. Furthermore, it is important to ensure that the surrounding skin is kept clean and dry and that care is taken to reduce trauma during dressing changes; the use of a barrier film may prove beneficial in protecting the skin and reducing the discomfort associated with dressing removal.

Pain management

It is important at this juncture to mention the key role of good pain management in wound care, which should aim to reduce and minimise the pain experienced in the provision of care. Nevertheless, several aspects of care provision may contribute to the pain experienced, including poor aseptic technique, choice of dressing or wound assessment skills (Jones, 2004). The timely and appropriate use of a pain assessment tool such as QUESTT (Baker and Wong, 1987) and management strategies should form part of the nursing care provided to the patient and should be incorporated in the plan of care (Clay and Chen, 2005). This is equally relevant in the case of the patient who has sustained an injury which will be treated in the A&E department or who has a chronic wound dressed by the community nurse. Pain assessment tools should be appropriate to the age and cognitive development of any infant, child or young person, and should be used regularly to assess the pain experiences and to evaluate the efficiency of any interventions used to manage the pain.

> **t**☆
> ### Practice tip
>
> Always administer analgesia prior to dressing changes to ensure the child benefits from its analgesic properties. Engage parents in using distraction techniques such as storytelling, reading, bubble blowing, singing or playing simple games, which can help children develop coping strategies.

Wound drains

On occasions, following surgical procedures it may be deemed necessary to insert a wound drain to allow drainage of any fluids collecting around the wound site. Various forms of drainage systems can be used to perform this function; however the principles of care, maintenance and observation remain similar in each situation. Nursing care should focus on observation of wound drainage – amount, type and characteristics; dressings around the site and security of the drain site until removal. Signs of infection at the site, such as redness, swelling, heat, pain and discharge, should also be monitored and noted (Jamieson, Whyte and McCall, 2007). Removal usually occurs within 24–48 hours after an operation, depending on the amount of drainage and the surgeon's preference. Upon removal, the drain site will require close observation for further discharge and the application of a dry dressing for the following 24 hours, and treatment will be dependent on the daily assessment of the wound (Pudner, 2001).

Wound closure

Wounds heal by one of two means, or a combination of both. Primary healing serves to manage wounds where an acute injury has occurred, no significant loss of tissue has taken place and the wound edges come together. Alternatively, with the loss of tissue the wound may heal by secondary intention, where the wound is supported in healing from the wound bed towards the surface, or if the wound is infected a combination of both. This is an area of wound management which requires consideration of the immediate requirements and of the long-term outcomes. Advances in wound management have seen the development of various primary closure products which include wound glue, steristrips, clips and sutures (including dissolvable and subcuticular as those most commonly used). The wound must be accurately assessed and thoroughly cleaned before the most suitable method of closure is chosen (Reynolds and Cole, 2006). For the infant, child or young person it is important to consider the cosmetic effect of using one type of closure over another, as non-dissolvable sutures, staples or infection can lead to permanent scarring or disfigurement. The infant's, child's or young person's compliance with the wound management plan is also integral to recovery, as attempts to remove dressings or suture materials may delay or interfere with wound healing process.

Procedure

Use the following guide to help you provide safe and effective wound care to children.

Support for child and family

1 Introduce yourself to the child and family.
2 Explain the procedure to the child and family and discuss each individual's role.
3 Gain consent to provide care.
4 Answer any queries or concerns.

Interventions

5 Clean the dressing trolley and assemble the equipment required.
6 Bring the trolley to the bedside and screen the area.
7 Ensure the child is positioned comfortably and is informed of what is going to happen.
8 Protect the child's dignity whilst examining and accessing the wound.

9 Wash hands and put on apron.
10 Open the dressing pack and additional requirements; remove the soiled dressing and place in the waste bag provided (if appropriate).
11 Wash hands and put on sterile gloves.
12 Clean the wound and surrounding area as appropriate, utilising evidence to support practice.
13 Apply the appropriate dressing, ensuring this is secured with additional dressings as required.
14 Check the child is comfortable.
15 Dispose of used equipment, including gloves and apron, in a clinical waste bin. Wash hands. Document the care provided and the child's response to it.

Care planning and documentation

It is important to support the continuity of care through the provision of factual, detailed prescriptions of care which accurately reflect the care delivered to the child and family. The Nursing and Midwifery Council (NMC, 2002) identify good record keeping as central to the communication of factual, contemporary and comprehensive information pertaining to the care, progress and treatments the patient has received, whilst denoting a skilled and safe practitioner. In delivering high-quality care for wound management, it is essential to develop prescriptions of care which reflect the care required and which are consistent with meeting the needs of the patient, while using evidence to develop and support plans (Owen, 2005).

In developing care plans relating to the wound it is vital to document accurately the stage of healing, the type of dressing used and any modifications required to the dressing, progress or deterioration, and the response to the dressing procedure. It is also important to document any instruction and teaching provided to the patient during the procedure as this will help to guide other practitioners' care delivery. This ultimately facilitates the continuity of care and collaboration between practitioners and patients (Kirrane, 2001; Singh et al, 2007).

Problems associated with wound management

Thus far we have examined the process of wound healing without considering impediments to its normal course. Indeed there are many intrinsic and extrinsic factors which inhibit the healing process and these will be briefly considered in this section of the chapter. First, it is important to note that for a lot of children, because of their body's general growth and development wounds heal rapidly and without any significant delay (Rossiter, 1997; Casey, 2002). Nevertheless, several factors may impact on the healing process and these include:

- the nature of the injury and its immediate management
- underlying diseases/conditions
- effects of medication on healing
- nutrition
- the presence of infection.

If the wound is sustained from a contaminated source, for example a fall on a dirty surface, a dog bite or an injury caused by a contaminated object, the site of the injury and the immediate first aid provided in cleaning the wound may alter the likelihood of the wound developing an infection. Immediate, thorough cleansing of the sustained injury and application of a clean or sterile dressing supports healing and reduces the risk of infection (Reynolds and Cole, 2006; Morgan and Palmer, 2007). If the injury is of a serious nature immediate medical advice should be sought.

Underlying conditions such as diabetes mellitus, renal disease or those associated with the injury (for example impaired circulation or malnutrition) may impact on the body's ability to respond to the injury and to heal itself. It is important for the nurse to assess these areas and their potential impact on wound healing during the assessment phase of wound management. The appropriate choice of dressings to provide an optimal healing environment and to support and protect the wound will also aid in the healing process.

Infants, children or young people receiving steroid therapy may experience delayed wound healing as these drugs can suppress the inflammatory response of the body and impact on wound healing (Timmons, 2003; Strodtbeck, 2005). Hence the children's nurse must assess the child in a holistic manner in order to identify and respond to any inhibiting factors and to support the tissues whilst healing occurs, including educating or informing the child and family about ways to support healing and what complications to look for. Additionally, consideration of allergies and current drug therapies may limit the choice of drugs used in the wound management plan of care (Reynolds and Cole, 2006).

Having examined the dynamic processes involved in wound healing, it is pertinent to consider the impact of nutrition on wound healing and how a healthy balanced diet supports repair and restoration to health. A diet should be rich in:

- proteins: for tissue repair
- carbohydrates: support increased metabolic rate
- fat: involved in cell formation
- vitamins and minerals: vitamins A, B, C, E and K; iron and zinc – support collagen production, tissue perfusion, skin formation and stimulate cell replication (Kemp, 2001).

For the nurse it is important to discuss with the patient the importance of a healthy, balanced diet in wound healing and to support their dietary intake. When dealing with children, the provision of small, frequent, appetising meals or snacks with attention to the likes and dislikes of the child are important aspects of the holistic nursing care required for the infant, child or young person with a wound.

The presence or subsequent development of infection in a wound has major implications for the patient in relation to healing, discomfort/pain, disability and costs – both personal and in terms of resources in dealing with the infection. Wound infection occurs in relation to the number of bacteria contaminating a wound and the resistance to infection, and may be linked to the type of wound as classified by the Medical Research Council (MRC, 1964, cited by Gould, 2001) as: clean; clean contaminated; contaminated and dirty wounds. The skill of the nurse in recognising the presence of infection (inflammation, discharge, delayed healing, pain, odour, wound breakdown [dehiscence], abscess formation) and ensuring early appropriate management is an essential element in wound care. Early identification of the contaminant and the appropriate antibiotic therapy to treat the infection effectively through wound swabbing and microbiological testing are integral to supporting wound healing. Effective use of standard precautions, including hand hygiene and the pertinent use of PPE, remains a central aspect in preventing, managing and treating wound infections (RCN, 2005).

Conclusion

This chapter has introduced you to the basic principles of aseptic technique and wound management – two of the pillars of quality healthcare delivery.

References

Baker, C. M. and Wong, D. L. (1987) 'A process of pain assessment in children', *Orthopaedic Nursing* **6**(1), 11–21.

Bastin, J. and Newton, H. (2007) 'Wound care', Chapter 4 in Chambers, M. and Jones, S. (eds), *Surgical Nursing of Children*, Edinburgh, Butterworth Heinemann.

Briggs, J. (2006) 'Solutions, techniques and pressure in wound cleansing', *Best Practice* **10**(2), 1–4.

Bryan, J. (2004) 'Moist wound healing: a concept that changed our practice', *Journal of Wound Care* **13**(6), 227–8.

Casey, G. (2002) 'Wound repair: advanced dressing materials', *Nursing Standard* **17**(4), 49–53.

Clay, C. S. and Chen, W. Y. J. (2005) 'Wound pain: the need for a more understanding approach', *Journal of Wound Care* **14**(4), 181–4.

Collier, M. (2003) 'Wound bed preparation: theory to practice', *Nursing Standard* **17**(36), 45–52.

Convatec (2004) *Aquacel Hydrofibre Dressing: Product data sheet*, Deeside, Convatec Limited.

Department of Health, Social Services and Public Safety (DHSSPSNI, 2007) *Northern Ireland Wound Care Formulary*, Belfast, DHSSPSNI.

Gound, D. (2001) 'Clean surgical wounds: prevention of infection', *Nursing Standard* **15**(49), 45–52.

Hampton, S. (2007) 'A focus on ActiForm Cool in the reduction of pain in wounds', *Wound Care*, September, S37–S42.

Jamieson, E. M., Whyte, L. A. and McCall, J. M. (2007) *Clinical Nursing Practices*, 5th edn, Edinburgh, Churchill Livingstone.

Jones, M. L. (2004) 'Minimising pain at dressing changes', *Nursing Standard* **18**(24), 65–70.

Kemp, S. (2001) 'The vital role of nutrition in wound healing', *Primary Health Care* **11**(1), 43–9.

Kingsley, A. (2002) 'Wound healing and potential therapeutic options', *Professional Nurse* **17**(9), 539–44.

Kirrane, C. (2001) 'An audit of care planning on a neurology unit', *Nursing Standard*, **24**(15), 36–9.

Medical Research Council (1964) 'Post operative wound infection', *Annals of Surgery 160–192*, cited in Gould, D. (2001) 'Clean surgical wounds: prevention of infection', *Nursing Standard* **15**(49), 45–52.

Molnlycke Healthcare, Wound care product guide.

Moffatt, C. J. (2002) *Pain at Wound Dressing Changes*, London, Halcyon Print.

Moffatt, C. J., Franks, P. J. and Hollinworth, H. (2002) *Understanding Wound Pain and Trauma: An international perspective*, London, Halcyon Print.

Morgan, M. and Palmer, J. (2007) 'Dog bites', *British Medical Journal* 334, 413–17.

National Institute for Health and Clinical Excellence (NICE) (2003) *Infection Control: Prevention of healthcare-associated infection in primary and community care*, London, NICE.

Nursing and Midwifery Council (NMC) (2002) *Guidelines for Records and Record Keeping*, London, NMC.

Owen, K. (2005) 'Documentation on nursing practice', *Nursing Standard* **19**(32), 48–9.

Oxford Mini-dictionary for Nurses (1998), 4th edn, Oxford, Oxford University Press.

Platt, C. (2005) 'Wound cleansing: is tap water best?' *Primary Health Care* **15**(5), 27–30.

Pudner, R. (2001) 'Post operative dressings in wound management', *Journal of Community Nursing* **15**(9) [online] http://www.jcn.co.uk/journal.asp?MonthNum=09&YearNum=2001&Type=backissie&Articleid=390 (accessed 10 February 2009).

Reynolds, T. and Cole, E. (2006) 'Techniques for acute wound closure', *Nursing Standard* **20**(21), 55–64.

Rossiter, G. (1997) 'Paediatric wound care (editorial)', *Journal of Wound Care* **6**(6), 255.

Royal College of Nursing (RCN) (2005) *Good Practice in Infection Prevention and Control Guidance for Nursing Staff*, London, RCN.

Singh, T., Arbuthnot, J.E., Stevenson, H. and Brown, L. (2007) 'The impact of introducing a care pathway for the treatment of minor paediatric burns', *Journal of Wound Care* **26**(2), 79–82.

Strodtbeck, F. (2005) 'Physiology of wound healing', *Newborn and Infant Nursing Reviews* **1**(1), 43–52.

Taylor, K. (2001) 'The management of minor burns and scalds in children', *Nursing Standard* **16**(11), 45–51.

Timmons, J. P. (2003) 'Factors that compromise wound healing', *Primary Health Care* **13**(5), 43–9.

Tortora, G. and Reynolds Grabowski, S. (2000) *Principles of Anatomy and Physiology*, 9th edn, New York, John Wiley.

Vuolo, J. C. (2006) 'Assessment and management of surgical wounds in clinical practice', *Nursing Standard* **20**(52), 46–56.

World Health Organization (WHO) (2005) *Global Patient Safety Challenge*, Geneva, WHO.

Chapter

33

Central venous catheters

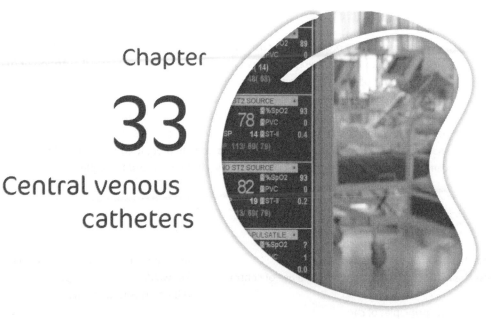

Janet Kelsey

Links to other chapters in *Foundation Skills for Caring*

28 Routes of medication administration
30 Universal precautions
32 Aseptic technique and wound management
38 Clinical holding for care, treatment or interventions

Links to other chapters in *Foundation Studies for Caring*

8 Healthcare governance
10 Nutritional assessment and needs
13 Infection prevention and control
14 Pharmacology and medicines

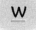

Don't forget to visit www.palgrave.com/glasper for additional online resources relating to this chapter.

Part
IV

Introduction

A central venous line provides long-term intravenous access and is used in a child or adult when their treatment includes therapy such as cytotoxic drugs, total parenteral nutrition or frequent administration of intravenous antibiotics. Insertion of the catheter is usually performed by a surgeon or an anaesthetist under general anaesthetic in children and local anaesthetic and sedation in adults. The procedure takes place using ultrasound imaging for insertion and accurate location of the final position of the catheter tip. This chapter discusses the care and management of central venous lines in adults and children. It considers the different types of central venous catheters, the risks associated with their use and principles of care.

Learning outcomes

This chapter will enable you to:

- discuss the rationale for using central lines
- discuss the risk factors associated with the use of central lines
- understand the principles of care
- underpin care with appropriate evidence-based knowledge
- reflect on your learning.

Concepts

- Central venous catheters
- Universal precautions
- General asepsis
- Risk factors
- Catheter-related bloodstream infections
- Wound dressings

A central venous catheter (CVC) is an intravenous device whose tip is placed in a large central vein, where it floats freely within the bloodstream in parallel to the vein wall. Types of CVC include short-term and long-term catheters such as tunnelled catheters (also known as Hickman lines), PICCs (peripherally inserted central catheters) and IPs (implantable ports, or portacaths). Single and multilumen catheters are available. The type to be used should be decided prior to insertion and depends on the range of uses anticipated (for example, multiple drug and fluid administration). As a general principle the lumen diameter and the number of lumens should be kept to a minimum, using single lumen catheters unless multiple ports are essential for the management of the patient (Pratt et al, 2007). Single lumen catheters are preferred for parenteral nutrition, however if multiple lumens are essential, then one lumen should be dedicated 'exclusively for that purpose' (except in neonates) (Pratt et al, 2007). Guidelines recommend considering the use of an antimicrobial or impregnated CVC for adults who require short-term (one to three weeks) CVC access and who are at risk of catheter-related bloodstream infections (CRBSI), where rates of CRBSI are high despite prevention strategies (CDC, 2002; Pratt et al, 2007).

Several factors are taken in to consideration when choosing the insertion site of CVC. These include patient-specific factors such as anatomic deformity, pre-existing CVC or bleeding diathesis, risk of mechanical complications such as bleeding, pneumothorax and thrombosis, and the risk of infection. Pratt and colleagues (2007) confirm that in adult patients the subclavian site is preferred for infection control purposes; however there is potential for mechanical complications and risk of subclavian vein stenosis. Catheters inserted into the internal jugular vein have a higher risk of catheter-related infection than those in either the subclavian or femoral veins; however femoral catheters have high colonisation rates in adults and should be avoided due to the higher risk of deep vein thrombosis. The use of ultrasound in placing catheters reduces mechanical complications and therefore may indirectly reduce the risk of infection by enabling uncomplicated catheter placement (NICE, 2002).

> ### Practice tip
>
> Choose a line with the least number of ports/hubs according to what is required.

Central venous lines have several uses:

- to monitor central venous pressure (CVP)
- diagnosis (for example, evidence of underlying cardiac pathology such as cardiac failure)
- drug administration of irritant, vesicant or hyper-osmolar drugs harmful to smaller lumen peripheral veins (for example, potassium chloride, noradrenaline/adrenaline, NahCO$_3$, parenteral nutrition, chemotherapy) or in the absence of suitable peripheral access
- fluid administration (for example, rapid infusion of a high volume of fluid)
- to provide long-term access for frequent or prolonged use (for example, chemotherapy, antibiotics, blood sampling, haemodialysis).

Centrally inserted non-tunnelled CVCs (Figure 33.1) are commonly used in the acute setting. They are not suitable for long-term use because they rarely remain free of infection for longer than seven to ten days; they are also uncomfortable and unsightly.

Tunnelled CVCs (Hickman lines) are intended for longer-term use in patients who require multiple infusions of fluids, blood products, drugs or parenteral nutrition. They are more comfortable and discreet than the non-tunnelled CVCs and can last for much longer. The tunnelled CVC (Figure 33.2) is inserted via the subclavian, jugular or femoral veins; it is tunnelled subcutaneously and exits at a convenient site (usually the chest wall) where it is secured with sutures. Tunnelled catheters have a 'cuff' within the tunnel to allow formation of fibrous tissue; this helps to prevent accidental dislodgement and helps to prevent infection tracking along the line.

PICCs (Figure 33.3) are intended for mid to long-term use in patients who require multiple infusions of fluids, blood products, drugs or parenteral nutrition. They are a common choice for central access in neonatal care. A PICC is a fine-bore CVC inserted into a peripheral vein, usually the basilic or cephalic vein, and threaded upwards towards the heart. PICCs are non-cuffed and therefore require securing to the skin of the patient using sutures, Steri-strips or a dedicated fixing device.

The implantable port (IP) (Figure 33.4) is similar to a tunnelled CVC but has no external parts. Instead of protruding from the patient's chest, the catheter ends in a rubber bulb or reservoir which is buried under the skin. The port is accessed through the skin using either a straight or angled non-coring needle. IPs are therefore more discreet and less intrusive than a tunnelled CVC. Ports require less maintenance when not in use than other types of catheter. They may also offer a lower risk of infection. They are suitable for patients who require long-term frequent and intermittent venous access.

CVCs used for blood processing (for example, haemodialysis, apheresis) may be known as permacaths (tunnelled) or vascaths (non-tunnelled). These catheters differ from other CVCs in the following respects:

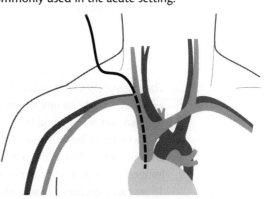

Figure 33.1 Centrally inserted non-tunnelled CVC

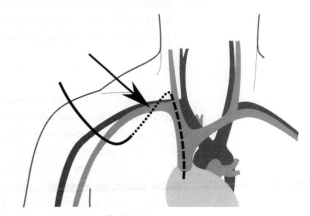

Figure 33.2 Tunnelled CVC

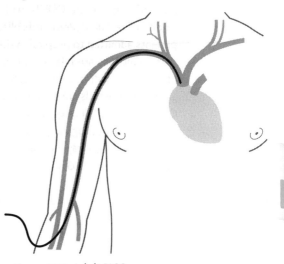

Figure 33.3 Adult PICC

Part

IV

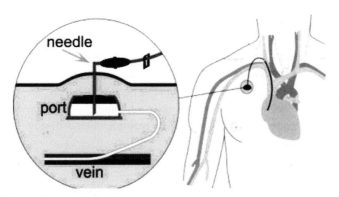

Figure 33.4. Implantable port

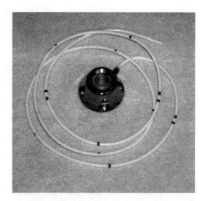

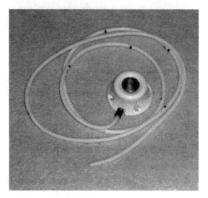

- They have a larger lumen size than other CVCs.
- The internal tip of the catheter is designed to allow blood to be withdrawn freely via one lumen and returned via the other lumen downstream of the blood being withdrawn (thus avoiding recycling of the treated blood). The lumens are often colour-coded red and blue and referred to as the 'arterial' and 'venous' lumens but both lumens lead into a vein and not an artery.
- These catheters may be locked between uses with a concentrated heparin solution to minimise the risk of occlusion. This varies depending on the patient's clinical status and local guidelines. If heparin is used as a lock it must be withdrawn from the catheter before use; otherwise the patient will receive a bolus dose of heparin.

Figure 33.5 Implantable port

Risk factors

Inserting a CVC into the circulatory system puts the patient at risk of local and systemic infections which can include insertion site infections that are spread either directly from the catheter, administration set or through intravenous fluids; CRBSI such as thrombophlebitis, endocarditis and septicaemia; or non-infectious complications such as mechanical or chemical phlebitis, infiltration or extravasation, haematoma, haemorrhage, thrombus, occlusion of blood vessels, air embolism, pneumothorax and fluid overload (CDC, 2002; CPHVA, 2007). Smythe (2006) reports that 42.3 per cent of bloodstream infections (BSI) are central line related and a significant cause of morbidity, estimating that up to 6000 patients a year in England may acquire CRBSIs, with additional costs incurred of £6209 per patient (National Audit Office, 2000). Pratt and colleagues (2007) report that approximately three in every 1000 patients admitted to hospital in the UK acquire a bloodstream infection, and nearly a third of these infections are related to central venous access devices (Coello et al, 2007). Most cases of CRBSI in children are caused by coagulase-negative staphylococci (37.7 per cent), although gram-negative rods are isolated in 25 per cent of PICU bacteraemia cases (Richards et al, 1999). CVC-associated BSI rates in paediatric intensive care units range from 7.7 to 46.9 infections per 1000 CVC-days (Yogari, Elward and Fraser, 2002; Pierce, Wade and Mok, 2000; Gray, Gossain and Morno, 2001; Stover et al, 2001; Urrea et al, 2003; CDC, 2002).

> **a Learning activity**
>
> Identify the main cause of CRBSI and what interventions are in place to reduce the number of CRBSIs in your area of practice?

Principles of care

Table 33.1 Interventions for CVC

Intervention	Recommendations
Education of patients, their carers and healthcare personnel.	→ Healthcare workers should be trained and assessed in catheter insertion. Paediatric specialists should insert catheters in children. → All healthcare personnel caring for a patient with a central venous catheter should be trained, and assessed as competent, in using and consistently adhering to the infection-prevention practices. → Audit of complications associated with central venous catheterisation should be in place. → Before discharge from hospital, patients and their carers should be taught any techniques they may need to use to prevent infection and safely manage a central venous catheter. → Follow-up training and support should be available to patients with central venous catheters and their carers.

Rationale

Organised educational programmes that enable healthcare staff to provide, monitor and evaluate care are critical to the success of reducing infection (CDC, 2002).

Risk of infection decreases with standardisation of aseptic care; insertion and maintenance of CVC by inexperienced staff increases the risk of CRBSI and catheter colonisation (CDC, 2002, 2005).

Intervention	Recommendations
General asepsis.	→ An aseptic technique must be used for catheter site care and for accessing the system. → Before accessing or dressing central vascular catheters, hands must be decontaminated either by washing with an antimicrobial liquid soap and water, or by using an alcohol hand rub. → Hands that are visibly soiled or contaminated with dirt or organic material must be washed with soap and water before using an alcohol hand rub. → Following hand antisepsis, clean gloves and a no-touch technique or sterile gloves should be used when changing the insertion site dressing, carrying out line manipulation or intravenous drug administration.

Rationale

CVCs carry a substantial risk of infection; therefore hand antisepsis and proper aseptic techniques are required for changing dressings and accessing the system (CDC 2002; NICE, 2003).

Intervention	Recommendations
Catheter site care. Monitoring catheter site. Using the right dressing to protect the catheter site.	→ Monitor catheter site visually or by direct palpation through the intact dressing on a regular basis. If patient has tenderness or raised temperature without an obvious source, remove dressing for thorough examination (CDC, 2002). → Monitor temperature, pulse and blood pressure at least daily when the patient is in hospital. → Encourage patients to report changes in catheter site or discomfort. → Use a sterile, transparent, semi-permeable polyurethane dressing to cover the catheter insertion site. → Transparent dressings should be changed every seven days, or sooner if they are no longer intact or moisture collects under the dressing. → If a patient has profuse perspiration or if the insertion site is bleeding or oozing use gauze dressing and replace when damp, loosened or soiled. Assess need for gauze dressing daily and change to transparent dressing as soon as possible. → Dressings used on tunnelled or implanted catheter insertion sites should be replaced every seven days until the insertion site has healed, unless there is an indication to change them sooner. → Do not submerge the CVC underwater; showering is permitted when it is protected by an impermeable cover. → Secure the catheter firmly to the skin away from the exit site with tape or with a dedicated device.

Rationale

The Healthcare Infection Control Practices Advisory Committee (HICPAC) found little difference in which type of dressing provided the greatest protection against infection (CDC, 2002). The choice of dressing is therefore a matter of preference. However, if blood is oozing from the catheter insertion site, a gauze dressing might be preferred. A NICE systematic review (2003) did not find any evidence to conflict with these conclusions.

Securing the catheter is more comfortable, helps to prevent tension or accidental dislodgement, and reduces 'to and fro' motion which may increases the risk of catheter-related sepsis (Haller and Rush, 1992).

Intervention	Recommendations
Catheter site care. Using an appropriate antiseptic agent for disinfecting the catheter insertion site during dressing changes.	→ An alcoholic chlorhexidine gluconate solution (preferably 2 per cent chlorhexidine gluconate in 70 per cent isopropyl alcohol) should be used to clean the catheter insertion site during dressing changes, and allowed to air dry. → Individual sachets of antiseptic solution or individual packages of antiseptic-impregnated swabs or wipes should be used to disinfect the dressing site. → Healthcare personnel should ensure that catheter-site care is compatible with catheter materials (tubing, hubs, injection ports, luer connectors and extensions) and carefully check compatibility with the manufacturer's recommendations. → An aqueous solution of chlorhexidine gluconate should be used if the manufacturer's recommendations prohibit the use of alcohol with the product. → Do not apply topical antibiotic ointment or creams on insertion sites as part of routine care.

Rationale

A recent meta-analysis assessed studies that compared the risk for CRBSI following insertion-site skin care with either any type of chlorhexidine gluconate (CHG) solution or povodine iodine (PI) solution (Chaiyakunapruk et al, 2002); the use of CHG rather than PI can reduce the risk for CRBSI by approximately 49 per cent in hospitalised patients who require short-term catheterisation: for every 1000 catheter sites disinfected with CHG rather than PI, 71 episodes of catheter colonization and 11 episodes of CRBSI would be prevented.

Alcohol and other organic solvents and oil-based ointments and creams may damage some types of polyurethane and silicon CVC tubing. The manufacturer's recommendations for using only disinfectants that are compatible with specific catheter materials must be followed. Topical ointments and creams may increase the rate of fungal infections and antimicrobial resistance (CDC, 2002; Pratt et al, 2007)

Intervention	Recommendation
Principles for catheter management. Accessing the system.	→ The injection port or catheter hub should be decontaminated with either alcohol or an alcoholic solution of chlorhexidine gluconate before and after it has been used to access the system.

Rationale

The risk of introducing infection should be minimised by decontaminating access ports before accessing the system (NICE, 2003).

Intervention	Recommendation
The use of in-line filters.	→ In-line filters, antibiotic lock solutions or systemic anticoagulants should not be routinely used for infection prevention.

Rationale

Although in-line filters reduce infusion-related phlebitis, no evidence was found to support their use in preventing infections associated with intravascular catheters and infusion systems (CDC, 2002). Filtration, in pharmacy, to reduce particulates is more practical and cost effective (Pratt et al, 2007).

Prophylactic use of antibiotic lock solutions is effective in neutropenic patients with long-term CVCs (CDC, 2002). However there is no evidence that routine use in all patients with CVCs reduces the risk of CRBSI and it may lead to increased antimicrobial resistance.

Intervention	Recommendations
The use of intermittent flushes.	→ 0.9 per cent sodium chloride for injection should be used to flush lumens in frequent use. → When recommended by the manufacturer, implanted ports or open-ended catheter lumens should be flushed and locked with heparin sodium flushes.

Rationale

Heparin at doses of 10 U/ml for intermittent flushing is no more beneficial than normal saline on duration of catheter patency or on prevention of complications associated with CVCs (Randolph et al, 1998; Goode et al, 1991; Peterson and Kirchoff, 1991).

Heparin flush solutions may be useful in maintaining patency in infrequently accessed catheter lumens, implantable ports and CVCs used for haemodialysis or apherisis (Pratt et al, 2007).

Intervention	Recommendation
The use of systemic anticoagulants.	→ Systemic anticoagulants should not be used routinely to prevent CRBSI.

Rationale

Heparin administered effectively reduces thrombus formation. However there is no definite evidence that it reduces CRBSI; this may be related to the type of heparin used and its administration (Pratt et al, 2007). Warfarin has been shown to reduce catheter-related thrombus but with the potential for extended prothrombin times.

Intervention	Recommendations
The use of needle-free devices. W —	→ Monitor and report any increase in the occurrence of device associated infection to Medicines and Healthcare Products Regulatory Agency (http://www.mhra.gov.uk). → Follow manufacturer's recommendations for changing the needle-free components and ensure that all components of the system are compatible and secured, to minimise leaks and breaks in the system. → Decontaminate the access port before and after use with a single- patient use application of alcoholic chlorhexidine gluconate solution unless contra-indicated by the manufacturer's recommendations, in which case aqueous povidone iodine should be used.

Rationale

Some of the devices may not be compatible with existing equipment.

Intervention	Recommendations
The use of administration sets.	→ Administration sets in continuous use need not be changed more frequently than every 72 hours unless they become disconnected or a central venous access device is replaced. → Administration sets for blood and blood products should be changed every 12 hours or when the infusion is complete, whichever is sooner, or according to manufacturer's guidelines. → Parenteral nutrition infusion sets should be changed every 24 hours unless the solution contains only glucose and amino acids, and are in continuous use; then this is reduced to every 72 hours.

Rationale

Replacing administration sets no more frequently than 72 hours after initiation of use is safe and cost-effective. When a fluid that enhances microbial growth is infused, more frequent changes are indicated as these products have been identified as independent risk factors for CRBSI.

Intervention	Recommendations
Routine flush of CVCs.	→ Use a brisk 'push–pause' flushing technique: i.e. flush briskly, pausing briefly after approximately each ml of fluid. → If the catheter possesses a clamp, clamp the line while the final ml of the flush is being injected to maintain positive pressure.

Rationale

The 'push–pause' technique causes turbulence within the catheter, which helps to flush away any debris and prevent occlusion of the lumen (RCN, 2003). Maintaining positive pressure may help prevent backflow of blood into the CVC.

⚠ **Professional alert!**

Do not allow untrained personnel to handle CVCs.

Table 33.2 **Complications with CVC**

Complications	Cause	Management
Infection and potential CRBSI indicated by pyrexia and or inflammation/tenderness at exit site.	Poor aseptic technique. Poor handwashing technique. Insufficient education and assessment of health care personnel. Inappropriate catheter and exit site care.	Refer to medical staff. Blood cultures. Exit site swabs. Increase frequency of monitoring TPR and BP. Intravenous antibiotics. In extreme cases the line may have to be removed.
Occlusion.	Catheter kinking. Catheter integrity impaired by thrombus formation or blood or drug precipitate.	Visually check external parts of line, alter patient's position and if line still appears blocked chest x-ray to exclude internal kinks. Consider using an antifibrinolytic agent such as urokinase to dissolve the clot. Consider regular heparinisation as a preventative measure. Can occur if some solutions are not infused correctly. Refer to experienced personnel for removal.
Catheter misplacement. Accidental pulls to the central line. Cuff protrudes from exit site.	 Check the exit site. If there is any drainage on the dressing (clear or bloody) put pressure on the dressing. The line appears to extend out from under the dressing farther than usual or there is a large amount of bleeding. Tissue has failed to adhere to cuff and catheter has migrated out.	There is evidence that ultrasound guided placement of central lines reduces the complication rate associated with this procedure (Dunning, 2003). Refer to experienced staff. Report the incident immediately. Stop infusions, tape catheter securely to skin near exit site; refer to medical staff.
Damage to the central line. Leakage from external portion of catheter when flushed. Pain or visible swelling when catheter is used or fluid leaks from exit site when catheter is flushed.	→ External catheter fracture causes. → Malposition of catheter. → Internal catheter fracture, fibrin sheath, separation of port and catheter (implantable ports). → Incorrect positioning of needle in implantable ports.	Clamp the line above the break close to the exit site. Report the incident immediately as the break may be able to be repaired under aseptic conditions. Report fractures under incident reporting procedures. Refer to medical staff and report fractures under incident reporting procedures.
Cardiopulmonary symptoms including any of the following: respiratory distress/failure apnoea, reduced oxygen saturation levels, tachycardia, bradycardia, hypotension, pallor, cyanosis, anxiety, chest pain, loss of consciousness.	Pneumothorax, air or catheter embolism, pulmonary embolism, cardiac tamponade or pericardial effusion.	Clamp the line close to the exit site. Turn patient so that he/she is lying on his/her heart side. Report the incident immediately. Call for medical assistance. Administer oxygen and monitor vital signs.

⚠ Professional alert!

CVCs carry a substantial risk of infection. Hand antisepsis and proper aseptic technique are therefore required for changing dressings and accessing the system (CDC, 2002; NICE, 2003). CVCs should only be inserted by trained personnel and in an environment which provides the optimal number of air exchanges to prevent infection.

ⓐ Learning activity

Locate the document 'Saving Lives: reducing infection, delivering clean and safe care', *High Impact Intervention No 1: Central venous catheter care bundle*, produced by the Department of Health. It can be downloaded from www.clean-safe-care.nhs.uk. Find out how the compliance tool is being implemented in your area of practice.

Equipment

The basic equipment required for accessing central lines is similar for each procedure, with variations according to the required task:

- trolley or medium-sized tray
- sterile dressing pack
- two sachets of cleaning fluid
- needles blue (23 g) or green (21 g)
- orange needle (25 g) or filter needle
- bare cannulae for tunnelled catheters
- gripper needles of appropriate size and length for use with implanted ports

- 10 ml syringes
- 5 ml Hepsal
- 10 ml normal saline 0.9 per cent
- appropriate blood bottles
- prescription chart
- sterile latex-free gloves
- dressing
- sharps container.

Taking blood

Table 33.3 Taking blood

Action	Rationale
Explain the procedure to the client. Expose the end of the line.	Gain consent and cooperation.
Decontaminate hands either by washing with an antimicrobial liquid soap and water, or by using an alcohol hand rub. Hands that are visibly soiled or contaminated must be washed with soap and water before using an alcohol hand rub.	To avoid microbial contamination.
Ensure appropriate blood bottles are available.	
Using aseptic technique, open dressing pack and empty equipment onto pack.	To provide a clean field to work from.
Gel hands.	To avoid microbial contamination.
Check expiry date and draw up normal saline 0.9 per cent or Hepsal, using filter needle if using glass ampoule, 10 ml syringe and expelling air bubbles. Discard needles.	Filter needle reduces the risk of drawing up glass particles. Pressure of fluids through a central line must not exceed 40 psi (2068 mm Hg); using a syringe smaller than 10 ml may rupture the line. Prevent injection of air.
Put on (sterile) gloves.	To prevent microbial contamination and protect against contamination from the patient's blood.
Place sterile towel on lap with line laid on it.	Maintain clean surface for procedure.
Wipe bung with cleaning fluid and allow to dry.	To prevent microbial contamination.

Part

IV

Action	Rationale
Hold bung with sterile gauze, unclamp line and withdraw 4–5 mls of blood slowly. Clamp line. Discard this blood unless it is required for blood cultures. If clotting studies are required, remove 10 mls of blood if line has previously been heparin locked.	To remove blood that contains previous flush.
Insert new syringe, unclamp line and withdraw blood required for samples. Clamp line and place syringe on tray.	To obtain uncontaminated blood sample.
Insert syringe containing normal saline 0.9 per cent flush into bung, unclamp line, flush with normal saline 0.9 per cent using brisk 'push–pause' flushing technique. Clamp line.	To flush line.
If Hepsal flush is being used, insert syringe into bung, unclamp line, flush and clamp whilst pushing in final 0.5 ml.	To heparin lock line and maintain positive pressure.
If accessing multiple lumens, clean and flush each lumen in the same manner.	To ensure all lumens are flushed.
Secure line into bag or fix to tag.	To prevent catheter misplacement.
Put blood in appropriate bottles following local policy for order of draw and transfer of blood into specimen bottles.	To ensure safe and appropriate sample transfer.
Dispose of all sharps and equipment as per local policy.	To prevent injury to self and others.
Document samples taken in client's records.	

> t☆ **Practice tip**
>
> Do not use central lines for blood sampling if a peripheral site is available.

Administering drugs

Table 33.4 Administering drugs

Action	Rationale
Explain the procedure to the client. Expose the end of the line.	Gain consent and cooperation.
Decontaminate hands either by washing with an antimicrobial liquid soap and water, or by using an alcohol hand rub. Hands that are visibly soiled or contaminated must be washed with soap and water before using an alcohol hand rub.	To avoid microbial contamination.
Using aseptic technique, open dressing pack and empty equipment onto pack.	To provide a clean field to work from.
Gel hands	To avoid microbial contamination.
Check expiry date and draw up medications, and normal saline 0.9 per cent or Hepsal, using filter needle if glass ampoule, 10 ml syringe and expelling air bubbles. Discard needles.	Filter needle reduces the risk of drawing up glass particles. Pressure of fluids through a central line must not exceed 40 psi (2068 mm Hg); using a syringe smaller than 10 ml may rupture the line. Prevent injection of air.
Put on (sterile) gloves.	To prevent microbial contamination and protect against contamination from the patient's blood.
Place sterile towel on lap with line laid on it.	Maintain clean surface for procedure.
Wipe bung with cleaning fluid and allow to dry.	To prevent microbial contamination

Action	Rationale
Hold bung with sterile gauze, unclamp line, flush with 5 ml normal saline 0.9 per cent, clamp line, discard flush syringe, attach syringe containing medication, unclamp line and administer medication according to manufacturer's recommendations, clamp line.	To administer medication according to local policy and manufacturers recommendations.
Insert syringe containing normal saline 0.9 per cent into bung, unclamp line, flush with normal saline 0.9 per cent. Clamp line.	To flush line.
If Hepsal flush is being used, insert syringe into bung, unclamp line, flush and clamp whilst pushing in final 0.5 ml.	To heparin lock line and maintain positive pressure.
If accessing multiple lumens clean and flush each lumen in the same manner.	To ensure all lumens are flushed.
Secure line into bag or fix to tag.	To prevent catheter misplacement.
Dispose of all sharps and equipment as per local policy.	To prevent injury to self and others.

Connecting or changing an infusion set

Table 33.5   Connecting or changing an infusion set

Action	Rationale
Explain the procedure to the client. Expose the end of the line.	Gain consent and cooperation.
Decontaminate hands either by washing with an antimicrobial liquid soap and water, or by using an alcohol hand rub. Hands that are visibly soiled or contaminated must be washed with soap and water before using an alcohol hand rub.	To avoid microbial contamination.
Check and prime appropriate administration set with prescribed intravenous fluid.	To ensure safe administration of intravenous fluid.
Using aseptic technique, open dressing pack and empty equipment onto pack.	To provide a clean field to work from.
Gel hands.	To avoid microbial contamination.
Put on sterile gloves.	To prevent microbial contamination and protect against contamination from the patient's blood.
Place sterile towel on lap with line laid on it.	Maintain clean surface for procedure.
Wipe bung with cleaning fluid and allow to dry.	To prevent microbial contamination.
Hold bung with sterile gauze, unclamp line, flush with 5 ml normal saline 0.9 per cent, clamp line, discard flush syringe, and attach intravenous administration set.	
If the line is already attached to an infusion, clamp the line, clean the connection, allow to dry, then remove and attach new set.	
Check whole system is complete and secure. Open clamp and set infusion to prescribed rate.	
Dispose of all sharps and equipment as per local policy.	To prevent injury to self and others.

Part

IV

Conclusion

This chapter has discussed the rationale for using a central venous line followed by the different types of central venous line available, the positions where they should be sited and their different uses. The risk factors and possible complications for a patient with a central venous line are clearly identified. The use of central venous lines is increasing and the skills required to care for patients with these devices in situ are essential. The general principles of care have been given in this chapter supported by a clear evidence base to help you to develop the knowledge required.

References

Centers for Disease Control and Prevention (CDC) (2002) *Guidelines for Hand Hygiene in Health-Care Settings: Recommendations of the Healthcare Infection Control Practices Advisory Committee and the HICPAC/SHEA/APIC/IDSA Hand Hygiene Task Force,* Morbidity and Mortality Weekly Report 2002;51(No. RR-16):1–45 [online] http://www.cdc.gov/mmwr/PDF/rr/rr5116.pdf (accessed 6 February 2008).

Chaiyakunapruk, N., Veenstra, D., Lipsky B. and Saint, S. (2002) 'Chlorhexidine compared with povidone-iodine solution for vascular catheter-site care: a meta-analysis', *Annals of Internal Medicine* 136, 792–801.

Coello, R., Charlett, A., Ward, V., Wilson, J., Pearson, A., Sedgwick, J. and Borriello, P. (2003) 'Device-related sources of bacteraemia in English hospitals: opportunities for the prevention of hospital-acquired bacteraemia', *Journal of Hospital Infection* 53, 46–57.

Dunnning, J. (2003) 'Ultrasonic guidance and the complications of central line', *Emergency Medicine Journal* 20, 551–2.

Goode, C. J., Titler, M., Rakel, B., Ones, D. S., Kleiber, C. and Small, S. (1991) 'A meta-analysis of effects of heparin flush and saline flush: quality and cost implications', *Nursing Research* 40, 324–30.

Gray, J., Gossain, S. and Morno, K. (2001) 'Three-year survey of bacteremias and fungemia in a pediatric intensive care unit', *Pediatr Infect Dis J* 20, 416–21.

Haller, L. and Rush, K. (1992) 'CVC infection: a review', *Journal of Clinical Nursing* 1, 61–6.

Community Practitioners' and Health Visitors' Association (CPHVA) (2007) 'Central venous catheters', CPHVA, [online] http://www.healthcarea2z.org/ditem.aspx/275/Central+venous+catheters (accessed 8 February 2008).

National Audit Office (NAO) (2000) *The Management and Control of Hospital Aquired Infection in Acute NHS Trusts in England,* London, The Stationery Office, NAO [online] www.nao.org.uk/publications/nao_reports/9900230.pdf.

National Institute for Clinical Excellence (NICE) (2002) 'Guidance on the use of ultrasound locating devices for placing central venous catheters (No. 49)', NICE [online] http://www.nice.org.uk.

NICE (2003) *Infection Control: Prevention of healthcare-associated infection in primary and community care,* Clinical guideline 2 [online] http://www.nice.org.uk (accessed 6 February 2008).

Peterson, F. Y. and Kirchoff, K. T. (1991) 'Analysis of the research about heparinized versus nonheparinized intravascular lines', *Heart and Lung* 20, 631–40.

Pierce, C. M., Wade, A. and Mok Q. (2000) 'Heparin-bonded central venous lines reduce thrombotic and infective complications in critically ill children', *Intensive Care Med* 26, 967–72.

Pratt, R .J., Pellowe, C., Loveday, H. P., Robinson, N., Smith, G. W. and the Epic Guideline Development Team (2007) 'The epic project: developing national evidence-based guidelines for preventing healthcare associated infections, phase 1: guidelines for preventing hospital-acquired infections', *Journal of Hospital Infection,* 47(Supplement), January, S1–S82.

Randolph, A., Cook, D., Gonzales, C. and Brun-Buisson, C. (1998) 'Tunneling short-term central venous catheters to prevent catheter-related infection: a meta-analysis of randomized controlled trials', *Critical Care Medicine* 26, 1452–7.

Royal College of Nursing (2003) IV Therapy Forum '*Standards for Infusion Therapy,* London, RCN.

Richards, M. J., Edwards, J. R., Culver, D. H. and Gaynes, R. P. (1999) 'Nosocomial infections in the pediatric intensive care units in the United States: national nosocomial infections surveillance system', *Pediatrics* 103, e39.

Rowley, S. (2001) 'Aseptic non touch technique (ANTT)', *Nursing Times* **97**(7) Infection Control Supplement VI–VIII.

Smythe, E. T. M. (2006) 'Healthcare acquired infection prevalence survey 2006', presented at the 6th international conference of the Hospital Infection Society, Amsterdam, Preliminary data available in Hospital Infection Society (2006) *The Third Prevalence Survey of Healthcare Associated Infections in Acute Hospitals* [online] www.his.org.uk (accessed 10 February 2009).

Stover, B. H., Shulman, S. T., Bratcher, D. F., Brady, M. T., Levine, G. L. and Jarvis, W. R. (2001) 'Nosocomial infection rates in US children's hospitals' neonatal and pediatric intensive care units', *Am J Infect Control* 29, 152–7.

Yogaraj, J. S., Elward, A. M. and Fraser, V. J. (2002) 'Rate, risk factors and outcomes of nosocomial primary bloodstream infection in pediatric intensive care unit patients', *Pediatrics* 110, 481–5.

Urrea, M., Pons, M., Serra, M., Latorre, C. and Palomeque, A. (2003) 'Prospective incidence study of nosocomial infections in a pediatric intensive care unit', *Pediatr Infect Dis J* 22, 490–4.

Chapter

34

Blood transfusion

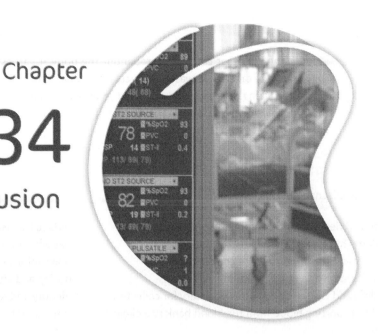

Siobhan MacDermott
and Karen Merrick

Links to other chapters in *Foundation Skills for Caring*

25 Intravenous therapy
28 Routes of medication administration
30 Universal precautions

Links to other chapters in *Foundation Studies for Caring*

4 Ethical, legal and professional issues
8 Healthcare governance
13 Infection prevention and control

Don't forget to visit www.palgrave.com/glasper for additional
online resources relating to this chapter.

Part

IV

Introduction

Blood is the fluid that circulates throughout the body. It carries oxygen and nourishment to the tissues and takes away waste products. It is made up of several different components. The blood circulating in your body is referred to as 'whole blood'. This chapter aims to highlight the principles of blood transfusion (transferring blood from one person into the veins of another).

Learning outcomes

This chapter will enable you to:

- outline different blood components and explain why they might be prescribed
- understand the importance of correct patient identification and sample labelling
- understand the safety measures necessary for collecting and transporting blood from the blood bank to a clinical area
- reduce the risks of transfusion by using appropriate patient and component identification checks
- make informed decisions about patient care before, during and after a blood transfusion
- identify and respond to an adverse reaction to transfused blood.

Concepts

- Blood components
- ABO blood group system
- Blood transfusion equipment
- Haemovigilance
- Adverse effects of blood transfusion
- Education and training

Composition of blood

Blood is basically composed of red cells and plasma in which other highly specialised cells are suspended. These include platelets, white blood cells and clotting factors.

An adult has about five litres of blood in circulation. The total blood volume is related to body mass.

Table 34.1 Total blood volume by body mass

Category	mL/kg	Approx blood volume
Adult male	70 mL/kg	90 kg = 6300 mL
Adult female	70 mL/kg	60 kg = 4200 mL
Child	80 mL/kg	30 kg = 2400 mL
Neonate	85–90 mL/kg	3 kg = 255–270 mL

Blood transfusion is an important and frequently lifesaving treatment and its use in clinical practice is common. However transfusion of blood products has only become commonplace in the last 100 years.

Historical review

The first human-to-human blood transfusion was carried out by James Blundell in 1818 in the United Kingdom (Giangrande, 2000). In 1901, ABO blood groups was discovered by Karl Landsteiner, who was awarded the Nobel prize for medicine in 1930. It was not until 1940 that the Rhesus antigens were identified in humans by Landsteiner and Wiener.

1818 First human-to-human blood transfusion – James Blundell.
1901 ABO blood group system discovered – Karl Lansteiner.

1940   Rhesus antigen system identified – Landsteiner and Wiener.

1948   National Blood Transfusion Service established in the UK.

1996   Serious Hazards of Transfusion (SHOT) – UK reporting scheme set up to identify blood component transfusion errors.

1999   National Haemovigilance Office (NHO) – Irish reporting scheme set up to identify blood component transfusion errors.

Approximately 2.5 million units of blood are supplied annually in the UK, of which 40–50 per cent are used in both elective and emergency surgery (Wells et al, 2002).

Transfusion can sometimes have serious and even fatal consequences, particularly when a haemolytic response occurs due to an incompatible transfusion (SHOT, 1998, 1999).

In the United Kingdom, Serious Hazards of Transfusion (SHOT) is a reporting scheme which identifies blood component transfusion errors also known as haemovigilance. Since its introduction the risks of receiving a blood transfusion have been highlighted. In 2005, EU Directive 2002/98 made reporting of serious transfusion reactions mandatory.

SHOT collated reports of serious transfusion hazards for the period 1996–2003, during which time 23 million units of blood components were supplied. The incidence of serious adverse reactions (per 100,000 units of blood supplied) was death, 0.2, and major morbidity, 1.1 (Stainsby et al, 2004).

Haemovigilance has been defined as:

> A set of surveillance procedures, from the collection of blood and its components to the follow-up of recipients, to collect and assess information on unexpected or undesirable effects resulting from the therapeutic use of labile blood products, and to prevent their occurrence or recurrence.
>
> (French Law, regulation no. 93–5, 4 January 1993)

In the United Kingdom, the chance that a unit of blood might transmit one of the viruses such as HIV or Hepatitis C for which blood is tested is lower, and estimated at HIV 0.14 per million, Hepatitis C virus 0.8 per million, and Hepatitis B virus 1.66 per million. Indeed more patients may be put at risk by receiving the wrong blood component (6:100,000) including ABO incompatible blood (1:100,000).

Similar haemovigilance programmes have been set up in other countries. In Ireland, the NHO is responsible for the collection and analysis reports of adverse events related to transfusion since 1999. In addition a 'near miss' programme was set up in the UK and Ireland to examine weaknesses and identify potential errors in the transfusion chain. In 2005, SHOT reported 1358 near-miss incidents, an increase of 26 per cent compared with 2004. Patient misidentification at the blood sampling stage resulting in 'wrong blood in tube' was the most common near-miss incident (SHOT, 2005).

The focus of SHOT in recent years has been on improving the safety of blood administration at the bedside. However, errors in hospital transfusion laboratories were responsible for 37 per cent of incorrect blood component transfused (IBCT) cases reported in 2005 in the United Kingdom. Haemovigilance programmes such as SHOT have clearly indicated that there are serious but avoidable risks to which recipients of blood transfusion are exposed (Wilkinson and Wilkinson, 2001).

Further, the UK Blood Safety and Quality Regulations 2005 and the EU Blood Safety Directive require that serious adverse events and serious adverse reactions related to blood and blood components are reported to the Medicines and Healthcare Products Regulatory Agency (MRHA), the UK Competent Authority for blood safety. Professionals involved in the transfusion process, such as blood banks/hospital transfusion teams, can use the MHRAs secure and confidential online reporting system. Reports of serious adverse event or serious adverse can be submitted electronically to the MHRA. This new reporting system is known as SABRE (Serious Adverse Blood Reactions and Events).

'Right patient–right blood' is an initiative aimed at reducing the risk of ABO-incompatible transfusions by improving the safety of blood administration (SHOT, 2005).

Part

IV

Blood groups

There are four major blood groups, O, A, B and AB.

Blood groups are also subdivided into Rhesus type, and are identified as Rhesus positive or Rhesus negative.

ABO system

- Group AB: has no ABO antibodies in its plasma.
- Group B: has Anti A antibody in its plasma.
- Group A: has Anti B antibody in its plasma.
- Group O: has Anti A + Anti B antibody in its plasma (McClelland, 2007).

Rhesus system

- Rhesus positive consists of positive Rhesus antigens on the red cell.
- Rhesus negative has no Rhesus antigens on the surface of the red cell.
- 80 per cent of Rhesus negative people readily produce Anti D upon stimulation.
- Anti D is an immune antibody.
- Antigenic stimulation includes:
  - blood transfusion
  - pregnancy
  - sharing needles (drug addicts).

Antibodies

- Antibodies can be formed within days of a transfusion.
- They can be formed up to six months after a transfusion.
- They are rare – usually not formed at all.

⚠ Professional alert!

Patients who have been transfused or have been pregnant can produce one or more immune antibodies.

A fresh sample (less than 24 hours) is required from patients who have previously been pregnant or if a transfusion has been received in the last 72 hrs (McClelland, 2007).

Table 34.2 ABO blood group compatibility

Patient blood group	Compatible with	Approximate percentage in the UK
O	O	47%
A	A and O	42%
B	B and O	8%
AB	AB, A, B and O	3%

Source: adapted from Contreras (1998).

Table 34.3 Red cells and plasma that can receive transfusions from specific blood groups

A B O Blood groups				
Patient's blood group	A	B	AB	O
Can receive red cells from	A and O	B and O	ALL	O only
Can receive plasma from	B	A	ALL	AB only

Table 34.4 Different types of blood products, usage, volume and storage

Component	Description	Indication for use	Average volume	Storage
Red cell concentrate	Made following the collection of whole blood, dividing it into separate components and removing most of the plasma (generally 20 ml of plasma remains per unit plus an additive solution).	Used to increase tissue oxygenation and for the treatment of anaemia or haemorrhage.	250–330 ml.	35 days @ between 2 °C and 6 °C (McClelland, 2007)
Pedi-packs	One unit of the above is divided into five separate parts.	To reduce donor exposure for infants under 12 months during the above episodes.	5 × 50 ml.	35 days @ +2 – +6 °C (McClelland, 2007).
Platelet concentrate	A unit of platelets from four or five donors, banked together from platelets removed from four or five donations of blood.	For the treatment of patients with platelet function defects.	198–250 ml.	5 days @ 22 °C +/– 2 °C (McClelland, 2007).
Platelets (apheresis)	A full unit of platelets collected from one donor only.	As above.	198–250 ml.	5 days @ 22 °C +/– 2 °C (McClelland, 2007).
Neonatal pack (apheresis platelets)	50 ml unit of platelets from a single donor – thus reducing the donor exposure.	As above.	50 ml.	5 days @ 22 °C +/– 2 °C (McClelland, 2007).
Frozen plasma (Octaplas/ Uniplas)	Imported plasma from United States where there is no evidence of Variant Creutzfeldt–Jacob disease (vCJD).	Treatment of thrombotic thrombocytopenia (TTP), plasma exchange.	200 ml.	1 year @ –30 °C.
Albumin 5 %	A protein in the plasma part of whole blood. Strength = 50 g per litre.	To restore and maintain blood volume depending on patients clinical condition (Baxter, 2007).	250–500 ml.	25 °C. Do not freeze. Check label expiry date.
Albumin 20%	A protein in the plasma part of whole blood. Strength = 200 g per litre.			8 °C. Do not freeze. Check label expiry date.
Cryoprecipitate	Prepared from plasma contents containing fibrinogen.	Given for haemorrhage and clotting disorders.	100 ml.	30 mins thawing in a water bath (McClelland, 2007).
Cryoprecipitate (apheresis)	As above.	As above.	15–20 ml.	15 mins thawing in a water bath.

Part

IV

Procedure for obtaining samples for blood groups and antibody screens

- To obtain approximately 1.5–2.0 ml blood for:
  - ABO group
  - Rh group
  - antibody screen.
- Sample can be used for up to 14 days (provided patient has never been transfused).
- Sample tube label MUST be *completed* and *signed* by the *sample taker*.
- Sample tube and request form should be *handwritten*.
- Sample tube should be labelled at the patient's side.
- Sample tube contains details such as the following, depending on *local guidelines*:
  - patient's surname
  - gender
  - patient's first name
  - date and time
  - hospital number
  - signature of sample taker
  - date of birth.

> ⚠ **Professional alert!**
>
> It is important to follow local guidelines when completing the details on a sample tube.

Storage

Blood is stored at 4 °C to avoid damage to the cells (Contreras, 1998). If the temperature is too high there is an increased tendency for bacterial growth, and if it is too low there is the risk of red cell damage, as freezing can result in cell breakdown. Blood must be stored in a monitored and alarmed blood bank fridge.

Prescription

- The prescription of blood is the responsibility of the medical officer, who should specify the date, correct product, quantity required, duration of transfusion, special requirements and any precautions related to patient care (Wilkinson and Wilkinson, 2001).
- In order to ensure safety in relation to blood transfusion, local guidelines should be followed and adhered to.
- The prescription should be handwritten by a medical officer on a prescription sheet.

PRESCRIPTION SHEET

	Date	Blood Component (include special requirements)	Reason for Transfusion	Pre-Transfusion Value	Volume to be infused & duration	Doctor's Prescribing Signature
1.	09/09/05	Red cells		Hb 6 g/dl ↓Hb	1 unit over 4°	
2.						
3.						
4.						
5.						
6.						

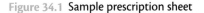

Figure 34.1 Sample prescription sheet

Administration

Each unit of blood should be checked against:

- blood compatibility report form
- blood compatibility label attached to the pack
- patient identification wristband (to include the full name of the patient, his or her date of birth and the hospital identity number)
- prescription.

When filling in blood transfusion observation charts:

- They should include observations (include temperature, heart rate, respiratory rate, blood pressure).
- A set of observations should be carried out: pre-transfusion; first 15 minutes following commencement of the transfusion; hourly (provided patient is stable) while the patient is being transfused; at end of transfusion.
- Two members of staff should sign the sheet and compatibility form (depending on local policy).
- Time commenced and time finished should be recorded.
- Information on reactions (yes or no) should be included.

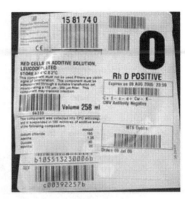

Figure 34.2 Blood compatibility label

Management

- Baseline observations should be recorded prior to the commencement of transfusion. They include temperature and pulse (McClelland, 1996), as well as respirations and blood pressure (BSCH, 1999, UK National Guidelines).
- There should be close monitoring during the first 15–30 minutes of each unit transfused. A haemolytic reaction can occur after just a few milliliters of incompatible blood (Mallett and Bailey, 1996).
- Observations should be documented separately from routine observations (NHO, 2002).
- Patients should be monitored in an easily observed area in the ward.
- Blood should be given via an infusion set with a 170–200 integral filter that removes micro-aggregates that can form during storage of the blood (see Figure 34.4) (McClelland, 2007).
- Only syringe drivers are suitable for infusing platelets, as platelets may be damaged by the roller pump systems in standard pumps (see Figure 34.5).
- Drugs should never be added to a transfusion as they can cause blood to clot or lyse (McClelland, 1996).
- The administration set should be changed on completion of the transfusion (Wilkinson and Wilkinson, 2001) or after three units of the same product.

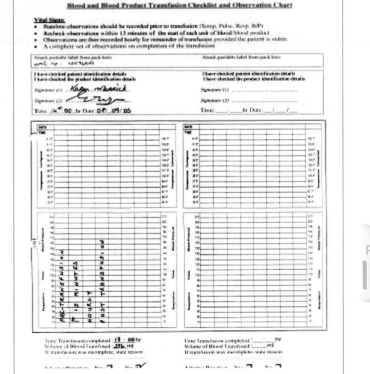

Figure 34.3 Transfusion compatibility chart

Part

IV

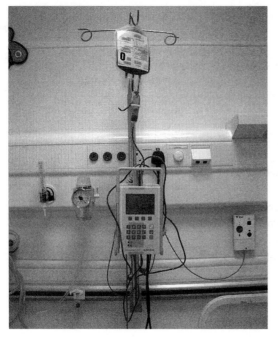

Figure 34.4 Braun Infusomat 170–200 integral blood filter

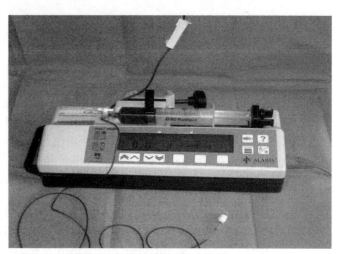

Figure 34.5 Alaris syringe driver

Complications

Complications related to blood transfusion largely relate to human error or failure to comply with policies (Wilkinson and Wilkinson, 2001). Some of the errors that can lead to adverse reactions include:

- incorrectly labelled blood samples
- incorrectly labelled blood units
- incomplete safety checks
- failure to recognise symptoms of adverse reactions during blood transfusion
- failure to respond appropriately to adverse reactions.

Incompatibility is recognised as the most important error that occurs in blood transfusion (Stainsby et al, 2008). SHOT (2007) revealed that 24 deaths in which transfusion reaction because of incorrect blood transfusion was a causal or contributory factor occurred between 1996 and 2007.

Table 34.5 Adverse reactions

Complications	Symptoms	Onset	Treatment
Nonhaemolytic febrile transfusion reaction (NFHTR)	Characterized by increase in temperature, chills, rigors. Most commonly occurs with platelets.	During or within hours of transfusion	Not generally medically dangerous but transfusion is discontinued, component wasted, lab investigations to exclude more serious complications (Eder and Chambers, 2007). Observe local guidelines.
Urticaria	Puritis and rash	1–3 per cent of transfusions. Less severe reactions can be delayed up to two or three hours post commencement of transfusion.	Give chloramphenermine, restart transfusion at a slower rate and observe patient closely (NBUG, 2004). Observe local guidelines.

Complications	Symptoms	Onset	Treatment
Severe allergic reaction	Puritis, rash, tachycardia, dyspnoea, cough, wheezing, malaise, swelling of lips, tongue and eyes	The shorter the interval from commencement to onset of symptoms the more severe the reaction	Stop transfusion, call for medical assistance, give oxygen, chloramphenermine, hydrocortisone +/- ventolin nebuliser (NBUG, 2004). Observe local guidelines
Anaphylaxis	Worsening of above symptoms plus stridor, wheeze, laryngeal oedema, abdominal pain, tachycardia, low blood pressure, +/- loss of consciousness	Anaphylaxis is very rare 1:47,000	Life-threatening. Give adrenaline, chloramphenermine, hydrocortisone and ventolin nebuliser. Send IgA levels. Seek haematology advice for future transfusions (NBUG, 2004). Observe local guidelines.
Transfusion associated circulatory overload (TACO)	Dyspnoea, hypoxaemia, central venous pressure, pulmonary oedema	During or within hours of completed transfusion. Incidence 1:3,000-14,000 units transfused. Up to 1 per cent of transfusions in elderly patients (NBUG, 2004).	Improves with diuretics. At-risk patients should be assessed prior to transfusion e.g. congestive heart failure, renal failure. Components can be given slowly (Eder and Chambers, 2007).
Acute haemolytic transfusion reaction (AHTR)	Agitation, nausea, chest or abdominal pain, fever, chills, dark urine, oozing from wound or puncture sites, generally unwell	Typically following accidental transfusion of ABO incompatible blood	Transfusion discontinued Symptoms treated Lab informed Component and patient lab investigations Haemovigilance/transfusion Officer and haematologist informed (NBUG, 2004).
Transfusion associated graft versus host disease (TAGvHD)	Progression of fever, rash, diarrhoea, raised liver function blood tests	Rare, 1–6 weeks post transfusion	Usually fatal. Seek medical advice. May require gamma irradiated blood products for future transfusions (NBUG, 2004).
Transfusion related acute lung injury (TRALI)	TRALI is associated with significant patient morbidity and the mortality rate may be as high as 25 per cent (NHO, 2003). Acute respiratory distress, hypotension, fever and rigors associated with bilateral pulmonary oedema with no evidence of cardiac failure or fluid overload (NBUG, 2004).	Symptoms typically begin within one or two hours of transfusion and always within six hours (Popovsky, 2001). Incidence 1:5,000 units transfused but probably underdiagnosed (NBUG, 2004).	May be life-threatening. Maintain airway, discontinue transfusion, commence oxygen, perform chest x-ray (NBUG, 2004). Generally patients will require O_2 support, with approximately 70 per cent requiring mechanical ventilation (NHO, 2003). Report TRALI as a serious adverse transfusion reaction.
Post-transfusion purpura (PTP)	Poor response to platelet transfusion and bleeding	Rare. Five to 12 days post transfusion	Seek expert haematology advice. Give high doses of Immunoglobulin G. Platelet transfusions may be required (NBUG, 2004).

Part

IV

More than 90 per cent of UK hospitals contribute to SHOT, which analysed 1630 events over the first six years. Of the reported events 64 per cent were errors in the transfusion process, leading to 193 instances of ABO incompatible transfusion.

Transfusion-related acute lung injury, bacterial contamination of platelets and transfusion-associated graft-versus-host disease were also identified as important preventable causes of mortality and morbidity. Data from SHOT has provided evidence to support the development of blood safety strategies in the UK.

Education and training

> **a Learning activity**
>
> Discuss in your learning group what is needed to ensure the safety of the transfusion process.

Some training suggestions are:

- Greater awareness and understanding of the blood transfusion process can help to reduce the incidence of adverse reactions.
- Up-to-date policies and guidelines should be disseminated to the multidisciplinary team involved in the transfusion process.
- Competency-based training must be implemented for all staff involved in the blood transfusion process (SHOT, 2003).
- There should be a haemovigilance/transfusion officer to monitor and keep detailed records of the transfusion audit trail within the healthcare system. In addition the haemovigilance officer/transfusion officer's role is to provide education and training on the transfusion process and to offer advice when required.
- Communication between the haemovigilance/transfusion officer, consultant haematologist and laboratory staff should provide best practice.
- A multidisciplinary hospital blood transfusion committee consisting of both clinical and non-clinical staff should be involved.

Alternative surgical blood therapies

Cell salvage

Blood aspirated from the operative field can be re-infused to the patient. This procedure is often used in cardiothoracic, vascular and spinal surgery, in which blood transfusions and the use of blood products have traditionally been high.

Autologous donation

Some patients can donate their own blood – up to four units – in advance of their own planned operation. It can be stored up to five weeks in controlled blood bank conditions. This may be useful in the case patients for whom it is difficult to provide compatible donor red cells. It is only practical if the operation scheduled is likely to need red cell transfusion. There should be sufficient time before surgery to donate at least two units of blood. The date for surgery must be fixed, so the blood does not become outdated. Iron replacement is required. This reduces the risk of developing red cell antibodies and of viral infection; however, it does not reduce the risk of bacterial contamination.

Erythropoetin

Administration of erythropoetin accelerates recovery of haemoglobin level before the operation or after major blood loss.

Iron supplements

Iron given pre-operatively is only likely to be effective if the patient's iron stores are low. Postoperatively, absorption of iron is probably good in patients without other chronic disease (McClelland, 2007).

Table 34.6 Competence assessment in blood and blood component management

	Goal	Actions	
Part 1 A	Collect and label a pre-transfusion blood sample.	Patient should wear an armband with a minimum of three patient identifiers: full name, hospital number and date of birth (observe local policy). If appropriate, patients should be asked to identify themselves prior to blood sampling; otherwise ask a parent/guardian. No armband, no blood sample! Blood request form should be handwritten only by a medical officer (see local policy). Check details on form correspond to patient's armband. Details on sample bottle should include full name, hospital number, date of birth, date and time of sampling, signature of sample taker (see local policy). Blood bottles must not be pre-labelled but labelled *at the bedside* immediately after blood sampling.	
Part 1 B	Critically evaluate the prescription, explaining why the patient is receiving a blood component.	→ low Hb → bleeding → lowered O$_2$ saturation	→ correct volume → correct duration → date and time of proposed transfusion.
Part 1 C	Demonstrate the correct procedure in collecting blood and blood components from the blood transfusion laboratory.	→ Patient correctly identified: i.e. armband. → IV cannula in patient prior to blood collection. → Pre-transfusion observations prior to blood component collection. → Blood collection docket correctly completed. The above checks will ensure that a unit of blood will not be removed from the blood transfusion laboratory unnecessarily. If involved in the transfusion chain, the collector must be certified competent (depending on local policy). Transport box to accompany collector. Procedure should take a maximum of 10–15 minutes. Patient identification must correspond to collection docket, compatibility report form and compatibility sticker on the blood component, as laid down in local policy. Place in collection box for transport back to clinical area. Sign collection docket when blood/blood component is removed from storage. Receiving staff member to sign collection docket on receipt of requisition (depending on local policy). A transfusion must commence within 30 minutes of its removal from storage. Blood/blood component must be returned to storage within 30 minutes in order to be re-used. Sign out or return components according to local guidelines.	
Part 1 D	Show where the policies/guidelines for safe transfusion are kept in the clinical area.	This should be done according to the policy of each individual clinical area. Should be stored at a central area to maintain maximum usage. Individual local guidelines must not be used as a substitute for local hospital policies/guidelines.	
Part 1 E	Demonstrate the pre-transfusion checks to include correct patient identification, the blood component and the compatibility.	Pre-transfusion observations prior to blood component collection will include: temperature, pulse, respiration rate and blood pressure. Ensure patient armband is on the patient, showing full name, hospital number and date of birth (see local policy). Ensure the blood group is identified on the blood component label (on the front of the pack), compatibility label (on the back of the pack) and compatibility report form.	

	Goal	Actions
Part 1 F	Identify the administration that is suitable for the blood component that is being transfused.	Ensure a suitable infusion pump is available for infusing the blood component. Only syringe drivers are suitable for infusing platelets, as platelets may be damaged by roller pump systems in standard pumps. A blood filter must be used for all blood components, except albumin due to its prior fractionation during the manufacturing process.
Part 2 G	Note the importance of baseline observations and vital signs during a transfusion.	Pre-transfusion observations give a baseline for the patient's observations prior to the commencement of a transfusion. This will identify any abnormalities with the patient's monitoring once a transfusion has started, thus identifying the start of a transfusion reaction. Observations to be carried out during a transfusion are: pre-transfusion, during the first 15 minutes (most likely time a reaction will occur), hourly (provided the patient is stable), end of the transfusion.
Part 2 H	Show where observations are recorded, along with the start and finish time, volume transfused, +/− transfusion reactions.	Documented separately from routine observations (NHO, 2002). Usually documented on the observation sheet of the blood/blood component prescription booklet if available (see local policy). Records should show signatures, date and time of transfusion commencement, patient vital signs, finish time, volume transfused and whether a reaction occurred.
Part 2 I	Identify the signs and symptoms of a reaction and demonstrate the course of action to be taken if one occurs.	Observe for any changes in baseline observations. These may include: heightened temperature, urticarial rash, eye +/−, tongue swelling, shortness of breath, difficulty in breathing, lowered O_2 saturation, rigors. Follow reaction guidelines as each one is different. Stop transfusion and call doctor immediately to review patient; NaCl IV infusion should be commenced; check vital signs; note the blood component details. In case of incorrect component transfused, complete reaction form and document all proceedings. Phone the blood transfusion laboratory to report the reaction. Follow local policy/guidelines to report reaction. Phone haemovigilance/transfusion officer for follow up.
Part 2 J	Use the correct documentation in recording a reaction and ensure hospital guidelines are followed.	Guidelines are followed in conjunction with doctor's orders. The local hospital reaction form is used. The form is then filed in the patient's notes for follow-up by the haemovigilance/transfusion officer and consultant haematologist.
Part 2 K	If a reaction has occurred, demonstrate the action to be taken in subsequent transfusions.	There should be an alert sticker on the inside of a patient's clinical notes highlighting any previous reaction. This should give directions from the consultant haematologist regarding precautions/instructions for future blood transfusions.
Part 2 L	Identify alternatives available for transfusion both pre and postoperatively.	→ Autologous donation: patients donate their own whole blood (pre-op) which is given back to them (intra-op/post-op) thus reducing donor exposure. → Cell salvage: patients' own blood is salvaged intra-op and returned to them, thus reducing donor exposure (intra-operatively). → Iron supplements: provide higher iron levels and higher oxygenation (pre-op). → Erythropoietin: boosts red cell growth thus increasing oxygenation (pre-op).

Conclusion

This chapter has introduced you to the components of blood, and the principles of best practice for blood transfusion.

References

Atterbury, C. and Wilkinson, J. (2000) 'Blood transfusion', *Nursing Standard* **14**(34), 47–52.

British Committee for Standards in Haematology Blood Transfusion (1999) 'The administration of blood and blood components and the management of transfused patients', *Transfusion Medicine* 9, 227–38.

Contreras, M. (ed.) (1998) *ABC of Transfusion*, 3rd edn, London, BMJ Books.

Eder, A. F. and Chambers, L. (2007) 'Noninfectious complications of blood transfusion', *Archives of Pathology and Laboratory Medicine* 131, 708–10.

Giangrande, P. L. (2000) 'The history of blood transfusion', *British Journal of Haematology* 110, 758–67.

McClelland, D. B. L. (ed.) (1996) *The Handbook of Transfusion Medicine*, 2nd edn, London, Stationery Office.

McClelland, D. B. L. (2001) *Handbook of Transfusion Medicine*, 3rd edn, London, Stationery Office.

McClelland, D. B. L. (2007) *Handbook of Transfusion Medicine*, 4th edn, London, Stationery Office.

Mallett, J. and Bailey, C. (1996) *Transfusion of Blood and Blood Products: The Royal Marsden NHS Trust manual of clinical nursing procedures*, London, Blackwell Science.

McClelland, D. B. L. (2007) *Handbook of Transfusion Medicine*, 3rd edn, London, Stationery Office.

National Blood Users Group (NBUS) (2004) *Guidelines for the Administration of Blood and Blood Components*, Dublin, National Haemovigilance Office.

National Haemovigilance Office (NHO) (2002) *National Haemovigilance Office Annual Report*, Dublin, NHO.

NHO (2003) *National Haemovigilance Office Annual Report*, Dublin, NHO.

Octapharma Limited (2002) *Octaplas: Summary of product characteristics*, Dublin, Specific Octapharma.

Popovsky, M. A. (2001) 'Transfusion-related acute lung injury (TRALI)', in M. A. Popovsky (ed.), *Transfusion Reactions*, 2nd edn, Bethesda, MD/AABB Press/London, Stationery Office.

Royal College of Nursing (2005) *Right Blood, Right Patient, Right Time: RCN guidance for improving transfusion practice*, London, Royal College of Nursing.

Serious Hazards of Transfusion (SHOT) (1998) *Annual Report 1996–1997*, Manchester, SHOT.

SHOT (1999) *Annual Report 1997–1998*, Manchester, SHOT.

SHOT (2003) *Annual Report 2003*, Manchester, SHOT.

SHOT (2004) *Annual Report 2002–2003*, Manchester, SHOT.

SHOT (2005) *Annual Report 2003–2004*, Manchester, SHOT.

Stainsby, D., Jones, H., Milkins, C., Gibson, B., Norfolk, D. R. and Revill, J. for the Serious Hazards of Transfusion Steering Group (2004). *Serious Hazards of Transfusion Annual Report 2003*, Manchester: SHOT.

Stainsby, D., Jones, H., Wells, A. W., Gibson, B and Cohen, H. (SHOT Steering Group) (2008) 'Adverse outcomes of blood transfusion in children: analysis of UK reports to the serious hazards of transfusion scheme 1996–2005', *British Journal of Haematology* **141**(1), 73–9.

Wells, A. W., Mounter, P.J., Chapman, C. E., Stainsby, D. and Wallis, J. P. (2002) 'Where does blood go? Prospective observational study of red cell transfusion in north England', *British Medical Journal* 325, 803–6.

Wilkinson, J. and Wilkinson, C. (2001) 'Administration of blood transfusions to adults in general hospital settings: a review of the literature', *Journal of Clinical Nursing* 10, 161–70.

Useful websites

Medicines and Healthcare products Regulatory Agency (MRHA): http://www.mhra.gov.uk

Serious Hazards of Transfusion: http://www.shotuk.org/

Chapter

35

Oxygen therapy and suction therapy

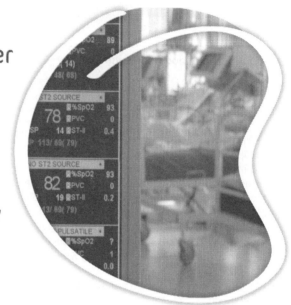

Neil Bloxham, Sharon Jones
and Gill McEwing

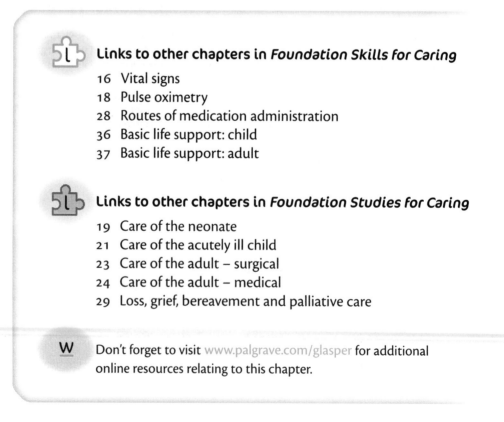

Links to other chapters in _Foundation Skills for Caring_

Links to other chapters in _Foundation Studies for Caring_

W   Don't forget to visit www.palgrave.com/glasper for additional
online resources relating to this chapter.

Introduction

If the body does not receive enough oxygen tissue damage will occur, which will eventually lead to brain damage and multi-organ failure. Maintaining a clear airway and/or administering oxygen can be a life-saving measure in some situations.

Oxygen requirements vary with each individual. Children have lower pulmonary reserves than adults and can decompensate more quickly (Giles, 2006).

The body's demand for oxygen can increase both in illness and following surgery. Acute hypoxaemia may be a result of a chest infection or an exacerbation of asthma, whereas chronic conditions, such as chronic obstructive pulmonary disease (COPD), may result in a slowly developing hypoxaemia. After surgery, this greater demand is due to an increased metabolism as a result of physiological stress and trauma, requiring the administration of supplemental oxygen (Torrance and Serginson, 2000).

Respiration can be compromised if the airway is blocked with secretions. Oropharyngeal and nasopharyngeal suction are methods that can help remove secretions from the respiratory tract and aid effective respiration when the patients are unable to do this for themselves.

The aim of this chapter is to facilitate your acquisition of knowledge with a sound rationale of the skills required in the provision of safe and effective practice pertaining to the administration of oxygen and suctioning of the oropharynx and nasopharynx.

Learning outcomes

This chapter will enable you to:

- describe, with evidence-based reasons, the procedures for the administration of oxygen via:
  - non re-breathe mask
  - nasal cannulae (or prongs)
  - facemask
  - head box

- discuss the potential hazards and complications that may occur with the administration of oxygen and how these may be minimised or prevented.
- describe the procedure of oropharyngeal and nasopharyngeal suction with an evidence-based rationale and discuss the indications and complications pertaining to the procedure.

Concepts

- Regulation of respiration
- Maintaining a clear airway
- Oxygen
- Personal safety
- Risks to the patient
- Complications of treatment

Administration of oxygen

Oxygen is a clear, colourless, tasteless and odourless gas. A constituent of atmospheric air – approximately 21 per cent – it readily supports combustion rather than having inflammable properties itself. It is vital in sustaining life, as it is an essential of aerobic cellular respiration, and a reduced amount of oxygen within the body is deleterious to health (Tortora, 1997; Porth, 2007). The brain particularly initiates clinically observable signs and symptoms. With brain cells continuing to function for approximately ten seconds without oxygen, unconsciousness occurs almost simultaneously with cardiac arrest, and brain cell death commences between four and six minutes.

Respiratory regulation is undertaken by chemoreceptors present in the respiratory centre in the medulla. These monitor blood levels of carbon dioxide and oxygen and are essential for the processes of supplying tissue oxygen demand and carbon dioxide removal (Porth, 2007). Such chemoreceptors are very sensitive to short-term changes in the level of carbon dioxide present; when the level is elevated this causes an increase in ventilation that peaks at about one minute; if carbon dioxide levels remain elevated then ventilation will decline. This physiological state has ramifications for those with chronically elevated levels of carbon

Part

IV

dioxide, such as COPD patients, as this stimulus for increased ventilation is minimal and there is a reliance on the stimulus provided by a decrease in blood oxygen level. In such cases an increase in oxygen, delivered in higher concentration by high flow, will lose the hypoxic drive mechanism (Marieb and Hoehn, 2007), with a consequent reduction in respiratory effort. This leads to a condition known as carbon dioxide narcosis, characterised by a confusional state, further deterioration and ultimately death (Smith, 2004). In managing such patients, low-concentration oxygen (24 to 28 per cent) should be administered until further assessment is achieved by arterial blood gas analysis. Continuing therapy aims to correct the hypoxia (maintaining SaO_2 above 90 per cent but not exceeding 94 per cent) without carbon dioxide retention or lowering of pH below 7.35 (NICE, 2004).

Practice tip

Oxygen saturation is referred to as: SaO_2. This is the ratio of actual haemoglobin oxygen content to the potential maximum oxygen-carrying capacity of the haemoglobin.

Learning activity

Review the patients in your practice area; are any of them prescribed oxygen therapy? Discuss with your mentor the reasons for their requiring oxygen and develop your understanding of their conditions or illness.

Procedural requirements and general considerations

Oxygen should be regarded as a drug (BNF, 2008), and consequently requires a prescription. However, it is important to note that in an emergency oxygen is often the first drug to be given, and exceptions to prescription may occur. It is essential that an appropriate clinician prescribe this for continued use as soon as the patient has stabilised.

Oxygen is given to hypoxaemic patients in order to decrease the work of breathing by increasing alveolar tension; the concentration required should be dependent upon the individual condition being managed. A detailed assessment of the patient is not usually made when prescribing oxygen, and clinical indicators are more readily used by medical and nursing staff (Bell, 1995). The amount of oxygen given is described as the fractional inspired oxygen concentration (FiO_2), which means the amount of oxygen a patient is breathing in. The flow rate required to achieve the prescribed FiO_2 will be determined by the type of apparatus being used to administer the oxygen (Timby, 2005).

Practice tip

There are risks associated with O_2 therapy and so the lowest possible concentration of O_2 should be delivered to maintain the FiO_2 within normal parameters. O_2 therapy should be discontinued as soon as possible (Toplis, 2007).

Complications of too high a concentration of oxygen include:

- Retinopathy of prematurity in preterm neonates (Bateman and Leach, 1998). It is thought that high O_2 concentrations can raise the partial pressure (PO_2) above 15 kPa resulting in retinopathy of prematurety. However there is some suggestion that this is due to wide swings in oxygen saturations rather than high oxygen concentrations (Kotecha and Allen, 2002).
- Pulmonary oxygen toxicity and permanent lung damage due to lengthy exposure to high levels of oxygen (Giles, 2006).
- Potential risk of respiratory failure in patients with chronic lung disease. A lower SaO_2 is accepted in these patients to prevent this (Toplis, 2007).

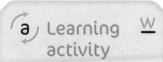

a Learning activity W

Visit the British Thoracic Society website and review the guidelines available for administration of emergency oxygen: 'Guidelines for emergency oxygen use in adult patients (2008)' www.brit-thoracic.org.uk.

⚠ Professional alert!

Oxygen supports combustion so there must be no smoking or naked flames in the vicinity of an oxygen cylinder/supply.

No oils or grease are to be used to lubricate any part of the cylinder or associated equipment.

Ensure hands are clean and free from oils or grease. If moisturising creams are required, ensure only approved creams are used and under no circumstances use oil-based creams.

Care should be taken when handling compressed medical oxygen cylinders (BOC Medical, 2008).

a Learning activity

Look at the oxygen cylinders available for patient use in your practice area; what colour are the cylinders and what precautions are advised?

Equipment required

- supply (ensure spanner available if needed for cylinder)
- flow meter appropriate to method of supply
- oxygen tubing
- humidifier and tubing
- delivery system appropriate for application (facemask or nasal cannulae).

Delivery systems

Different methods of oxygen delivery result in different amounts of achievable FiO_2, so this should be taken into account when choosing the method of delivery.

Table 35.1 Delivery of oxygen by different methods

Maximum achievable FiO_2 at 6L/min of O_2	
Nasal prongs	50 per cent
Simple mask without reservoir bag	50 per cent
Mask without reservoir bag (partial rebreathing)	70 per cent
Mask with reservoir bag (non rebreathing)	90 per cent
Head box	95 per cent

Source: Toplis (2007).

Nasal cannulae

These are sometimes referred to as nasal prongs or nasal spectacles.

This delivery system is generally well tolerated and does not require extra humidification as the nasal passages warm and moisten the oxygen.

At one end the clear plastic tubing is attached to the oxygen flow meter, and at the other there are two short tapered prongs, approximately 1 cm in length, that sit just inside the anterior nares. The prongs can be cut shorter if required. The tubing can be secured to the cheeks with a suitable adhesive, ensuring that a protective film is placed on the cheeks before securing with tape.

- *Neonatal nasal cannulae*: can deliver a maximum flow rate 2 litre/min.
- *Paediatric nasal cannulae*: can deliver a maximum flow rate 3 litre/min.
- *Adult nasal cannulae*: flow rates above 6–8 litres/minute may cause discomfort and drying of nasal mucosal lining. Healthcare staff should ensure nasal toilet is carried out regularly.

Nasal cannulae have been demonstrated to achieve equivalent oxygenation to that of facemasks. This method of oxygen administration is beneficial for patients whose condition precludes facemask application or for those who are unable to tolerate a facemask (Eastwood and Dennis, 2006). The World Health Organisation recommends that nasal cannulae are a safe and efficient means of oxygen administration, particularly for use in developing countries where an inexpensive method of oxygen administration is favoured (Frey and Shann, 2003).

⚠ Professional alert!

Caution: if the prongs fit too tightly in neonates or infants it may result in accidental administration of continuous positive airway pressure (CPAP).

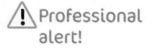

Part

IV

Application of nasal cannulae

1   Connect to appropriate oxygen supply by flow meter set at prescribed flow rate.
2   Confirm flow of gas by listening; if nothing is heard increase flow temporarily and when flow detected reduce to that prescribed.
3   Locate cannulae on patient's face; insert prongs into nares.
4   Pass tubing over ears and behind head.
5   Caution: the head should not rest on any part of the cannula if the patient is lying down.
6   Move the sliding collar towards the head to ensure secure fit.
7   For adults and larger children:
    ● Pass cannula tubing over and behind each ear. Gently secure by moving sliding collar towards chin. Tape may also be used to secure cannulae.

Tape may be fixed to cheek to secure cannula

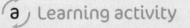

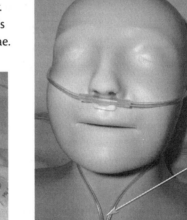

Sliding collar

Figure 35.1 Nasal cannula

Figure 35.2 Nasal cannula with a sliding collar

(a) Learning activity

Find the different types of nasal cannulae available on your ward/unit; look at the size and instructions for use. If any patients are having oxygen administered through nasal cannulae, ask them if they find them uncomfortable in any way and if they can compare them with other forms of oxygen administration.

Facemasks

There are a variety of different types of facemasks available; usually they are made of soft rigid plastic with ventilation holes in the sides to dilute the oxygen. The oxygen concentration is adjusted by altering the flow rate, either via the flow meter or with the use of fixed-concentration masks. These masks deliver a known percentage of oxygen concentration in accordance with the advised flow rate of oxygen delivery. High concentrations of oxygen can be given using these masks, but attempts to deliver a low concentration entail a risk of carbon dioxide accumulation. Some patients will not tolerate masks for long periods, as they can make the patient feel as though they are being suffocated (and they interfere with communication) (Timby, 2005).

If this form of delivery of oxygen is used for more than four hours then humidification should be added to prevent drying of the mucosa and to aid loosening of any secretions (Toplis, 2007).

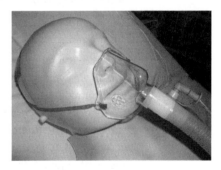

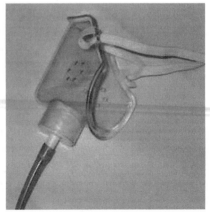

Figure 35.3 Delivery of oxygen

Application of an oxygen facemask

1 Collect required equipment:
   - oxygen flow meter
   - green oxygen tubing
   - correct size/type of oxygen mask.
2 Wash your hands to avoid cross infection.
3 Explain to the patient that they require oxygen therapy to assist their breathing and gain consent to apply the mask.
4 Place the mask over the patient's nose and mouth. Secure the elastic around the back of the head to hold the mask in place. Make sure the mask is comfortable.
5 Connect the oxygen tubing to the flow meter at one end and the mask at the other, allowing a suitable length for patient movement and comfort.
6 Adjust the dial on the flow meter to provide the prescribed amount of oxygen.
7 Observe the patient regularly to assess condition.

Non rebreathing mask

This is a semi-rigid facemask available in both adult and child sizes which has the addition of a reservoir with a one-way valve between the facemask and the reservoir bag. This acts to prevent the accumulation of expired gases and consequently the retention of carbon dioxide (Pierce, 1995). These masks are usually used in an emergency situation when very high doses of oxygen are required; the flow rate should be set at 15 litres and the bag should be inflated before the mask is fitted to the patient (Chandler, 2001).

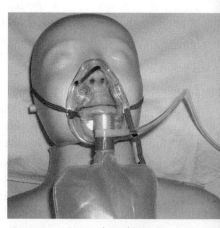

Figure 35.4 Non-rebreathing mask

Head box

A head box is a clear Perspex box which comes in different sizes and is placed over the head/upper body of an infant. It can only be used with babies less than 8 months old and should not be used for long periods as it limits movement.

Head boxes can deliver oxygen effectively and are non-invasive. The FiO_2 can be easily monitored using an oxygen analyser placed inside the box; to ensure accuracy the analyser needs to be calibrated frequently (Frey and Shann, 2003).

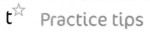

t☆ Practice tips

- The tubing should be positioned to avoid it blowing directly onto the baby's face.
- The oxygen should be warmed to prevent cooling the baby and if the therapy is prolonged the oxygen should be humidified (Giles, 2006).
- A total gas flow of 10 litres is advisable to prevent the infant rebreathing carbon dioxide.

One of the problems with this method of oxygen delivery is that the carer cannot cuddle the infant without removing him or her from the box, and so losing the oxygen therapy.

Figure 35.5 Head box

Care of an infant in a head box

1 Make sure the parents understand why the infant requires to be nursed in a head box and how it works.
2 Prepare the correct sized head box for use.

Part

IV

3 Set up the humidification system and monitor and maintain the water level while in use.

4 Prepare the oxygen analyser for use by calibrating first in air and then in 100 per cent oxygen. Test the alarm is working. Place the probe through the small hole in the head box designed for this purpose.

5 Locate the oxygen supply to be used.

6 With the baby positioned either on its back or side, place the head box over the baby's head; where possible the shoulders should be outside the box, but in very small babies the shoulders may also be positioned inside the box. Ensure that the arched hole over the baby's neck or upper body is not occluded as this may lead to carbon dioxide retention.

7 Pass the elephant tubing into the head box through the larger hole. Position it so that the oxygen does not blow onto the baby's face, either to the side of the face or behind the head.

8 Make sure the oxygen analyser is positioned near the baby's face but away from the end of the tubing delivering the oxygen.

9 Attach an oxygen saturation monitor to the baby; set the upper and lower limits for oxygen levels and heart rate.

10 Set the humidifier dial to provide the required oxygen concentration.

11 Using the oxygen analyser regulate the oxygen flow until the required oxygen concentration is achieved.

12 Monitor the baby's oxygen saturations and respiratory rate. Check that these are within the predetermined levels set by the medical staff. Report any changes in recordings that may suggest the treatment is not successful.

> ## (a) Learning activity
>
> If you are involved in the care of an infant in a head box for the administration of oxygen, ask the parent how they feel their baby is coping with the experience and any problems they have encountered.
>
> Ask the nurse responsible for the care of the infant about the advantages and disadvantages of using this method of oxygen administration.

> ## (c) Professional conversation
>
> Anisha, children's nurse, says, 'Harry was a 6-month-old baby admitted with bronchiolitis and nursed in a head box with continuous oxygen saturation (SaO_2) monitoring being undertaken by pulse oximetry. I noticed an irregular and haphazard waveform and erratic readings, from the observation chart I could see that baby Harry had a trend of readings above 97 per cent and that the probe had recently been changed. Harry was alert, and looked well and settled. Such readings are a possible indicator that the probe containing the two light-emitting diodes is not opposite the probe containing the photo-detector, so I repositioned the probes on Harry's foot –a good position for infants – ensuring that the probe with the diodes was on top and that with the photo-detector opposite and beneath his foot which was warm and well perfused. I secured the probe as indicated by the manufacturer. Within a couple of minutes there was a good waveform and a consistent reading could be taken.'

Humidification

Indications for humidification (Hufton, 2007):

- When more than 2 litres (28 per cent) of oxygen is used for more than five hours.
- Where there are thick retained secretions.
- When the upper respiratory tract is bypassed by an endotracheal tube or tracheostomy.
- It should be used in babies with respiratory problems as their immature respiratory system and smaller airways are functionally inefficient.
- When the patient is dehydrated.

- When direct trauma to the respiratory system has occurred, for example burns or smoke inhalation.
- Where there is reduced mucociliary clearance, for example anaesthetic or sedation induced.

Inhaled air is normally warmed and humidified by the nose and upper respiratory tract; this increases its capacity to hold vapour. It is recognised that when tracheal temperature falls below 37 °C, airway mucoid secretions become thicker and there is a reduction in cilia mobility.

Without humidification in the inspired air, heat and moisture are taken from the mucociliary epithelium. This leads to mucosal drying, which causes cilial dysfunction, leading to an accumulation of secretions, an increased risk of infection and retained secretions blocking small airways. When this occurs atelectasis (alveolar collapse) can happen, with a decrease in lung function and potential hypoxaemia (Carrol, 1997; Fell and Boehm, 1998; Ward and Park, 2000; Dougherty and Lister, 2004). When administering oxygen, supplementary humidification is beneficial to the patient. Warm humidification is optimum when delivered at a temperature 32–36 °C with 100 per cent humidity (Pilkington, 2004).

Humidification chambers can be attached to the oxygen equipment to moisten the oxygen before it is inhaled (Alexander, Fawcett and Runciman, 2006). The method of humidification depends on the method of oxygen administration, and the equipment available in the clinical setting.

The heated passover humidifier is the most efficient as the particle size/vapour is smaller than in cold systems and saline nebulisers. Increased particle size allows for more pathogens to be carried, therefore increasing infection risk (Hufton, 2007).

To set up humidification apparatus

1 Connect the green oxygen tubing from the oxygen flow meter to the humidifier.
2 Position the humidifier securely close to the bed and below bed level.
3 Hang the water bag approximately 50 cm above the chamber.
4 Turn on the humidifier and make sure the temperature is set correctly; it will take about 20–30 minutes for the temperature to be achieved.
5 The dial on the humidifier will state the flow rate required to achieve the prescribed concentration of oxygen from the humidifier.
6 Check the water level in humidifier water; ensure the water bottle is replaced as required.
7 If there is condensation in the circuit, drain back to chamber.
8 Ensure circuit is changed every seven days, or according to manufacturer's instructions.

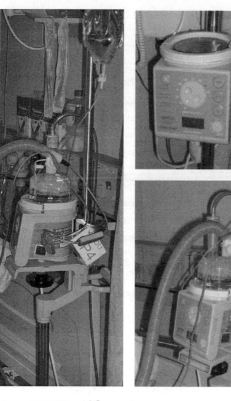

Figure 35.6 Humidifier equipment

t ☆
Practice tip

Water will collect in the wide bore tubing; this should be emptied by disconnecting the tubing, emptying out the water into a bowl or draining back into the chamber and then reattaching the tubing (Nicol et al, 2004; Hufton, 2007).

Part

IV

Flow meters

These vary in design and flow rate, common types include:

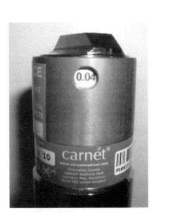
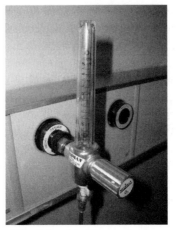
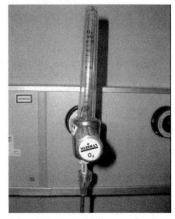

1 litre/minute – 0.01 litre graduations   15 litre/minute – 1 litre graduations   1 litre/minute – 0.1 litre graduations

Figure 35.7 Flow metering

Maintaining a clear airway

Healthy adults and children keep their airways clear by the normal processes of coughing, sneezing, blowing their noses and the gag reflex. There are times when this process becomes compromised and suction may be required to retain patency of the airway. This can occur following an anaesthetic or during periods of disease when there is an overproduction of mucous and secretions, or in small babies when the respiratory tract is immature.

Suctioning is the procedure used to aspirate secretions through a catheter connected to suction apparatus; this can be a portable machine or a wall-mounted connection. Suctioning is performed to remove potentially dangerous secretions from the oropharynx, trachea and bronchi (Alexander et al, 2006). Suctioning may be required when the patient demonstrates any of the following symptoms and is unable to clear their airway naturally (Carey and Kelsey, 2008):

- increased respiratory rate, possibly with irregular respirations
- noisy respirations, rattling, bubbling sounds
- visible signs of bubbling from the mouth or nose
- signs of pallor or cyanosis
- use of accessory muscles of respiration including nasal flaring
- decreased oxygen saturation.

The two main routes for suctioning are via the oropharyngeal/nasopharyngeal path or via a tracheostomy.

Oropharyngeal and nasopharyngeal suction

Oropharyngeal suction is when a catheter is inserted into the mouth, pharynx and trachea, and suction is applied to remove secretions. In nasopharyngeal suction the catheter is inserted into the nose, pharynx and trachea through the nose.

⚠ Professional alert!

Oropharangeal suction is not recommended in patients who have or may have a basal skull fracture, or with intranasal trauma or severe intranasal disease.

Caution should be taken when the patient has pulmonary oedema, severe bronchospasm and/or recent lung, tracheal or oesophageal surgery and raised intracranial pressure (Donaldson and Holliday, 2007).

Nasal suction is not recommended for patients who may have a frontal skull fracture or nasal leakage of cerebrospinal fluid.

Using the correct size of catheter is important; select one that is large enough to remove the aspirate but will not obstruct or cause trauma to the airway (Carey and Kelsey, 2008). There are different types of catheters. Some have the main opening at the end of the catheter and others have it at the end of the catheter but positioned on the side of the tubing; both have additional openings further up the side of the catheter. The catheters with the hole at the end of the tube are more effective when removing thick mucous but can cause more irritation to the respiratory mucosa than the side-opening catheter (Kozier et al, 2008). When secretions are required to be removed from the mouth this is usually achieved successfully with a Yankauer suction catheter, although care must be taken to avoid damaging the oral cavity.

Suction catheters usually have a suction control port to enable control of the suction pressure by the user; this is achieved by the user placing a thumb over the port.

Table 35.2 Catheter sizes and pressures for suctioning of non-intubated patients

Age	Sizes of catheter (French gauge)	Pressures
Newborn infant	5–6½	60–80 mmHg (8–10 kPa)
6 months	8	60–80 mmHg (8–10 kPa)
1 year	8–10	80–100 mmHg (10.6–13.3 kPa)
2 years	10	80–100 mmHg (10.6–13.3 kPa)
5 years	12	80–100 mmHg (10.6–13.3 kPa)
10 years to adult	12–14	Max 120 mmHg (16 kPa)

Source: Carey and Kelsey (2008).

ⓐ Learning activity

When on placement, look at the different types and sizes of suction catheters available. Think of a variety of patients and decide which catheter would be most suitable to meet each patient's needs.

Performing oropharyngeal or nasopharyngeal suction

Equipment required:

- portable suction machine or piped source of vacuum with calibrated pressures
- suction tubing to connect from the wall or portable suction unit to the suction catheter
- collection jar
- appropriate sized sterile suction catheters
- sterile disposable gloves
- plastic apron
- sterile water/normal saline
- sterile bowl
- sterile towel
- facemask and goggles if there is a risk of infection
- towel
- ambu bag and oxygen: emergency equipment will be required if the condition of the child becomes unstable and suffers hypoxaemia or respiratory distress (Carey and Kelsey, 2008).

Part

IV

Procedure

Each hospital will have its own policy regarding suctioning which should be followed in practice. The guidelines below are an example of good practice:

1 If the patient is conscious, explain the procedure and gain consent. It is important to gain patients' co-operation and ensure that they understand their role in the procedure. Informing patients that the procedure will relieve their breathing problem is often reassuring. Explain that it is a painless procedure but may be uncomfortable and cause them to cough or gag (Kozier et al, 2008). If the patient is unconscious it is important to give this information to any relatives or carers present as suction can be distressing to watch if unprepared.

2 Organise the practice area to protect the patient's dignity and privacy.

3 Collect the equipment required.

4 Pre-oxygenation may be required to avoid hypoxaemia in patients that are having oxygen therapy. This is achieved by increasing the oxygen intake and asking the patient to take deep breaths.

5 Wash hands and dry thoroughly.

6 Put on a disposable apron.

7 Goggles should be worn if there is a risk of airborne infection.

8 If possible the patient should be sitting up if conscious; if not then position the patient on his or her side to reduce the risk of aspiration. If oropharyngeal suction is to be performed the head should be turned to one side; if nasopharyngeal suction is required then the neck should be hyper extended (Kozier et al, 2008).

9 An unconscious patient can be placed lateral or supine for better access and removal of vomit (Dixon, 2006).

10 Place towel under the patient's chin/cheek.

11 Connect tubing to suction unit and switch on; select the correct pressure for the patient.

12 Set up equipment for the procedure, open sterile towel, carefully open sterile bowl and place on towel, pour sterile water/saline into sterile bowl.

13 Open suction catheter pack and place catheter onto sterile towel.

14 Put on sterile gloves.

15 Attach the catheter to the suction tubing.

16 For nasopharyngeal suction, pre-measure the catheter from the nose to the suprasternal notch. For oral suction measure from the mouth to the suprasternal notch. Mark this using the fingers of the dominant hand.

17 Lubricate the end of the catheter with sterile water or saline to reduce friction.

18 Gently introduce the suction catheter into the airway without applying suction.

19 For oropharyngeal suction insert the catheter along the side of the mouth as this prevents gagging (Kozier et al, 2008).

20 For nasopharyngeal suction insert the catheter along the floor of the nasal cavity as this helps avoid the nasal turbinates (Kozier et al, 2008). If any resistance occurs, withdraw catheter and try again. If further resistance is met try the other nostril, then consider using a smaller catheter (Donaldson and Holliday, 2007).

21 When the catheter has reached the required depth, apply suction by placing thumb over suction port control and gently withdraw the catheter. Try to avoid rotating the catheter as this can cause trauma (Donaldson and Holliday, 2007).

22 The whole procedure should take no longer than ten seconds to prevent hypoxia (Kozier et al, 2008; Mallet and Dougherty, 2000).

23 Wrap the catheter around the gloved hand then pull back the glove over the used catheter and discard according to universal precautions.

24 Observe the patient for any signs of discomfort and respond appropriately.

25 If the patient was previously having oxygen therapy, reapply and monitor oxygen saturations if required and allow patient time to recover.

26 If further suction is required, repeat the procedure using a new catheter and glove.

27 Flush the suction tubing with sterile water to remove secretions from the tube (Mallet and Dougherty, 2000).

28 Clean the patient's mouth, remove the towel and attend to the patient's comfort needs.

29 Dispose of the remaining glove, water and waste container according to universal precautions.

30 Wash and dry hands thoroughly.

31 Replace any equipment required for next suction procedure.

32 Document procedure and any significant findings.

33 The suction tubing and container should be changed every 24 hours or according to local policy guidelines.

⚠ Professional alert!

There are a number of potential complications of oro/nasopharyngeal suction and therefore it should only be performed when clinically indicated:

- trauma to the tracheal or bronchial mucosa
- laryngospasm when the larynx is touched
- hypoxia
- suctioning-induced hypoxaemia (insufficient oxygen reaching the body tissues)
- raised intracranial pressure
- cardiac arrhythmias, bradycardia, tachycardia
- respiratory arrest
- infection
- hypertension
- hypotension
- vaso-vagal nerve stimulation
- pulmonary atelectasis (alveolar collapse)

(Thompson, 2000; Dixon, 2006; Donaldson and Holliday, 2007.

Conclusion

The continuous supply of oxygen to the tissues is essential for survival. The need for oxygen therapy occurs when either the respiratory or the circulatory system are not functioning effectively. The healthcare professional should be able to provide oxygen by the most appropriate method to meet the patient's needs. Respiration can be compromised by the accumulation of secretions in the oropharynx, trachea or bronchi, and by performing oropharyngeal or nasopharyngeal suctioning the healthcare professional can remove these potentially dangerous secretions.

References

Alexander, M., Fawcett, J. and Runciman, P. (2006) *Nursing Practice Hospital and Home*, adult 3rd edn, Edinburgh, Churchill Livingstone.

American Association for Respiratory Care (2004) *Respiratory Care Journal* 49(9).

American Thoracic Society (2006) Online. http://www.thoracic.org (accessed May 2008).

Bateman, N. and Leach, R. (1998) 'Acute oxygen therapy', *British Medical Journal*, 317, 798–801.

Bell, C. (1995) 'Is this what the doctor ordered? Accuracy of oxygen therapy prescribed and delivered in hospital', *Professional Nurse* 10(5), 297–300.

BNF (2008) *British National Formulary* 55, London, BMJ Group and RPS Publishing.

BOC Medical (2008) 'Medical gas data sheet: medical oxygen', BOC [online] http://www1.boc.com/uk/sds/ (accessed 26 December 2008).

Carey, M. and Kelsey, J. (2008) 'Suctioning', pp. 214–20 in Kelsey, J. and McEwing, G. (eds), *Clinical Skills in Child Health Practice*, Edinburgh, Churchill Livingstone Elsevier.

Caroll, P. (1997) 'When you want humidity', *RN* (May), 31–5.

Chandler, T. (2001) 'Oxygen administration', *Paediatric Nursing* 13(8), 37–42.

Dixon, M. (2006) 'Practices in children's nursing', pp. 273–6 in E. Trigg and T. Mohammed, *Guidelines for Hospital and Community*, 2nd edn, London, Churchill Livingstone.

Donaldson, P. and Holliday, L. (2007) 'Oropharyngeal and nasopharyngeal suctioning', pp. 306–9 in Glasper, E., McEwing, G. and Richardson, J. (eds), *Oxford Handbook of Children's and Young*

Part
IV

People's Nursing, Oxford, Oxford University Press.

Dougherty, L. and Lister, S. (eds) (2004) *The Royal Marsden Manual of Clinical Nursing Procedures*, 6th edn, Oxford, Blackwell Publishing.

Eastwood, G. M. and Dennis, M. J. (2006) 'Nasopharyngeal oxygen (NPO) as a safe and comfortable alternative to facemask oxygen therapy', *Australian Critical Care* **19**(1), 22–4.

Fell, H. and Boehm, M. (1998) 'Easing the discomfort of oxygen therapy' *Nursing Times* **94**(38), 56–8.

Frey, B. and Shann, F. (2003) 'Oxygen administration in infants', *Arch. Dis Child. Fetal Neonatal Ed* 88, 84–8.

Giles, R. (2006) 'Oxygen therapy', pp. 257–63 in Trigg, E. and Mohammed, T. (eds), *Practices in Children's Nursing: Guidelines for hospital and community*, 2nd edn, Edinburgh, Churchill Livingstone.

Hufton, R. (2007) 'Using a humidifier', pp. 316–17 in Glasper, E., McEwing, G. and Richardson J. (eds), *Oxford Handbook of Children's and Young People's Nursing*, Oxford, Oxford University Press.

Kotecha, S and Allen, J. (2002) 'Oxygen therapy for infants with chronic lung disease', *Archives of Diseases in Childhood* **87**(1), 11–14.

Kozier, B., Erb, G., Berman, A., Snyder, S., Lake, R. and Harvey, S. (2008) *Fundamentals of Nursing Concepts, Process and Practice*, Harlow, UK, Pearson Education.

Mallet, J. and Dougherty, L. (2000) The Royal Marsden NHS Trust Manual of Clinical Nursing Procedures, 5th edn, Oxford, Blackwell Science.

Merieb, E. and Hoehn, K. (2007) *Human Anatomy and Physiology*, 7th edn, San Francisco, Pearson Education.

NICE (2004) *Guideline 12: Chronic obstructive pulmonary disease*, London, National Institute for Clinical Excellence.

Nicol. M., Bavin, C., Bedford-Turner, S., Cronin, P. and Rawlings-Anderson, K. (2004) *Essential Nursing Skills*, Edinburgh, Mosby.

Pierce, L. N. N. (1995) *Guide to Mechanical Ventilation and Intensive Respiratory Care*, London, W.B. Saunders.

Pilkington, F. (2004) 'Humidification for oxygen therapy in non-ventilated patients', *British Journal of Nursing* **13**(2), 111–15.

Porth, C.M. (2007) *Essentials of Pathophysiology: Concepts of altered health states*, 2nd edn, Philadelphia, Lippincott, Williams and Wilkins.

Resuscitation Council UK (RCUK) (2005) [online] http://www.resus.org.uk/pages/pbls.pdf (accessed 28 March 2008).

Smith, T. (2004) 'Oxygen therapy for older people', *Nursing Older People* **16**(5), 22–8.

Thompson, L. (2000) 'Suctioning adults with an artificial airway', *The Joanna Briggs Institute for Evidence-based Nursing and Midwifery Systematic Review* 9.

Timby, B. (2005) *Fundamental Nursing Skills and Concepts*, 8th edn, London, Lippincott Williams and Wilkins.

Toplis, D. (2007) 'Administration of oxygen', pp. 298–9 in Glasper, E., McEwing, G. and Richardson, J. (eds), *Oxford Handbook of Children's and Young People's Nursing*, Oxford, Oxford University Press.

Torrance, C. and Serginson, E. (2000) *Surgical Nursing*, London, Bailliere Tindall.

Tortora, G. (1997) *Introduction to Human Biology*, 4th edn, Harlow, UK, Addison Wesley Langman.

Ward, B. and Park, G. R. (2000) 'Humidification of inspired gases in the critically ill', *Clin Intensive Care* 11(4), 169–76.

Chapter

36

Basic life support: child

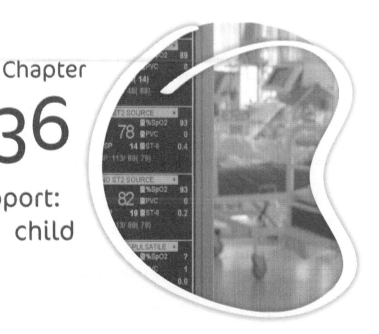

Janet Kelsey and Gill McEwing

Links to other chapters in *Foundation Skills for Caring*

Links to other chapters in *Foundation Studies for Caring*

W Don't forget to visit www.palgrave.com/glasper for additional online resources relating to this chapter.

Part

IV

Introduction

It is unusual for infants and children to require basic life support. However accidents are still the commonest cause of death in children, and children with chronic illnesses who are surviving are more likely to require emergency interventions. For these reasons it is important that health professionals, parents and members of the public are confident that they can react competently in such cases. This chapter considers the emergency response to a child requiring basic life support. It takes the reader through the stages of recognising and responding to this critical situation using the structured approach to care.

Learning outcomes

This chapter will enable you to:

- be aware of some of the causes of cardiorespiratory arrest in infants and children

- recognise when a cardiac arrest occurs in infants and children

- identify the keys stages in delivering basic life support for an infant and a child.

Concepts

- Emergency care
- Communication
- Assessment

- Decision making
- Safety
- Team working

- Family support

Causes of cardiorespiratory arrest

The underlying cause of cardiorespiratory arrest in infants and children is different from that in adults. Progressive respiratory insufficiency accounts for 60 per cent of all paediatric arrests (secondary cardiorespiratory arrest). Upper airway disease may include croup or foreign body aspiration and lower airway bronchiolitis, pneumonia and asthma. Also respiratory depression can be caused by, for example, prolonged convulsions, raised intracranial pressure, neuromuscular disease or drug overdose. Secondary cardiorespiratory arrest is due to the body's inability to cope with the underlying illness or injury. The preterminal rhythm is bradycardia, which leads to asystole or pulseless electrical activity (Kelly, 2007). This can be preceded by either respiratory or circulatory failure. Respiratory failure leads to inadequate oxygenation, hypoxia and hypercapnia that cause acidosis, cell damage and cell death, leading to cardiac arrest. Circulatory failure, causing deprivation of essential nutrients and oxygen and the inability to remove waste products, leads to hypoxia and acidosis. Inadequate circulation will also result in vital organs being under-perfused and cell damage will result. Respiratory and circulatory failure can occur separately or together, but as the condition becomes worse both will occur (Kelly, 2007). Other important causes include sepsis, anaphylaxis, dehydration and hypovolaemia caused by, for example, gastroenteritis or burns.

ⓐ Learning activity

Find out the incidence of admissions to hospital due to respiratory illness in young children in your area of practice.

As the pathologies that affect children usually cause a secondary cardiorespiratory arrest, primary cardiac arrest in children is rare and ventricular fibrillation has been reported in less than 10 per cent of cases. Children often have a relatively long 'pre-arrest' phase where cardiac arrest is preceded by a prolonged physiological deterioration.

> ### t☆ Practice tip
>
> Impending cardiopulmonary arrest may be averted by early recognition of the child's distress and prompt intervention.
>
> Once cardiac arrest occurs the outcome is poor, with survival rates of between 3–17 per cent (Anaesthesia UK, 2005).

Outcomes

The National Audit of Paediatric Resuscitation (2006) is collecting data for all children under the age of 16 years who have a respiratory or cardiac arrest event (not newborn resuscitation). Over 120 centres have reported 1491 events from 72 centres; of these 1127 occurred out of hospital and 364 in hospital. Of the 364 in hospital the majority occurred on the ward (239), 16 in paediatric intensive care units, 98 in accident and emergency and 11 in other locations. Survival rates in hospital are as follows:

- Of the 50 children in asystole, 16 had a return of spontaneous circulation (ROSC) and 9 were either sent to other centres or returned home.
- Of the 109 children in bradycardia, 88 had an ROSC and 67 were either sent to other centres or returned home.
- 32 children presented in pulseless electrical activity (PEA), of whom 16 had an ROSC and eight were either sent to other centres or returned home.
- Ten children were in ventricular fibrillation/ventricular tachycardia (VF/VT); three had an ROSC and two were either sent to other centres or returned home.
- The remaining 148 children had an unspecified rhythm; 137 had an ROSC and 108 were either sent to other centres or returned home.

Out of hospital events numbered 1127, with 80 per cent occurring at home, 9 per cent in a public place or the street, 1 per cent at school and 1 per cent at a recreational place (for example, a park or swimming pool). For 642 of the out-of-hospital events the primary diagnosis was: 27 per cent cardiac, 25 per cent respiratory, 12 per cent trauma, 9 per cent sudden infant death syndrome (SIDS), 5 per cent drowning, 5 per cent threatened airway, 1 per cent fitting, 16 per cent others. In 485 events the primary diagnosis was either not documented or unknown. Of the 978 children (83.4 per cent) who had chest compressions, 62 per cent were in asystole, 6 per cent were in PEA, 5 per cent were in VF and 2 per cent were in bradycardia.

In the out-of-hospital group:

- 606 children were in asystole, but only 42 of this group had an ROSC, with 12 being discharged home or sent to another centre.
- 49 children were in ventricular fibrillation; nine had an ROSC, with four being discharged home or sent to another centre.
- PEA accounted for 68 children; 18 had an ROSC, with five being discharged home or sent to another centre.
- Only 29 children had a bradycardia diagnosed. However, the survival profile of this group was the best, with 20 having an ROSC and seven being discharged home or sent to another centre.

> ### a Learning activity
>
> Identify the data for cardiac and respiratory arrest in your local paediatric high-dependency unit (HDU) or paediatric intensive care unit (PICU) audit. This information is part of a national audit and is available on the internet. Your local HDU or PICU will be able to direct you to where this information is available.

Basic life support (BLS)

> The full paediatric BLS sequence is for healthcare professionals with a duty to respond to paediatric emergencies (e.g. A&E staff, paediatric doctors and nurses, paramedics). These people usually work in teams of two or more rescuers. Lay providers who are particularly likely to attempt resuscitation of a child should be taught the adult sequence with the paediatric modifiers.
>
> (RCUK, 2006)

With the introduction of Guidelines 2000, the Resuscitation Council (UK) defined a healthcare professional as:

> a person who holds a recognised vocational qualification in a medical or related discipline whose employment of work includes at least some degree of clinical responsibility. A first aider is not a healthcare professional.
>
> (RCUK, 2006)

It is broadly accepted that cardiopulmonary resuscitation, including compressions and/or ventilations, should be undertaken in children who have arrested, and although there are few systematic reviews most clinicians regard bystander cardiopulmonary resuscitation as an important intervention in out-of-hospital cardiopulmonary arrest.

Blood pressure will fall with any lapse in chest compressions, and it will take several chest compressions to restore blood perfusion to cardiac tissue; with more interruptions in cardiac compressions the survival rate is reduced. The new BLS guidelines therefore place greater emphasis on uninterrupted chest compressions, with a resultant ratio of 30 compressions to two breaths for non-healthcare responders; however healthcare responders with a duty to respond should initiate 15 compressions to two breaths. In addition, no more than two attempts should be made at achieving effective breaths before compressions are recommenced.

The paediatric modifiers to the adult BLS algorithm are:

- Give five initial breaths before starting chest compressions.
- If on your own, perform one minute of CPR before going for help.
- Compress the chest by approximately one-third of its depth. Use two fingers for an infant under 1 year; use one or two hands for a child over 1 year as needed to achieve an adequate depth of compression.

⚠ Professional alert!

The 2005 International Liaison Committee on Resuscitation's consensus recommendation on science treatment encourages 'trained rescuers to provide both ventilations and chest compressions'. The consensus recommendation goes on to encourage those rescuers who are reluctant or unable to perform ventilations to institute and continue chest compressions without interruption.

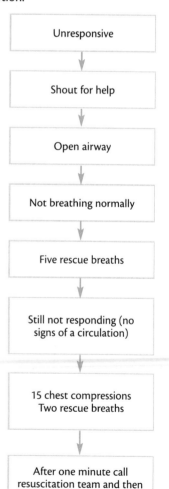

⟳ Learning activity

What is the recognised number in your hospital to call the resuscitation team? If you were working in the community how would you call for help?

Figure 36.1 Paediatric basic life support (for healthcare professionals with a duty to respond)

Basic life support in infants and children follows the airway, breathing and circulation sequence:

1 Ensure the safety of the rescuer and child. It is essential that the rescuer does not become a victim and the child is removed from further danger as quickly as possible. This should precede all further actions.

2 Assess the child's responsiveness. Gently stimulate the child by speaking loudly and asking, 'Are you all right?' Shake by the shoulders or pinch gently. Do not shake children with suspected cervical spine injuries. Young children are unlikely to respond in a meaningful way, but may make some sound or open their eyes.

3 If children respond but are struggling to breathe, leave them in the position in which you find them unless they are in further danger. Children with respiratory distress often position themselves to maintain patency of a partially obstructed airway. Unless advanced support is available, attempts to improve a partially maintained airway are potentially dangerous as total occlusion may occur. Check the child's condition regularly and get help if needed. If the child does not respond, the rescuer should shout for help and then provide basic life-support for one minute before going for assistance. It may be possible to take a small child or infant with you whilst summoning help. Check first to see if there is evidence of trauma. The likelihood of injury may be evident from the child's location or position; for example, a child found at the foot of a tree is more likely to have suffered trauma than one found in bed. If more than one rescuer is present, then one should go for help whilst the other commences resuscitation. After shouting for help, open the child's airway. Use the appropriate technique for the age of the child. Try to do this with the child in the position in which you find him/her. If this is not possible, then carefully turn the child on to his/her back and open the airway. Again if trauma is suspected, turn the child with head and neck firmly supported. Do not allow the head to twist, roll or tilt. Avoid head tilt if cervical spine injury is suspected.

4 Keep the airway open and check breathing. Look for chest and abdominal movement. Listen at the mouth and nose for breath sounds. Feel for expired air movement on your cheek. Look, listen and feel for up to ten seconds before deciding that breathing is absent. If children are breathing, place them in the recovery position and continue to assess them.

5 If the child is not breathing or there is ineffective, gasping or obstructed breathing, carefully check for and remove any obvious airway obstruction, but do not perform a blind finger sweep. Give up to five rescue breaths. With each breath, the child's chest should move. Take a breath before each rescue breath to optimise the amount of oxygen delivered to the child. Breathe slowly and steadily for between one and one and a half seconds. This minimises the risk of gastric distension, which can reduce the effectiveness of rescue breathing by pushing up the diaphragm and reducing lung volume. If the chest either does not rise or any rise is inadequate, then the airway may be obstructed. Recheck the child's mouth for obvious obstructions. Readjust the airway position. Five attempts should be made to achieve two effective breaths. If you are still unsuccessful, then consider foreign body obstruction and move on to the airway obstruction sequence.

6 Assess the child's circulation. Take no more than ten seconds to check the pulse, using the correct technique for the age of the child (infants, brachial or femoral; children, carotid). At the same time look for signs of life such as any movement, including swallowing or breathing. If you can detect signs of circulation within the ten seconds but no breathing, then continue rescue breathing for one minute before going for help. If somebody else has gone for help, continue rescue breathing until the child starts breathing effectively on his/her own. If at this point the child remains unconscious, then turn him/her onto the side into the recovery position.

7 If there is no palpable pulse or it is less than one beat per second, or if you are not sure, then start chest compressions using an age-appropriate technique, and combine the chest compressions with rescue breathing. Remember the ratio of compressions to breaths for infants and children is 30:2 for lay rescuers but for two or more rescuers with a duty to respond it is 15:2. The recommended rate of compressions is the same for all: 100 times per minute. However, this is the rate and not the number of compressions to be given in a minute, as there will be interruptions for ventilation.

8 You should continue to resuscitate until the child demonstrates spontaneous respiration and pulse, or help arrives, or you become exhausted.

a) Learning activity

Find out the anatomical differences between adults and children that will affect the resuscitation of infants and children.

There are some specific differences in technique for different sizes of children and you must be aware of these in order to give the optimum support.

The major differences in technique for an infant

- To open the airway the head and chin should be tilted to the 'sniffing position'. This is achieved by placing one hand on the forehead and tilting the head back into a neutral position, avoiding excessive neck extension and taking care not to press on the soft issues under the chin. A jaw thrust may be used if cervical spine injury is suspected.

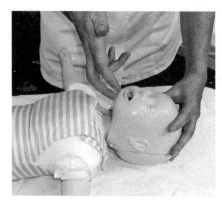

Figure 36.2   Opening the airway

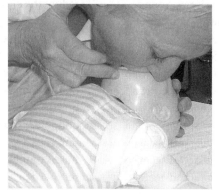

Figure 36.3   Rescue breaths

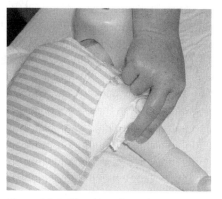

Figure 36.4   Checking the pulse

- Deliver five rescue breaths. When delivering rescue breaths, cover the mouth and nose with your mouth, ensuring you have a good seal, blow steadily into the mouth and nose for between one and one and a half seconds.
- If you are trained and experienced check the circulation. The brachial pulse is easiest to feel on the inner aspect of the upper arm between the elbow and the shoulder. Gently press with index and middle fingers until you feel the pulse.

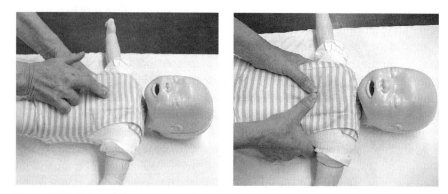

Figure 36.5   External chest compression

- If the pulse rate is less than 60 beats per minute, that is less than one per second, external chest compressions should begin without delay.
- If you are alone, perform chest compressions by using two fingers of one hand to compress the lower third of the sternum; this is one finger's breadth above the xiphisternum, the angle where the lowest ribs join in the middle. If there are two rescuers, use the encircling technique: place your thumbs flat side by side on the lower third of the sternum, with the tips pointing towards the infant's head. Spread the rest of both hands, with fingers together, encircling the lower part of the infant's rib cage with the tips of the fingers supporting the infant's back. Depress the lower sternum with your thumbs to approximately one-third of the depth of the infant's chest (RCUK, 2005).

The major differences in technique for a child

- To open the airway, place one hand on the forehead and tilt the head back into a neutral or slightly extended position (Figure 36.6). Lift the lower jaw with the tips of two fingers of the other hand. Avoid excessive neck extension and take care not to press on the soft issues under the chin. A jaw thrust may be used if cervical spine injury is suspected.

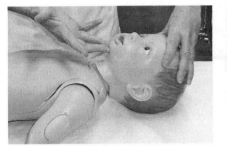

Figure 36.6 Opening the airway

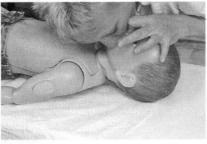

Figure 36.7 Rescue breaths

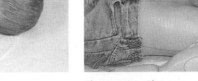

Figure 36.8 Chest compression

- To deliver rescue breaths, make a mouth-to-mouth seal and pinch the soft part of the child's nose tightly with your thumb and index finger, maintaining head tilt (Figure 36.7).
- If you are trained and experienced, check the circulation. In children the carotid pulse should be palpated.
- If the pulse is absent, then external chest compressions should begin without delay.
- For children, the heel of one hand is used to compress the lower third of the sternum, which is one fingers breadth above the xiphisternum, ensuring that the fingers are lifted to prevent pressure being applied over the child's ribs (Figure 36.8). Position yourself vertically above the child's chest, with your arms straight; compress the sternum by one-third of the depth of the child's chest (RCUK, 2005).
- In larger children or when the rescuer is small, it may be better to use both hands: locate the lower half of the sternum and place the heel of one hand in position, then place the other hand directly on top of the first hand and interlock fingers. Raise the fingers off the chest to ensure that pressure is not applied to the child's ribs.

Conclusion

This chapter has set out the structured approach for the resuscitation of infants and children. It outlines the different approaches required for the two age groups. The probable causes of arrest have been outlined and the outcomes discussed. The need for prompt, competent action has been stressed and it is the responsibility of all healthcare professionals to be able to respond to this situation within their level of expertise.

References

Anaesthesia UK (2005) 'Cardiorespiratory arrest in children', Anaesthesia UK [online] http://www.anaesthesiauk.com (accessed 28 March 2008).

Kelly, M. (2007) 'Reasons why children arrest', in Glasper, E., McEwing, G. and Richardson, J. (eds), *Oxford Handbook of Children's and Young People's Nursing*, Oxford, Oxford University Press.

National Audit of Paediatric Resuscitation (2006) Resuscitation Council UK [online] http://www.resus.org.uk/pages/naprfaq.htm (accessed 28 April 2008).

Resuscitation Council UK (RCUK) (2005) [online] http://www.resus.org.uk/pages/pbls.pdf (accessed 28 March 2008).

RCUK (2006) [online] http://www.resus.org.uk/pages/faqPBLS.htm (accessed 26 March 2008).

Chapter

37

Basic life support: adult

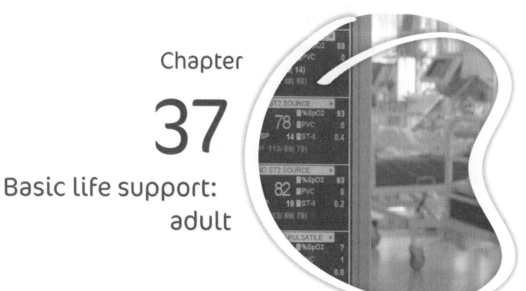

Jan Heath

Links to other chapters in *Foundation Skills for Caring*

Links to other chapters in *Foundation Studies for Caring*

W   Don't forget to visit www.palgrave.com/glasper for additional online resources relating to this chapter.

Introduction

The outcome from cardiac arrest is poor. Survival figures range from 3–44 per cent depending on the location and help available. Survival rates will clearly be better if the victim collapses in the presence of people who know what to do, and especially if the event takes place where a defibrillator is available. The results from first responder schemes and statistics from hospital cardiac arrests have shown that patients who collapse in hospital are more likely to survive, (particularly where the presenting rhythm is ventricular fibrillation and staff trained to use the defibrillator are attending the patient) than those collapsing outside hospital. Basic life support (BLS) provided by bystanders will improve the survival of victims of cardiac arrest, but only a small percentage of the population in the UK can perform cardiopulmonary resuscitation (CPR).

This chapter considers the emergency response to an adult requiring basic life support. It takes you through the stages of recognising and responding to this critical situation using the structured approach to care.

Learning outcomes

This chapter will enable you to:

- recognise a cardiac arrest
- call for help and identify key facts required by the telephone operator
- follow the basic life support algorithm
- discuss and understand the reasons for the recommended ratio for BLS
- identify the possible causes of an anaphylactic reaction
- list the signs and symptoms of anaphylaxis
- be aware of the need for regular resuscitation training
- identify the drug dosages and route of administration for adrenaline in anaphylaxis.

Concepts

- Recognition of a medical emergency
- Empowerment
- Knowing when and how to call for expert help
- Principles of basic life support

There are many reasons that adults collapse. The degree of intervention depends on many factors, including:

- location
- help available
- circumstances contributing to the collapse
- the ability of people attending.

Any intervention should be in accordance with the Resuscitation Council *Guidelines* (RCUK, 2005), based on the 2005 International Consensus on Cardiopulmonary Resuscitation and Emergency Cardiovascular Care Science with Treatment Recommendations (CoSTR), which was published in November 2005.

a Learning activity

Find out the incidence of admissions to hospital as a result of cardiac arrest in your area. How many had received basic life support skills while waiting for the paramedics?

t Practice tip

The following activities are based on the Resuscitation Council Guidelines 2005. The interventions should be practised on a regular basis in the skills laboratory using appropriate training mannequins under the supervision of resuscitation officers or trained instructors.

Up-to-date information is available from the Resuscitation Council website: www.resus.org

Cardiopulmonary resuscitation (CPR)

This is a simple but important skill. If more people knew how to perform basic life support more lives would be saved. In the United Kingdom up to 260,000 people suffer a heart attack each year. It is estimated that 30 per cent die before they get to hospital.

Basic life support

The Resuscitation Council *Guidelines* (RCUK, 2005) describe the steps outlined in Figure 37.1, which must be followed to perform BLS.

BLS follows simple steps which can be most effective if applied promptly at the time of collapse. BLS may be performed by a single rescuer with no equipment, or using simple devices such as a face shield if they are available. Some rescuers are unwilling to perform mouth-to-mouth rescue breathing even though there is no evidence that they are putting their own health at risk. If the would-be rescuer fails to perform mouth-to-mouth resuscitation, the rescuer should be encouraged to perform chest compressions alone. It is important to act quickly, and to avoid or keep to a minimum any pauses in the procedure.

The recommendations in the 2005 guidelines place the emphasis on looking for signs of life rather than spending time trying to assess for the presence of a carotid pulse. The rationale is that attempting to feel the carotid pulse can waste precious time and is unreliable when attempted by untrained individuals. Absence of normal breathing is important but nonhealthcare professionals can mistake irregular gasping (agonal breathing patterns) for normal breathing, and have failed to provide BLS when it is required as a result. Forty per cent of victims of cardiac arrest have agonal respirations, and therefore reliance on recognising abnormal breathing patterns when deciding whether to perform BLS puts many victims at risk. The guidelines (RCUK, 2005) now state that collapsed individuals who are unresponsive with irregular gasping breathing should have life support intervention.

BLS is exhausting both physically and mentally, so help must be called for promptly. If you are alone with the victim, shout for help. If this is unlikely to raise a response, go to a telephone or find help yourself.

We can all imagine desperate situations where we could be alone with a collapsed individual with no prospect of help, but in reality these are rare events, and it is more likely that there will be access to a phone, or other people can be alerted to the emergency.

Clear sensible communication is essential in these circumstances. Asking for help requires you to communicate by dialling an appropriate number (now 2222 in all hospitals: National Patient Safety Agency), and tell the person answering what the emergency is and what help is required.

If the emergency takes place out of hospital someone must go to a telephone and call 999 or 112, report the emergency and state clearly where the victim is located, what the problem is and which emergency service is required.

Performing chest compressions is extremely tiring. If more than one rescuer is present, the person delivering the chest compressions should change over approximately every 2 minutes. This should be done with the minimum of disruption to the resuscitation, since disruptions can seriously affect the outcome.

Adult basic life support

There is a mandatory checklist of steps to take when dealing with a collapsed adult.

Safety

Is it safe to approach the victim? Check for danger. Is the situation safe for the victim, yourself and any bystanders?

> ⚠ **Professional alert!**
>
> It is important to try to ensure the safety of the victim and the rescuer before attempting resuscitation.

Response

Check the victim for responsiveness. Gently shake their shoulders and ask loudly, 'Are you all right?'

If they respond:

- Leave the victim where they are if they are not in danger.
- Do not move the victim if there is a suspicion of trauma.
- Try to find out what has happened to the victim.
- Give appropriate reassurance.
- If they are breathing turn them into the recovery position.
- Send for help.

If there is no response:

- Assess the situation and get appropriate help.
- Ask someone to get an ambulance if you are out of hospital, or call the cardiac arrest team if you are in a hospital.
- If you are on your own, go to make this call at this point.

Airway

Turn the victim onto their back. Open the airway using a chin lift. Put your fingers under the victim's chin, place one hand on their forehead and tilt their head back while lifting their chin. This aims to move the tongue back from the posterior pharyngeal wall.

Breathing

Once the airway is open, look, listen and feel for signs of normal breathing and signs of life such as swallowing, gasping, movements.

- Look at the victim's chest for any movement.
- Listen at the victim's mouth for sounds of breathing.
- Feel for any expired air on your cheek.
- Do this for no longer than 10 seconds. If in doubt, act as though breathing is not normal.

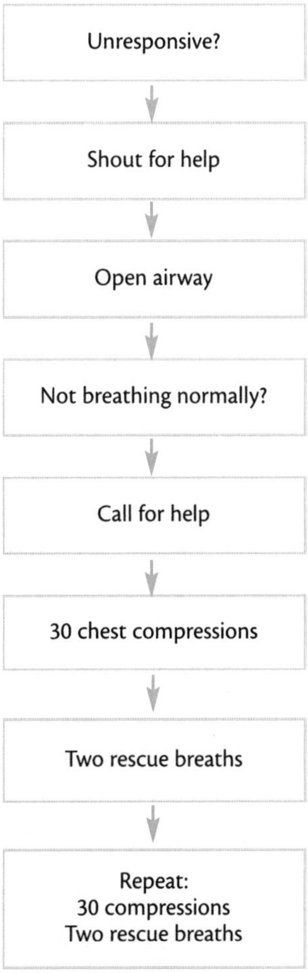

⚠ Professional alert!

In approximately 40 per cent of cases, immediately after cardiac arrest the victim takes noisy gasps. These are agonal gasps. This is not normal breathing. Therefore nonhealthcare professionals are advised to proceed with CPR if the victim is unconscious, unresponsive and not breathing normally.

If the victim is breathing normally:

- Place the victim in the recovery position.
- Ask someone to go for help. If you are alone, go for help yourself and call an ambulance.
- Monitor the victim's breathing while waiting for assistance.

If the victim is not breathing normally:

- Get help: either ask someone else to raise the emergency services, or if you are alone, do this yourself.
- This is a seriously ill person and resuscitation must be started.
- Begin chest compressions.

Initially patients who have collapsed suddenly with no previous respiratory problems will have reasonable oxygen concentrations in their blood, which makes chest compressions more important than ventilation.

Some rescuers are unwilling to perform mouth-to-mouth ventilation, because of

---

Unresponsive?

↓

Shout for help

↓

Open airway

↓

Not breathing normally?

↓

Call for help

↓

30 chest compressions

↓

Two rescue breaths

↓

Repeat:
30 compressions
Two rescue breaths

Figure 37.1 Adult basic life support (for healthcare professionals with a duty to respond)

Part

IV

either the perceived risk of infection or dislike of the procedure. Therefore by emphasising the importance of initially providing chest compressions in adults, you will encourage nonhealthcare professionals to begin some form of resuscitation.

Performing chest compressions

1   Kneel by the side of the victim's chest.
2   Place the heel of one hand on the centre of the victim's chest in line with the armpits. Avoid the upper abdomen and the bottom end of the sternum.
3   Place the heel of the other hand on top of the first hand.
4   Interlock your fingers to avoid applying pressure over the victim's ribs.
5   Position yourself so that your shoulders are over the victim's chest, with your arms straight.
6   Press down on the breast bone to a depth of 4–5 cm.
7   After each compression release the pressure and repeat without changing position, at a rate of 100 compressions per minute.
8   Compression and release should take equal amounts of time.
9   After 30 compressions begin rescue breaths.

⚠ Professional alert!

Chest-compression-only CPR is only effective for a limited period of about 5 minutes. It is not recommended as the standard procedure for out-of-hospital cardiac arrest, but nonhealthcare professionals should be encouraged to do this if they are unwilling to perform rescue breaths. Combined chest compression and ventilation is the better method of CPR.

Rescue breaths

1   Open the airway again using the head tilt, chin lift procedure.
2   Using the hand that is on the victim's forehead, close the victim's nose by pinching the soft part of the nose using your thumb and index finger.
3   Continue with the chin lift but allow the victim's mouth to open.
4   Breathe in normally.
5   Place your lips around the victim's mouth and with a good seal blow steadily into their mouth watching the victim's chest rise. This should take about 1 second, and constitutes an effective rescue breath.
6   Maintaining the victim's position, take your lips away. Allow the air to come out and watch the chest wall fall.
7   Take another breath and repeat to give a total of two effective breaths.
8   Go back to the landmarks on the chest and repeat the 30 chest compressions.

⚠ Professional alert!

Some rescuers are worried that it might be possible to transmit HIV during mouth-to-mouth rescue breathing. As yet there is no evidence that this has ever occurred. There have been some isolated reports of transmission of tuberculosis and severe respiratory distress syndrome (SARS) (RCUK, 2005).

Specific filters and barrier devices with one-way valves can prevent oral bacteria transmission during mouth-to-mouth rescue breathing. If these devices are available, they should be used as a precautionary measure.

t☆
Practice tip

If the rescuer is unable or unwilling to perform rescue breaths, they should proceed with chest compressions only at a rate of 100 per minute.

Only stop if the victim begins to breathe normally.

t☆
Practice tip

In a confined space BLS can be performed by leaning over the victim's head if one person is involved. When two rescuers are present, a rescuer may straddle the victim.

t☆
Practice tip

If the victim's mouth is damaged, preventing a good seal, mouth-to-nose rescue breaths should be given.

t☆
Practice tip

If rescue breaths do not make the chest rise as in normal breathing, then before your next attempt at rescue breaths:

1 Make sure there is no visible obstruction in the victim's mouth which can be removed.
2 Make sure there is adequate head tilt and chin lift.
3 Only attempt two rescue breaths each time before continuing with chest compressions.

⚠ **Professional alert!**

Interruptions in chest compressions are linked with a reduced chance of survival for the victim. BLS should continue without interruptions until one of the following occurs:

● Help arrives to take over.
● The victim starts to respond, shown by movement or breathing normally.
● You are physically too exhausted to continue.

t☆
Practice tip

If you have assistance, either perform both compressions and rescue breaths for 2 minutes then change over with the other rescuer, or work together, with one person delivering compressions and the other giving the breaths. This will help prevent exhaustion. Try to ensure a minimum delay at handover.

Rescue breaths should be performed after the 30 compressions. Do not perform chest compressions while the breathing is delivered, as there is an unprotected airway which is at risk of gastric regurgitation if the chest is being compressed during the inflation breaths. If the person doing chest compressions is pressing on the chest while the other person is attempting to do respirations, the person breathing is actually trying to inflate the chest and lift the weight of the chest-compressing person!

Rescue breathing is not a pleasant activity, but it is essential to get breath (expired air contains approximately 16 per cent oxygen) into the victim (RCUK, 2005).

There are many devices available to provide a barrier between you and the victim.

After each 30 compressions return to the airway. Repeat the airway-opening manoeuvre, then after taking a normal breath yourself, make a seal around the victims' mouth with your mouth and blow your expired air into the victim enough to see their chest rise.

Continue at a ratio of 30 compressions to two breaths.

Summary

Danger	Check for danger
Response	Check for response
Shout	Shout for help
Airway	Open the airway
Breathing	Check for normal breathing
CPR	Start CPR
Ratio	30 compressions to two breaths
Rate	100 compressions over 1 minute

ⓐ **Learning activity**

When in the skills laboratory, practise CPR on the mannequins to ensure you are competent and confident to perform this activity.

Part

IV

Recovery position

There are a variety of guidelines to assist you in putting an individual into the recovery position. The intention is to put the patient in a stable near-lateral position with the head independent and with no pressure on the chest to restrict breathing.

The recommendation from the Resuscitation Council (RCUK, 2005) is:

1 Remove the victim's spectacles, if they are wearing any.
2 Kneel beside the victim and make sure that both their legs are straight.
3 Place the arm nearest to you out at right angles to their body, elbow bent with the hand palm uppermost.
4 Bring the far arm across the chest, and hold the back of the hand against the victim's cheek nearest to you.
5 With your other hand, grasp the far leg just above the knee and pull it up, keeping the foot on the ground.

6 Keeping the hand pressed against their cheek, pull on the far leg to roll the victim towards you onto their side.
7 Adjust the upper leg so that both the hip and knee are bent at right angles.
8 Tilt the head back to make sure the airway remains open.
9 Adjust the hand under the cheek if necessary, to keep the head tilted.
10 Check breathing regularly.

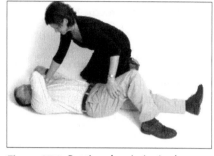
Figure 37.3 Putting the victim in the recovery position

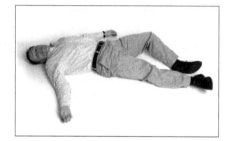
Figure 37.2 The recovery position

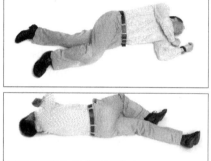
Figure 37.4 The recovery position

If the victim is required to remain in this position for more than 30 minutes they should be turned onto the opposite side at the 30-minute point.

Bag mask ventilation

Training is vital to support the use of bag mask devices. These are advantageous, and are used in hospital to allow supplementary oxygen to be delivered. Many different types are available. The majority are designed for single patient use and should be disposed of afterwards.

> **ⓐ Learning activity**
>
> Take the opportunity to practise putting someone into this position, so you will feel confident of how to do it in an emergency.

Anaphylaxis

Anaphylaxis is a rare but life-threatening reaction to an allergen. There is not a conclusive definition for anaphylaxis, but it should be considered when more than two of the skin, respiratory, circulatory, neurological and gastroenterology systems are affected. Other features that are usually present are:

- erythema
- generalised pruritis
- urticaria
- angio-odema
- wheeze
- rhinitis
- conjunctivitis
- itching of palate/external auditory meatus
- nausea, vomiting, abdominal pain
- palpitations
- sense of impending doom.

What happens during anaphylaxis?

An anaphylactic reaction occurs following exposure to an allergen to which a person has been sensitised. People who have asthma and allergies are at high risk of anaphylaxis (Pumphrey and Gowland, 2007). Repeated exposure results in specific IgE antibodies recognising the allergen and creating a reaction to it. This encourages mast cells to release inflammatory mediators, which cause an anaphylactic reaction. It is the rapid release of large quantities of mediators that causes leakage of capillaries, mucosal swelling which results in cardiovascular and respiratory shock.

> **a) Learning activity**
>
> Find out the most common causes of an anaphylactic reaction in an adult or child.

When dealing with patients presenting with difficulty with breathing, severe rashes and/or circulatory problems following exposure to elements that can cause anaphylaxis, urgent action is required.

Procedure

1 Act immediately.
2 Remove the item causing the event if possible. For example, if antibiotics are the cause, stop administering them. If it is an insect sting, immediately scrape away any insect parts at the site of the sting. Avoid squeezing. Unfortunately nothing can be done if the cause is something the person has eaten.
3 Put the victim in a position where they are able to breathe more easily if possible.
4 The victim may feel very faint or look very pale. If so lie the victim down.
5 Give 100 per cent oxygen if possible.
6 An experienced anaesthetist is mandatory if the event occurs in hospital.

Medication for anaphylaxis in adults

Intramuscular adrenaline 0.5 ml 1:1000 solution (500 mcg).
If there is no improvement after five minutes repeat the dose.
Chlorphenamine 4 mg orally or 10 mg by slow intravenous injection.
Fluids given intravenously are usually necessary.
Salbutamol 5 mg given by nebuliser can be used to relieve bronchospasm.

There should never be any delay in the treatment of anaphylaxis, but the guidelines changed in 2008. This could lead to some confusion until everyone who might treat victims is fully aware of the new guidelines, particularly as this is a relatively rare medical emergency. Full details of the new version of the guidelines to treat anaphylaxis are available at www.resus.org.uk/pages/whatsnew.htm

In-hospital resuscitation

The resuscitation team

Each organisation will have its own action plan to attend to individuals who collapse. There should be a team that responds to victims of cardiac arrest. Its composition varies but there should be a minimum of two doctors trained to deal with such emergencies.

The team should collectively have the skills to deal with:

- airway interventions
- routes for drug administration
- monitoring and defibrillation
- knowledge of drugs and fluids
- post resuscitation management
- team leader skills.

Ideally there should be a separate paediatric team with appropriately trained individuals. Some other points to consider include:

- Cardiopulmonary resuscitation is a medical emergency which occurs infrequently with little or no warning. There is a greater likelihood of dying from a cardiac arrest than there is of survival.
- Since you must act urgently in these situations, you cannot rely on looking up the guidelines from a textbook. You should aim to memorise the steps, but posters and algorithms can be useful.
- Cardiac arrest is an emergency for which annual or more frequent updates are mandatory for all individuals who have the privilege of looking after patients.
- Guidelines and equipment must be simple to use and accessible.
- You should identify facilities and personnel which will help you practise the skills required to manage medical emergencies and CPR.

Conclusion

Emergency life support is rarely a predicted event out of hospital. It is important to be able to recall basic principles of resuscitation which may be of benefit to the victim if you are in a position to give assistance within your capabilities.

After dealing with a medical emergency there should be the opportunity to have debriefing if required.

References

Ashton, A., McCluskey, A., Gwinnutt, C. L. and Keenan, A. M. (2002) 'Effect of rescuer fatigue on performance of continuous external chest compressions over 3 minutes', *Resuscitation* 55, 151–5.

Bahr, J., Klingler, H., Panzer, W., Rode, H. and Kettler, D. (1997) 'Skills of lay people in checking the cartoid pulse', *Resucitation* **35**(1), 23–6.

European Resuscitation Council (2005) *European Resuscitation Council Guidelines for Resuscitation 2005*, Resuscitation 2005; 67 (Suppl.1): S1–S190.

Handley, A. J. (2002) 'Teaching hand placement for chest compression: a simpler technique', *Resuscitation* 53, 29–36.

Pumphrey, R. S. and Gowland, M. H. (2007) 'Further fatal allergic reactions to food in the United Kingdom, 1999–2006', *Journal of Allergy and Clinical Immunology* **119**(4),1018–19.

Resuscitation Council UK (RCUK) (2005) *Guidelines for Adult Life Support*, London, RCUK.

Useful websites

www.alsg.org.uk
Epipen: www.epipen.co.uk
RCUK: www.resus.org.uk

Chapter

38

Clinical holding for care, treatment or interventions

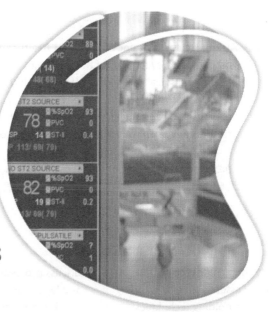

Philomena Morrow and
Patricia McGuinness

Links to other chapters in *Foundation Skills for Caring*

3 Communication
4 Communicating with adolescents
5 Anxiety
6 Sign language
28 Routes of medication administration

Links to other chapters in *Foundation Studies for Caring*

3 Evidence-based practice and research
4 Ethical, legal and professional issues
5 Communication
9 Moving and handling
16 Safeguarding children
17 Safeguarding adults
21 Care of the acutely ill child

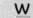

W Don't forget to visit www.palgrave.com/glasper for additional online resources relating to this chapter.

Introduction

The need for restraint of clients in healthcare environments varies according to the area of practice. However, many of the principles that relate to this issue are applicable to all, or most, health and social care settings (Horsburgh, 2004).

Restraint may involve the physical containment of one individual by another person or persons and can range from activities which are subtly applied, for example locking doors to restrict movement out of a prescribed area, to physical and/or chemical interventions.

Professionals who engage in holding or restraining practices must be mindful of the professional and legal implications of the situation.

Learning outcomes

This chapter will enable you to:

- identify the significance of individual assessment and planning appropriate holding techniques for children, young people and vulnerable adults

- discuss professional, ethical and legal issues that require consideration for holding and restraining practices

- identify the skills required through out each stage when engaging holding techniques for care, treatment or interventions.

Concepts

- Restraining
- Immobilisation
- Clinical holding
- Consent
- Accountability
- Partnership
- Participation
- Multidisciplinary collaboration

Technological advances invariably increase the likelihood of children and young people being the subject of medical examinations and treatments which are painful and invasive. Physical restraint or holding down of children and vulnerable adults has been generally accepted where this is necessary to ensure success in carrying out various therapeutic and diagnostic procedures (Tomlinson, 2004). It is seen as a common component of nursing practice to promote safety and prevent potential adverse responses (Selekman and Snyder, 1997).

However, this does not imply that holding or restraining practices should be undertaken without careful assessment and planning of techniques and options tailored to suit individual needs. The circumstances under which restraint is justified and the acceptable means by which it is to be achieved, as well as alternative methods sought, should be clearly reviewed and documented. In each situation it is important to consider the physical and psychological effects, as well as ethical, legal and safety issues. The justification in practice is that the use of restraint is in the child or vulnerable adult's best interest and is carried out to prevent the patient or others from suffering or being likely to suffer significant harm.

The role of parents is implicit in all aspects of care treatment or interventions involving children and young people. Parents require support and understanding when making decisions which may involve them in the act of holding their child during medical or nursing procedures, as this experience may be emotionally and physically distressing (Tomlinson, 2004). Parents

⚠ Professional alert!

Accountability requires a demonstration that the actions or inactions have been those of a reasonable and competent practitioner. If this is not proved, the nurse may attract penalties of varying gravity depending on the seriousness and consequences of the action or inaction (Horsburgh, 2004).

should have the opportunity of expressing their desired level of participation and you ought not to assume that they should assist.

Restraint and immobilization of children, young people and vulnerable adults are significant issues for health professionals who are involved in their care. Hardy and Armitage (2002) argue that professional guidance and healthcare law are ambiguous in this regard, failing to offer direct objective guidance. They further contend that a degree of complexity is added when having to consider the child's wishes, particularly if the child's views differ from those of the parents.

Legal and ethical issues

Professional regulatory bodies for healthcare professionals have standards of conduct performance and ethics which clearly articulate that registered practitioners are accountable for promoting and protecting the rights and best interests of their patients. Therefore where the use of restraint, holding still and containing children and young people and vulnerable adults is concerned, health professionals must consider patients' rights and the legal framework surrounding them. This includes the Human Rights Act, the European Convention on the Rights of the Child (1989) and Consent and Capacity Assessment (DHSSPS, 2007). In addition health professionals must be proficient in assessing risk, making appropriate clinical judgments and managing situations where physical restraint or holding may have potential adverse effects. There is increasingly an emphasis on avoiding restrictive interventions through staff training and patient education (Mohr, Petti and Mohr, 2003).

Under general UK law, a person is deemed to be a child until the age of 18 years – see the Children (Northern Ireland) Order and the Children Act. Crucial to child development and contemporary healthcare, is the child's ability to make informed choices (Hardy and Armitage, 2002). Despite the increasing number of publications discussing children's capabilities to be involved and exercise choice in decision-making processes, the notion that their rights should be invested in those with parental responsibility still dominates the attitudes and practices of health professionals. Hardy and Armitage (2002), the Children Northern Ireland Order (1995) and the Children Act (1989) recognise the need to act in the best interests of the child as his/her welfare is paramount, but also refer to the rights of children to have their wishes and feelings considered. This places a responsibility on the healthcare professional to develop competencies and skills necessary to enable children to express treatment preferences, while at the same time acting in their best interest. However when treatment is considered to be in the best interests of children but does not concur with their wishes, then immobilisation or restraint may be considered necessary if medical examination or treatment is to be undertaken (Hardy and Armitage, 2002).

Invasive, painful procedures are difficult for patients; examples include venous blood sampling, insertion of venous access devices, subcutaneous or intramuscular injections, insertion of enteral feeding tubes, lumbar punctures and bone marrow aspirations. These procedures may be equally distressing for a vulnerable adult, particularly one who is unable to comprehend the need for specific care, treatment or investigations. It is often the restraint during procedures rather than the pain that causes distress and trauma.

The term restraint is defined as the positive application of force with the intention of overpowering the individual (DH, 2002), whereas immobilisation is rendering someone fixed or incapable of moving. It is clear that the difference between the two terms is the use of force in order to accomplish restriction (Hardy and Armitage, 2002). Immobilisation may therefore be referred to as restriction to which the child, young person or vulnerable adult has consented, and restraint as that to which consent has not been given. It would appear that the terms are used synonymously in practice. Lambrenos and McArthur (2003) introduced the term 'clinical holding' to describe positioning the individual so that a medical procedure could be carried out in a controlled manner, wherever possible with their consent.

Part

IV

⚠ Professional alert!

Involuntary restraint of patients who are competent to consent to or refuse treatment is both unethical and illegal (Van Norman and Palmer, 2001). Intervention without consent in adults constitutes battery in law unless the patient is incapable of giving consent.

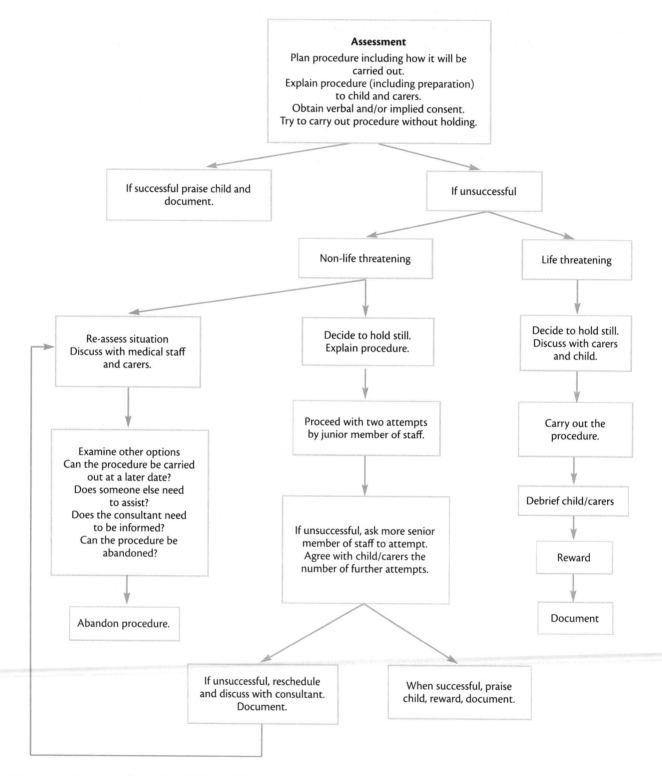

Figure 38.1 Framework for holding children still for clinical procedures

Source: by kind permission of Mrs D. Dooley (Director of Nursing) and Staff Nurse P. McGuinness, Children's Ward, Daisy Hill Hospital, Newry, Southern Health and Social Care Trust.

In the United Kingdom, the age of consent for care, treatment or interventions has been established as 16 years of age (DH, 2003b). However Gillick competency, which was implemented following the House of Lords decision in the *Gillick v West Norfolk and Wisbech Area Health Authority* (1985), rules that children under the age of 16 could give consent provided they had reached a sufficient understanding and intelligence regarding proposed interventions. Refusal of treatment, on the other hand, may be overruled by a person with parental responsibility (DH, 2003b). Ideally, consent should involve the child or young person, parents and health professionals acting in partnership, so that participation by all in the decision-making process is respected.

Ethical considerations arise in situations where treatment interventions are invasive, painful and frightening but are paramount for the welfare of the child, young person or vulnerable adult. Forcing patients to undergo treatment without negotiating with them or finding other ways of achieving the same outcome is unacceptable professional behaviour and may constitute abuse. Even where there is justification for holding a child or young person, this may be resisted by persons with parental responsibility. This may present conflicts relating to welfare of the child or young person and the values and parental choices.

⚠ Professional alert!

The need to communicate and cooperate in the implementation of policies and procedures and the responsibility of management in ensuring that staff are adequately prepared, and updated in practices in restraint and holding techniques are the standard recommendations issued by the European Committee for the Prevention of Torture and Inhuman or Degrading Treatment or Punishment (2005). In addition concerns about practices should be actively addressed and staff at all levels should feel comfortable in discussing issues which may have implications for the child, young person or vulnerable adult.

Framework for practice

Skills required throughout each stage of the implementation of care, treatment or intervention include verbal and non-verbal communication to ensure effective negotiation, facilitation, and participation by all involved. Multidisciplinary collaboration is essential, as there must be careful consideration of whether a procedure is really necessary. In an emergency, there may not be time to explore alternative strategies to holding a patient for necessary care, treatment or interventions. McGuinness's framework (2007) presents a strategy for informing the decision-making process in relation to clinical holding for care, treatment or interventions. This framework should be included within a policy and procedure document which has been developed in conjunction with members of the multidisciplinary team.

During the procedure it is important to ensure that all involved in carrying out the treatment or care face the individual and explanations are given throughout.

Careful individualised assessment and planning is required to support decision making, with reference to relevant guidelines and locally developed policies (Folkes 2005) during the preintervention, intervention and post intervention periods

Pre-intervention care

Good preparation for procedures may prevent the need for holding. Assessment of the individual's needs in relation to the intended care, treatment or intervention should be undertaken within the context of the multidisciplinary team, and within an environment of care and respect and include the following:

- age, developmental stage of child, young person or vulnerable adult and their ability to understand why the intervention is necessary, how and where it will be undertaken and who will be involved
- prior experiences and outcomes of painful procedures

- child, young person's or vulnerable adult's expressed concerns and attention to wishes and feelings regarding the procedure and they should be given time to internalise information
- understanding of the risks and benefits of the proposed intervention before consent is sought
- parental wishes in relation to their involvement and their understanding of the needs, risks and benefits of proposed intervention before consent is sought
- necessary psychological preparation to include play therapists to support appropriate behavioural strategies aimed at reducing anxieties
- discussion and agreement regarding positions to be maintained during the intervention period

Where necessary, consider pharmaceutical strategies such as the use of conscious sedation – this should be prescribed, administered and monitored by experienced medical and nursing staff. You should also:

- assess the risk of, and anticipate, situations that may arise during the procedure (Mohr et al 2003)
- prepare the environment and all necessary equipment to ensure that once the care, treatment or intervention is commenced it is carried out as quickly and efficiently as possible
- where procedures are planned, and pain can be predicted, the opportunity should be taken to prepare children through play and education, and to plan pain relief for use during the procedure (DOH 2003).

Intervention

Agreements made during the preintervention period should be adhered to as far as is possible and should include:

- sufficient staff members and equipment such as appropriate toys are available for children to effectively engage in distraction techniques
- support for parents to participate as planned
- sensitive support for child, young person or vulnerable adult who are unaccompanied by family member.

During clinical holding there should be an avoidance of:

- pressure against joints
- restricting breathing
- inflicting added pain (Tomlinson 2004).

During the procedure it is important that all involved in carrying out the treatment or care face the individual and explanations are given throughout.

Post-intervention care

The following should be considered in the post-intervention phase:

- Immediately inform the child, young person or vulnerable adult when the care, treatment or intervention is complete.
- Praise and give rewards for having endured a difficult or painful procedure.
- Ensure the individual is made comfortable and provide appropriate follow-up support and necessary information.
- Monitor for complications that may arise as a result of physical or psychological effects of the intervention.
- The assessment, care plan and evaluation of the care, treatment or intervention should be carefully documented (Nursing and Midwifery Council, 2005; Health Professions Council, 2003; General Medical Council, 2006).

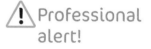 Professional alert!

The holds developed should be biomedically approved for stress points and may include positions which are prone, semi recumbent and seated (Lambrenos and McArthur 2003).

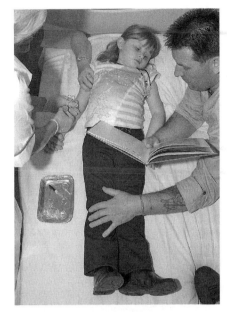

Figure 38.2 Appropriate positioning, holding and distraction during venepuncture

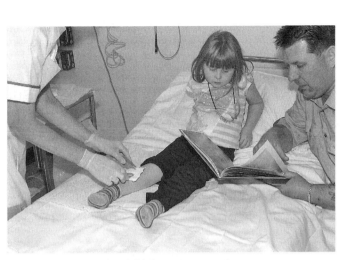

Figure 38.3 Facing the child during interventions

> ## (a) Learning activity
>
> In each of the scenarios below discuss the pre, inter and post-intervention care required.

> ## (s) Scenario: an uncooperative patient
>
> John is a 32-year-old who has sustained a laceration to the left leg following an accident due to excess alcohol intake. The laceration needs to be sutured and he requires an x-ray to ascertain additional injuries. John is very agitated and refuses to cooperate.

> ## (s) Scenario: illness in an infant
>
> Polly, a 3-year-old, has been admitted to hospital with a history of vomiting for the past 24 hours. She requires fluids administered intravenously so has to have a cannula inserted. However Polly is very distressed and irritable. Mum is very anxious about her daughter's condition and feels that she is 'very unwell'.

Conclusion

This chapter has introduced you to the key principles of clinical holding. It is important that all clinical holding interventions are undertaken after due consideration of the professional and legal implications.

References

Department of Health (DH) (2002) *Guidance for Restrictive Physical Intervention*, London, Stationery Office.

DH (2003a) *Getting the Right Start: National service framework for children. Standard for hospital services*, London, DH.

DH (2003b) *Good Practice in Consent*, London, DH.

DH, Social Services and Public Safety (DHSSPS) (2007) *Consent and Capacity Assessment*, Belfast, DHSSPS.

Folkes, K. (2005) 'Is restraint a form of abuse?' *Paediatric Nursing* **17**(6), 41–4.

General Medical Council (2006) *Good Medical Practice*, London, GMC.

Hardy, M. and Armitage, G. (2002) 'The child's right to consent to x-ray and imaging investigations; issues of restraint and immobilization from a multidisciplinary perspective', *Journal of Child Health Care* **6**(2), 107–19.

Health Professions Council (2003) *Standards of Conduct, Performance and Ethics*, London, HPC.

Horsburgh, D. (2004) 'How, and when, can I restrain a patient?' *Postgraduate Medicine* 80, 7–12.

Lambrenos, K. and Mc Arthur, E. (2003) 'Introducing a clinical holding policy', *Paediatric Nursing* 15, 30–3.

McGuinness, P. (2007) *Framework for Holding Children Still for Clinical Procedures*, Children's Ward, Daisy Hill Hospital, Newry, Southern Health and Social Care Trust.

Mohr, W. K., Petti, T. A. and Mohr, B. D. (2003) 'Adverse effects associated with physical restraint', *Canadian Journal of Psychiatry* **48**(5), 330–6.

Nursing and Midwifery Council (2004) *The NMC Code of Professional Conduct: Standards for conduct, performance and ethics*, London, NMC.

Nursing and Midwifery Council (2005) *Guidelines for Records and Record Keeping*, London, NMC.

Royal College of Nursing (2003) *Restraining, Holding Still and Containing Children: Guidance for good practice*, London, RCN.

Selekman, J. and Snyder, B. (1997) 'Institutional policies on the use of physical restraints on children', *Paediatric Nursing*, **23**(5), 531–7.

Tomlinson, D. (2004) 'Physical restraint during procedures: issues and implications for practice', *Journal of Paediatric Oncology Nursing* **21**(5), 258–63.

United Nations (1989) *United Nations Convention on the Rights of the Child*, London, Children's Rights Office.

Van Norman, G. A. and Palmer, S. K. (2001) 'The ethical boundaries of persuasion: coercion and restraint in clinical anaesthesia practice', *International Anaesthesiology* 39, 117–29.

Legislation

Children Act 1989.
Children (Northern Ireland) Order 1995.
Human Rights Act 1998. Children Act 1989.
Children (Northern Ireland) Order 1995.
Human Rights Act 1998.

Chapter

39

Orthopaedic procedures

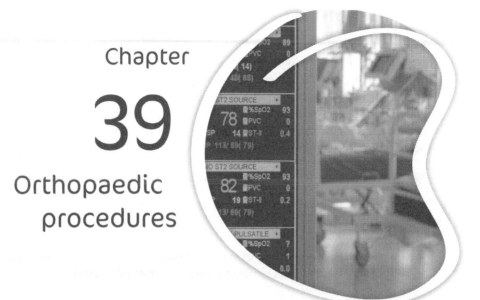

Ross Sherrington

Links to other chapters in *Foundation Skills for Caring*

Links to other chapters in *Foundation Studies for Caring*

W   Don't forget to visit www.palgrave.com/glasper for additional online resources relating to this chapter.

Part

IV

Introduction

The aim of this chapter is to provide the reader with an insight into some of the technical skills involved in caring for an adult orthopaedic patient. The areas of plaster care, pin site care and traction form the basis for the technical competencies listed in the RCN (2005) framework for orthopaedic and trauma nursing. The utilisation of slings and plaster of Paris casts is common across a range of musculoskeletal disorders, so the healthcare worker could potentially encounter them in many areas of practice. The use of skin traction and pin site care may be encountered in specific care circumstances.

Learning outcomes

This chapter will enable you to:

- describe, with evidence-based reasons, the procedure for the following orthopaedic skills: slings, plaster of Paris, pin site care, application of skin traction.

Concepts

- Insight
- Adult orthopaedic technical skills
- Evidence-based practice
- Patient information
- Scoped practice
- Competencies

Slings

Slings are used to support an injured arm or shoulder. The type of sling used will depend on the nature of the injury and on any medical advice.

Table 39.1 Three types of slings in common use

Sling		Use
Broad arm sling Figure 39.1 **Broad arm sling**		Used to support the forearm and elbow.
Collar and cuff Figure 39.2 **Collar and cuff**		The upper arm hangs free with the weight of the arm aiding the alignment of the upper arm with humeral injuries (Dandy and Edwards, 2004).
High arm sling Figure 39.3 **High arm sling**		Useful when elevating the forearm and hand injuries.

⚠ Professional alert!

Encourage patients to remove all rings and constricting jewellery from the injured limb as soon as possible, thus avoiding potential restriction and compromise to their circulation (Miles, 2004).

Procedure when applying a broad arm sling

> ### [S] Scenario: undiagnosed wrist injury
>
> Nikki, aged 55, has fallen while out shopping, onto her outstretched arm. She is complaining of a painful wrist. The application of a broad arm sling will help support the forearm until further investigations are completed.

You will require:
- a triangular bandage
- a safety pin.

Procedure

Table 39.2 Application of a broad arm sling

Action	Rationale
Explain procedure to ensure the patient understands the need for broad arm sling to be applied and help gain their compliance.	To gain verbal consent (DH, 2001). Provide opportunity for patient to ask questions.
Check if patient requires any analgesia and offer as prescribed.	Ensure effective and safe administration of analgesia to the patient (NMC, 2004).
Ensure the patient is positioned comfortably and support the injured forearm approximately parallel to the ground with the wrist slightly higher than the elbow. Carefully position the triangular bandage by sliding it between the injured arm and the chest, carrying the point behind the elbow of the injured arm (St Johns Ambulance et al, 2006). Take the top point of the bandage around the back of the patient's neck. **Figure 39.4** Application of a broad arm sling	Ideally the patient is sitting or standing in an upright position to aid alignment of the triangular bandage. See Figure 39.4.
Bring the lower end of the bandage up and over the patient's injured forearm to meet the other end over the shoulder of the uninjured arm.	Ensure the forearm is raised slightly by checking the angle at the elbow is less than 90 degrees before securing the sling, to reduce any potential swelling of the forearm and hand.
Tie a non-slip knot.	A reef knot is ideal as it is a flat knot that will not press into the skin, thus avoiding potential discomfort around this site.
Ensure the elbow is secured by folding the excess bandage at the point over the front of the elbow, and secure with a safety pin.	
Check the comfort of the patient.	Ensure the broad arm sling is effectively supporting the forearm.
Regularly check the neurovascular observations of the affected arm.	Ensure there is no compromise to the circulation or any neurological compression.

Part

IV

Procedure when applying a collar and cuff

> **[S] Scenario: undiagnosed injury to upper arm**
>
> Masani, aged 40, has slipped on her kitchen floor and fallen. She is complaining of a painful upper arm. The application of a collar and cuff sling will help support the upper arm in alignment until further investigations are completed.

You will require:
- a collar strip (commercial available kit)
- a fastener band.

Procedure

Table 39.3 Applying a collar and cuff

Action	Rationale
Explain procedure to ensure the patient understands the need for a collar and cuff to be applied and help gain their compliance.	To gain verbal consent (DH, 2001). Provide opportunity for patient to ask questions.
Check if patient requires any analgesia and offer as prescribed.	Ensure effective and safe administration of analgesia to the patient (NMC, 2004).
Ensure the patient is positioned comfortably and arm is supported. Allow the elbow to hang at the side of the body. Place collar strap around back of the patient's neck. Figure 39.5 Applying a collar and cuff 1	Ideally in an upright position to aid alignment of upper arm. Allow sufficient room for the patient's head to be able to slip through the hoop.
Position the other end of the strap around the wrist of the patient's affected arm. Figure 39.6 Applying a collar and cuff 2 	Allow sufficient room for the arm to slip through this second hoop.
The two hoops are then held at a mid point with a fastening band.	
When the collar and cuff is secured, ensure the forearm is held in a position slightly raised above 90° from the elbow.	Ensures the upper arm is allowed to hang free under the effect of gravity; thus the gravitational force will aid the alignment of the upper arm. The slightly elevated forearm helps reduce any potential swelling of the forearm and hand.
Check the comfort of the patient.	Ensure the collar and cuff are effectively supporting the upper arm.
Regularly check the neurovascular observations of the affected arm.	Ensure there is no compromise to the circulation or any neurological compression.

Procedure when applying a high arm sling

> **S** Scenario: undiagnosed injury to wrist and hand
>
> Shannon, aged 29, has taken a tumble on a dry ski slope near her house. She fell on to her outstretched hand and is now complaining of a painful hand. The application of a high arm sling will help support the forearm and elevate the hand to reduce potential swelling until further investigations are completed.

You will require:

- a triangular bandage.

Procedure

Table 39.4 Applying a high arm sling

Action	Rationale
Explain procedure to ensure the patient understands the need for a high arm sling to be applied and help gain their compliance.	To gain verbal consent (DH, 2001). Provide opportunity for patient to ask questions.
Check whether patient requires any analgesia and offer as prescribed.	Ensure effective and safe administration of analgesia to the patient (NMC, 2004).
Ensure the patient is positioned comfortably and hand is supported by placing the arm on the affected side across the chest and encourage the fingertips to touch the opposite shoulder (St Johns Ambulance et al, 2006).	Ideally in an upright position to aid alignment of triangular bandage.
Carefully position the bandage over the patient's affected arm/hand with the upper tip over the shoulder that is supporting the hand and the point of the bandage beyond the elbow.	
Supporting the arm, tuck the base under the forearm and behind the elbow.	
Bring the lower end up diagonally across the patients back to meet the other end at the shoulder. Figure 39.7 Applying a high arm sling	Tie a non-slip knot such as a reef knot, beyond the collarbone.
Check the comfort of the patient.	
Regularly check the neurovascular observations of the affected arm and hand.	Ensure there is no compromise to the circulation or any neurological compression.

> ⚠ **Professional alert!**
>
> There is a potential risk of joint stiffness of the arm if the limb remains immobile in a sling. Advise patients to move their fingers, wrists, elbows and shoulders as their injuries allow. Advice sheets explaining potential exercises of the arm will help reduce this potential problem.

Part

IV

Monitoring the neurovascular observations of the affected arm

Check how the patient feels; it is important to monitor the circulation in the injured arm on a regular basis. Love (1998) feels the frequency between observations should reflect a situation in which time could be critical if neurovascular compromise is detected in the affected limb. The ability to detect a compromised limb through careful observation enables prompt referral and subsequent treatment (Judge, 2007).

Assess the affected limb for:

- pain (out of proportion to injury)
- pain (on passive movement)
- lack or reduced ability to complete active movement
- altered sensation, onset of pins and needles (Tucker, 1998).

In addition to your observations, ask the patient to report immediately any changes in the pain, sensation, swelling or movement.

When checking the neurovascular observations of the injured arm, remember to compare them with those in the opposite limb (Dykes, 1993).

If possible, check the patient's peripheral pulses in the affected limb normally over the radius.

Accurately record these observations (NMC, 2008) and notify the medical team of any concerns or changes in these observations.

> **t** ☆
> ## Practice tip
>
> A patient with arm injuries will probably require assistance to maintain personal hygiene under both arms. Check if patients need assistance with buttons and bra straps. Offer advice on loose fitting clothing which may be easier to cope with when dressing.

Plasters and casts

The aim of the following section is to care safely for a patient who has had a plaster of Paris cast applied. Casting incorporates a range of technical skills that involve the application, adaptation and removal of casts. All of these areas require knowledge and clinical judgement (Prior, 2001). Healthcare practitioners must hold appropriate competencies as recognised by their employer and work within their code of conduct.

> **S** ## Scenario: a fractured wrist
>
> Julia Jones, aged 49 has tripped on a grating outside her house and fallen onto her outstretched arm. An x-ray has confirmed the clinical indications of a fractured wrist. Most injuries to the distal radius occur as a result of a fall onto the outstretched hand (Larsen, 2002). The medical team have assessed her injury and wish to admit her in order to manipulate the wrist, with the possibility that internal fixation may be required. Whilst awaiting surgery the medical team have requested a below-elbow plaster of Paris back slab to be applied to support the injured arm and aid Julia's comfort.

> **a** ## Learning activity
>
> List any possible reasons for Julia to be prone to such injuries.

Reasons for casting

Casts are applied for a variety of reasons. Some of the principle reasons are listed in *A Framework for Casting Standards* published by the RCN Society of Orthopaedic Nursing and Trauma (2000).

Table 39.5 Reasons for applying a cast

Reason for cast	Function
For the treatment of fractures.	To support the fracture site, control movement of fragments and damaged tissue.
After surgery.	To support and immobilise joints and limbs.
For the management and correction of deformities.	By inserting a wedging or application of serial plasters.
For support and to aid pain relief.	To ensure rest of damaged soft tissue.

Learning activity

Describe the possible signs and symptoms Julia might experience with such an injury.

Practice tip

With the patient's permission, carefully remove all rings and watches from the injured limb as soon as possible (Miles, 2004). The limb extremities are likely to swell, so any restricting bands could compound the situation and compromise circulation.

We shall now look at an example of a below-elbow back slab (referred to as metacarpal back slab), which is required for Julia.

You will require:

- a basic plaster trolley with bucket of water
- a tape measure
- a plastic apron and sheeting
- one 10-cm roll of padding
- a 10-cm plaster of Paris slab cut to shape. Eight layers for small arms and ten layers for adult arm
- a 10-cm-wide crepe bandage
- a triangular bandage
- a plaster strip to finish.

The aim of the back slab is to maintain the arm in the correct position, with a smooth inner surface that provides adequate support and does not cause any constriction to blood supply or nerves.

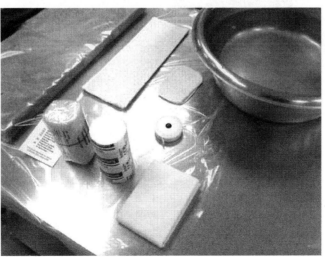

Figure 39.8 Material for a plaster cast

Procedure

Table 39.6 Applying a back slab

Action	Rationale
Check the medical notes for written instructions for the reason why the cast or back slab is being applied (Prior and Miles, 1999a).	To ensure the instructions state the extent of the plaster and position of the limb is to be held (RCN/SOTN, 2000).
Explain the proposed procedure to the patient.	To gain their consent and compliance.
Aid the patient's comfort by supporting her affected limb. Offer analgesia as prescribed.	If a painful limb is to be positioned successfully, the patient must be relaxed and comfortable. Ensure effective and safe administration of analgesia to the patient (NMC, 2004).
Check the skin is intact around the hand and forearm (Prior and Miles, 1999a, 1999b).	Check for any abrasions or signs of infection.
Apply the under cast padding, starting from the knuckles up to the just below the elbow. The padding must be applied without any ceases or ridges. When the plaster slab is applied the padding can be pulled over to provide additional padding at the plaster ends.	Stockinette should not be used in an acute injury such as Mrs Jones's because of the possibility of post-trauma swelling; if this occcurs the stockinette can be constrictive (Prior and Miles, 1999a, 1999b).
Measure the arm to calculate the length of plaster slab required to accommodate a backslab 2 cm proximal to the knuckles and 3 cm distal to the elbow. Figure 39.9 Applying a back slab	To allow free movement of the fingers (metacarpo phalangeal joints) and sufficient distance to allow free flexion of the elbow joint (Miles, 2004).
Cut required length of plaster of Paris.	Shape and round off corners of slab to ensure these do not press into the skin when applied.
Usually a dorsal slab is applied using 10 cm plaster of Paris in eight layers (ten layers for large arms).	
Submerge the cut plaster into a bucket with tepid water (according to manufacturer's instructions, normally around 25 °C) until the bubbles have ceased (three seconds). Remove and gently squeezed to remove excess water. Figure 39.10 Preparing cut plaster	The water temperature will affect the setting time of the plaster and may adversely affect the patient if too hot or cold
The slab is applied on the dorsal aspect of the arm without tension.	Ensure the plaster is smooth by using the palms of the hands to ensure the inner surface reflects the smooth outer surface and is without any creases (RCN/SOTN, 2000). Figure 39.11 Smoothing the cast

Action	Rationale
Pre-wet the crepe bandage and gently apply around the arm with back slab in situ.	A dry crepe bandage would absorb the moisture from the wet plaster, which may cause the crepe to shrink and lead to the limb being constricted (Miles, 2004).
Use plaster strip to secure end of crepe bandage.	Ensure the strip is positioned over the top of the back slab; if it is over the soft bandage areas it may lead to pressure and discomfort.
Clean the fingers and exposed skin of any plaster. Leave the plaster to dry naturally. Support on a pillow or broad arm sling.	Plaster of Paris requires 48 hours to gain its full strength.
Complete relevant documentation (NMC, 2008).	Good record keeping is essential to provide evidence of care delivered.

When caring for a patient who has a cast applied it is important to offer appropriate advice and to follow the actions in Table 39.7.

Table 39.7 Applying a cast

Action	Rationale
Keep a frequent and careful check upon the state of the circulation of the affected limb.	Careful monitoring enables early detection of any signs or symptoms of neurovascular compromise (Middleton, 2003).
Support the affected limb, normally with a broad arm sling or on a pillow (Miles, 2004). Figure 39.12 **Supporting the arm**	To allow the cast to dry naturally without the risk of indenting or cracking the plaster (Prior and Miles, 1999b).
Examine the fingers for signs of swelling. If possible elevate the encased limb.	Gravity can assist the venous return from the limb.
Encourage finger and toe movements and other joints not immobilised by plaster (RCN/SOTN, 2000). Figure 39.13 **Movement in joints not immobilised by plaster**	To assist venous return and avoid stiffness of the unaffected joints.
Enquire about the presence and site of any pain.	The pain could indicate an area of pressure created by: → uneven bandaging → insufficient padding → too tight or loose cast → rough edges of cast (Prior and Miles, 1999b). Investigate possible cause and inform medical team.

Part

IV

Action	Rationale
If not obscured by the cast or bandages, palpate the peripheral pulses.	To check for any changes in arterial circulation.
If the position of the back slab leaves the pulse inaccessible, then consider performing a capillary refill test by pressing on the fingernail then releasing to observe the nail bed return to its original colour.	Check capillary refill on both limbs. Normal capillary refill of two seconds indicates good perfusion (Judge, 2007). Prolonged capillary refill time could indicate diminished capillary perfusion and should be reported.
Examine the extremities for the presence of altered skin sensibility.	It is important to see all the fingers move as each digit has a separate nerve supply (Nicol et al, 2004). A 'pins and needles' sensation, numbness or inability to move extremities may indicate nerve compression and should be reported.

Many patients will go home wearing casts from either the wards, the emergency department or fracture clinic, so be sure to give them clear verbal and written instructions together with any additional information relating to their specific treatment

It is important to reaffirm verbal instructions with written information. Patients can refer to this to aid their understanding and compliance with treatment (Taylor and Cameron, 1999). Any advice should be written in clear and accessible language.

Written advice that could be given regarding the care of the plaster, may look like this:

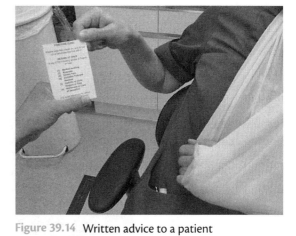

Figure 39.14 Written advice to a patient

You should:

- Keep the limb elevated when resting.
- Move the joints (not in the cast) through their full range of movement, especially your fingers and toes.

You should not:

- Allow the cast to get wet, but keep it clean and dry.
- Heat the plaster, as it is a good conductor and retainer of heat. Heating could cause a burn.
- Scratch the skin beneath the plaster, or stick anything such as knitting needles inside the cast.

Go to your nearest emergency department at once if:

- There is an increase in pain in the limb.
- Your limb becomes numb.
- There is an increase in swelling.
- Your fingers or toes are discoloured.
- The plaster is cracked or breaking; do not try to fix the cast yourself or remove the cast.

Skeletal pins

Metal pins and wires have been designed and used in a variety of different orthopaedic treatments. A percutaneous skeletal pin is a metal pin which has been inserted through a skin incision into the bone (Temple and Santy, 2004). A range of different pins have been designed for specific purposes, which may include the application of skeletal traction or external fixation devices.

(a) Learning activity

A patient who was being treated with a circular frame commented, 'My leg feels like the hub of a bicycle wheel with the pins coming out holding the leg in position like the spokes of the wheel.' Consider this within your learning group. Discuss the concerns a patient in a circular frame may have and how you might deal with these.

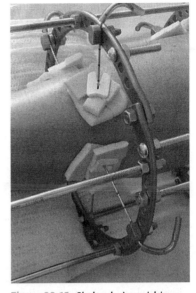

When skeletal pins are attached to a rigid external frame this is referred to as an external fixator. Holmes and Brown (2005) note that various types of external systems (unilateral, bilateral or circular) are used, depending on the anatomical site and problem being treated. Often the external fixator is used to position broken bone segments in their correct position and alignment until adequate healing has occurred.

Figure 39.15   Skeletal pins within a Ilizarov frame

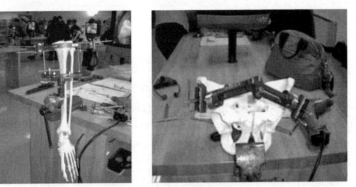

Figure 39.16
a) Tibia and fibula: circular system.
b) Pelvis: unilateral external fixator system

External pin site care refers to the care given by the healthcare practitioner to the area immediately surrounding the point where the pin or wire enters the skin. One of the risks associated with wearing an external fixator is an infected pin site (Sims and Saleh, 2000; Brereton, 1998). The aim of pin site care is to prevent any infection and prevent overgrowth of tissue/skin around the pin (United Bristol Healthcare NHS Trust, 2003).

(e) Evidence-based practice box

A Cochrane review (2004) by Temple and Santy to assess the effect on infection rates of different methods of cleansing and dressing orthopaedic percutaneous pin sites concluded there appeared very little evidence as to which pin site care regimen best reduces infection rates.

Care of the pin site

A literature review on pin site care indicates that opinions on the appropriate management vary (Temple and Santy, 2004). Refer to local policies when considering assessment and delivery of care in relation to immediate postoperative care, further management of exudates and ongoing pin site care. Walker (2007) has divided the evidence for skeletal pin care into three sections: cleansing, dressings and removal of exudates/crusts from around the pins.

You will need:

- a dressing pack
- a cleansing solution (dependant on local policy)
- sterile gloves
- sterile scissors
- gauze swabs
- a keyhole dressing (local policy).

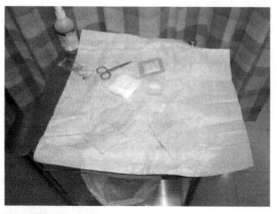

Figure 39.17 Materials for pin site care

Table 39.8 Care of the pin site

Action	Rationale
Refer to local protocols regarding pin site care. The essential outcomes in caring for pin sites are the reduction of inflammation and the prevention of infection (Santy and Newton-Triggs, 2006).	Adhere to evidence-based local protocols.
Explain the pin site care procedures to the patient.	To gain consent (DH, 2001). To provide an opportunity for the patient to ask questions.
Ensure the patient's privacy is maintained by only exposing the area of the body with the external fixator.	To ensure the patient's dignity and help maintain warmth throughout the procedure.
Check if patient requires any analgesia and offer as prescribed before commencing any pin site care procedures.	Ensure effective and safe administration of analgesia (NMC, 2004).
Apply principles of aseptic technique which must be rigorously maintained at all times during pin site care and observation (Lee-Smith et al, 2001).	To reduce the risk of cross-infection.
Considerations regarding cleaning of the pin sites: ➜ when to commence cleaning pin sites after insertion ➜ subsequent frequency of cleaning pin sites ➜ type of cleaning solution to be used ➜ what materials to use when cleaning around pin site ➜ technique used when cleaning the pin sites.	Refer to local protocol. Observe for any local skin reaction; document and report to medical team.
Considerations regarding pin site dressings: ➜ initial post operative dressing ➜ how the dressing should be applied ➜ to use a dressing or leave exposed once the haemoserous fluid has stopped.	Refer to local protocol. Initial post operative dressings are used to absorb haemoserous fluid (Holmes and Brown, 2005); non-stick absorbent dressing for the first 48 hours. Opinion is divided whether pin sites should be dressed or left exposed once the initial drainage has subsided (Walker, 2007).
Considerations regarding the easing skin away from pin site and crust removal: ➜ Observe for exudates and crust formation around pin sites. The management of crust around pin sites will vary depending on local protocol. ➜ Observe for any signs of infection around individual pin sites. Sites should be inspected daily (Sims et al, 2000).	Refer to local protocol. Treat each pin site as an individual wound. Pin site infection is a potential risk so monitoring of the pin sites is an important part of the treatment (Sims et al, 2000).
Documentation the procedure and any observations made (NMC, 2008).	Good record keeping is essential to provide clear evidence of the care delivered and allows for the planning of the future management of the pin sites and external fixator.

It is not always possible to say how long the frame will be on. The length of time depends upon the type of injury or condition being treated (United Bristol Healthcare NHS Trust, 2005). Patient compliance is an important factor as the pins and frame are often in place for many months (Sims and Saleh, 2000).

It is important to draw up a treatment plan which encourages the patient to take 'ownership' and care for the frame and pin sites. As soon as possible, patients should be encouraged to become involved in the care of their pin sites with the goal of continuing their care if discharged home with their fixator in situ. This skill must be taught effectively to ensure patient compliance (RCN, 1999) and the patient is to be given a written copy of the pin site care plan to reinforce the verbal information given (Brereton, 1998).

It is important that both the healthcare practitioner and patient are able to recognise any signs of pin site infection and report any concerns to the medical team.

> ### t⭒
> ### Practice tip
>
> It is important to recognise any potential signs of pin site infection. Observe for any of the following:
> - red inflamed area around the pin
> - increased pain and tenderness around the pin
> - thick fluid discharge (note any change in colour or smell of the discharge)
> - swelling around the pin (RCN, 1999).

Skin traction

The fundamental principle of skin traction is the application of a traction force over the adjoining skin, which is then transmitted via the soft tissues to the underlying bone (Davis and Barr, 1999). Nonadhesive skin traction is sometimes referred to as Buck's traction.

The application of non-adhesive skin traction will be described in the following section. It can potentially be used as a temporary measure in the treatment of acetabular and hip fractures (Nichol, 1995). Skin traction rarely reduces the fracture but its aim is to reduce the pain experienced through attaining normal anatomical alignment and reducing muscle spasm around the injury site (Styrcula, 1994b).

The procedure of applying skin traction is used in setting up more complex traction systems, for example in the use of a Thomas splint or Hamilton Russell traction system.

[S] Scenario: leg injury requiring possible skin traction

Amy (86) has just been admitted to your ward. She has caught her foot on a door threshold, fallen on her side and sustained a fractured left neck of femur. There is a delay in commencing the required surgery to the hip until all the requested pre-operative investigations have been completed.

In an effort to alleviate the muscle spasm and associated pain that Amy appears to be experiencing, it has been suggested that her prescribed analgesia should be reviewed and skin traction applied to the affected leg.

For the application of adult skin traction, you will need:
- A commercially available skin application kit, each kit contains a foam-lined stirrup, retaining straps and cord.
- 2–3 kg (5 lb) weight with suitable holder (refer to weight limits recommended by the manufactures of the traction appliance).
- Traction system pulley.
- Tape.
- A traction system that allows the suspension of the traction weight.

Part

IV

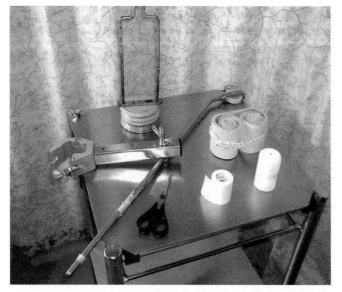

Figure 39.18 Equipment for adult skin traction

⚠ Professional alert!

There are some potential contra-indications associated with the application of skin traction which are summarized by Jerre, Doshe and Karlsson (2000):

- skin damage or sepsis in the area where the skin traction is to be applied
- pressure sores
- distal oedema
- vascular compromise
- peroneal nerve palsy
- blisters secondary to mechanical shearing forces applied to the skin.

Table 39.9 The application of non-adhesive skin traction to an adult

Action	Rationale
Explain the procedure to ensure the patient understands the purpose of the application of skin traction.	To gain consent (DH, 2001). To provide an opportunity for the patient to ask questions.
Wash hands and put on a disposable apron (DH, 2003).	Universal precautions and control of infection.
Before traction application is commenced, it is important to check skin integrity.	Refer to the alert section describing the potential contra-indications to skin traction (Jerre, Doshe and Karlsson, 2000).
Only expose the area of the lower limb as required to check skin and successfully apply skin traction.	To ensure the patient's dignity and help maintain warmth throughout the procedure.
Check if patient requires any analgesia and offer as prescribed before handling the affected limb.	To ensure effective and safe administration of analgesia (NMC, 2004).
Carefully support the limb normally around the ankle and knee joints. Assistance will be needed to hold the extension strips in position whilst application of retention bandages is completed (Love, 2000). Begin wrapping at distal end of the limb starting above the malloelas.	This will allow you to position the skin traction straps along each side of the leg on the lateral and medial aspects of the limb, using an imaginary line between the malleolus and the greater trochanter as a guide to where the straps should lie (Stewart and Hallett, 1983). Avoid pressure on the Achilles tendon. The encircling bandage must be firmly applied, but must not embarrass the circulation (Stewart and Hallett, 1983).
Position the foam-lined stirrup to allow enough room below the foot (normally around 10 cm) for the patient to be able to flex it without restriction and so that the proximal end of the stirrup protects the bony prominences of the malleoli. Figure 39.19 Position of stirrup	Encourage the patient to dorsiflex the foot. This acts as a method of checking for any potential compression on the peroneal nerve which could lead to symptoms of foot drop.

Action	Rationale
Continue wrapping by applying an even pressure until the landmark of the tibial tuborosity is reached. Check the comfort with the patient, ensuring the bandaging is smooth and evenly applied (Styrcula, 1994b). Secure wrapping bandage with a piece of tape. **Figure 39.20 Wrapping the limb**	Figure 39.21 indicates where the upper limit of the wrapping bandage should lie. This is the small notch where the distal patella tendon attaches to the tibia. The purpose is to avoid pressure being exerted on the common peroneal nerve, which may result in peroneal nerve palsy (Love, 2000). Depending on local policy the retaining strips can be held out straight to run up to the thigh and the wrapping bandage continued above the knee. Alternatively these retaining strips can be cut to finish at the level of the knee or folded back onto themselves. **Figure 39.21 Finding the upper limit of the wrapping**
Support the affected leg on a pillow.	Ensure the heel is free from pressure by placing the heel below the pillow end.
Feed the traction cord through and secure at the base of the foot section with a non-slip knot such as the bowline.	To ensure weights remain securely attached to the traction cord. A step-by-step illustration of tying the knot is included on the companion website. **W**
Attach the pulley and its supporting mechanism at the foot of the bed.	This will depend on the type of bed and local traction system available.
Feed the traction cord through the now suspended pulley. The cord must run freely over the pulley (RCN SOTN, 2002b). The weight must hang free and not rest on the floor (RCN SOTN, 2002b). Adjust the required length of the cord so that when the weight is tied to the end it will be suspended distal from the pulley and off the floor (Davis and Barr, 1999). **Figure 39.22 Cord and pulley**	To ensure that the appropriate pulling force is applied for optimal therapeutic effect at all times. The line of pull of the cord should be correct and regularly checked (Styrcula, 1994a). To check the weights are free running and do not catch, particularly on the bed ends when the patient moves. **Figure 39.23 Position of weight**
Elevate the bed end to an angle of 5°. **Figure 39.24** **Bed elevation**	Any force needs an opposing force. Skin traction pulls the limb distally with the resulting effect of sliding the patient down towards the bed end. To provide an opposing force use the tilting mechanisms of the bed to raise the bed end up (Nichol, 1995).
Check the neurovascular observations of the limb.	Refer to relevant sling sections which discusse neurovascular observations of a limb.

Part

IV

Action	Rationale
Check the comfort of patient by following these guidelines: → The traction system must be inspected at least at the beginning of each shift (RCN SOTN, 2002b). → The skin traction should be removed and reapplied at least once a day (Love, 2000). → Inspect the traction bandages and straps frequently, checking there has been no slippage of these or any signs of wrinkles. Check with the patient for any tender areas and inspect the skin area.	Skin care for the client in skin traction requires special attention to skin and bony prominences as there is a potential for any of the contra-indications developing as noted in the previous alert section. Inspection ensures early detection of signs of pressure or friction to the patient's skin.
Remove apron and wash hands (DH, 2003).	Universal precautions for control of infection.
Document the procedure and any observations made, and note the patient's response to the application of the skin traction (NMC, 2008).	Good record keeping is essential to provide clear evidence of care delivered.

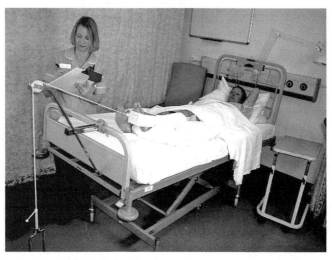

Figure 39.25 Completing documentation

⚠ Professional alert!

A frequent check on the position of the retaining bandaging is required as there is a tendency for the strapping to be pulled down towards the foot and this will compromise the circulation and effectiveness of the traction system. Reapplication will be required, and rechecking of the patient's skin condition.

t☆ Practice tip

Be aware of your own posture whilst completing this procedure; adjust the bed height to a safe working height, thus minising the need to stoop.

Love (1997) notes the risk of musculoskeletal injury associated with prolonged static stooping.

ⓔ Evidence-based practice

There is no agreement on the use of pre-operative skin traction and practice may vary according to local policy or specific patient need. A recent Cochrane review (Parker and Handoll, 2001) of pre-operative traction for fracture of the proximal femur in adults concluded from the evidence available that routine use of traction prior to surgery for hip fracture does not appear to have any benefit. Parker and Handoll felt the evidence is also insufficient to rule out the potential for specific fracture types or to confirm additional complications due to traction use.

Conclusion

This chapter has shown you some of the most common skills required when dealing with an adult orthopaedic patient. You should always act in accordance with your employer's local procedures and the scope of your own role.

References

Brereton, V. (1998) 'Pin-site care and the rate of local infection', *Journal of Wound Care* **7**(1), 42–4.

Dandy, D. J. and Edwards, D. J. (2004) *Essential Orthopaedics and Trauma*, 4th edn, Edinburgh, Churchill Livingstone.

Davis, P. and Barr, L. (1999) 'Principles of traction', *Journal of Orthopaedic Nursing* 3, 222–7.

Department of Health (DH) (2001) *Consent – What you have a Right to Expect: A guide for adults*, London, DH.

DH (2003) *Winning Ways: Working together to reduce healthcare associated infection in England*, London, DH.

Dykes, P. C. (1993) 'Minding the five P's of neurovascular assessment', *American Journal of Nursing* **93**(6), 38–9.

Holmes, S. and Brown, S. J. (2005) 'Skeletal pin site care: National Association of Orthopaedic Nurses, Guidelines for orthopaedic nursing', *Orthopaedic Nursing* **24**(2), 99–107.

Jerre, R., Doshe, A. and Karlsson, J. (2000) 'Preoperative skin traction in patients with hip fractures is not useful', *Clinical Orthopaedics and Related Research* 378, 169–73.

Judge, N. L. (2007) 'Neurovascular assessment', *Nursing Standard* **21**(45), 39–41.

Larsen, D. (2002) 'Assessment and management of hand and wrist fractures', *Nursing Standard* **16**(36), 45–53.

Lee-Smith. J., Santy, J., Davis, P., Jester, R. and Kneale, J. (2001) 'Pin site management, towards a consensus: Part 1', *Journal of Orthopaedic Nursing* 5, 37–42.

Love, C. (1997) 'An update of the evidence into the cause and prevention of prolapsed intervertebral disc: Part 1', *Journal of Orthopaedic Nursing* **1**(4), 199–205.

Love, C. (1998) 'A discussion and analysis of nurse-led pain assessment for the early detection of compartment syndrome', *Journal of Orthopaedic Nursing* **2**(3), 160–7.

Love, C. (2000) 'Bandaging skills for orthopaedic nurses', *Journal of Orthopaedic Nursing* **4**(2), 84–91.

Mandzuk, L. L. (1991) 'External pin site care: a review of the literature and nursing practice', *Canadian Orthopaedic Nurses Association* **13**(1), 10–15.

Middleton, C. (2003) 'Compartment syndrome: the importance of early diagnosis', *Nursing Times* **99**(21), 30–2.

Miles, S. (2004) 'Slabs for emergency applications, below elbow slabs', *Journal of Orthopaedic Nursing* 8, 136–41.

Nichol, D. (1995) 'Understanding the principles of traction', *Nursing Standard* **9**(46), 25–8.

Nicol, M., Bavin, C., Bedford-Turner, S., Cronin, P. and Rawlings-Anderson, K. (2004) *Essential Nursing Skills*, 2nd edn, Edinburgh, Mosby.

Nursing and Midwifery Council (NMC) (2004) *Guidelines for the Administration of Medicines*, London, NMC.

NMC (2008) Section 4:4 *The NMC Code of Professional Conduct: Standards for conduct, performance and ethics*, London, NMC.

Parker, M. J. and Handoll, H. H. G. (2001) 'Pre-operative traction for fracture of the proximal femur in adults', *The Cochrane Library* 1, 1–26.

Prior, M. (2001) 'Education and training in casting: the whim of managers', *Journal of Orthopaedic Nursing* 5, 116–19.

Prior, M. and Miles, S. (1999a) 'Casting part 1', *Emergency Nurse* 7, 2

Prior, M. and Miles, S. (1999b) 'Principles of casting', *Journal of Orthopaedic Nursing* **3**(3), 162–70.

Royal College of Nursing (RCN) (2005) *Competencies – An Integrated Career and Competencies: framework for orthopaedic and trauma nursing*, London, Royal College of Nursing.

RCN, Society of Orthopaedic and Trauma Nursing (1999) *External Fixators*, London, Royal College of Nursing.

RCN, Society of Orthopaedic and Trauma Nursing (2000) *A Framework for Casting Standard*, London, Royal College of Nursing.

RCN, Society of Orthopaedic and Trauma Nursing (2002a) *A Traction Manual*, London, Royal College of Nursing.

RCN, Society of Orthopaedic and Trauma Nursing (2002b) 'Traction update', *Journal of Orthopaedic Nursing* 6, 230–5.

Santy, J. and Newton-Triggs, L. (2006) 'A survey of current practice in skeletal pin site management', *Journal of Orthopaedic Nursing* 10, 198–205.

Sims, M. and Saleh, M. (2000) 'External fixation, the incidence of pin site infection', *Journal of Orthopaedic Nursing* **4**(2), 59–63.

Sims, M., Bennett, N., Broadley, L., Harris, B., Hartley, J., Lake, S. and Pagdin, J. (1999) 'External fixation: part 1', *Journal of Orthopaedic Nursing* **3**(4), 203–9.

Sims, M., Bennett, N., Broadley, L., Harris, B., Hartley, J., Lake, S. and Pagdin, J. (2000) 'External fixation: Part 2', *Journal of Orthopaedic Nursing* 4, 26–32.

St Johns Ambulance, St Andrews Association, British Red Cross (2006) *First Aid Manual*, London, Dorling Kindersley.

Stewart, J. D. M. and Hallett, J. P. (1983) *Traction and Orthopaedic Appliances*, Edinburgh, Churchill Livingstone.

Styrcula, L. (1994a) 'Traction basics: part 1', *Orthopaedic Nursing* **13**(2). 71–4.

Styrcula, L. (1994b) 'Traction basics: part IV traction for lower extremities', *Orthopaedic Nursing* **13**(5), 59–68.

Taylor, D. and Cameron, P. (1999) 'Discharge instructions for emergency department patients: what should we provide?' *Journal of Accident and Emergency Medicine* **17**(2), 86–90.

Temple, J. and Santy, J. (2004) 'Pin site care for preventing infections associated with external bone fixators and pin (Cochrane Review)', *The Cochrane Library* 1.

Tucker, K. R. (1998) 'Compartment syndrome: the orthopaedic nurse's vital role', *Journal of Orthopaedic Nursing* 2, 33–6.

United Bristol Healthcare NHS Trust (2003) *Information for Patients and Carers: Pin site protocol*, Bristol, The United Bristol Healthcare NHS Trust.

United Bristol Healthcare NHS Trust (2005) *About your Circular Frame*, Bristol, The United Bristol Healthcare NHS Trust.

Walker, J. A. (2007) 'Evidence for skeletal pin site care', *Nursing Standard* **21**(45), 70–6.

Part

IV

Chapter

40

Last offices

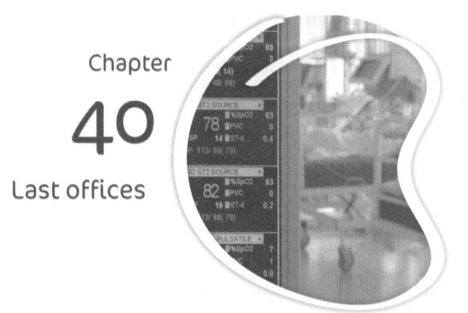

Deborah Heron and Lucy Smith

Links to other chapters in *Foundation Skills for Caring*

- 3 Communication
- 7 Breaking significant news
- 9 Patient hygiene

Links to other chapters in *Foundation Studies for Caring*

- 4 Ethical, legal and professional issues
- 5 Communication
- 6 Culture
- 9 Moving and handling
- 29 Loss, grief, bereavement and palliative care
- 31 Child emergency care and resuscitation
- 32 Adult emergency care and resuscitation

Don't forget to visit www.palgrave.com/glasper for additional online resources relating to this chapter.

Introduction

This chapter considers the practical aspects of dealing with the death of a patient. For the purposes of this chapter only the aftermath of an adult dying in hospital will be considered. It is a rarity in contemporary healthcare for a child to die in hospital, although the unexpected death of a child presents inevitable difficulties for all concerned. Such deaths usually occur in an emergency or intensive care department environment. Following the death of a child, wherever that may occur, the principal role of the healthcare professional is to provide support for the child's family.

Last offices is the care given to a deceased patient which demonstrates our respect for the dead; it is focused on fulfilling religious and cultural beliefs as well as health and safety and legal requirements (Dougherty and Lister, 2008). Approximately 80 per cent of deaths occur in National Health Service hospitals (NHS), care homes or hospices: regardless of the place of death healthcare professionals will have an important role to play (DH, 2008).

Despite there being documented evidence of nurses caring for the dead dating back to the nineteenth century (Wolfe, 1988), the emphasis of the care has changed. Pearce (1963) discussed how plugging, packing and tying patient orifices to prevent the leakage of body fluids were important aspects of last offices. Today the emphasis principally centres on the legal aspects of death, timely care and consideration for the patients' and relatives' cultural, spiritual, emotional and religious views (DH, 2008).

Nurses spend more time caring for dying patients than any other healthcare professionals (Ferrell, Grant and Viriani, 1999), and within the hospital setting such care is often delivered by student nurses (Cooper and Barnett, 2005). Dealing with death and dying can be an emotional and at times stressful experience for all healthcare professionals. Johnson (1994) and Kiger (1994) highlight how emotions such as anxiety and fear can surround seeing a dead person for the first time, and as a healthcare student this might be the first time you have ever experienced death in any context. Cooper and Barnett (2005) support this view but also add that the procedural aspects of last offices can cause individuals anxiety. This chapter aims not only to identify and discuss the procedure of last offices but also to highlight some of the other aspects you may need to consider.

Learning outcomes

This chapter will enable you to:

- demonstrate through discussion an understanding of the procedure of last offices
- demonstrate through discussion an understanding of the legal, professional, health and safety issues that are involved in last offices
- seek information that supports and guides practice of last offices.

Concepts

- Care procedures following the death of an adult
- Sensitivity and respect
- Religious and cultural requirements following death
- Safe and effective care following death
- Legal aspects of post-mortem care

⟨S⟩ Scenario: death and a student nurse

Rebbeca, a first-year student nurse, is working in an elderly care ward.

A woman named Phillippa, whom Rebecca has cared for over the last couple of weeks, has died. Rebecca's mentor Ayesha, a registered nurse, asks if she would like to assist her in performing last offices. Rebecca has never undertaken this task but recognises that it is an important aspect of patient care.

Part

IV

Cultural religious and spiritual issues

Prior to performing last offices it is important to acknowledge the patient's cultural and spiritual beliefs and to seek guidance from the family or relevant religious leaders. Be mindful of the fact that not all patients will have strong beliefs that will necessitate strict adherence to a specific religious or cultural practice. Also, consider that beliefs within cultures or religions may differ and may be more dynamic for some people than for others, and therefore are not necessarily predictable.

Procedure

- Maintain privacy and dignity (DH, 2001); for example draw curtains.
- Inform a senior nurse and request him or her to verify that the patient is dead.

S Scenario continued

Rebecca was quite worried and anxious about how the relatives might react and what if any support she would be able to offer.

Ayesha said that all relatives react differently when they experience loss; some may be quite tearful or angry while others will be quiet and subdued, and that there is no right or wrong way to react. The most important thing the healthcare professional can do is listen and be there for the family.

---

e Evidence-based practice   W

The Department of Health (2005) published a paper to develop bereavement services within the National Health Service. Principally, the paper recognised that grief is normal after bereavement but that the lay public often lacked any real understanding of grief, and as such they needed information and support. This has led to the development by a number of hospitals of information leaflets that offer guidance and support for the relatives at the time of death. The chaplaincy team also offers a very useful source of support. If, however, the relatives need a more formal opportunity for discussion, they can be advised to contact a number of both local and national organisations such as:

- Bereavement advice:
  www.crusebereavementcare.org.uk.
- Bereavement UK: www.bereavementuk.co.uk.

- Provide information and support to next of kin as appropriate.
- Allow the family quiet time with the patient to say their goodbyes without unnecessary interruption.
- Contact medical staff for certification of the death.

S Scenario continued

Rebecca asked Ayesha what was the difference between verification and certification.

Ayesha stated that within the End of Life Care Strategy published by the Department of Health (2008), the following definitions were given.

Verification concerns confirming that death has occurred. It can be performed by any healthcare professional specifically trained in this procedure; within nursing this would fall under the remit of an expanded role (Dimond, 2008).

Certification is a legal requirement and must be undertaken by a medical practitioner and involves identifying, documenting and certifying the reason for death.

- Establish any legal or health and safety issues (for example the patient may need to have a post-mortem or may have had a potentially contagious illness that requires special precaution protocols to be followed).

a Learning activity

Prior to performing the physical act of last offices it is important to consider the legal, cultural and religious implications or beliefs. For example does the nature of the patient's death need referral to a coroner, as in the case of an accident?

Access www.dh.gov.uk and establish when to refer to a coroner or when a post-mortem is necessary (type in the words coroner or post-mortem).

t Practice tip

Moving and handling
When handling the patient it is important to undertake a moving and handling risk assessment using for example ELIOT (Environment, Load, Individual, Other, Task) (Smith, 2005).

t Practice tip

Infection control
Body fluids may leak after death and the use of body bags may be required as a special precaution. This may also be the case for specific infectious diseases (Higgins, 2008).

The Department of Health has an advisory committee that provides guidance on dangerous pathogens (Dimond, 2008). You might be required to wear full protective clothing; the body may need to be wrapped in a special cadaver bag which should be clearly labelled as a high-risk infectious body. For further guidance please read your local policy guidelines (Public Health Act, 1984).

- If appropriate the senior staff may discuss tissue donation with the next of kin.

S Scenario continued

Rebecca was a little confused to learn patients who had died would still be considered suitable to donate organs. Ayesha explained to Rebecca that even after a person had died other people may benefit from their death as patients can donate tissue such as their skin, corneas, sclera and other optical material, bone, and heart valves; tissue can often be transplanted days or weeks after the donation has taken place (Kent, 2007). Sque, Long and Payne (2003) showed that relatives who were comfortable with their decision to donate a person's organs tended to have less complicated bereavement issues or unresolved grief reactions. This issue needs to be broached very carefully and sensitively by an experienced qualified healthcare professional. Donation needs to be agreed either by the patient in the form of an advanced directive prior to the death or by the patient's next of kin.

More detailed information about organ donation can be accessed at www.uktransplant.org.uk.

- Ascertain from the next of kin or patient's notes as to whether or not there are any specific wishes that the patient expressed for actions after their death, such as cultural or religious practices.

S Scenario continued

Rebecca asked Ayesha where she could access information about specific religious and cultural practices relating to patients who have died.

Ayesha suggested talking to the family, reading the patient's notes or contacting the local religious leaders. In some hospitals this list is held and can be accessed via the hospital's switchboard or local chaplaincy team.

Part

IV

- Gather appropriate equipment, which may include linen, linen trolley, wash bowl and personal protective clothing such as gloves and apron, in line with local policy.
- Discontinue any infusions such as intravenous fluids and nasogastric feeds.
- Lay the patient flat and place the palms so that they are flat.
- Close the patient's eyes (which may be achieved by applying gentle pressure for 30 seconds or placing damp gauze on the eyes once they are closed).
- Attend to personal hygiene needs as required and according to the local protocol.
- Put in false teeth, or if this is not possible place them in a named pot with the patient's hospital number evident so that they can go with the patient. Ensure mouth care is provided.
- Ensure any open wounds are covered and clean.
- Clean and reapply stoma bags where necessary.
- Remove venflons, catheters, naso-gastric tubes and drains if the patient does not need to go for a post-mortem.

t⭑ Practice tip

If the patient is to go for a post-mortem then venflons and catheters should be left in situ, although any bags of fluid should be disposed of in accordance with the local policy guidelines. The venflons should have a bung applied and the catheter should be spigotted in order to minimise any seepage.

Patients might need to go for a post-mortem if for example:
- The cause of death appears unclear.
- The deceased has not been seen by a medical practitioner during their last illness.
- The cause of death may be deemed to be unnatural or caused by violence or neglect.

- The death may have been as a result of an industrial disease such as mesothelioma.
- The death may have occurred during an operation or before the patient has had a chance to recover from the anaesthetic.

(Coroners Act, 1988 Section 8(1); Section 19(3))

- Remove jewellery in the presence of a second nurse and document unless specifically agreed by the family, and store in a secure place following the local protocol. If jewellery is left on the body, tape any rings and ensure that the information is documented on the patient's paperwork and countersigned.
- Dress the patient according to the local policy and according to the patient and family's wishes.
- Apply two identity labels containing the patient's name, date of birth, date of death and any other information and documentation as required by the local protocols such as notification of death paperwork.
- Wrap a sheet around the body, ensuring that the face and feet are covered, and secure this with either tape or a bandage.
- If the patient is leaking fluid from orifices or wounds, place in a body bag to prevent cross-infection.
- Ensure that patient identification is evident on either the sheet or body bag.
- Request removal of the body by either portering staff or the funeral directors, depending upon the place in which you are working.
- Clear and clean the area in accordance with the local trust protocol.
- Document all actions in the nursing notes.
- Pack and document the patient's property and store or transfer it as appropriate.
- Inform other relevant health and social care professionals.

t ✰ Practice tip

When performing last offices nurses often talk to the patient as though they were still alive, as they feel less awkward doing so and find this process comforting and respectful (Cooper and Barnett, 2005). However, if this makes you feel uncomfortable, it is not essential.

Discussing and reflecting upon the emotional aspects of last offices can be helpful alongside focusing upon the procedure itself.

S   Scenario continued

Rebecca asked Ayesha if it was permissible for the family of the deceased to assist with last offices.

Ayesha replied that if the family wished to be involved in last offices then there was no reason why they could not be. However, it is important to inform the family that if they feel uncomfortable or unhappy with performing last offices then they can stop at any time.

Professional responsibilities

- Ensure procedure is carried out in accordance with local protocols.
- Maintain privacy and dignity throughout.
- Offer appropriate support to the family.
- Ensure all documentation is completed with the relevant dates and times, and is legible and signed.
- Be mindful of confidentiality.
- Respect the patient's and their family's wishes and advocate on their behalf.
- Work within the NMC Code of Professional Conduct (2008).

Cooke (2000) emphasises that from the nurse's point of view care of the deceased can offer a point of closure on the nurse–patient relationship. Last offices is often the 'last thing' a nurse can do for a patient.

What happens to the patient's body after leaving the ward?

It is usual in a hospital setting for the body to be taken to the morgue to be stored before transfer to the funeral home. The morgue is maintained at a low temperature, which is essential for preserving the body before burial or cremation.

Once transferred to the funeral home, the main aim is to care for the body, maintaining respect and dignity and fulfilling patient and family wishes. Arrangements for either a cremation or burial will be made with the family, and support will be given in decision making at this often difficult time. Viewings of the body can take place if the family wish for this. Embalming is also an option, which again preserves the body until cremation or burial, and is an alternative to a 'cool' room.

Conclusion

The procedure of last offices is one which requires sensitivity and understanding. This chapter not only outlines the process of last offices, to act as a guide and reference for practice, but also highlights additional aspects that could and should be considered at this time. These include organ donation, cultural, spiritual, religious, legal and professional, and health and safety issues. Alongside the practical aspects of care, it is also pertinent to consider the emotional element that some nurses may experience at this time. Reflecting on and discussing both practical and emotional elements of this procedure may well help develop skills and knowledge for the future.

Part

IV

References

Cooke, H. (2000) *When Someone Dies. A practical guide to holistic care at the end of life*, Oxford, Butterworth-Heinemann.

Cooper, J. and Barnett, M. (2005) 'Aspects of caring for dying patients which cause anxiety to first year student nurses', *International Journal of Palliative Nursing* 11(8): 423–30.

Department of Health (DH) (2001) *Essence of Care*, London, DH.

DH (2005) *When a Patient Dies: Advice on developing bereavement services in the NHS*, London, DH.

DH (2008) *End of Life Care Strategy: Promoting high quality care for adults at the end of life*, London, DH.

Dimond, B. (2008) *Legal Aspects of Death*, London, MA Healthcare.

Dougherty and Lister (2008) *The Royal Marsden Hospital Manual of Clinical Nursing Procedures*, 7th edn, Oxford, Wiley and Blackwell.

Ferrell, B. R., Grant, M. and Viriani, R. (1999) 'Strengthening nursing education to improve end of life care', *Nursing Outlook* 47, 252–6.

Higgins, D. (2008) 'Carrying out last offices', *Nursing Times* 104(38), 24–5.

Johnson, G. R. (1994) 'The phenomenon of death: a study of diploma in higher education nursing students' reality', *Journal of Advanced Nursing* 19, 1151–61.

Kiger, A. (1994) 'Student nurses' involvement with death: the image and the experience', *Journal of Advanced Nursing* 20, 679–86.

NMC (2008) *The Code: Standards for conduct, performance and ethics of nurses and midwives*, London, NMC [online] www.nmc-uk.org (accessed 10 February 2009).

Pearce, E. (1963) *A General Textbook of Nursing* (first published 1937), London, Faber & Faber.

Smith. J., (2005) *The Guide to the Handling of People*, 5th edn, Teddington, Middlesex, Backcare.

Sque, M., Long, T., and Payne, S. (2003) *Organ and Tissue Donation: Exploring the needs of families*, final report of a study for the British Organ Donor Society and the National Lottery Community Fund, Southampton, University of Southampton.

Wolfe, Z. (1988) *Nurses' Work: The sacred and the profane*, Philadelphia, University of Pennsylvania Press.

Further reading (multicultural awareness)

Akhtar, S. (2002) 'Nursing with dignity. Part 8. Islam', *Nursing Times* 98(16), 40–2.

Baxter, C. (2002) 'Nursing with dignity. Part 5: Rastafarianism', *Nursing Times* 98(13), 42–3.

Christmas, M. (2002) 'Nursing with dignity. Part 3: Christianity 1', *Nursing Times* 98(11), 37–9.

Collins, A. (2002) 'Nursing with dignity. Part 1: Judaism', *Nursing Times* 98(9), 34–5.

Gill, B. (2002) Nursing with dignity. Part 6. Sikhism', *Nursing Times* 98(14), 39–41.

Jootun, D. (2002) 'Nursing with dignity. Part 7. Hinduism', *Nursing Times* 98(15), 38–50.

Northcott, N. (2002) 'Nursing with dignity. Part 2: Buddhism', *Nursing Times* 98(10), 36–8.

Papadopoulos, I. (2002) 'Nursing with dignity. Part 4: Christianity 2', *Nursing Times* 98(12), 36–7.

Simpson, J. (2002) 'Nursing with dignity. Part 9. Jehovah's Witness', *Nursing Times* 98(17), 36–7.

The local hospice is also a place to access advice and support regarding last offices and procedures surrounding death.

Useful websites

Organ donation: www.uktransplant.org.uk
Bereavement advice: www.crusebereavementcare.org.uk
Bereavement UK: www.bereavementuk.co.uk/

Chapter

41

Specimen collection

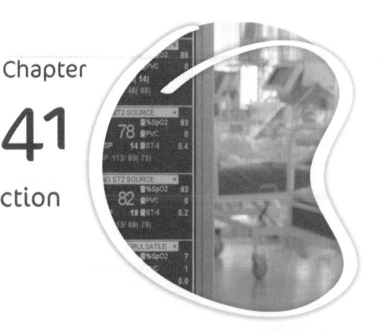

Yvonne Corcoran

Links to other chapters in *Foundation Skills for Caring*

3 Communication
9 Patient hygiene
13 Catheterisation and catheter care
30 Universal precautions
38 Clinical holding for care, treatment or interventions

Links to other chapters in *Foundation Studies for Caring*

4 Ethical, legal and professional issues
5 Communication
6 Culture
13 Infection prevention and control

Don't forget to visit www.palgrave.com/glasper for additional
online resources relating to this chapter.

Part
IV

Introduction

This chapter aims to provide you with knowledge and understanding of the skills required to collect specimens for microbiological, biochemical or other laboratory investigations from patients in the healthcare setting.

Specimen collection can be defined as the collection of a required amount of body fluid or tissue for examination in a laboratory in order to isolate or identify the possible presence of pathogenic microrganisms (Mims et al, 1998). The results may be used for screening purposes, to confirm a diagnosis, to treat a patient appropriately or for research.

Specimen collection is often the first and most important step undertaken when investigating the nature of a disease, determining a diagnosis and applying the appropriate treatment (Dougherty and Lister, 2004).

Although general principles of specimen collection apply, you will need to refer to local policy and be familiar with local protocols regarding the collection of specimens and issues relating to their collection, storage and transport.

Learning outcomes

This chapter will enable you to:

- understand the importance of laboratory investigations
- know the appropriate procedure for the collection of specimens with regard to timing, method/technique, equipment required and patient needs
- know the correct method of transporting specimens to the laboratory following collection

- understand the importance of universal precautions with regard to specimen collection (refer to Chapter 30)
- be aware of the complications that might arise as a result of specimen collection.

Concepts

- Diagnostic specimen collection
- Skills in specimen collection

- Safety in specimen collection
- Infection control and biosecurity in specimen collection

Specimen collection

Specimen collection is a fundamental aspect of clinical practice. The healthcare practitioner plays an important role in the collection of specimens, including:

- identifying the need for and the importance of specimen collection
- initiating the procedure for taking a specimen where appropriate, for example if signs of wound infection are present during a dressing change (Papasian and Kragel, 1997)
- collecting the required specimen in the correct volume and in the correct container
- deploying the correct collection technique and ensuring safe practice in order to avoid contamination or cross-infection and to ensure the validity of test results
- establishing good communication among all members of the multi-disciplinary team involved, which is essential in this process.

In older children specimens for laboratory investigation are collected in a similar manner to adults once their understanding and cooperation regarding the procedure have been established. However, infants and younger children may be unable to follow directions or control their bodily functions (Hockenberry and Wilson, 2007). Collecting specimens from children may be further complicated by their cognitive ability/developmental stage. This will have a direct impact on their ability to understand what is being asked of them. Specific procedures are required in order to collect specimens from this group of patients.

Parents should be encouraged to assist the healthcare practitioner during the procedure and the practitioner should be conscious of the language used to communicate with the child and family.

Universal precautions

Universal precautions are a set of guidelines that aim to protect healthcare workers against the risk of becoming contaminated with potentially infectious blood or body secretions (Bennett and Mansell, 2004). Since a medical history and examination cannot identify all patients with blood-borne infectious agents, standard precautions should be consistently used for all patients. Therefore blood and body fluids of every patient must be considered to be potentially infectious. Universal precautions should be adhered to by all healthcare practitioners during the collection of specimens, to protect both the patient and the healthcare professional.

⚠ **Professional alert!**

Human tissue and body fluids are potential health hazards to all staff handling them. Gloves should be worn at all times when collecting and handling specimens.

Documentation

All specimens must be clearly labelled to identify their source. Unlabelled or incorrectly labelled specimens are normally discarded (Health Services Advisory Committee, 1991). Specimens collected should be labelled clearly with at least the following details:
- patient's first name and surname
- patient's date of birth
- date and time of sampling
- ward.

A laboratory request form must also accompany all specimens. A request to take a specimen is normally made by a doctor and should include the following details:
- patient's first name and surname
- patient's date of birth
- patient's hospital number
- ward/department
- type of specimen
- date and time collected
- relevant patient history/diagnosis
- any antimicrobial drugs being taken by patient
- name of requesting doctor
- biohazard label, if required.

⚠ **Professional alert!**

Correct and complete information is required on all laboratory request forms. The requisition must be legible and completed in indelible ink. Incomplete information results in delays, difficulty in reporting or possible rejection.

Transportation of specimens

All healthcare professionals involved in the transport of specimens should be trained in the proper procedures. The specimen container used must be appropriate for the purpose and properly closed, and should not be externally contaminated with its contents (Health Services Advisory Committee, 1991). Specimens should be placed in a double self-sealing plastic bag with one compartment for the request form and the other the specimen (Dougherty and Lister, 2004). Specimens need to arrive in the laboratory as soon as possible in order to maximise the chance of any organisms that are present surviving and being identified. They should be transported in a washable transport container designated for this procedure, and any spillages must be dealt with appropriately at once. If there is a delay in specimens being sent to a laboratory the following procedure should take place:
- Blood culture samples should be kept in a 37 °C incubator.
- All other specimens should be stored in a specially designated specimen refrigerator at a temperature of 4 °C. This low temperature will slow down bacterial growth (Higgins, 1995).

⚠ **Professional alert!**

The temperature of specimen fridges should be monitored to ensure they are at the correct temperature. Only specimens awaiting delivery to the laboratory should be stored in these fridges.

General principles

1 Always gain consent verbally from the patient prior to collecting a specimen. In order to gain consent and cooperation the procedure should be explained in full and the patient allowed time to ask questions about the procedure. In the case of a child, parental consent should also be secured. If specimens are being collected for research purposes, a written consent is required and patients can refuse with prejudice.

2 Ensure the patient's privacy and dignity are maintained during the procedure in order to maintain self-esteem and trust.

3 Wash and dry hands in accordance with hospital guidelines before and after the procedure to reduce the risk of cross-infection (DH, 2001).

4 Standard precautions should be followed strictly during the collection and transportation of all specimens, including the wearing of disposable gloves and plastic apron.

5 Common principles apply to specimen collection, but knowledge of local policy with regards to specimen collection is essential. Guidelines regarding the collection and transport of specimens should be in place locally (COSHH, 1999).

6 Specimen collection should take place at the most appropriate time in order to obtain the most accurate results. Attention must be paid to the risk of contamination of the specimen.

7 Requests for specimen collection are normally made by a doctor and should be collected where possible prior to commencing treatment. Antimicrobial treatment should not commence prior to specimen collection (Baillie, 2001).

8 Specimens should be obtained using safe techniques and practices (Higgins, 2000).

9 All specimens collected should be inspected for apparent abnormalities such as colour, consistency and odour.

10 Once collected all specimens must be labelled in full with the correct patient details and accompanied by a laboratory request form. Patient identity should be confirmed verbally and by checking details on the patient's ID band.

11 Be sure to collect an adequate sample size. Otherwise samples may not be suitable for analysis or results may be inaccurate.

12 Once collected, specimens should be dispatched to the laboratory by the appropriate transport method, or placed in a specimen fridge for collection. Always refer to local policy regarding transport methods for specimens. Some specimens will need to be transported in special mediums or sent to external laboratories for analysing.

13 Ensure the patient is comfortable after the procedure.

14 Equipment used should be disposed of safely or cleaned in accordance with hospital infection control guidelines.

15 Document the procedure and any observations noted in the patient's hospital notes. Nurses are accountable for their actions and record keeping is essential (Nursing and Midwifery Council, 2004).

16 If you are uncertain about any issues relating to specimen collection, refer to local policy or contact laboratory personnel.

> ## (a) Learning activity
>
> Investigate the policy of your local health authority on specimen collection.

Practical aspects of collecting specimens

The next section will describe the procedure/skills required to collect the most commonly requested specimens at clinical level including:

- nasal swab
- throat swab
- wound swab
- eye swab
- sputum specimen
- urine specimen
  - MSU
  - 24-hour urine collection
  - catheter specimen
  - bag specimen (infant)
- faeces specimen.

⚠ Professional alert!

Disposable gloves and apron should be worn at all times when collecting or handling specimens to avoid cross-contamination of the specimen and the nurse (Camm, 2004; Hilton and Baker, 2003; Hockenberry and Wilson, 1996).

Nasal swab: to establish the presence of pathogenic micro-organisms in the nose

Table 41.1 Procedure for taking a nasal swab

Equipment required	Procedure/skill	Rationale
Sterile swab Disposable gloves and apron Sterile water (2 ml) Laboratory request form	Explain the procedure to the patient and ensure privacy.	To ensure patient understands the procedure and gives their consent.
	Wash hands and dry in accordance with hospital policy before and after obtaining the specimen.	To reduce the risk of cross-infection (Gould, 1994).
	Ensure patient is in a suitable position to allow access to the nasal cavity.	
	Moisten the sterile swab prior to insertion into the nose (if the nose is dry).	The nasal cavity can be dry.
	Insert the swab into the anterior nares and then upwards towards the tip of the nose and rotate. Both nares should be swabbed by the same swab. Replace swab into cover and label appropriately.	In order to acquire an adequate specimen.
	Ensure patient is comfortable post procedure. Document procedure in patient's nursing notes. Dispose of all waste appropriately.	

> t ☆
> ### Practice tip
> If area to be swabbed appears dry, always moisten the swab with sterile water before collecting a sample.

Throat swab: to establish the presence of pathogenic micro-organisms in the throat

Table 41.2 Procedure for taking a throat swab

Equipment required	Procedure/skill	Rationale
Sterile swabs Spatula Disposable gloves and apron Laboratory request form	Explain the procedure to the patient and ensure privacy.	To ensure patient understands the procedure and gives his/her consent.
	Wash hands and dry in accordance with hospital policy before and after collecting the specimen.	To reduce the risk of cross infection (Wilson, 2006).
	Assist the patient to a position appropriate to view the tonsilliar bed.	Extra light may be required.
	Use a spatula, applied gently to the tongue if required, to optimise access to the faucial tonsils. Gently rub the swab over the pillars of the fauces.	This may cause a gagging reflex in the patient.
	Avoid touching other areas of the mouth with the swab.	Contamination of the specimen can occur.
	Ensure the patient is comfortable after the procedure. Document procedure in patient's hospital notes.	

Part

IV

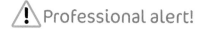 Professional alert!

Always consider the need for analgesia prior to the collection of specimens where necessary.

Wound swab: a sample of exudate from a wound

Table 41.3 Procedure for taking a wound swab

Equipment	Procedure/skill	Rationale
Sterile swabs Disposable gloves and apron Laboratory request form	Explain the procedure to the patient and ensure privacy.	To ensure patient understands the procedure and gives his/her consent.
	Wash hands and dry in accordance with hospital policy before and after collecting the specimen.	To reduce the risk of cross-infection (Horton, 1995).
	Inspect the wound for signs of infection. Swab should be obtained before any dressing or cleaning of the wound takes place. Gently rotate a sterile swab over the wound in order to collect an adequate sample of wound exudate. Replace swab into cover and label appropriately. Dispatch specimen to laboratory for analysis.	It may be appropriate in certain circumstances to use more than one swab.
	Ensure the patient is comfortable after the procedure. Document procedure in patient's hospital notes.	

Eye swab: to identify the organisms responsible for the presence of exudate from the eye

Table 41.4 Procedure for taking an eye swab

Equipment	Procedure/skill	Rationale
Sterile swab Disposable gloves and apron Laboratory request form	Explain the procedure to the patient and ensure privacy.	To ensure patient understands the procedure and gives his/her consent.
	Wash hands and dry in accordance with hospital policy before and after collecting the specimen.	To reduce the risk of cross-infection (Horton, 1995).
	Ask the patient to look upwards and gently pull the lower lid down. Apply a sterile swab gently over the conjunctival sac (inside the lower lid). Replace swab into cover and label appropriately. Ensure the patient is comfortable after collecting the specimen. Document procedure in patient's hospital notes.	

Urine specimen collection

A urine specimen is sometimes called a clean-catch, urine-culture or midstream specimen of urine, and is a method of collecting a quantity of urine for testing. In the infant, a bag specimen of urine is often the collection method of choice.

A specimen of urine may also be collected for urinalysis purposes at ward/local level.

Table 41.5 Procedure for collection of a mid-stream urine specimen (adult and older child)

Equipment	Procedure/skill	Rationale
Universal sterile specimen container Disposable gloves and apron Bedpan/urinal Sterile receiver Laboratory request form	Explain and discuss the procedure to the patient.	To ensure patient understands the procedure and gives their consent.
	Wash and dry hands in accordance with hospital policy before and after collecting the specimen.	To reduce the risk of cross-infection (Horton, 1995).
	Ask patient to begin passing urine and collect a mid-stream specimen directly into the container or a sterile receiver for females. Remove container before patient finishes passing urine.	To reduce the risk of contamination of the specimen with organisms normally present on the skin.
	Label specimen and dispatch to laboratory for analysis.	Urine specimens should be analysed within 2 hours of collection or within 24 hours if kept refrigerated at 4 °C.
	Ensure the patient is comfortable after collecting the specimen. Document procedure in patient's hospital notes.	

t☆

Practice tip

Mid-stream specimens of urine should be collected first thing in the morning where possible.

Table 41.6 Procedure for 24-hour urine collection

Equipment	Procedure/Skill	Rationale
24-hour urine collection container Disposable gloves and apron Laboratory request form	Explain the procedure to the patient and ensure privacy.	To ensure patient understands the procedure and gives their consent.
	Wash hands and dry in accordance with hospital policy before and after collecting the specimen.	To reduce the risk of cross-infection (Horton, 1995).
	Ask the patient to empty their bladder at the time appointed to commence the collection. This specimen should be discarded.	Only urine produced within the appointed 24-hour period should be collected.
	All urine voided by the patient during the next 24 hours is collected. The collection will end with the patient voiding their bladder exactly 24 hours after the collection commenced.	Results will be invalid if all urine is not collected during the appointed 24-hour period.
	Label specimen and dispatch to the laboratory for analysis. Document procedure in patient's hospital notes.	

t☆

Practice tip

Carefully explain to the patient/family that all urine voided during the appointed 24-hour period is collected in the collection receptacle which has been labelled with the patient's details.

Part

IV

Table 41.7 Procedure for collection of a catheter specimen of urine

Equipment	Procedure/skill	Rationale
Swab saturated with isopropyl 70% Sterile needle and syringe Universal sterile specimen container Disposable gloves and apron Laboratory request form	Explain the procedure to the patient and ensure privacy.	To ensure patient understands the procedure and gives their consent.
	Wash hands and dry in accordance with hospital policy before and after collecting the specimen.	To reduce the risk of cross-infection (Horton, 1995).
	Clean the access point with alcohol swab. Collect required amount of urine using a sterile syringe and needle (not always required – needleless port system).	Reduce the risk of needle stick injury.
	Place specimen in sterile container. Label specimen and dispatch to laboratory. Ensure the patient is comfortable after collecting the specimen. Document procedure in patient's hospital notes.	

⚠ **Professional alert!**

Never disconnect the drainage bag or collect a specimen from the outlet tap of the urine drainage bag.

Table 41.8 Procedure for collection of a bag specimen of urine (infant)

Equipment	Procedure/skill	Rationale
Sterile urine bag of suitable size for the child Sterile container Disposable gloves and apron Laboratory request form	Wash hands and dry in accordance with hospital policy before and after collecting the specimen.	To reduce the risk of cross-infection (Horton, 1995).
	Explain procedure to the child and parents.	To ensure child and parents understands the procedure and gives their consent.
	Wash and dry the genitalia with soap and water prior to collection of the specimen.	Normal hygiene of the genitalia is considered sufficient to minimise contamination from the skin prior to collection (Trigg and Mohammed, 2006).
	Remove protective seal from the urine bag. In the female infant the adhesive urine bag should be placed over the vulva, starting from the perineum and working upwards. In the male infant the adhesive urine bag is placed over the penis. Observe the bag frequently until urine is passed. Remove the bag gently and place the urine specimen in the sterile container. Label specimen and dispatch to the laboratory.	*t*☆ **Practice tip** Place the urine bag on the infant prior to a feed in order to increase the likelihood of collecting a sample.
	Wash the nappy area after collecting the specimen. Ensure the infant is comfortable. Document procedure in patient's hospital notes.	

Collection of a faeces specimen

Table 41.9 Procedure for collection of a faeces specimen

Equipment	Procedure/skill	Rationale
Sterile container Disposable gloves Sterile spatula and container Bedpan Laboratory request form	Explain the procedure to the patient and ensure privacy.	To ensure patient understands the procedure and gives their consent.
	Wash hands and dry in accordance with hospital policy before and after collecting the specimen.	To reduce the risk of cross-infection (Horton, 1995).
	Ask the patient to defecate into a clean bedpan. Using a spatula or scoop enough faecal material to fill a third of the specimen container.	To avoid contamination from other organisms.
	Label specimen and dispatch to laboratory. Document procedure in patient's hospital notes.	

t☆
Practice tip

A faeces specimen is frequently requested to test for faecal occult blood (FOB). This test can be performed at ward level using a test card specially designed for this purpose.

Sputum specimen

Table 41.10 Procedure for collection of a sputum specimen

Equipment	Procedure/skill	Rationale
Suitable universal container Sputum trap Disposable gloves Laboratory request form	Explain the procedure to the patient and ensure privacy.	To ensure patient understands the procedure and gives their consent.
	Wash hands and dry in accordance with hospital policy before and after collecting the specimen.	To reduce the risk of cross-infection (Horton, 1995).
	Encourage patient to cough deeply in order to expectorate sputum. If patient has difficulty producing sputum, a physiotherapist may be called to assist. In some situations a sputum trap may be used to collect a specimen.	First thing in the morning may facilitate the process.
	Once specimen is collected, label with patient details and send to laboratory for analysis. Ensure patient is comfortable. Document procedure in patient's hospital notes.	

t☆
Practice tip

Avoid collecting the specimen after the patient has eaten as the specimen may be contaminated with food particles.

Conclusion

Specimen collection is an important part of the healthcare professional role, and this chapter has introduced you to the main techniques you will require in practice. Remember to abide by the universal precautions for infection prevention when collecting specimens.

Bibliography

Baillie, L. (2001) *Developing Practical Nursing Skills*, London, Arnold.

Bennett, G. and Mansell, I. (2004) 'Universal precautions: a survey of community nurses experience and practice', *Journal of Clinical Nursing* **13**, 413–21.

Camm, J. (2004) 'What does it take to ensure safe hand decontamination by nurses?', *Professional Nurse* **19**(12), 26–8.

COSHH (1999) *The Control of Substances Hazardous to Health Regulations: Code of practice*, London, Stationery Office.

Department of Health (2001) 'Standard principles for preventing hospital acquired infection', *Journal of Hospital Infection* **47**(suppl), 21–37.

Dougherty, L. and Lister, S. (2004) *The Royal Marsden Hospital Manual of Clinical Nursing Procedures*, 6th edn, Oxford, Blackwell.

Gould, D. (1994) 'Nurses' Hand Decontamination Practice: Results of a local study', *The Journal of Hospital Infection*, **28**(11), 15–30.

Health Services Advisory Committee (1991) *Safety in Health Services Laboratory: The labelling, transport and reception of specimens*, London, Stationery Office.

Hilton, S. and Baker, F. (2003) 'Transmission of infection', *Professional Nurse* **18**(9)

Higgins, C. (1995) 'Microbiological examination of urine in urinary tract infection', *Nursing Times* **91**(11), 33–5.

Higgins, C. (2000) 'Microbiology testing', pp. 295–325 in Higgins, C. (ed), *Understanding Laboratory Investigations*, Oxford, Blackwell Science.

Hockenberry, M. J. and Wilson, D. (2007) *Wong's Nursing Care of Infants and Children*, 8th edn, Missouri, Mosby Elsevier.

Horton, R. (1995) 'Handwashing: the fundamental infection control principle', *British Journal of Nursing*, **4**(16), 926–33.

Mackintosh, C. A. and Hoffman, P. N. (1984) 'An extended model for the transfer of micro-organisms via the hands: differences between organisms and the effect of alcohol disinfection', *Journal of Hygiene* **92**, 345–55.

Mims, C. A. et al (1998) 'General principles and specimen quality', Chapter 13 in Mims, C. A. et al (eds), *Medical Microbiology*, St. Louis, C.V. Mosby.

Nursing and Midwifery Council (2004) *Medication Policy for Nurses*, London, NMC.

Papasian, C. J. and Kragel, P. J. (1997) 'The microbiology laboratory's role in life threatening infections', *Critical Care Nurse*, **20**(3), 44–59.

Royal College of Nursing (1997) 'Universal precautions', *Nursing Standard* **11**(32).

Trigg, E. and Mohammed, T. A. (2006) *Practices in Children's Nursing*, London, Elsevier.

Wilson, M. L. (1996) 'General principles of specimen collection', *Clinical Infectious Diseases*, **22**(5), 766–77.

Index